Glaucoma Handbook

Glaucoma Handbook

Edited by

Anthony B. Litwak, O.D., F.A.A.O.

Adjunct Associate Professor, Pennsylvania College of
Optometry, Philadelphia; Assistant Clinical Professor,
Pacific University College of Optometry, Forest Grove,
Oregon; Assistant Clinical Professor, New England College
of Optometry, Boston; Assistant Clinical Professor, State
University of New York State College of Optometry,
New York; Residency and Student Program Director,
Department of Veterans Affairs, Maryland Health Care
System, Baltimore

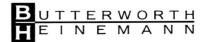

Boston • Oxford • Auckland • Johannesburg • Melbourne • New Delhi

Library of Congress Cataloging-in-Publication Data
Glaucoma handbook / [edited by] Anthony B. Litwak
    p. ; cm.
  Includes bibliographical references and index.
  ISBN 0-7506-9776-8
   1. Glaucoma—Handbooks, manuals, etc. I. Litwak, Anthony B.
  [DNLM: 1. Glaucoma—Handbooks. WW 39 G552 2001]
  RE871 .G547 2001
  617.7'41—dc21

                                                                    00-031220

British Library Cataloguing-in-Publication Data
A catalogue record for this book is available from the British Library.

The publisher offers special discounts on bulk orders of this book.
For information, please contact:

Manager of Special Sales
Butterworth–Heinemann
225 Wildwood Avenue
Woburn, MA 01801-2041
Tel: 781-904-2500
Fax: 781-904-2620

For information on all Butterworth–Heinemann publications available,
contact our World Wide Web home page at: http://www.bh.com

10 9 8 7 6 5 4 3 2 1

Printed in the United States of America

This book is dedicated to Lisa, Lauren, Diane, and my mom for their love, understanding, and support.

Contents

Contributing Authors

Paul C. Ajamian, O.D., F.A.A.O.
Center Director, Omni Eye Services of Atlanta

Steven J. Boeyink, O.D.
Roswell Eye Clinic, Roswell, Georgia

Anthony A. Cavallerano, O.D.
Staff Optometrist, Beetham Eye Unit, Joslin Diabetes Center, Boston

Kelliann Dignam, O.D.
Adjunct Clinical Professor, State University of New York State College of Optometry, New York; New England College of Optometry, Boston; Pennsylvania College of Optometry, Philadelphia; Attending Optometrist, Baltimore/Fort Howard Veterans Administration Medical Center, Baltimore

Mitchell W. Dul, O.D., M.S.
Chairman and Director of Clinical Sciences, Glaucoma Institute, State University of New York State College of Optometry, New York

Judith E. Goldstein, O.D.
Staff Optometrist, Department of Ophthalmology, University of Maryland Medical Center, Baltimore

Jimmy Jackson, M.S., O.D., F.A.A.O.
Director of Clinical Development, TLC Laser Eye Centers, Denver, Colorado

Peter A. Lalle, O.D.
Adjunct Faculty, Pennsylvania College of Optometry, Philadelphia; Chief of Optometry, Veterans Administration Maryland Health Care System, Baltimore

Anthony B. Litwak, O.D., F.A.A.O.
Adjunct Associate Professor, Pennsylvania College of Optometry, Philadelphia; Assistant Clinical Professor, Pacific University College of Optometry, Forest Grove, Oregon; Assistant Clinical Professor, New England College of Optometry, Boston; Assistant Clinical Professor, State University of New York State College of Optometry, New York; Residency and Student Program Director, Department of Veterans Affairs, Maryland Health Care System, Baltimore

Bruce E. Onofrey, R.Ph., O.D., F.A.A.O.
Adjunct Assistant Clinical Professor of Optometry, Clinical Programs, University of California, Berkeley, School of Optometry; Clinical Staff, Department of Eye Services, Lovelace Medical Center, Albuquerque, New Mexico

Thomas R. Stelmack, O.D.
Associate Professor, Illinois College of Optometry, Chicago; Assistant Professor, Department of Ophthalmology, University of Illinois at Chicago College of Medicine; Chief of Optometry, Veterans Administration Health Care System—West Side Division, Chicago

Robert S. Stutman, O.D.
Omni Eye Specialists, Baltimore; Adjunct Clinical Instructor, Illinois College of Optometry, Chicago, State University of New York State College of Optometry, New York, and University of Waterloo College of Optometry, Waterloo, Ontario, Canada; Consultant, Eye Clinic, Baltimore Veterans Administration Medical Center

J. James Thimons, O.D., F.A.A.O.
Adjunct Clinical Professor, New England College of Optometry, Boston; Clinical Director, TLC Laser Centers, Fairfield, Connecticut

Kelly H. Thomann, O.D.
Adjunct Assistant Clinical Professor of Clinical Science, State University of New York State College of Optometry, New York, New England College of Optometry, Boston, and Illinois College of Optometry, Chicago; Chief of Optometry Service, Veterans Administration Hudson Valley Health Care System, Montrose, New York

Preface

I have had the privilege of working in a large urban VA hospital in downtown Baltimore for more than 15 years. The majority of our patients are elderly men with a multitude of systemic problems. More than one-half of our patient population is African American. These demographics represent a population at high risk for the development of glaucoma, and as such, the diagnosis of either glaucoma or glaucoma suspect is among our top three clinical diagnoses. Glaucoma is a complex disease that is often oversimplified because we do not understand its pathophysiology. A further complication is the fact that the clinical course of patients with similar risk factors can vary greatly. I have found the intricacies of glaucoma diagnosis and management to be both fascinating and challenging. Over the years, my clinical skills have been shaped by the instruction of some of the leading experts in the field of glaucoma. For this I am grateful, and I am excited to have the opportunity to share this knowledge with others.

Why another glaucoma textbook?

The most obvious reason is that there have been significant technological and therapeutic advances since the mid 1990s in glaucoma diagnosis and treatment. New technologies for imaging the optic nerve and nerve fiber layer are now available. The perimetric science of short wavelength automated perimetry (SWAP) allows for the early detection of glaucoma damage. The introduction of the Swedish Interactive Thresholding Algorithm (SITA) represents a more efficient means of gathering data than does standard white on white perimetry. Frequency doubling perimetry (FDT) is a unique perimetric test that may allow the clinician to screen for glaucoma in a large population with both high accuracy and efficiency. The clinician must learn to incorporate these technological advances into practice to better manage glaucoma patients. On the therapeutic front, the glaucoma treatment paradigm continues to expand. Topical prostaglandins, alpha agonists, and carbonic anhydrase inhibitors offer potent intraocular pressure–lowering effects with better side-effect profiles than some of the more established glaucoma medications. This has resulted in a restructuring of the glaucoma treatment hierarchy. It is important that the clinician understand the potential side effects of each of the therapeutic agents, as well as their placement in the glaucoma treatment regime.

Another objective for writing this book was so that I could express my philosophy on glaucoma management. Detecting early glaucoma damage and deciding when to initiate treatment in the glaucoma suspect is a topic of much controversy, and although diagnosing advanced glaucomatous optic neuropathy is rarely a dilemma, managing and determining progression in patients with advanced disease often is. Many remedies and management schemes are based on anecdotal experience. This handbook is a compilation of academic literature and clinical experience. I try to incorporate practice guidelines and clinical experience and explore other philosophies on glaucoma management so that each practitioner can make informed clinical decisions. My approach is constantly being modified based on new information released. This book is designed to be clinically oriented while incorporating the academic information that is available.

Finally, I wanted to design a textbook that clinicians could refer to on a daily basis to assist in glaucoma diagnosis and treatment decisions. This book is not intended to replace the classic academic textbooks of glaucoma; it is designed to give practical clinical information and guidelines. The contributing authors are all seasoned clinicians, and I am grateful to each of them for sharing their insights on this enigmatic disease. I hope that this book will aid students, residents, and doctors to improve their diagnostic and management skills for the benefit of their glaucoma patients.

There are many individuals who participated directly and indirectly in the production of this book. Thanks to all of the authors who contributed their time and expertise. I am especially indebted to Jim Thimons, Paul Ajamian, Tony Cavallerano, and Alan Robin for their help and guidance. Special thanks to Kelliann Dignam for her encouragement and humor. Rick Sharpe and Peter Lalle were fantastic mentors and role models for teaching and educating students and residents. Thanks to all the persons who assisted with the book illustrations, including the folks from the Maryland VA Health Care System's Medical Media Department—Rick Milanich, Jordan Denner, and Richard Bauer. Laurel Cook Lowe is a superb illustrator and very receptive to making modifications to get the art just right. Barbara Murphy was the visionary who initiated the whole project. Thanks to all the people at Butterworth–Heinemann—Leslie Kramer, Jodie Allen, and Karen Oberheim—and at Silverchair Science + Communications—Nancy Bishop and Lisa Cunningham. Special gratitude to Sophia Battaglia at Silverchair—it has been a real pleasure. Finally, thanks to Cindy Metrose and Eric Schmidt and the many students and residents I have had the pleasure to interact with.

A. B. L.

PART

I

Introduction

CHAPTER 1

Introduction

Anthony B. Litwak

Complex diseases rarely yield simple solutions. Glaucoma is often a complex disease. The pathophysiology is not well understood. Similar individuals of age, race, and ocular risk factors can have wide variation in the development of glaucoma, the rate of progression, and the response to treatment. It is arduous to define a typical glaucoma patient, and therefore management and treatment choices must be individualized for each patient.

Glaucoma is a leading cause of blindness in the elderly and the African-American population. Glaucoma cannot be prevented, but treatment can reduce the rate of optic nerve damage, allowing patients to visually function in their daily life routines. Management of glaucoma patients should never be cookbooked. The decision-making process develops for each doctor from academic knowledge, clinical experience, personal philosophies of the disease, and the individual characteristics of each patient. This book was written to share some personal philosophies on glaucoma, and the proceeding chapters incorporate knowledge of the literature and clinical expertise to provide a template for effective glaucoma management that can and should be modified for each individual patient.

Early to moderate and sometimes even severe glaucoma damage rarely gives the patient signs or symptoms of their disease. This allows most patients with even advanced glaucoma damage to perform daily tasks that require visual function. However, the lack of visual symptoms often leads to considerable optic damage before the patient seeks medical attention. It is estimated that more than one-half of the patients with glaucoma are undiagnosed. In the past, screening for glaucoma was

difficult. Tonometry was popularized in the past as a screening mechanism, but no matter what cut-off number is selected, tonometry yields poor sensitivity and specificity.[1] Tonometry used as an isolated test should be abandoned as a screening device. Even combining risk factors with quantitative data does not separate patients affected and unaffected by glaucoma.[1,2] The current philosophy for glaucoma screening is routine periodic comprehensive eye examination targeted at high-risk groups. However, this approach is not necessarily time- or cost-efficient. New technology, such as frequency doubling perimetry, may provide a better cost- and time-efficient screening technique for glaucoma.[3,4]

When developing a logical approach to glaucoma diagnosis and management, it is important to remember that glaucoma is a chronic, progressive optic neuropathy. Many risk factors are associated with the development of glaucoma (see Chapter 2), but none of these risk factors or combinations of risk factors defines glaucoma. Glaucoma may or may not be associated with elevated intraocular pressure (IOP). Elevated IOP is a strong risk factor for glaucoma, and the higher the IOP, the greater the risk of developing glaucoma; however, elevated IOP alone does not define the disease. The majority of patients who have statistically elevated IOP never develop glaucoma neuropathy, and a sizable minority of glaucoma patients never exhibit statistically elevated IOP (see Chapter 14). Risk factors for glaucoma should not be ignored, but at the same time, the diagnosis should not be made based solely on elevated IOP.

Gonioscopy is a diagnostic skill that should be performed on all glaucoma and glaucoma-suspect patients (see Chapter 4). The majority of glaucoma patients in North America have primary open-angle disease, but angle-closure glaucomas and secondary glaucomas must be ruled out to make this diagnosis. This is a foremost distinction because many of the treatment modalities are quite different for angle-closure (see Chapters 16 and 17) and secondary open-angle glaucoma (see Chapter 15).

Glaucoma is a disease of the optic nerve, and therefore the evaluation of the optic nerve and nerve fiber layer deserves scrutinous attention (see Chapters 5 and 6). Optic nerve evaluation represents the most important clinical piece of information in the diagnosis of glaucoma. The optic nerve should be evaluated and photographed in stereopsis through a dilated pupil. A direct ophthalmoscope should be reserved for situations in which using a stereoscopic method is not feasible. The degree of cupping or lack of neural-retinal rim tissue is underestimated with a monocular technique, such as use of a direct ophthalmoscope. This misjudgment results from using color contour change rather than topographic contour change.

The simple recording of a cup-to-disc ratio neglects other useful optic nerve signs characteristic of optic nerve damage. The clinician should pay attention to the amount of neuro-retinal rim tissue, asymmetry of rim tissue, size of the optic disc, presence of acquired pits of the optic nerve, peripapillary atrophy, and disc hemorrhages. The clinician should also learn how to examine the retinal nerve fiber layer, because the nerve fiber layer evaluation gives objective information concerning optic nerve status and can lead to an earlier diagnosis of glaucoma damage than conventional automated perimetry. Serial photographs of the optic nerve and nerve fiber layer can be inspected to determine glaucoma progression.

Automated perimetry is an integral tool in diagnosing glaucoma (see Chapter 7), however, it is common for many visual field defects to disappear on subsequent testing because of a learning-curve phenomenon, and many patients are simply unable to produce accurate visual fields no matter how many attempts are made. The visual field results should collaborate the optic nerve and nerve fiber layer status. If the two don't match, one should repeat the field test. If the visual field still does not match the optic nerve test, and the field test does not suggest a vertical midline defect from a neurologic etiology or other explainable nonglaucomatous etiology, then the accuracy of the field test should be questioned.

My general approach to glaucoma management is to treat patients with IOP-lowering agents if they exhibit signs of glaucoma damage to the optic nerve, nerve fiber layer, or visual field. It is important to set a target pressure (a theoretical level of IOP at which the rate of further damage to the optic nerve is unlikely to affect the patient's quality of visual function during his or her lifetime). The target pressure is calculated from the baseline IOP (based on at least three IOP readings) and the degree of optic nerve damage, based on stereoscopic

assessment of the optic nerve, nerve fiber layer, and visual field testing. The greater the degree of damage, the lower the target pressure (see Chapter 11). In general, patients with mild damage have their IOP lowered 20–30%; patients with moderate damage, 30–40%; and patients with severe damage, 40–50% from the baseline highest IOP reading. These target reductions are starting guidelines and should be adjusted on an individual case analysis. The age of the patient should also be considered in the aggressiveness of treatment. Younger patients theoretically have more years to become impaired from glaucoma than an elderly patient. Target pressures are reanalyzed based on the clinical course of the disease. Follow-up schedule and repeat visual field testing are determined by the degree of damage, the achievement of a desired target pressure, stability of progression, and the duration of control (see Chapter 12).

The doctor should attempt to diagnose and treat glaucoma at the first sign of optic nerve compromise. Although the majority of patients with glaucoma do not go blind, knowing the future rate of glaucoma progression is impossible. The visual field should collaborate the optic nerve findings but may be normal in the early stages of the disease.[5] Blue-yellow perimetry has been shown to be more sensitive in identifying early damage,[6] but it has the disadvantages of higher patient variability and a longer testing time than white-on-white perimetry. I only use blue-yellow testing in a patient who has a normal white-on-white visual field test whom I strongly suspect has optic nerve damage from glaucoma. After discussing the options with the patient, I recommend lowering the IOP by 20–30% in patients with early signs of optic nerve damage, even though the white-on-white visual field test appears normal.

I am less inclined to treat elevated IOP in the absence of optic nerve or nerve fiber damage or visual field defects. I will treat most patients who maintain IOP of 30 mm Hg or above, because of the greater risk of developing glaucoma and also the potentially greater risk of developing venous occlusive disease. I consider treatment for patients with IOP in the high 20s if other glaucoma risk factors (strong family history or African American) are present. However, if the optic nerve appears healthy and the IOP is in the low to mid 20s, I rarely initiate treatment unless the patient is overly anxious without it. My target IOP is 20% from the baseline IOP or less than 30 mm Hg, whichever is lower.

Newer medications have been introduced that have had a significant impact on the way we treat glaucoma. However, I still use beta blockers as a first line of therapy in patients without medical contraindications because they are generally well tolerated and cost-effective. Newer medications, such as topical prostaglandins (latanoprost [Xalatan]), alpha agonists (brimonidine tartrate [Alphagan]), and topical carbonic anhydrase inhibitors (dorzolamide [Trusopt], and brinzolamide [Azopt]), have limited the use of pilocarpine, epinephrine, and oral carbonic anhydrase inhibitors as adjunctive medications. Latanoprost and brimonidine tartrate can also be used as primary agents in glaucoma therapy. It is important to become familiar with the advantages, side effects, and contraindications of these medications (see Chapter 8). Likewise, the clinician must develop a treatment protocol that fits these newer medicines into the daily treatment triage (see Chapter 11).

The rate of glaucoma progression is difficult to estimate from the initial evaluation. If a patient presents with glaucomatous damage and no prior medical records are available, it is impossible to know how long the disease has been present, what the rate of vision loss has been, or what the future loss will be. Determining glaucoma progression is perhaps the most difficult aspect of glaucoma management. Serial visual field testing is probably the best tool for determining glaucoma progression; however, visual field testing can show marked variability in areas of damaged ganglion cell receptor fields (long-term fluctuation [LTF]). Differentiating between normal glaucoma visual field fluctuation and actual glaucoma progression can be arduous. True progression may take up to six visual fields to validate (see Chapter 7). At a minimum, visual field progression should be confirmed with at least one additional visual field, especially when surgical intervention is being contemplated.

Lack of patient education leading to noncompliance can be a major cause of progression in many glaucoma patients. Monitoring for side effects or noncompliance with medications is an important aspect of glaucoma management. Techniques to determine and rectify poor compliance are discussed in Chapter 13. Use of multiple topical medications may contribute to poor compliance and I generally recommend argon laser trabeculoplasty (see Chapter 9) for patients after they are on two or three topical medications. Argon laser trabeculoplasty can also be used as primary therapy in a patient who has contraindications to medical therapy, is unable to instill eyedrops, cannot afford medications, or is unlikely to be compliant with medications. If a patient is compliant with medications and still progresses in the disease, then aggressive intervention is warranted. Filtering surgery (see Chapter 10) should be considered in the treatment regimen of a patient with confirmed progression on medical therapy. Filtering surgery can be also considered for a patient who presents with severe glaucoma damage on initial presentation. Of course, the benefits of filtering surgery must be weighed against the potential complications (cataract development, hypotony, and infection).

These recommendations are general guidelines for glaucoma management. Each patient must be evaluated individually, and these guidelines can be incorporated to tailor-make an effective management plan (see Chapter 18). Modification of these guidelines is acceptable based on the treatment response. I look forward to the not-so-distant future, in which doctors will directly treat the optic nerve in glaucoma therapy (neuroprotection, axonal rescue), and lowering IOP will serve as an adjunctive therapy for some patients. Genetic screening may allow the diagnosis of glaucoma before the patient develops glaucomatous damage. Gene therapy may cure the patient of glaucoma before optic nerve damage occurs. I welcome the new technologies that will assist us in better diagnosis and treatment of our patients.

REFERENCES

1. Tielsch JM, Katz J, Singh K, et al. A population-based evaluation of glaucoma screening: The Baltimore Eye Survey. Am J Epidemiol 1991;134:1102–1110.

2. Wang F, Tielsch JM, Ford DE, et al. Evaluation of screening schemes for eye disease in a primary care setting. Ophthalmic Epidemiol 1998;5(2):69–82.

3. Johnson CA, Samuels SJ. Screening for glaucomatous visual field loss with frequency doubling perimetry. Invest Ophthalmol Vis Sci 1997;38:413–425.

4. Quigley HA. Identification of glaucomatous visual field abnormality with the screening protocol of frequency doubling perimetry. Am J Ophthalmol 1998; 6:819–829.

5. Quigley HA, Dunkelberger GR, Green WR. Retinal ganglion cell atrophy correlated with automated perimetry in human eyes with glaucoma. Am J Ophthalmol 1989;107:453–464.

6. Johnson CA, Adams AJ, Casson EJ, et al. Blue on yellow perimetry can predict the development of glaucomatous visual field loss. Arch Ophthalmol 1993; 111(15):645–650.

PART

II

Diagnosing Glaucoma

Epidemiology and Risk Factors for Glaucoma

Kelliann Dignam and Robert S. Stutman

EPIDEMIOLOGY

Prevalence of Glaucoma Worldwide

It is estimated that at the start of the twenty-first century, 66.8 million people worldwide will have glaucoma. More than one-half of individuals with glaucoma are unaware that they have the disease. This places glaucoma second only to cataracts as the leading cause of blindness in the world.[1,2] The ratio of open-angle to closed-angle glaucoma cases worldwide is 1 to 1, or approximately 33 million cases each. An additional 6 million people will have secondary glaucoma. In a comprehensive review of published epidemiologic data, Quigley[1] estimated the prevalence of both open-angle and angle-closure glaucoma as a function of age for different ethnic groups throughout the world (Table 2-1). It is interesting to note that in whites, the ratio of open-angle to angle-closure glaucoma is 11 to 1. Among those of African descent, this ratio is significantly higher at 150 to 1. However, in China, the prevalence of angle-closure glaucoma is three times greater than that of open-angle glaucoma.

Open-Angle Glaucoma

The mean age-adjusted prevalence of open-angle glaucoma for adults of *European descent* (United States, Canada, Europe, former Soviet states, Australia, and New Zealand) is approximately 2.42%. The prevalence increases exponentially with age. Among *African-* (including African Americans) and *Asian-derived* persons, the relationship between prevalence and age is a linear one, with Africans having the highest prevalence of open-angle glaucoma with increasing age (Figure 2-1). It

is presumed that the prevalence of open-angle glaucoma in *Latin America* and the *Near East* is similar to that of the European population.

Angle-Closure Glaucoma

The average prevalence of angle-closure glaucoma in *European-derived* persons older than 40 years is 0.2%. The relationship between age and prevalence for angle-closure glaucoma is assumed to follow the same exponential function as open-angle glaucoma, but at a rate that is 11 times lower than that of open-angle glaucoma. Unlike open-angle glaucoma, angle-closure glaucoma is rare among those of *African* descent. The prevalence rate for angle-closure glaucoma in African Americans is approximately one-half that of Europeans, or 0.1%.[1] There is some evidence to suggest that the rate of angle-closure glaucoma among *Latin Americans* and people from the *Near East* is five times higher than among those of European descent.[1] Angle-closure glaucoma is the most prevalent form of glaucoma among adults in the *Philippines*.[3] Age-specific data derived from *Asian* populations support a linear relationship between the prevalence of glaucoma and age. It is important to note that angle-closure glaucoma appears to be more common among the *Chinese* than among any other ethnic group. The ratio of angle-closure glaucoma to open-angle glaucoma in this ethnic group is approximately 3 to 1.[1,4] A higher ratio of angle-closure glaucoma to open-angle glaucoma also exists among the *Eskimos* of Canada, Alaska, and Greenland. In these ethnic groups, 2–3% of the general population older than 40 years suffers from angle-closure glaucoma.[5–7]

TABLE 2-1. Number of People with Glaucoma Worldwide

Group	Open-angle glaucoma	Angle-closure glaucoma	Total population	Ratio of open-angle glaucoma to angle-closure glaucoma	Percentage of population with open-angle glaucoma	Percentage of population with angle-closure glaucoma
China	7,444,663	22,333,990	1,288,704,314	0.33	0.58	1.73
India	5,591,042	5,591,042	1,435,699,181	1.00	0.39	0.39
South Asia	4,224,819	4,224,819	769,979,570	1.00	0.55	0.55
European derivation	6,945,870	609,287	1,116,845,880	11.4	0.62	0.06
Africa	7,026,081	46,285	723,834,244	151.8	0.97	0.01
Latin America	1,278,751	560,856	506,533,880	2.28	0.25	0.11
Near East	640,040	280,719	323,624,981	2.28	0.20	0.09
Total	33,151,266	33,646,997	6,165,222,154	0.98	0.54	0.55

Total with primary glaucoma   66,798,263

Source: Modified from HA Quigley. Number of people with glaucoma worldwide. Br J Ophthalmol 1996;80:389–393.

Secondary Glaucoma

It is difficult to predict an accurate prevalence rate for the secondary glaucomas because many epidemiologic studies fail to make the distinction between primary open-angle glaucoma and the secondary glaucomas. Another confounding variable is the lack of a universal definition for each of the specific secondary glaucomas. In Quigley's review of epidemiologic data, he included pigmentary and exfoliation glaucoma in the prevalence calculations for primary open-angle glaucoma. A review of studies including *European, African,* and *Asian* populations suggests that the prevalence of the remaining secondary glaucomas is 0.44%.[1]

Pediatric Glaucoma

All forms of glaucoma in infants and children are very rare. As a result, few population-based studies exist from which an accurate estimate of prevalence might be made. A list of conditions associated with the developmental glaucomas, as well as causes of secondary glaucoma in this population, can be found in Table 2-2.

Prevalence in the United States

In the United States, it is estimated that 2.47 million Americans (1.84 million white and 619,000 African American) will have glaucoma by the start of the twenty-first century.[8] Glaucoma is the second leading

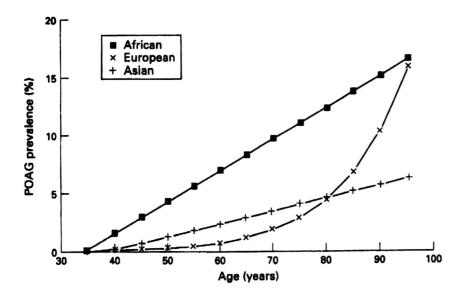

FIGURE 2-1. The prevalence of primary open-angle glaucoma (POAG) in European, African, and Asian people by age. (Reprinted with permission from HA Quigley. Number of people with glaucoma worldwide. Br J Ophthalmol 1996;80:389–393.)

TABLE 2-2. Conditions Associated with Developmental Glaucomas

Aniridia

Sturge-Weber syndrome

Neurofibromatosis

Goniodysgenesis syndromes

Axenfeld's anomaly

Rieger's syndrome

Peter's anomaly

Rubella

Turner syndrome

Trisomy 21

Trisomy 13

Trisomy 18

Trisomy 29

Marfan syndrome

Pierre Robin syndrome

Congenital iris hypoplasia

Weill-Marchesani syndrome

Oculodentodigital dysplasia

Lowe syndrome

Microcornea

Microspherophakia

Broad thumb syndrome

Homocystinuria

Congenital ectropion uveae

Zellweger syndrome

Anomalous superficial iris vessels

Secondary pediatric glaucomas

Tumors

   Retinoblastoma

   Juvenile xanthogranuloma

Inflammation

   Rubella

   Juvenile rheumatoid arthritis

   Herpes simplex

Retinopathy of prematurity

Trauma

Persistent hyperplastic primary vitreous

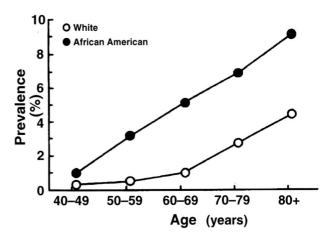

FIGURE 2-2. Age-prevalence relationship of open-angle glaucoma among African Americans and whites. Primary open-angle glaucoma begins earlier in life and is more prevalent at every age older than 40 years among African Americans than among whites. (Reprinted with permission from JM Tielsch, A Sommer, J Katz, et al. Racial variations in the prevalence of primary open angle glaucoma: The Baltimore Eye Survey. JAMA 1991;226[3]:369–374.)

cause of blindness in the United States and the most common cause of blindness among *African Americans*. This increased prevalence among African Americans was evident in the 1990 population data from the U.S. Department of Commerce Bureau of the Cen-

sus. They reported a 1.7% prevalence rate of glaucoma among *whites* (including *Hispanics, Asians,* and *Native Americans*) and a 5.6% rate among African Americans. The age-prevalence relationship of open-angle glaucoma for African Americans is a linear one that starts to rise at 40 years of age[9] (Figure 2-2). Although acute angle-closure glaucoma is extremely rare among African Americans, the frequency of chronic angle-closure glaucoma is significant and is believed to equal that of whites.[10]

Of those estimated to have glaucoma, 50% are unaware that they have the disease.[9,11] This is due in large part to the symptomless nature of open-angle glaucoma, inefficient screening methods for detection, and a lack of public awareness regarding the disease.[12] In most cases, blindness from glaucoma is preventable and is dependent on early detection and treatment. Risk factors associated with glaucoma have varying degrees of significance (Table 2-3). It is important to determine patients at risk for developing glaucoma, and to identify the glaucoma patients most likely to progress to visual impairment.

RISK FACTORS

Given that disease is not randomly distributed in the population, and considering the multicausal nature of disease, isolating specific risk factors for a given condition can be difficult. Such is the case with glaucoma. Although associations do not imply causation, they might provide insight into disease mechanisms

TABLE 2-3. Risk Factors for the Development of Glaucoma

Intraocular pressure (IOP)	Elevated IOP is a strong risk factor
Age	Increased risk with increasing age
Race	African American: strong risk factor for primary open-angle glaucoma (POAG)
	Chinese: strong risk factor for angle-closure glaucoma (ACG)
Family history	First-degree relatives of persons with POAG estimated to be four to eight times more likely to develop glaucoma
Refractive error	Increased risk of POAG with high myopia
	Increased risk of ACG with high hyperopia
Gender	Gender difference not a risk factor for POAG
	Increased prevalence of pigment dispersion syndrome among men
	Increased prevalence of ACG among women
Trauma	Late-onset glaucoma after trauma estimated at 2–10%
Diabetes	Possible increased risk, thought to be related to small-vessel disease and/or systemic blood abnormalities, resulting in compromised vascular perfusion to the optic nerve
Hypertension	Complex association
	Possible protective effect in younger patients
	Increased risk in older patients
Hypothyroidism	Possible association
Steroid use	Increased IOP in response to steroid use is more common in persons with glaucoma, their first-degree relatives, myopes, and persons with diabetes
Migraine	Possible association with normal-tension glaucoma
Alcohol use	Unclear; further investigation is warranted
Smoking	Unclear; further investigation is warranted

and can help to identify high-risk populations at whom screening methods should be directed. Recognized associations can result in the earlier detection and better management of glaucoma. Potential risk factors for the development of glaucoma are listed in Table 2-3.

Intraocular Pressure

Elevated intraocular pressure (IOP) is probably the most significant ocular risk factor for developing glaucomatous optic nerve damage.[13] Although no conclusive evidence supports this direct correlation,[14] a number of reports demonstrate that the incidence or prevalence of glaucomatous optic nerve damage rises as IOP increases.[15–17] Patients with bilateral open-angle glaucoma tend to have more damage in the eye that has higher IOP. Patients with unilateral glaucoma tend to have a secondary cause of increased IOP in the eye with glaucomatous damage.[18,19]

The incidence of glaucomatous optic nerve damage increases from approximately 3% in patients with an IOP between 21 and 25 mm Hg, to more than 50% in patients whose IOP is higher than 35 mm Hg (Table 2-4).[20,21] The incidence of open-angle glaucoma (OAG) is five times greater in patients with an IOP higher than 21 mm Hg than in those patients with IOP lower than 21 mm Hg.[22] Patients with an IOP higher than 25 mm Hg have twice the incidence of glaucomatous damage compared with patients with an IOP lower than 25 mm Hg.[23]

Despite these data, the majority of patients with IOP higher than 21 mm Hg never develop glaucomatous optic nerve damage. Many investigators have attempted to define the incidence rate of glaucoma among those with untreated ocular hypertension. This incidence rate tends to vary from study to study, largely as a result of study design and patient demographics (Table 2-5). It is generally believed that the incidence rate of a visual field defect among those with elevated IOP is 1% per year.[24] Conversely, a significant minority of patients with IOP consistently less than or equal to 21 mm Hg have glaucomatous optic nerve damage. In fact, one-half of the

TABLE 2-4. Incidence of Optic Nerve Damage Relative to Intraocular Pressure

Intraocular pressure (mm Hg)	Incidence with optic nerve damage (%)
20–24	3
25–29	7
30–34	14
35–39	52
40–44	61
45–49	75
50–54	83
55–59	83
<60	70

Source: HA Quigley, S Vitale. Models of open-angle glaucoma prevalence and incidence in the United States. Invest Ophthalmol Vis Sci 1997;38(1):83–91.

TABLE 2-5. Incidence of Chronic Open-Angle Glaucoma Among Persons with Ocular Hypertension

Investigator(s)	Number of patients with ocular hypertension	Observation period (years)	Number of patients who developed open-angle glaucoma (%)
Perkins[91,92]	124	5–7	4 (3.2)
Walker[93]	109	11	11 (11)
Wilensky et al.[94]	50	Average, 6	3 (6)
Norskov[95]	68	5	0
Linner[96]	92	10	0
Kitazawa et al.[97]	75	Average, 9.5	7 (9.3)
David et al.[98]	61	Average, 3.3; range, 1–11	10 (16.4)
Hart et al.[99]	92	5	33 (35)
Armaly et al.[13]	5,886	13	(1.7)
Lundberg et al.[100]	41	20	14 (34)
Schulzer et al.[71]	73	6	21 (29)

Source: Modified from MB Shields (ed). Textbook of Glaucoma (4th ed). Baltimore: Williams & Wilkins, 1988;155.

patients classified in the Baltimore Eye Survey as having reproducible, demonstrable glaucomatous field loss had an initial IOP below 21 mm Hg.[25] Many of these patients showed an elevated IOP on follow-up visits. However, approximately 20% of these glaucoma patients never exhibited an IOP greater than 21 mm Hg. Elevated IOP, therefore, does not define glaucoma, and "normal" IOP does not exclude glaucoma.

Consequently, IOP is only one of many risk factors contributing to glaucomatous optic nerve damage. The correlation between IOP and development of glaucomatous optic nerve excavation is more likely a continuum: the higher the pressure, the greater the risk of damage. Glaucoma patients demonstrate different levels of susceptibility to IOP. A "safe" or "normal" level of IOP therefore differs from one patient to another, depending on the vulnerability of the optic nerve and the presence and degree of other risk factors.

Normal Distribution of Intraocular Pressure

Several investigators have determined that the IOP in an adult population with no known eye disease is, in general, normally distributed in a pattern resembling a Gaussian curve. Leydhecker's classic investigation of 10,000 individuals without glaucoma revealed a mean IOP of 15.5 mm Hg ± 2.57 mm Hg. The upper limit of this "normal" distribution was approximately 20.5 mm Hg, which represents 2 SD above the mean.[26] Thus, *statistically healthy individuals* were defined as having IOP less than or equal to 21 mm Hg. *Patients with IOP greater than 21 mm Hg* were defined as having glaucoma or as being at greater risk for developing glaucoma. Closer inspection of these data, however, revealed that this distribution was not Gaussian, but skewed to the right (Figure 2-3).[27,28] This means that an upper limit for IOP cannot be determined by simply adding 2 or 3 SD to the mean.

Age

The risk of developing glaucoma increases with age (see Figures 2-1 and 2-2). Armaly and associates reported that the risk of developing primary open-angle glaucoma in persons older than 60 years was seven times greater than that of those younger than 40 years.[29] The overall prevalence of primary open-angle glaucoma among whites is approximately 2%. In whites between the ages of 43 and 54, the reported prevalence is 0.9%. Among those 75 years and older, the prevalence rate is significantly higher at 4.7%.[30] Increasing prevalence rates with increasing age have been also reported among African Americans. African Americans tend to develop glaucoma at a younger age than whites and have the disease approximately 27% longer. Patients diagnosed with glaucoma at an early age may warrant more aggressive therapy because a longer life span with the disease could translate into a greater probability of significant vision loss during that patient's lifetime. In contrast, the older patient with a shorter life expectancy may not need to be treated as aggressively.

Although angle-closure glaucoma can occur at any age, it is most often diagnosed in the 50- to 65-year-old age group.[31] However, when the age-specific incidence is calculated, the risk of acute angle-closure glaucoma is found to increase progressively with age.[32] Angle-closure glaucoma occurs in eyes that have a

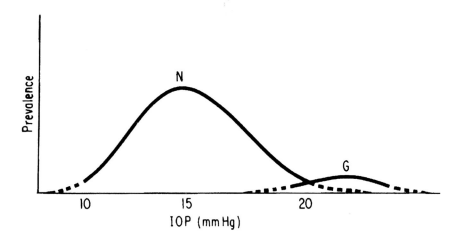

FIGURE 2-3. Theoretical distribution of intraocular pressures (IOP) in nonglaucoma (N) and glaucoma (G) populations shows overlap between the two groups (*dotted lines* represent uncertainty of extreme values in both populations). (Reprinted with permission from MB Shields [ed]. Textbook of Glaucoma [4th ed]. Baltimore: Williams & Wilkins, 1998;47.)

smaller than normal axial length and a decreased anterior chamber angle depth.[33] With age, thickening of the lens and its forward displacement is believed to cause a further shallowing of the anterior chamber depth. When the amount of narrowing results in critically narrow angles, the likelihood of chronic angle-closure and acute angle-closure attacks increases. Persons who have undergone cataract surgery are at a decreased risk of angle-closure attack due to a deeper postsurgical anterior chamber depth.

Race

The Baltimore Eye Survey found the prevalence of glaucoma in African Americans to be four to five times greater than that of whites. African Americans were found to have higher prevalence rates of glaucoma in every age category, with elderly African Americans having the highest prevalence rate at 11.26% for those 80 years and older (see Figure 2-2).[9] Glaucoma occurs at a younger age in African Americans than in whites, and at the time of diagnosis, the cup-to-disc ratio tends to be greater, IOP higher, and visual field loss more significant in African Americans than in whites.[9,34,35] African Americans are not only more likely to have glaucoma, but they progress at a more rapid rate, are more resistant to treatment, and are more likely to go blind from the disease. Studies estimate the rate of blindness among whites to be between 2.5% and 4.4% per case of glaucoma. The rate of blindness for African Americans is significantly higher at 8%.[1] Javitt and associates demonstrated that the undertreatment of African Americans with glaucoma may be an important factor contributing to this higher rate of blindness. They calculated the expected rate of glaucoma surgery for African Americans based on reported rates of surgery for white Medicare patients, and the conservative estimate that glaucoma is at least four times more prevalent among African Americans. They observed that African Americans were 45% less likely to undergo necessary laser or

incisional surgery for glaucoma than would be expected.[36] This may be related to the fact that African Americans report only two-thirds the number of office visits for glaucoma as whites.[37]

Approximately 0.2% of whites will suffer an angle-closure attack. The incidence of angle-closure attacks among African Americans is rare, but the incidence of chronic angle-closure glaucoma is equal to that of whites.[1] The risk of developing angle-closure glaucoma is higher than the risk of primary open-angle glaucoma in Southeast Asians, Japanese, North American Eskimos, and adults in the Philippines.[3,6,38]

It has been reported that *Japanese* persons, and *Asians* in general, have a higher prevalence of normal-tension glaucoma. It is important to note, however, that the mean IOP among Asians is 13 mm Hg, 2–3 mm Hg lower than in people of European descent.[39] Therefore, an IOP of 18 mm Hg is 2 SD above the normal mean IOP in Asians. Publications from Asia and Japan that report this higher prevalence of normal-tension glaucoma are using 21 mm Hg as the defining limit for normal-tension glaucoma, likely resulting in an inflated number of normal tension glaucoma patients.[40]

Family History of Glaucoma

The relevance of a positive family history of glaucoma is not yet completely understood. It has been estimated that first-degree relatives of patients with primary open-angle glaucoma are four to eight times more likely to develop glaucoma.[41,42] Glaucoma may be present in as many as 16% of first-degree relatives of those with primary open-angle glaucoma, as compared with less than 2% of the general population.[43] A confirmed strong family history of glaucoma should raise suspicion and might prompt earlier treatment of a glaucoma suspect. A family history of blindness caused by glaucoma is of particular interest, as it may signal the need for more aggressive therapy or closer follow-up. Substantiating a family history of glaucoma and blindness is often difficult. Many patients tend to confuse cataracts for glaucoma, and might attribute vision loss from diabetic retinopathy, macular degeneration, or other pathology to glaucoma. Asking the patient whether a relative might have had cataracts rather than glaucoma, or inquiring about topical eyedrop use or a history of diabetes might help to clarify the family history.

The genetic factors involved in the inheritance patterns of glaucoma are under investigation. Some forms of juvenile open-angle glaucoma (onset between the age of 3 years and early adulthood) have been shown to be genetically determined. The mode of inheritance in these cases is autosomal dominant with high penetrance. The phenotype has been mapped to chromosome 1 in the region q21-q31.[44] This disorder is caused by mutations in the trabecular meshwork–induced glucocorticoid response protein (TIGR) gene.[44,45] Adult-onset primary open-angle glaucoma has been mapped to three gene loci (chromosomes 2cen-q13, 3q21-q24, and 8q23).[45,46] A fourth locus (10p15-p14) has been identified for the normal tension form of primary open-angle glaucoma.[47] As the genetic mystery surrounding glaucoma continues to unravel, it is not implausible to speculate that simple blood testing might someday replace or supplement current methods of glaucoma screening. Genetic screening might identify persons predisposed to the development of glaucoma before optic nerve damage occurs.

Refractive Error

High myopia and high hyperopia have been associated with an increased risk of developing glaucoma. Perkins and Phelps found that, in a select group of patients with primary open-angle glaucoma, there were four times as many myopes (more than 1 D) than in a similar age-matched sample of the U.S. population.[48] They also found a higher incidence of ocular hypertension and normal-tension glaucoma in patients with myopia.[48] The Blue Mountain Eye Study found an increased risk of glaucoma among patients with moderate to high myopia (greater than or equal to 3 D), and a borderline risk for low myopia (less than 3 D).[49] Lotufo and coworkers found that persons younger than 35 years with more than 3 D of myopia had a higher prevalence rate of primary open-angle glaucoma. They also found that young African-American patients, especially when myopic, were more susceptible to elevated IOP than whites.[50] Perhaps the most intriguing observation regarding the relationship between glaucoma and refractive error is that patients with myopia are more likely to develop progressive glaucomatous damage than are hyperopes or emmetropes.[51] Chihara and coworkers found this increased risk of progressive visual field loss only among persons with severe myopia (greater than or equal to 4 D).[52] It is important to note that many clinic-based studies have an inherent study design flaw, in that myopes in general are more likely to report for ocular examination than are hyperopes or emmetropes. This represents an increased likelihood of glaucoma detection among myopic patients. Taking this into consideration, it is still generally accepted that an increased risk of glaucoma exists among high myopes. Perhaps defective connective tissue elements in the optic nerve, lamina cribrosa, and scleral shell may result in a shared pathogenetic pathway.

Pigmentary dispersion syndrome and pigmentary glaucoma usually occur in eyes with a moderate degree of myopia that have a greater than normal anterior chamber depth and volume.[53,54] It is believed that peripheral iris concavity in these eyes facilitates iridozonular contact, thereby increasing pigment liberation. Angle-closure glaucoma occurs more frequently in hyperopic eyes that have a shorter than average axial length; a shallow anterior chamber; a thicker, more anteriorly placed lens; and a smaller than normal radius of corneal curvature.[55-57]

Gender

Gender difference is not thought to be a significant risk factor for the development of primary open-angle glaucoma. Most studies support a greater prevalence of pigment dispersion syndrome among males than females, with the male-to-female ratio being approximately 2 to 1.[53,58] Females are two to three times more likely to experience primary angle-closure glaucoma than their male counterparts.[57,59] The reason for this increased prevalence among women has yet to be explained, except in the case of Eskimo women. These women have an unusually high prevalence of shallow anterior chambers and narrow angles, thus predisposing them to angle-closure glaucoma.[60]

Trauma

A past history of blunt ocular injury can lead to the development of secondary glaucoma and has clinical implications for treatment and management. Although it is possible for glaucoma to develop soon after trauma, it may not manifest for several years.[61] Establishing accurate prevalence and incidence rates for traumatic glaucoma is difficult, because many individuals do not seek medical attention at the time of the incident, and remote traumas often go unreported. The severity of past ocular trauma is also difficult to substantiate. The occurrence of late-onset glaucoma after ocular trauma is estimated to be 2–10%.[62,63]

The most common causes of post-traumatic elevated IOP are angle recession (Color Plate 14) and hyphema (Color Plate 13). IOP is more likely to be elevated if 270 degrees or more of the angle are affected.[62]

If the clinical examination is suggestive of unilateral glaucoma, suspicion of a traumatic etiology should increase, and further investigation is warranted. Inquiring about facial or periocular scars might provide clues to significant past ocular trauma. Clinical findings in support of a traumatic etiology might include:

- Traumatic corneal scarring
- Irregular pupils
- Anisocoria
- Iris sphincter tear
- Iridodialysis
- Asymmetric or rosette cataract (Color Plate 12)
- Phakodonesis
- Lens subluxation or dislocation
- Angle recession
- Pigment clumping in the angle (see Color Plate 15)

Diabetes

There has been much debate as to whether a positive association between diabetes and glaucoma exists. Although the Baltimore Eye Survey[64] and the Barbados Eye Study[65] found no significant and consistent association between diabetes and glaucoma, several other studies have. The Rotterdam Eye Study[66] found that diabetes mellitus was associated with an overall mean IOP increase of 0.31 mm Hg in each eye, and a threefold increase in the presence of high-tension glaucoma. The Beaver Dam Eye Study[67] found glaucoma to be more prevalent among persons with older-onset diabetes than in those without diabetes (4.2% versus 2.0%). When persons with a history of glaucoma treatment were included in the analysis, the number of persons with diabetes was two times higher than in those without (7.8% versus 3.9%). The Blue Mountain Eye Study[68] of Australia also supports a positive association between glaucoma and diabetes. It showed a 5.5% prevalence of glaucoma in those with diabetes compared with a 2.8% prevalence in those without, with the age-gender-adjusted odds ratio being approximately 2 to 1. Ocular hypertension was also more common in persons with diabetes (6.7%) than in those without (3.5%). Of those persons with glaucoma, 13.0% had diabetes compared with 6.9% without. Among those with untreated glaucoma, the age-gender-adjusted mean IOP was 0.6 mm Hg higher in people with diabetes than in those without. It has been hypothesized that small-vessel disease or systemic blood abnormalities can result in compromised vascular perfusion to the optic nerve, which increases the risk of glaucomatous optic neuropathy.[69] It should be noted that persons with diabetes are more likely to be referred for or to seek an eye examination because of the risk of diabetic retinopathy. This might result in a clinical bias towards the detection of glaucoma among persons with diabetes in the general clinic population.

Hypertension

Just as with diabetes mellitus, there have been many conflicting reports regarding the possible association between hypertension and glaucoma. Whereas Jonas and Grundler[70] and Schulzer and Drance[71] found no positive association between hypertension and primary open-angle glaucoma, Tielsch and associates did.[72] This association may be more complex than previously assumed. Tielsch and coworkers found that young people with hypertension are less likely than nonhypertensive people of the same age group to develop glaucoma.[72] Among the elderly, however, hypertension does become a significant risk factor for the development of glaucoma (Figure 2-4). It has been suggested that in the early stages of systemic hypertension, the higher head of blood pressure increases vascular flow and decreases the chance of atrophy of the optic nerve. After years of chronic hypertension, compromises in vascular integrity result in a decreased ability of the head of blood pressure to overcome the resistance of increased IOP, thus increasing the chance of optic nerve compromise.[73] Tielsch and coworkers also demonstrated that persons with a diastolic perfusion pressure (diastolic blood pressure–intraocular pressure) below 30 mm Hg had six times the age-race-adjusted risk of primary open-angle glaucoma of persons with perfusion pressures greater than 50 mm Hg. They suggest that compromised ocular blood flow and autoregulation may be important factors in primary open-angle glaucoma. Nocturnal reduction in blood pressure represents an additional risk for glaucomatous optic neuropathy,[74] particularly in normal-tension glaucoma.

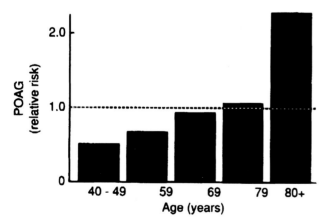

FIGURE 2-4. Relationship between hypertension and primary open-angle glaucoma (POAG) as a function of age. Early in life, systemic hypertension reduces the risk for POAG. Later in life, it increases the risk. (Reprinted with permission from JM Tielsch, J Katz, A Sommer, et al. Hypertension, perfusion pressure, and primary open-angle glaucoma. A population-based assessment. Arch Ophthalmol 1995;113[2]:216–221.)

TABLE 2-6. Indications for Use of Corticosteroids in Ocular Disease

Eyelids
  Allergic blepharitis
  Contact dermatoblepharitis
  Herpes zoster dermatoblepharitis
  Chemical burns
  Neonatal hemangioma
Conjunctiva
  Allergic conjunctivitis
  Vernal conjunctivitis
  Herpes zoster conjunctivitis
  Chemical burns
  Mucocutaneous conjunctival lesions
Cornea
  Immune reaction after keratoplasty
  Herpes zoster keratitis
  Disciform keratitis
  Marginal corneal infiltrates
  Superficial punctate keratitis
  Chemical burns
  Acne rosacea keratitis
  Interstitial keratitis
Uvea
  Anterior uveitis
  Posterior uveitis
  Sympathetic ophthalmia
Sclera
  Scleritis
  Episcleritis
Retina
  Retinal vasculitis
Optic nerve
  Optic neuritis
  Temporal arteritis
Globe
  Endophthalmitis
  Hemorrhagic glaucoma
Orbit
  Pseudotumor
  Graves' ophthalmopathy
Extraocular muscles
  Ocular myasthenia gravis

TABLE 2-7. Systemic Conditions That May Require the Use of Systemic Corticosteroids

Chronic obstructive pulmonary disease

Asthma

Sarcoidosis

Systemic lupus erythematosus

Rheumatoid arthritis

Giant cell arteritis

To prevent transplant rejection

Hypothyroidism

Smith and associates[75] reported a statistically significant association between hypothyroidism and primary open-angle glaucoma. It is hypothesized that hypothyroidism results in the accumulation of hyaluronic acid in the trabecular meshwork, which may increase outflow resistance, thereby increasing IOP. This may be reversible with systemic treatment for the hypothyroidism.[76] Further investigation into a possible association between hypothyroidism and glaucoma is warranted.

Steroid Use

Certain individuals are prone to elevations in IOP with prolonged steroid use. (See Tables 2-6 and 2-7 for indications of ocular and systemic steroid use.) The exact mechanism responsible for this increase in IOP is not well understood. There are steroid-sensitive receptors on the cells of the trabecular meshwork; steroid interaction with these receptors may somehow alter aqueous outflow facility. Trabecular meshwork cells of eyes treated with dexamethasone have been shown to exhibit decreased phagocytic ability.[77] Electron microscopy has shown that steroid treatment can result in the accumulation of glycosaminoglycans and other extracellular materials in the trabecular meshwork, which may increase resistance to aqueous outflow.[78,79] This ocular hypertensive effect has been reported with various steroid preparations, including topical, oral, and inhaled preparations; periocular injections; and dermatologic creams. Although increases in IOP are possible in all patients, those most likely to exhibit a steroid response include persons with primary open-angle glaucoma, their first-degree relatives, myopes, and persons with diabetes or collagen vascular disease.[80–82] Increases in IOP usually develop within 2–8 weeks of steroid initiation and tend to reverse within 1–3 weeks of discontinuation. In some cases, however, permanent increases in IOP have occurred despite discontinuation of steroid use.[83,84]

Migraine

It has been suggested that individuals who suffer from migraines may be at an increased risk of developing open-angle glaucoma, especially normal-tension glaucoma. The vasoconstriction associated with migraines and Raynaud's disease may lead to decreased vascular perfusion to the optic nerve head and an increased risk of glaucomatous optic neuropathy. Studies attempting to substantiate this association have been conflicting. Phelps and Corbett noted an increased frequency of both migraine and other types of headaches in patients with normal-tension glaucoma as compared with healthy individuals, persons with ocular hypertension, and persons with primary open-angle glaucoma.[85] Data from the Blue Mountain Eye Study suggest a possible association between typical migraine headache and open-angle glaucoma.[86] Both the Beaver Dam Eye Study[87] and a study by Usui and coworkers[88] failed to confirm this association. These differences may be a factor of the specific populations studied, variations in the accepted definition of migraines, or both.

Smoking and Alcohol Consumption

Whether smoking or alcohol consumption represents an increased risk for glaucoma is uncertain. Morgan and Drance[89] showed a positive relationship between smoking and increased IOP, but an association between smoking and glaucoma could not be made. The Beaver Dam Eye Study[90] found no difference in the frequency of glaucoma as a function of either smoking or alcohol consumption. Larger epidemiologic studies need to be performed so that the effects of these variables with respect to IOP and glaucoma can be better understood.

REFERENCES

1. Quigley HA. Number of people with glaucoma worldwide. Br J Ophthalmol 1996;80:389–393.

2. Thylefors B, Negrel AD, Pararajasegaram R. Epidemiologic aspects of global blindness prevention. Curr Opin Ophthalmol 1992;3:824–834.

3. Genio CA, Gavino BC. Glaucoma profile in the Philippines General Hospital. Philipp J Ophthalmol 1983;15:1–2.

4. Congdon NG, Quigley HA, Hung PT, et al. The impact of age, cataract and visual acuity on whole-field scotopic sensitivity screening for glaucoma in rural Taiwan. Arch Ophthalmol 1995;113:1138–1143.

5. Drance SM. Angle closure glaucoma among Canadian Eskimos. Can J Ophthalmol 1973;8:252.

6. Arkell SM, Lightman DA, Sommer A, et al. The prevalence of glaucoma among Eskimos of Northwest Alaska. Arch Ophthalmol 1987;105:482.

7. Clemmesen V, Alsbirk PH. Primary angle-closure glaucoma in Greenland. Acta Ophthalmol 1971;49:47.

8. Quigley HA, Vitale S. Models of open-angle glaucoma prevalence and incidence in the United States. Invest Ophthalmol Vis Sci 1997;38(1):83–91.

9. Tielsch JM, Sommer A, Katz J, et al. Racial variations in the prevalence of primary open angle glaucoma: the Baltimore Eye Survey. JAMA 1991;226(3):369–374.

10. Alper MG, Laubach JL. Primary angle-closure glaucoma in the American Negro. Arch Ophthalmol 1963;79:663j–668.

11. Wang F, Ford D, Tielsch JM, et al. Undetected eye disease in a primary care clinic population. Arch Intern Med 1994;154:1821–1828.

12. Yen MT, Wu CY, Higginbotham EJ. Importance of increasing public awareness regarding glaucoma. Arch Ophthalmol 1996;114:635.

13. Armaly MF. Ocular pressure and visual fields. A ten-year follow-up study. Arch Ophthalmol 1969; 81:25–40.

14. Krakau CET. Intraocular pressure elevation—cause or effect in chronic glaucoma? Ophthalmology 1981;182:141–147.

15. Hollows FC, Graham PA. Intraocular pressure, glaucoma, and glaucoma suspects in a defined population. Br J Ophthalmol 1966;50:570–586.

16. Kahn HA, Milton RC. Revised Framingham Eye Study: prevalence of glaucoma and diabetic retinopathy. Am J Epidemiol 1989;111:769–776.

17. Mason RP, Kosoko O, Wilson MR, et al. National survey of the prevalence and risk factors of glaucoma in St. Lucia, West Indies. Part I: prevalence findings. Ophthalmology 1989;96:1363–1368.

18. Cartwright MJ, Anderson DR. Correlation of asymmetric damage with asymmetric intraocular pressure in normal-tension glaucoma (low-tension glaucoma). Arch Ophthalmol 1988;106:898–900.

19. Crichton A, Drance SM, Douglas GR, Schultzer M. Unequal intraocular pressure and its relation to asymmetric visual field defects in low-tension glaucoma. Ophthalmology 1989;69:1312–1314.

20. Pohjanpelto PEJ, Palva J. Ocular hypertension and glaucomatous optic nerve damage. Acta Ophthalmol 1974;52:194.

21. Kass MA, Hart WM Jr, Gordon M, Miller JP. Risk factors favoring the development of glaucomatous visual field loss in ocular hypertension. Surv Ophthalmol 1980;25:155.

22. Armaly MF, Krueger D, Maundes L, et al. Biostatistical analysis of the Collaborative Glaucoma Study. I. Summary report of the risk factors for glaucomatous visual-field defects. Arch Opthamol 1980; 98(12):2163–2171.

23. Odberg T, Riise D. Early diagnosis of glaucoma. II. The value of the initial examination in ocular hypertension. Acta Ophthalmol 1987;65:58.

24. Schulzer M, Drance SM, Douglas GR. A comparison of treated and untreated glaucoma suspects. Ophthalmology 1991;98:301–307.

25. Van Buskirk EM, Shields MB (eds). 100 Years of Progress in Glaucoma. Philadelphia: Lippincott–Raven, 1997.

26. Shields MB (ed). Textbook of Glaucoma (3rd ed). Baltimore: Williams & Wilkins, 1992;53–54.

27. Armaly MF. On the distribution of applanation pressure. I. Statistical features and the effect of age, sex, and family history of glaucoma. Arch Ophthalmol 1965;73:11.

28. Kashgarian M, Packer H, Deutsch AR, et al. The frequency of distribution of intraocular pressure by age and sex groups. JAMA 1966;197:611.

29. Armaly MF, Krueger DE, Maundir L, et al. Biostatistical analysis of the Collaborative Glaucoma Study. I. Summary report of the risk factors for glaucomatous visual field defects. Arch Ophthalmol 1980;98:2163–2171.

30. Klein BEK, Klein R, Sponsel WE, et al. Prevalence of glaucoma. The Beaver Dam Eye Study. Ophthalmology 1992;99:1499–1504.

31. David R, Tessler Z, Yassur Y. Epidemiology of acute angle closure glaucoma: incidence and seasonal variations. Ophthalmologica 1985;191:4–7.

32. Teikari J, Raivio I, Nurminen M. Incidence of acute glaucoma in Finland from 1973–1982. Graefe's Arch Clin Exp Ophthalmol 1987;225:357–360.

33. Congdon N, Wang F, Tielsch JM. Issues in the epidemiology and population-based screening of primary angle-closure glaucoma. Surv Ophthalmol 1992;36:411–423.

34. Martin MJ, Sommer A, Gold EB, et al. Race and primary open angle glaucoma. Am J Ophthalmol 1985;99:383–387.

35. The advanced glaucoma intervention study (AGIS). 3. Baseline characteristics of black and white patients. Ophthalmology 1998;105(7):1137–1145.

36. Javitt JC, McBean M, Nicholson GA, et al. Undertreatment of glaucoma among black Americans. N Engl J Med 1991;325:1418–1422.

37. Javitt JC. Universal coverage and preventable blindness. Arch Ophthalmol 1994;112:453.

38. Lowe R. The problems of glaucoma in Singapore. Singapore Med J 1968;9:76.

39. Shiose Y, Kitazawa Y, Tsukahara S, et al. Epidemiology of glaucoma in Japan—a nationwide glaucoma survey. Jpn J Ophthalmol 1991;35:133–155.

40. Quigley HA. Mechanisms of Glaucomatous Optic Neuropathy. In EM Van Buskirk, MB Shields (eds), 100 Years of Progress in Glaucoma. New York: Lippincott–Raven, 1997;79–98.

41. Miller SJH. Genetics of glaucoma and family history studies. Trans Ophthalmol 1978;98:290–292.

42. Tielsch JM, Katz J, Sommer A, et al. Family history and risk of primary open angle glaucoma. The Baltimore Eye Survey. Arch Ophthalmol 1994; 112(1): 69–73.

43. Leske MC. The epidemiology of open-angle glaucoma: a review. Am J Epidemiol 1983;188:166–191.

44. Sheffield VC, Stone EM, Alward WL, et al. Genetic linkage of familial open angle glaucoma to chromosome 1q21-q31. Nat Genet 1993;4:47–50.

45. Trifan OC, Traboulsi EI, Stoilova D, et al. A third locus (GLC1D) for adult-onset primary open-angle glaucoma maps to the 8q23 region. Am J Ophthalmol 1998;126(1):17–28.

46. Sarfarazi M. Recent advances in molecular genetics of glaucomas. Hum Mol Genet 1997;6:1667–1677.

47. Sarfarazi M, Child A, Stoilova D, et al. Localization of the fourth locus (GLC1E) for adult-onset primary open-angle glaucoma to the 10p15-p14 region. Am J Hum Genet 1998;62:641–652.

48. Perkins ES, Phelps CD. Open-angle glaucoma, ocular hypertension, low-tension glaucoma, and refraction. Arch Ophthalmol 1982;100:1464–1467.

49. Mitchell P, Hourihan F, Sandbach J, Wang JJ. The relationship between glaucoma and myopia: the Blue Mountain Eye Study. Ophthalmology 1999; 106(10):2010–2015.

50. Lotofo D, Ritch R, Szmyd L Jr, Burris JE. Juvenile glaucoma, race, and refraction. JAMA 1989; 261(2):249–252.

51. Phelps CD. Effect of myopia on prognosis in treated primary open-angle glaucoma. Am J Ophthalmol 1982;93:622–623.

52. Chihara E, Liu X, Dong J, et al. Severe myopia as a risk factor for progressive visual field loss in primary open-angle glaucoma. Ophthalmologica 1997; 211(2):66–71.

53. Scheie HG, Cameron JD. Pigment dispersion syndrome: a clinical study. Br J Ophthalmol 1981; 65:254–269.

54. Davidson JA, Brubaker RF, Ilstrup DM. Dimensions of the anterior chamber in pigment dispersion syndrome. Arch Ophthalmol 1983;101:81–83.

55. Tomlinson A, Leighton DA. Ocular dimensions in the heredity of angle-closure glaucoma. Br J Ophthalmol 1973;57:475–486.

56. Lee DA, Brubaker RF, Ilstrup DM. Anterior chamber dimensions in patients with narrow angles and angle-closure glaucoma. Arch Ophthalmol 1984; 102:46–50.

57. Lowe RF. Causes of shallow anterior chamber in primary angle closure glaucoma. Am J Ophthalmol 1969;67:87–93.

58. Farrar SM, Shields MB, Miller KN, Stoup CM. Risk factors for the development and severity of glaucoma in the pigment dispersion syndrome. Am J Ophthalmol 1989;108:223.

59. Lowe RF. Angle-closure glaucoma: acute and subacute attacks: clinical types. Trans Ophthalmol Soc Aust 1961;21:65–75.

60. Alsbirk PH. Anterior chamber depth and primary angle-closure glaucoma. 1. An epidemiologic study in Greenland Eskimos. Act Ophthalmol 1975;53:89–104.

61. Kaufman JH, Tolpin DW. Glaucoma after traumatic angle recession. Am J Ophthalmol 1974; 78:648–654.

62. Herschler J. Trabecular damage due to blunt anterior segment injury and its relationship to traumatic glaucoma. Trans Am Acad Ophthalmol Otolaryngol 1977;83:239–248.

63. Tonjum AM. Intraocular pressure and facility of outflow late after ocular contusion. Acta Ophthalmol 1968;46:886–908.

64. Tielsch JM, Katz J, Quigley HA, et al. Diabetes, intraocular pressure, and primary open-angle glau-

coma in the Baltimore Eye Survey. Ophthalmology 1995;102:(1):48–53.

65. Leske MC, Connell AMS, Wu Suh-Yuh, et al. Risk factors for open-angle glaucoma. Arch Ophthalmol 1995;113:918–924.

66. Dielemans I, de Jong PT, Stolk R, et al. Primary open-angle glaucoma, intraocular pressure, and diabetes mellitus in the general elderly population. The Rotterdam Study. Ophthalmology 1996;103(8):1271–1275.

67. Klein BEK, Klein R, Jensen SC. Open-angle glaucoma and older-onset diabetes. The Beaver Dam Eye Study. Ophthalmology 1994;101(7):1173–1177.

68. Mitchell P, Smith W, Chey T, Healey PR. Open-angle glaucoma and diabetes: the Blue Mountain Eye Study, Australia. Ophthalmology 1997;104(4): 712–718.

69. Wilson MR. Epidemiologic features of glaucoma. Int Ophthalmol Clin 1990;30:153–160.

70. Jonas JB, Grundler AE. Prevalence of diabetes mellitus and arterial hypertension in primary and secondary open-angle glaucomas. Graefe's Arch Clin Exp Ophthalmol 1998;236(3):202–206.

71. Schulzer M, Drance SM. Intraocular pressure, systemic blood pressure and age: a correlational study. Br J Ophthalmol 1987;71:245–250.

72. Tielsch JM, Katz J, Sommer A, et al. Hypertension, perfusion pressure, and primary open-angle glaucoma. A population-based assessment. Arch Ophthalmol 1995;113(2):216–221.

73. Sommer A, Tielsch JM. Primary Open-Angle Glaucoma. A Clinical-Epidemiologic Perspective. In ME Van Buskirk, MB Shields (eds). 100 Years of Progress in Glaucoma. New York: Lippincott–Raven,1997:136.

74. Graham SL, Drance SM, Wijsman K, et al. Ambulatory blood pressure monitoring in glaucoma. The nocturnal dip. Ophthalmology 1995;102(1):61–69.

75. Smith KD, Arthurs BP, Saheb N. An association between hypothyroidism and primary open-angle glaucoma. Ophthalmology 1993;100(10):1580–1584.

76. McDaniel D, Besada E. Hypothyroidism—a possible etiology of open-angle glaucoma. J Am Optom Assoc 1996;67(2):109–114.

77. Matsumoto Y, Johnson DH. Dexamethasone decreases phagocytosis by human trabecular meshwork cells in situ. Invest Ophthalmol Vis Sci 1997; 38(9):1902–1907.

78. Francois J. Corticosteroid glaucoma. Ophthalmologica 1984;188:76–81.

79. Godel V, Rogenbogen L, Stein R. On the mechanism of corticosteroid-induced ocular hypertension. Ann Ophthalmol 1978;10:191–196.

80. Armaly MF. Effect of corticosteroids on intraocular pressure and fluid dynamics: I. The effect of dexamethasone in the normal eye. Arch Ophthalmol 1963;70:482–491.

81. Becker B, Podos SM. Elevated intraocular pressure following corticosteroid eye drops. JAMA 1963;185:884.

82. Becker B, Hahn KA. Topical corticosteroids

and heredity in primary open angle glaucoma. Am J Ophthalmol 1964;57:543.

83. Armaly MF. Effect of corticosteroids on intraocular pressure and fluid dynamics: the effect of dexamethasone in the normal eye. Arch Ophthalmol 1963;70:482–491.

84. Becker B, Mills DW. Corticosteroids and intraocular pressure. Arch Ophthalmol 1963;70:500–507.

85. Phelps CD, Corbett JJ. Migraine and low-tension glaucoma: a case-control study. Invest Ophthalmol Vis Sci 1985;26:1105.

86. Wang JJ, Mitchell P, Smith W. Is there an association between migraine headache and open-angle glaucoma? Findings from the Blue Mountain Eye Study. Ophthalmology 1997;104(10):1714–1719.

87. Klein BE, Klein R, Meuer SM, Goetz LA. Migraine headache and its association with open-angle glaucoma: the Beaver Dam Eye Study. Invest Ophthalmol Vis Sci 1993;34(10):3024–3027.

88. Usui T, Iwata K, Shirakashi M, Abe H. Prevalence of migraine in low-tension glaucoma and primary open-angle glaucoma in Japanese. Br J Ophthalmol 1991;75:224.

89. Morgan RW, Drance SM. Chronic open-angle glaucoma and ocular hypertension: an epidemiological study. Br J Ophthalmol 1975;59:211–215.

90. Klein BE, Klein R, Ritter LL. Relationship of drinking alcohol and smoking to prevalence of open-angle glaucoma. The Beaver Dam Eye Study. Ophthalmology 1993;100(11):1609–1613.

91. Perkins ES. The Bedford glaucoma survey. I. Long-term follow-up of borderline cases. Br J Ophthalmol 1973;57:179.

92. Perkins ES. The Bedford glaucoma survey. II. Rescreening of normal population. Br J Ophthalmol 1973;57:186.

93. Walker WM. Ocular hypertension. Follow-up of 109 cases from 1963 to 1974. Trans Ophthalmol Soc UK 1974;94:525.

94. Wilensky JT, Podos SM, Becker B. Prognostic indicators in ocular hypertension. Arch Ophthalmol 1974;91:200.

95. Norskov K. Routine tonometry in ophthalmic practice. II. Five-year follow-up. Acta Ophthalmol 1970;48:873.

96. Linner E. Ocular hypertension. I. The clinical course during ten years without therapy. Aqueous humor dynamics. Acta Ophthalmol 1976;54:707.

97. Kitazawa Y, Horie T, Aoki S, et al. Untreated ocular hypertension. A long-term prospective study. Arch Ophthalmol 1977;95:1180.

98. David R, Livingstone DG, Luntz MH. Ocular hypertension—a long-term follow-up of treated and untreated patients. Br J Ophthalmol 1977;61:668.

99. Hart WM Jr., Yablonski M, Kass MA, et al. Multivariate analysis of the risk of glaucomatous visual field loss. Arch Ophthalmol 1979;97:1455.

100. Lundberg L, Wettrell K, Linner E. Ocular hypertension. A prospective twenty-year follow-up study. Acta Ophthalmol 1987;65:705.

Clinical Examination for Glaucoma

Kelliann Dignam and Robert S. Stutman

The clinical examination to diagnose glaucoma follows the same protocol as the comprehensive routine eye examination. After a careful patient history is taken, visual acuity, pupils, confrontation visual fields, slit lamp evaluation, tonometry, and a dilated evaluation of the optic nerve are performed. When glaucoma is suspected or diagnosed, gonioscopy and automated visual field testing should also be performed. Supplemental testing of color vision and contrast sensitivity as they relate to glaucoma can also be incorporated into the examination.

PATIENT HISTORY

Given the typically asymptomatic nature of primary open-angle glaucoma (POAG), the initial patient history is directed at uncovering risk factors for glaucoma (Table 3-1). If subsequent clinical findings are suspicious for either primary or secondary glaucoma, an expanded history is used to aid in the differential diagnosis and to guide management and treatment decisions.

The case of the new patient with previously diagnosed glaucoma can be a challenging one. Inquire as to what led the previous doctor to diagnose glaucoma (elevated intraocular pressure [IOP], documented optic nerve damage, or visual field loss). Knowledge of pretreatment IOP is important for the determination of a target IOP. A history of medication use and possible intolerance or allergy is crucial. If and when laser or filtration surgery was performed and whether it was monocular or binocular should be determined. The patient should be asked whether his or her glaucoma and visual fields were thought to be stable. If optic nerve photographs were taken, the doctor should ask whether they

are obtainable. Review of past optic disc photos is more accurate than relying on a past clinician's written cup-to-disc ratios because interobserver variability can be high. Whenever possible, past ocular records should be obtained to supplement current clinical findings and to avoid unnecessary duplication of testing or the reinstitution of ineffective or harmful treatment modalities.

An established glaucoma patient should be asked, at each follow-up visit, what ocular or oral medications have been taken, how many times a day they were taken, and the time of the last drop instillation or oral medication. It is best to have the patient state the medication names and dosing regimens because the patient's unprompted response can lend valuable information regarding patient compliance. Side effects of the specific medications should be elicited and addressed to ensure patient safety and to maintain medication compliance.

VISUAL ACUITY

Glaucoma preferentially affects the superior and inferior arcuate bundles of the retinal nerve fiber layer. The papillomacular bundle, which is responsible for central visual acuity, remains relatively spared until late in the disease process. Therefore, good visual acuity is usually preserved until the advanced stages of the disease, at which time visual field loss can affect central vision. Many unsuspecting patients with glaucoma, and even patients diagnosed with glaucoma, mistake good visual acuity for good ocular health. Professional eye care might not be sought, or poor compliance with medications or follow-up appointments might result. Therefore, the importance of patient education cannot be overemphasized.

TABLE 3-1. Diagnosing Glaucoma: Relevant Patient History

Age

Race

Ocular symptoms

Past history of injury or trauma

Past history of surgery, including laser surgery

Past history of increased intraocular pressure

Previously diagnosed and/or treated glaucoma

Positive family history of glaucoma

Positive family history of blindness

Relevant systemic history

    Hypertension

    Diabetes

    Thyroid disease

    Migraine

    Vascular disease

    Medication use

As with any ocular examination, monocular visual acuity measurements should be taken. If the best-corrected visual acuity is reduced, it must be explained by the clinical findings. Unless the glaucomatous damage is severe, the initial assumption is that the vision loss is due to some other cause.

One exception to this rule of preserved visual acuity occurs when a sudden rise in IOP forces fluid into the cornea at a rate that exceeds the ability of the endothelial pumps to detergess the cornea. Corneal edema, microcysts, and bullae can result, producing blurred vision and the symptom of colored halos around light (as opposed to the white halos around light that accompany uncorrected refractive error) (Figure 3-1). These symptoms most commonly occur with angle-closure glaucoma, but any acute rise in IOP can produce such symptoms.

Vision loss due to advanced glaucoma must be differentiated from that caused by cataracts, macular degeneration, diabetic retinopathy, or any number of other conditions to which this population is susceptible. The effect of a cataract or media opacity on vision can be estimated during the dilated examination by grading the clarity of the view on funduscopic examination (i.e., a 20/80 cataract should result in a 20/80 view of the fundus). The laser interferometer or a potential acuity meter (PAM) may also be used to assess the contribution of media opacity to decreased visual acuity. Asbell and colleagues[1] compared best-corrected Snellen visual acuity with that measured by the PAM in patients with clear media. They found that PAM visual acuity is a reliable indicator of Snellen visual acuity in eyes with normal ocular health, eyes with mild-moderate glaucoma, and when PAM visual acuity is better than 20/60. However, when visual field loss is severe or when PAM visual acuity is worse than 20/60, Snellen visual acuity and PAM visual acuity may not correlate each other.

If the media do not match the visual acuity, another disease process is likely at work. The fundus should be evaluated for conditions that explain the decreased vision. Examples of such conditions include age-related macular degeneration, diabetic retinopathy with macular edema, and branch and central retinal vein or artery occlusions. Ischemia, inflammation, or compression of the optic nerve can also lead to visual acuity or visual field loss. Optic disc edema or disc pallor due to optic atrophy can result in visual field loss that must be differ-

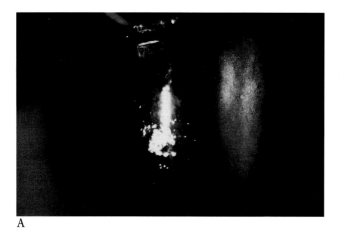
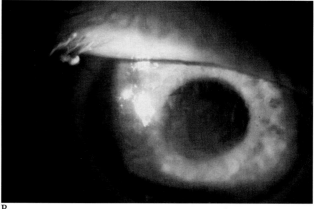

A   B

FIGURE 3-1. Corneal edema can result when a significant or sudden rise in intraocular pressure forces fluid into the cornea at a rate that exceeds the ability of the endothelial pumps to detergess the cornea. Slit-lamp appearance of microcystic corneal edema in a patient with an acute rise in intraocular pressure (**A**). The accumulation of fluid under intact epithelium can result in the formation of bullae (**B**).

entiated from that caused by glaucoma. All of these observations are critical as they can affect both visual acuity and visual fields. The clinician must keep this in mind when interpreting the visual fields and setting the course of therapy.

Having ruled out other causes of decreased visual acuity, it may be considered that the glaucomatous optic neuropathy is responsible. Although, as stated above, central visual acuity is usually preserved until the late stages of glaucoma, it can be affected if visual field loss encroaches fixation. Pickett and colleagues[2] showed that decreased vision with associated central field loss can be a relatively early finding in a minority of glaucoma patients (Figure 3-2). Anctil and Anderson[3] also found a subtle reduction in visual acuity in patients with mild glaucoma damage who exhibited a scotoma impinging on fixation or a depression in the central visual field. Levene[4] showed a gradual decrease in Snellen visual acuity with progressive central visual field loss. (*Sensitivity loss* was defined as a visual field defect of at least 10 decibels from normal at the most central point of 1.4-degree eccentricity. Visual acuity dropped 1.5 lines per quadrant for one and two affected quadrants, and 2.0–2.5 lines for three and four quadrants affected.)

The subjective worsening of vision is especially relevant in those patients with endstage disease in whom objective signs of progression can be very difficult to measure. Such symptomatology might warrant more aggressive therapy, closer observation, or both. Patients in whom fixation is threatened should be followed with central 10-2 threshold visual field testing (see Figure 7-4).

PUPILS

Pupillary testing is performed to evaluate the integrity of the afferent and efferent visual pathways. The afferent neural pathway runs from the retinal ganglion cells to the pretectal area. Abnormalities in the afferent neural pathway may result in abnormalities in the pupillary light reflex, but they do not produce anisocoria. Defects of the efferent visual pathway, which runs from the central nervous system to the iris musculature, often produce anisocoria. Careful pupillary evaluation should be performed on all patients, taking care to note differences in size, shape, reactivity, and the presence or absence of a relative afferent pupillary defect (APD, Marcus Gunn pupil).

When pupil size is unequal, physiologic anisocoria, Adies tonic, and Horner's pupils should be considered. Trauma causing a sphincter tear (Figure 3-3) or past inflammation with posterior synechia of the iris might also result in a difference in pupil size, shape, and reactivity. This information is useful in the differential diagnosis of the secondary glaucomas.

In patients currently being treated for glaucoma, differences in pupil size and reactivity might be explained by topical medication use. Sympathomimetics, such as Iopidine, epinephrine, and dipivefrin, can result in pupillary dilation, whereas miotics, such as carbachol and pilocarpine, constrict the pupil. These reactions can provide an objective measure of compliance. If a patient is on miotic therapy and the pupils are still reactive to light, the patient may be noncompliant or may have problems with dexterity and instillation of medication. Heavily pigmented irides, however, may still show some reactivity, especially with bright illumination and under the magnification of the slit lamp.

The presence or absence of a relative APD is assessed using the swinging-flashlight test (Figure 3-4). This test is performed in a dimly lit room using a bright light source (transilluminator or indirect ophthalmoscope) while the patient fixates on a distance target. If both the afferent and efferent visual pathways are intact, the pupils will react as follows: The clinician initially shines a bright light into the right eye, and the right pupil should constrict. This is called the *direct response*. The pupil in the left eye will simultaneously constrict as a result of the consensual pupillary response. The light is then quickly swung over to the left eye. If the transition from right eye to left eye is rapid enough, the left pupil will maintain constriction from the consensual response. More often, the slight delay in light presentation to the left eye results in both pupils dilating slightly, and then both constricting as the light source is presented to the left eye. The light is then swung back to the right eye, which should be constricted as a result of the consensual response from stimulus presentation to the left eye. This process is repeated, observing the pupillary response in the eye to which the stimulus is presented. As the light source is swung back and forth between the two eyes, each pupil should be seen to either constrict or maintain constriction as the light source is presented. This is noted as a *negative APD*, or a *negative Marcus Gunn pupil*.

A positive APD results when a unilateral defect along the afferent visual system leads to an inability of that pathway to perceive the full strength of the stimulus. Assuming a significant left optic neuropathy, the pupillary response will be as follows: When the light is presented in front of the right eye, both pupils constrict. When the light source is presented to the left eye, the left optic nerve (afferent pathway) perceives the light source as being less bright as the right eye, and the left pupil (efferent system) will dilate. The consensual response dictates that the right pupil will also simultaneously dilate. When the light source is again presented to the right eye, it will perceive the full strength of the stimulus and will constrict. As the light source is repeatedly presented to each eye, the pupils will be seen to constrict when the light source is presented to the eye with the intact afferent pathway, and to dilate when presented to the eye with compromised afferent pathway.

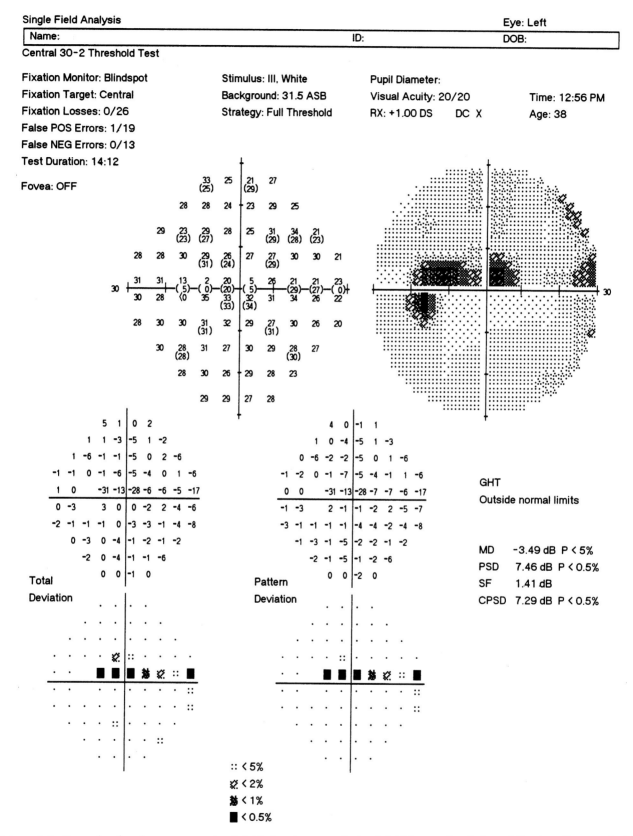

Single Field Analysis   Eye: Left

Name: ID: DOB:

Central 30-2 Threshold Test

Fixation Monitor: Blindspot   Stimulus: III, White   Pupil Diameter:
Fixation Target: Central   Background: 31.5 ASB   Visual Acuity: 20/20   Time: 12:56 PM
Fixation Losses: 0/26   Strategy: Full Threshold   RX: +1.00 DS   DC X   Age: 38
False POS Errors: 1/19
False NEG Errors: 0/13
Test Duration: 14:12

Fovea: OFF

GHT
Outside normal limits

MD   -3.49 dB P < 5%
PSD   7.46 dB P < 0.5%
SF   1.41 dB
CPSD   7.29 dB P < 0.5%

Total Deviation

Pattern Deviation

:: < 5%
⬩ < 2%
⬚ < 1%
■ < 0.5%

FIGURE 3-2. Example of a glaucomatous visual field showing central visual field loss and splitting of fixation. Decreased vision with associated central field loss can be a relatively early finding in a minority of glaucoma patients.

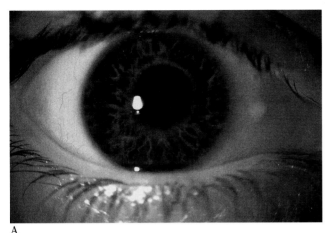 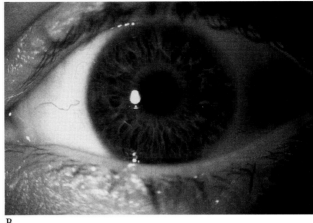

A   B

FIGURE 3-3. Anisocoria secondary to trauma. Note the iris sphincter tear in the right eye (**A**) at 1 o'clock. (**B**) Normal left pupil.

If a patient presents with only one functioning iris sphincter or only one visible pupil (e.g., if dense corneal opacity is present), testing for the presence of a relative APD is still possible. The examiner needs only to observe the response of the one visible or functioning pupil. If the reactive pupil dilates when light is presented to the nonreactive pupil, the eye with the nonreactive pupil is diagnosed as having a positive APD by reverse (Figure 3-5).

Asymmetric optic nerve and chiasmal lesions tend to produce a relative APD. Retinal lesions should not produce an APD unless the lesion is extensive or grossly asymmetric. Unilateral cataracts as a rule do not produce an APD. In fact, it has been shown that a dense unilateral cataract may produce a small relative APD in the other eye.[5] While this occurrence is not well understood, it has been hypothesized that an adjustment in the gain of the visual system might result in a heightened sensitivity on the side with the cataract. In general, if a relative APD is demonstrated in an eye with a dense cataract, it should be assumed that underlying retinal or optic nerve damage is present.

In POAG, pupillary reflexes tend to be normal and without a relative APD because the disease process is bilateral. In cases of asymmetric glaucoma or secondary glaucoma, a relative APD may be present on the side with more advanced damage. Approximately 20%–30% more damage in one eye is necessary to produce a relative APD. With endstage disease and light perception or no light perception vision, the pupil may not react to direct light stimulation.

CONFRONTATION VISUAL FIELD TESTING

Confrontation visual field testing is a poor screening method for the detection of early or moderate visual field loss. A person with extensive visual field loss by automated perimetry may also appear normal by confrontation visual field testing. This is because the size of the stimulus used with automated perimetry is much smaller (typically 3 mm) compared with fingers, which subtend a larger visual angle and are therefore more easily seen. Confrontation visual field testing is, however, a simple and rapid means to screen for gross, advanced visual field defects. Shahinfar and coworkers[6] showed that when visual field defects are identified by confrontation visual field testing, the specificity that those defects are real is 97%.

The visual field is divided into four quadrants that are separated by a vertical and a horizontal hemianopic line. The intersection of these hemianopic lines projects to the fovea. Given the anatomy of the visual pathway, lesions anterior to the optic chiasm should be monocular, whereas lesions posterior to the chiasm should be binocular and respect the vertical meridian. Therefore, confrontation visual field testing can be particularly useful in detecting hemianopic or quadrantanopic visual field loss secondary to postchiasmal lesions (cerebrovascular accidents, trauma, tumor). In the case of the glaucoma patient, the superior or inferior nasal visual field is typically affected first. Endstage glaucoma damage may present as binasal (superior and inferior) or a complete altitudinal field defect by confrontation testing.

Technique

In confrontation testing, the examiner is seated directly opposite and on eye level with the patient. The two should be separated by a distance of approximately 60 cm, and there should be good uniform room illumination. Except in the case of extreme refractive error, the patient's spectacles should be removed because the frame or bifocal may produce

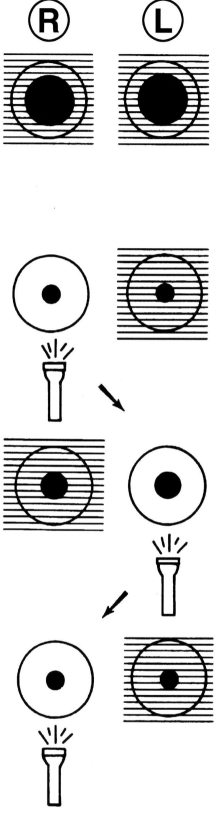

FIGURE 3-4. Swinging flashlight test performed in dim illumination in a patient with a left relative afferent pupillary defect. (Reprinted with permission from SH Thompson. The Pupil. In Adler's Physiology of the Eye [9th ed]. St. Louis: Mosby–Year Book, 1992;423.)

artifactual defects in the visual field. This test is performed monocularly; when testing the patient's right eye, the patient's left eye is covered and the examiner's right eye is closed (and vice versa for testing the patient's left eye). The patient is instructed to look only at the open eye of the examiner. This provides a central fixation target for the patient while allowing the examiner to monitor the patient's gaze. The examiner uses the limitations of his or her own visual field as a reference guide for the patient's visual field. The examiner then tells the patient, "I am going to show you either one, two, or five fingers. You continue to look straight into my open eye and tell me how many fingers you see." The four quadrants in each eye are tested in this manner, with the fingers of the examiner being presented in an arc, as in a bowl perimeter, approximately 30 degrees (approximately 30 cm) from fixation (Figure 3-6). If the patient reports that they don't see a stimulus presented, the examiner should move his or her fingers gradually closer to fixation until the patient sees it. In this manner, the extent of visual field constriction can be determined. This method can be further modified by using a technique called simultaneous hand perception. Here, the examiner holds up both hands separated by a distance of 3–4 inches. With the two hands straddling the vertical meridian, the examiner asks the patient whether one hand appears to be clearer than the other. Using this technique, a relative hemianopic visual field defect may be discovered. The same technique can be applied while the examiner straddles the horizontal meridian to uncover anterior chiasmal defects that might be more advanced in either the superior or inferior visual field. The results of this test are recorded monocularly. If each eye is normal, the result is recorded as "full to finger counting." Abnormal findings are recorded from the patient's perspective (Figure 3-7).

COLOR VISION

Although conventional color vision testing is not considered part of the current glaucoma screening protocol, many studies have shown that color perception is defective in glaucoma patients.[7] It is important to distinguish between congenital and acquired color vision deficits. Congenital color vision defects occur as a result of an inherited abnormality in photopigment composition. They are binocular and symmetric, and do not change over time. Acquired color vision loss, or *dyschromatopsia*, can result from demyelinating disease, trauma, vascular compromise, neoplasias, and degenerative disease. Therefore, acquired dyschromatopsia can be asymmetric and monocular or binocular, and can change over time.[8] Many investigators have turned to the study of acquired color vision defects associated

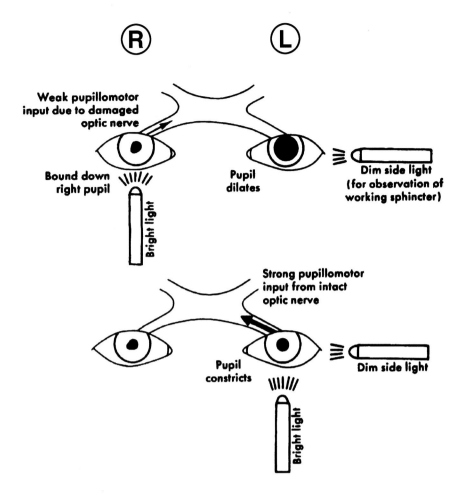

FIGURE 3-5. This figure demonstrates an afferent pupillary defect when one eye has an immobile pupil. When one pupil is immobilized, it is still possible to demonstrate an afferent defect by observing the direct and consensual response of the intact pupil. (Reprinted with permission from SH Thompson. The Pupil. In Adler's Physiology of the Eye [9th ed]. St. Louis: Mosby–Year Book, 1992;424.)

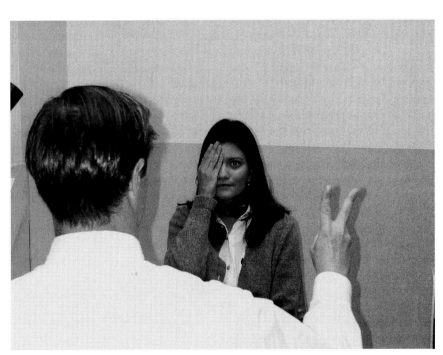

FIGURE 3-6. Confrontation visual field testing. The examiner sits opposite from and on eye level with the patient. The examiner's fingers are presented in an arc around the patient.

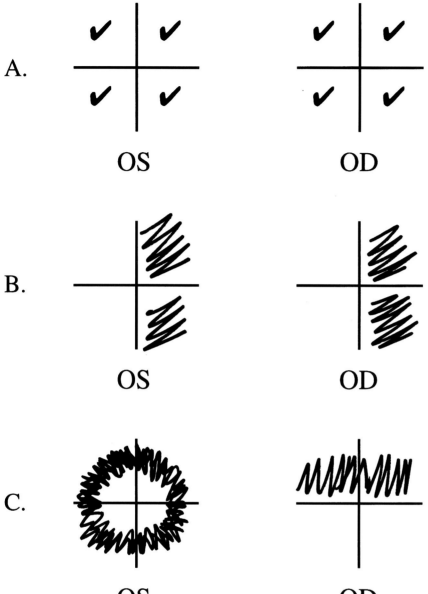

FIGURE 3-7. Confrontation visual field testing is recorded with respect to the patient's visual field. (**A**) Visual fields full to finger counting right eye (OD) and left eye (OS). (**B**) Shaded areas depict a right homonomous hemifield defect. (C) Superior altitudinal field loss OD and peripheral constriction OS.

with glaucoma to aid in the early diagnosis and treatment of this condition.

Drance and associates[9] were among the first to report that compromise to the blue-yellow pathway is linked with early glaucomatous damage. Their findings have since been corroborated by numerous other investigators.[10–13] Jonas and Zach[14] used Roth's Besancon anomalometer, the Farnsworth 100 hue test, and Nagel's anomaloscope to compare color vision in people with normal vision to that of patients with chronic open-angle glaucoma. They found that decreased blue sensitivity was correlated with a decrease in nerve fiber layer visibility, increased glaucomatous optic neuropathy, and larger perimetric defects. They found no difference in red-green color discrimination between those

with normal eyes and those with glaucomatous optic nerve damage.

Many of the early studies on glaucoma and acquired color vision defects were performed using conventional color vision tests that were designed to evaluate congenital dyschromatopsias. Congenital dyschromatopsias result from an absence or alteration in one or more of the cone photopigments.[15] Damage due to acquired disease is not as selective and therefore produces variable results when conventional color vision testing is applied. Another fault of conventional color vision testing with glaucoma is that the majority of color vision tests, such as the Farnsworth-Munsell 100 hue test, test only the central visual field (the central 2 degrees).

Given that the extrafoveal field is affected earlier than the central visual field in glaucoma, investigators have incorporated color vision testing into automated perimetric tests. Since then, it has been shown that blue-on-yellow perimetry (where a blue stimulus is presented on a yellow background) is capable of detecting glaucomatous visual field loss and progression earlier than is possible with white-on-white perimetry.[13,16,17] These defects in short-wavelength sensitivity have been shown to correspond with retinal nerve fiber layer defects, and can precede white-on-white visual field defects by 3–4 years.[17]

Sample and colleagues[16] conducted a 5-year follow-up study that compared the results of color visual fields in normal eyes, suspect eyes, and eyes that had developed glaucoma. A 440-nm blue test target on a bright-yellow background was used. The eyes that developed glaucoma over the course of the follow-up period, as well as those labeled as *high-risk glaucoma suspects*, showed a higher mean defect and more defective points than both low-risk suspects and normal eyes. There was no statistically significant difference found between low-risk suspects and normal eyes.

Yamagami and coworkers[18] used color perimetry to compare extrafoveal color vision deficits in subjects with normal-tension glaucoma (NTG) versus subjects with POAG. They developed a color vision analyzer wherein blue-yellow saturation discrimination could be measured without being affected by luminance. Subjects had visual field defects confined to either the upper or lower hemifield with conventional white-on-white perimetry. In the spared hemifield (as tested with white-on-white perimetry), a defect on blue-yellow perimetry was discovered in only 11% of NTG eyes versus 52% of POAG eyes. The hemifield that showed a defect with white-on-white testing showed a blue-yellow defect in 75% of eyes with either NTG or POAG. These findings may suggest that a different subset of ganglion cell axons are initially damaged in NTG compared with high-tension POAG.

Blue-on-yellow testing, or short-wavelength automated perimetry (SWAP), has been incorporated into perimetric testing. However, because of increased test time and high normal variation, it is not useful as a general screening tool. Short-wavelength automated perimetry is used to examine high-risk glaucoma suspects who test normal on conventional white-on-white perimetry (see Chapter 7).

CONTRAST SENSITIVITY

It is well established that contrast sensitivity is compromised in a number of acquired ocular diseases.[19,20] Although a patient may exhibit good Snellen visual acuity, the quality of vision as it relates to contrast sen-

sitivity might be reduced. Several investigators have demonstrated that glaucoma damage affects contrast sensitivity function before conventional visual field loss or loss of visual acuity occurs.[21,22] It appears that low and middle spatial frequencies are affected initially by glaucoma.[23,24] Low and middle spatial frequency deficits contribute to mobility problems and the inability to recognize faces and large objects.[25] Loss of the higher spatial frequencies translates to reduced Snellen visual acuity.

A concept known as *frequency-doubling technology* (FDT) has now been incorporated into perimetric testing, and it shows promise as a screening method for the detection of glaucoma.[26,27] When a low spatial frequency sinusoidal grating (less than 1 cycle per degree) undergoes high temporal frequency counterphase flicker (less than 15 Hz), it appears to have twice as many light and dark bands as are actually present (Figure 3-8). This is called the *frequency-doubling illusion*.[28] The low spatial frequency, when coupled with the high temporal frequency, is thought to preferentially stimulate a subset of retinal ganglion cells in the magnocellular pathway. This subset is made up of large-diameter fibers that have nonlinear response properties. It is hypothesized that early glaucomatous damage has a predilection for these large-diameter fibers,[29] and the frequency-doubling effect could be used to detect damage in these cells. Another hypothesis, referred to as the *reduced redundancy theory*,[30] states that early glaucomatous loss can be more easily detected by selectively testing visual systems that have minimal redundancy. The magnocellular cells (M-cells) responsible for the perception of the frequency-doubling illusion represent only 3–5% of the total number of retinal ganglion cells, and there-

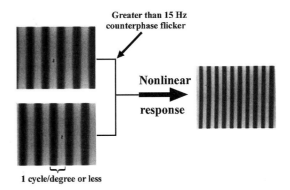

FIGURE 3-8. Diagram shows frequency-doubling effect. Vertical light and dark bars are flickered back and forth so the light bars become dark and the dark bars become light. The patient appears to see twice the number of vertical bars, hence the term *frequency doubling*. It is proposed that a special subset of ganglion cell axons are sensitive to the frequency-doubling phenomenon. (Photo courtesy of Zeiss Humphrey Systems, Dublin, CA.)

TABLE 3-2. Anterior Segment Findings Relevant to Glaucoma Diagnosis

Location	Findings
Conjunctiva	Hyperemia, dilated episcleral veins
Cornea	Edema, endothelial pigment, exfoliation material on endothelium, keratic precipitates, scarring, high peripheral anterior synechiae
Anterior chamber	Pigment, inflammatory cells, flare, hyphema
Iris	Pigment dusting, heterochromia, defects in the pupillary ruff, exfoliation flakes, transillumination defects, rubeosis irides, iris atrophy, posterior synechiae, corectopia, sphincter tear, iridodialysis, peripheral anterior synechiae
Lens	Thickening, pigmentation, exfoliation material, traumatic/asymmetric cataract, iridodonesis, dislocation/subluxation

fore they are an ideal target for a focused screening technique.

Frequency-doubling technology (FDT) has been incorporated into a portable, lightweight screening device known as the *Humphrey FDT perimeter* (see Chapter 7). This device is capable of rapid screening (approximately 1 minute per eye) or threshold testing (approximately 4 minutes per eye). It has been shown to have high test-retest reliability, as well as high sensitivity and specificity for the detection of glaucomatous visual field loss. Quigley demonstrated that the FDT screening strategy was capable of detecting glaucomatous visual field loss in 91% of eyes (30 out of 33) with an abnormal glaucoma hemifield test by Humphrey 24-2 threshold testing. Of eyes with normal glaucoma hemifield tests, 94% (31 out of 33) also tested normal using FDT perimetry.

EXTERNAL EVALUATION/SLIT-LAMP EXAMINATION

Although the external and slit-lamp evaluations of the patient with glaucoma are often unremarkable, the presence of certain external and anterior segment abnormalities can have significant diagnostic and management implications. Careful pre- and postdilation inspection of the anterior segment aids in the differential diagnosis of the primary, secondary, and mixed-mechanism glaucomas. Slit-lamp biomicroscopy, in combination with gonioscopy, allows the clinician to make the crucial differentiation between primary open-angle, closed-angle, and secondary glaucoma. The following is a discussion of the clinically relevant external and slit-lamp findings in the adult glaucoma patient (Table 3-2).

External Evaluation

The observation of facial or periocular scars and ptosis resulting from trauma may lend support to a diagnosis of traumatic glaucoma. It is important to specifically question the patient regarding these scars, as patients often fail to mention remote trauma when questioned during the taking of their history.

Sturge-Weber syndrome is characterized by a hamartoma (a congenital tumor arising from tissue normally present in the involved area) of vascular tissue that runs along the distribution of the trigeminal nerve. This hamartoma produces a characteristic skin lesion termed a *port-wine stain*. If the port-wine stain is distributed along both the ophthalmic and maxillary divisions of the trigeminal nerve, the chance that glaucoma is present is approximately 50%.[31] The mechanism for the development of glaucoma associated with Sturge-Weber syndrome is not well understood. Proposed theories include an associated congenital anomaly of the anterior chamber angle[32] and increased episcleral venous pressure related to episcleral hemangiomas.[33]

Various conditions associated with glaucoma might result in iris heterochromia. These include Fuch's heterochromic iridocyclitis, pigmentary glaucoma, chronic uveitis, and glaucomatocyclitic crisis. A possible association between congenital Horner's syndrome and glaucoma has also been reported in the literature.[34] Iris heterochromia is best observed outside the slit lamp with gross observation.

Slit-Lamp Examination

Conjunctiva, Sclera, and Episclera

The conjunctiva, sclera, and episclera tend to be normal in the chronic open-angle glaucoma patient. Diffuse injection or circumlimbal flush may be evident in the patient with iritis (Color Plate 6) or scleritis. This patient may have trabecular meshwork debris, peripheral anterior synechia, or trabeculitis, resulting in an IOP spike and possible uveitic glaucoma. In the case of acute angle-closure attack or neovascular glaucoma, conjunctival and ciliary injection occur in response to iris ischemia and the accompanying inflammation. Conjunctival injection can also be a sign of elevated episcleral venous pressure, which can be associated with blood reflux in Schlemm's canal (Color Plate 16) and a rise in IOP.

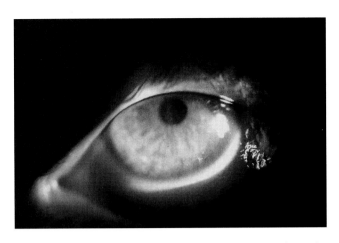

FIGURE 3-9. Deposition of fine pigment granules on the endothelial surface of a patient with pigmentary glaucoma. The pigment is typically oriented in an elongated vertical pattern and is called a *Krukenberg's spindle*.

TABLE 3-3. Grading Scale for Anterior Chamber Inflammation Using a 1-by-1-mm Slit Beam

Classification	Cells	Flare
Grade 0	0	Absent
Trace	1–4	Barely noticeable
Grade 1	4–8	Mild
Grade 2	9–15	Moderate
Grade 3	Too many to count	Marked
Grade 4	Obscures iris details	Severe

Cornea

Corneal opacities may be indicative of a past traumatic event or possible herpetic infection, both of which may result in elevated IOP from anterior chamber inflammation and its sequelae. Pigment deposition on the corneal endothelium may result from pigment dispersion syndrome, pigmentary glaucoma, or exfoliation. The typical pattern for this pigment accumulation is that of a vertically elongated line, termed a *Krukenberg's spindle* (Figure 3-9). In the case of exfoliation syndrome or glaucoma, a flake-like deposition of a grey fibrilogranular material can occur on the corneal endothelium. Keratic precipitates on the endothelial (Color Plate 7A) are a sign of past or present anterior chamber inflammation. In the case of acute angle-closure glaucoma, the patient may present with corneal edema because of the dysfunction of the corneal endothelial cell pumps (see Figure 3-1).

Anterior Chamber

The anterior chamber should routinely be evaluated for the presence of pigmentary or inflammatory cells and flare (Color Plate 7B). In the setting of iris neovascularization or trauma, red blood cells or a hyphema may also be observed (Color Plate 13). Inspection of the anterior chamber should be performed before the instillation of fluorescein, which diffuses into the anterior chamber and mimics the appearance of flare. The anterior chamber should again be evaluated after dilation for postdilation pigment release. This may occur more frequently in cases of pigment dispersion and exfoliation. In such cases, postdilation IOP measurements should be performed to evaluate for a possible IOP spike. It should be

noted that postdilation pressure rises can also occur in the absence of pigment release in both open- and narrow-angle glaucoma patients and in patients without glaucoma.

Proper inspection of the anterior chamber is carried out as follows: The patient is positioned at the slit lamp and is instructed to look straight ahead. The room lights should be turned off, so the examination room is completely dark. The slit lamp's illumination is turned up to the highest setting, and the lamp is positioned at a 30- to 40-degree angle from the microscope. Using an initial slit beam 1-mm wide and 3 mm in length and under high magnification, the clinician inspects the anterior chamber for the presence of cells or flare. If cells or flare are observed, the beam height should then be decreased to 1 mm to grade the amount of anterior chamber inflammation (Table 3-3). When grading the anterior chamber reaction, the examiner should make the distinction between inflammatory cells (white), pigmentary (brown) cells, and red blood cells.

Before dilation, the depth of the anterior chamber should also be assessed so that eyes at risk of chronic or acute angle-closure attack might be identified. The van Herick angle estimation technique (Figure 3-10) compares the apparent depth of the peripheral anterior chamber with the apparent width of the slit-lamp beam as it passes through the cornea. The light source is narrowed to an optic section and is placed at a 60-degree angle to the microscope. The light beam is focused at the limbus and should be moved slightly so that the shadow of the anterior chamber is just visible. The width of the optic section as it traverses the cornea is then compared with the width of the dark shadow behind it. This shadow represents the apparent depth of the anterior chamber. The depth at both the temporal and nasal limbus is assessed and graded on a scale of 1–4, with 1 being narrow and 4 being the most open (Table 3-4). Angles judged to be narrow (grades 1–2) by van Herick estimation warrant gonioscopy before dilation (Figure 3-11). It should be noted that van Herick angle estimation is not a substitute for gonioscopy

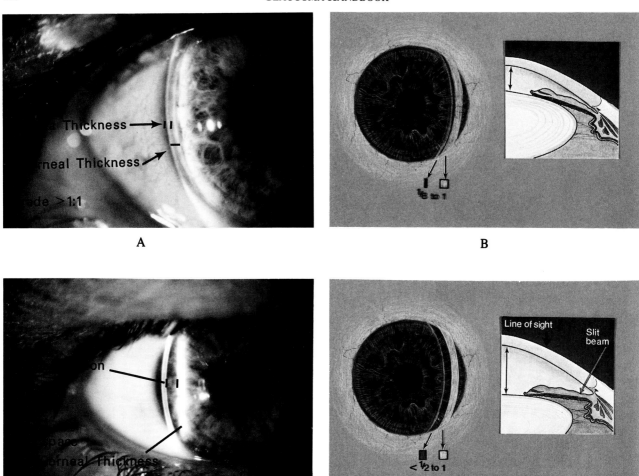

FIGURE 3-10. van Herick angle estimation technique. Slit lamp angled 60 degrees. Use optic section. The thickness of the space between the posterior cornea and the iris is judged in relation to the corneal thickness at this location. (A) Angle width is closed. (B) Artist's representation. Note that the central chamber is shallow as well. (C) Angle width is open normal appearance more than $\frac{1}{2}$:1. (D) Artist's representation. Note normal depth of central chamber. (Reprinted with permission from B Fisch. Gonioscopy and the Glaucomas. Boston: Butterworth–Heinemann, 1993;23.)

in the evaluation of a glaucoma patient or a patient suspect for glaucoma.

When positioning of the patient at the slit lamp is not possible, the depth of the anterior chamber angle can be approximated using the penlight shadow test (Figure 3-12). This test is performed under dim illumination while the patient fixates a distance object. A transilluminator or penlight is held at an angle of approximately 100 degrees temporally and in the same horizontal plane of the eye to be examined. The light source is then rotated forward. As the angle of the light source approaches 90 degrees (perpendicular to the cornea), the temporal half of the iris should illuminate. The nasal limbus should also glow as a result of sclerotic scatter. A certain percentage of the nasal aspect of the iris will also become illuminated, depending on the depth of the anterior chamber. The deeper the anterior chamber angle, the greater the amount of nasal iris illumination. By grading the percentage of nasal iris illumination, the clinician can estimate the likelihood of angle closure (Table 3-5).

TABLE 3-4. Grading Scheme for van Herick Angle Estimation

Classification	Anterior chamber depth
Grade 4	PAC ≥ 1 CT
Grade 3	PAC .25–.50 CT
Grade 2	PAC = .25 CT
Grade 1	PAC < .25 CT

PAC = shadow created by the peripheral anterior chamber; CT = apparent corneal thickness.

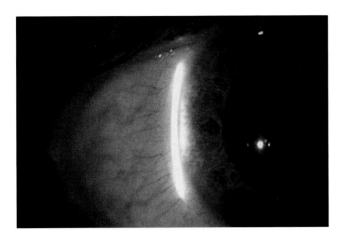

FIGURE 3-11. Clinical example of a grade 1 anterior chamber angle by van Herick angle estimation.

Iris

The surface of the iris should be evaluated for the presence of pigment dusting, which can result from pigment dispersion or exfoliation syndrome. Exfoliation material can also be found on the iris surface or at the pupil border (Color Plate 4). The presence of iris transillumination defects should be noted. Spoke-like transillumination defects that occur in the midperipheral iris corroborate the diagnosis of pigment dispersion syndrome (Color Plate 3),[35] whereas pupillary border defects are more commonly associated with exfoliation syndrome.[36] Diffuse transillumination defects have been associated with diabetes, and localized defects have been linked to long-standing open-angle glaucoma and uveitis.[35] Posterior synechiae, or adhesions between the posterior iris and the anterior lens surface, are the result of chronic or recurrent iritis or pupillary block (Figure 3-13). During an acute angle-closure attack, the anterior chamber angle may be so shallow as to permit iridocorneal touch. The pupil is typically vertically oval and fixed in the mid-dilated position (see Figure 16-3). The iris vessels are generally engorged.

Iris sphincter tears (see Figure 3-3) or iridodialysis (Figure 3-14) may result from past ocular trauma, which represents an increased risk of trabecular meshwork dysfunction and elevated IOP. The iris should also be carefully inspected for neovascularization, particularly in patients with diabetes, vaso-occlusive disease, or ocular ischemic syndrome. Iris neovascularization is most likely to occur around the pupil border, or around the borders of a peripheral iridotomy/iridectomy (Color Plate 10).

Iridocorneal endothelial (ICE) syndrome is a primary disorder of the corneal endothelium that usually presents in young adulthood. The main ocular findings in ICE syndrome are unilateral corneal edema, corectopia (distortion of the pupil, or a "second" pupil in a previously normal eye), broad-based peripheral anterior synechiae (high peripheral anterior synechiae; Color Plate 9), and iris atrophy. The ICE syndrome is composed of a specific subset of ocular disorders, including Chandler's syndrome, progressive iris atrophy, and iris nevus (Cogan-Reese) syndrome (see Chapter 17). These disorders all result from an abnormal proliferation of the corneal endothelial cell layer. This cell membrane can migrate across the anterior chamber angle and surface of the iris. Contracture of this membrane can result in synechial closure of the anterior chamber angle, elevated IOP, and iris stretching or atrophy. Each of the ICE syndromes has a prominent clinical feature: Chandler's syndrome has more prominent corneal changes (edema) and fewer iris abnormalities, progressive iris atrophy has more prominent iris changes (corectopia, iris atrophy, and hole formation) and fewer corneal abnormalities, and Cogan-Reese syndrome has nodular, pigmented iris lesions with various degrees of corneal and iris involvement. Frequently, there is overlap in corneal and iris features in the three disorders. Posterior polymorphous dystrophy can also be associated with corneal abnormalities and glaucoma, but this condition is inherited and bilateral.

Lens

Examining the lens after dilation is important, because it may provide additional diagnostic clues to the presence of secondary glaucoma. Posterior synechiae are most commonly the result of chronic or recurrent iritis and

TABLE 3-5. Penlight Estimation of the Anterior Chamber Angle and Likeliness of Angle Closure

Angle type	Percentage of nasal iris illumination	Angle subtended between iris and cornea (degrees)	Grading of anterior chamber angle	Probability of angle closure
Wide open	100	45	4	No risk
Open	75	30	3	Low risk
Narrow	50	20	2	Moderate risk
Extremely narrow	25	10	1	High risk
Closed	0	0	0	100%

Source: Modified from JC Townsend. Clinical Procedures in Optometry. Philadelphia: JB Lippincott, 1991;37–38.

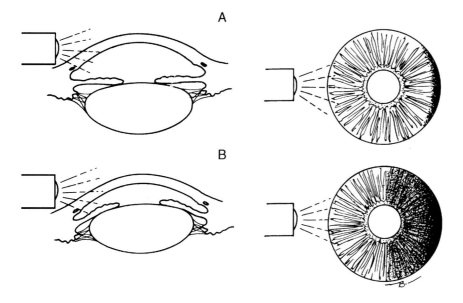

FIGURE 3-12. Penlight shadow test for anterior chamber depth estimation. (**A**) Illumination of the nasal aspect of the iris in eye with a deep anterior chamber. (**B**) Lack of illumination of the nasal aspect of the iris in an eye with a shallow anterior chamber. (Reprinted with permission from MB Shields. Textbook of Glaucoma [2nd ed]. Baltimore: Williams & Wilkins, 1987.)

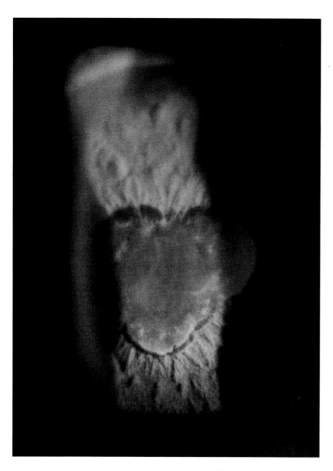

FIGURE 3-13. Posterior synechiae are adhesions between the posterior iris and the anterior lens surface. They are most commonly the result of chronic or recurrent iritis and can cause poor or irregular pupil dilation.

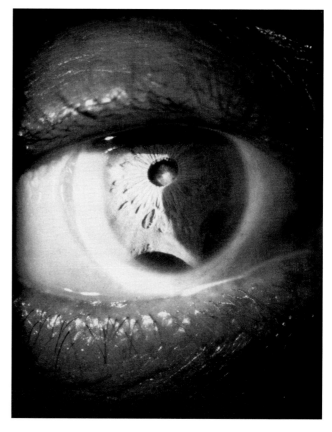

FIGURE 3-14. Iridodialysis may result from past ocular trauma, which represents an increased risk of trabecular meshwork dysfunction and elevated intraocular pressure.

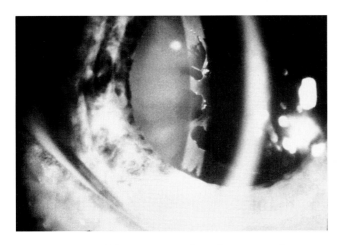

FIGURE 3-15. Exfoliation material on the anterior lens capsule after dilation.

can cause poor or irregular pupil dilation (see Figure 3-13). If the entire circumference of the iris is synched to the lens, then the patient will develop a secondary angle-closure attack. A peripheral iridotomy should be performed prophylactically in a patient approaching 360 degrees of posterior synechiae (see Chapter 17).

Specific types of cataracts can act as historical markers of past ocular trauma or relevant systemic medication use. Rosette or asymmetric cataracts may be the result of ocular trauma (Color Plate 12), whereas posterior subcapsular cataracts may be a side effect of long-term oral steroid use. Glaukomflecken are irregular white opacities in the anterior portion of the lens that result from acute elevations in IOP. These acute elevations in IOP can result from intermittent or acute angle-closure glaucoma, or from steroid-induced IOP spikes. The anterior lens surface and lens zonules should be evaluated for the presence of exfoliation material (Figure 3-15). Phakodonesis and iridodonesis may be suggestive of exfoliation or trauma. This can be assessed by having the patient rapidly shift fixation. Under these conditions, the iris and lens will appear to shake. A dislocated or subluxed lens may migrate forward and become entrapped in the pupil, leading to angle-closure glaucoma.

Phacolytic glaucoma should be suspected when white debris is seen floating in the anterior chamber of an eye with a hypermature cataract with elevated IOP. This whitish material is a high-molecular-weight protein capable of dissolving through the intact lens capsule and blocking aqueous outflow through the trabecular meshwork. Phacomorphic glaucoma is a form of secondary angle-closure glaucoma. It occurs when an intumescent cataractous lens, or age-related growth change to the lens, results in the anterior movement of the lens and a shallowing of the anterior chamber angle. Comparing gonioscopy findings between the two eyes aides in the differentiation of phacomorphic glaucoma from primary angle-closure glaucoma. In phacomorphic glaucoma, gonioscopy of the unaffected eye should reveal a deep anterior chamber angle, whereas eyes at risk of primary angle-closure attack have narrow anterior chamber angles bilaterally.

TONOMETRY

Clinical measurement of IOP is accomplished by tonometry. Two basic types of tonometers obtain this information by relating a deformation of the globe to the responsible force: applanation (flattening) and indentation tonometry. Applanation tonometry relies on a flattening of the globe, which keeps the shape of deformation constant, allowing IOP to be calculated mathematically. Indentation tonometry consists of using a fixed weight to deform the globe. Conversion charts based on empirical data are used to estimate the IOP.

Goldmann Applanation Tonometry

Goldmann applanation tonometry, the standard of reference in clinical measurement of IOP, is based on the Imbert-Fick law, which states that an external force against a sphere (F) equals the pressure in the sphere multiplied by the area flattened by the external force (A):

$$F = IOP \times A$$

The pressure (IOP) is calculated from the force applied to applanate the globe divided by the fixed area of the applanation probe. Although it is a relatively uncomplicated law of physics, practical application of this principle requires consideration of several complicating factors. These variables include the effect of capillary action between the tonometer probe and the cornea, variable corneal curvature, corneal astigmatism, varying amounts of fluid on the cornea, corneal thickness, and varying scleral rigidity. Goldmann experimented with different tonometer designs and determined that the probe with 3.06-mm diameter flattening for the human eye effectively balances the capillary force of the cornea. Additionally, the Goldmann tonometer has a generally well-defined range of insensitivity to the other factors listed.[37]

Procedure for Goldmann Tonometry

The Goldmann tonometer is mounted on the slit lamp so that the examiner views directly through the center of a plastic biprism used to applanate the cornea. The biprism is placed in contact with the apex of the cornea. The two prisms in the tonometer probe optically convert the circular area of corneal contact into semicircles (Figure 3-16). When the examiner

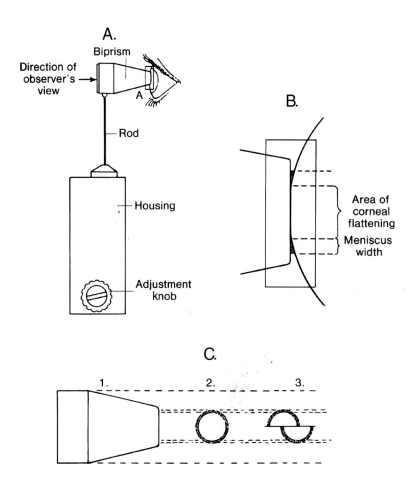

FIGURE 3-16. Goldmann-type applanation tonometry. (**A**) Basic features of tonometer, shown in contact with patient's cornea. (**B**) Enlargement shows tear film meniscus created by contact of biprism and cornea. (**C**) View through biprism (1) reveals circular meniscus (2), which is converted into semicircles (3) by prisms. (Reprinted with permission from MB Shields. Textbook of Glaucoma [4th ed]. Baltimore: Williams & Wilkins, 1998;56.)

performs Goldmann tonometry, the cornea is anesthetized, stained with sodium fluorescein (or a combination such as Fluress), and brightly illuminated with the cobalt-blue light source from the slit lamp. The examiner visualizes the fluorescent semicircles thorough the biprism and adjusts the force against the cornea until the inner margins of the semicircles just overlap (Figure 3-17). The IOP measurement is then read off the dial markings in millimeters of mercury (mm Hg), and the time the test was performed should be noted.

The width of the semicircles may influence the reading in Goldmann applanation tonometry. A wider meniscus (too much fluorescein dye) results in falsely elevated IOP measurement, whereas a thinner meniscus (insufficient amount of fluorescein dye) results in an underestimation of the IOP. Additionally, improper vertical alignment of the mires, so that one semicircle is larger than the other, leads to an overestimation of the IOP.

Immobilizing the lids during tonometry is a decision that the practitioner should make based on each individual patient. If the tonometer tip is allowed to touch the patient's upper lid, capillary action will draw a reservoir of tears down from underneath the upper eyelid, resulting in thicker semicircles and an overestimation of the IOP. Furthermore, a blink or blepharospasm can also affect the tonometry reading. A patient who squeezes his or her eyelids can cause an artificially increased IOP reading. Properly bracing the patient's lids against the bone of the orbital rim should eliminate this variable, but the clinician must be sure not to apply pressure to the globe when holding the eyelids (Figure 3-18).

The examiner must also remember that corneal astigmatism can influence Goldmann tonometry. More than 3 D of corneal astigmatism results in IOP underestimation for with-the-rule astigmatism and an overestimation of IOP for against-the-rule astigmatism.[38] The IOP reading should be adjusted 1 mm Hg for every 3 D of corneal astigmatism.[39]

Schiøtz Indentation Tonometry

The body of the Schiøtz tonometer (Figure 3-19) consists of a footplate, which rests on the cornea. A plunger moves unhindered within the footplate to indent the cornea. The movement of a needle on a scale indicates the degree of indentation of the globe. A 5.5-g weight is fixed to the plunger and can be increased to 7.5, 10,

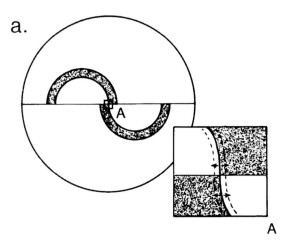

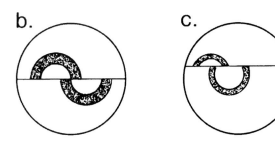

FIGURE 3-17. Semicircles of Goldmann-type applanation tonometry. Photograph (**a**) shows the proper width and position. Enlargement (**A**) depicts excursions of semicircles caused by ocular pulsations. (**b**) Semicircles are too wide. (**c**) Vertical and horizontal alignment is improper. (Reprinted with permission from MB Shields. Textbook of Glaucoma [4th ed]. Baltimore: Williams & Wilkins, 1998;57.)

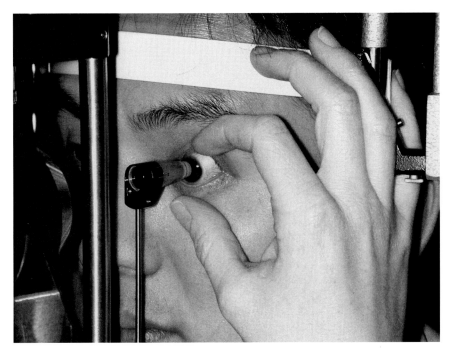

FIGURE 3-18. Technique for immobilizing the lids during Goldmann applanation tonometry. The upper and lower lids are retracted and held against the orbital rim. Care should be taken to avoid exerting pressure on the globe and inducing artifact.

and 15 g by adding weights. The higher weights are used to more accurately measure higher levels of IOP.

The procedure for Schiøtz tonometry is to first anesthetize the cornea. The patient is then placed in a supine position and asked to fixate a target overhead. The footplate rests on the center of the cornea to allow free vertical movement of the plunger (Figure 3-20).

The tonometry reading is obtained from the scale, which measures the extent of indentation on the globe. The more the plunger indents the cornea, the higher the scale reading, and the lower the IOP. Generally, the examiner starts with the 5.5-g weight. If the scale reading is less than or equal to 4, additional weight should be used to obtain a more accurate reading. A conversion table is used to determine the IOP in mm Hg from the scale and plunger weight. When recording, the scale reading, weight, IOP, and conversion chart should all be noted. For example, a scale reading of 6.0 was obtained using a 5.5-g weight. This corresponds to 14.6 mm Hg of pressure, according to the 1955 conversion chart. It should be documented as 6/5.5 = 14.6 mm Hg ('55) (Table 3-6). The Schiøtz tonometer is portable, sturdy, relatively inexpensive, and easy to operate. Its versatility makes it ideal for obtaining IOP measurements on patients who are unable to maneuver into a slit lamp or patients restricted to stretchers.

Tono-Pen

The Tono-pen (Mentor, Norwell, MA)(Figure 3-21) is a self-contained, handheld, battery-operated tonometer. It contains a central plunger surrounded by a footplate, which connects to a sensing element. The force exerted on the plunger is transmitted as a voltage wave that is analyzed by a microprocessor. The voltage-wave configuration adequacy is evaluated and 4–10 IOP readings are collected and averaged. The digital mean value is displayed on a liquid crystal display along with a coefficient of variation. The range of variation is given as 5%, 10%, 20%, or more than 20%. The 5% coefficient represents the most accurate measurement and is therefore generally accepted to be the most clinically valuable.

In clinical comparisons with Goldmann tonometry readings, the Tono-pen was accurate in the normal IOP range (11–20 mm Hg). However, the Tono-pen can underestimate Goldmann IOP readings in the higher range (21–30 mm Hg) and overestimates in the

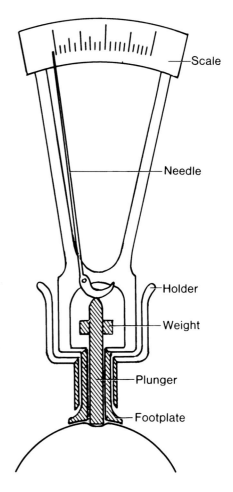

FIGURE 3-19. Schiøtz tonometer. (Reprinted with permission from MB Shields. Textbook of Glaucoma [4th ed]. Williams & Wilkins: Baltimore, 1987;52.)

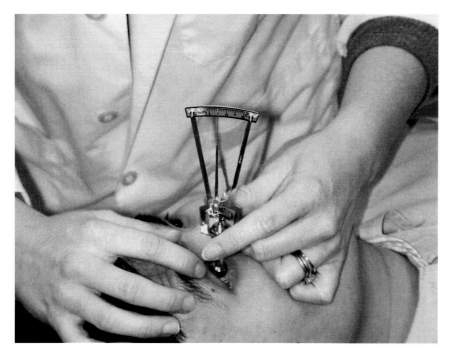

FIGURE 3-20. Technique of indentation tonometry with the Schiøtz tonometer.

TABLE 3-6. Schiøtz Tonometry Conversion Table

Tonometry reading	Pressure (mm Hg)			
	Load (5.5 g)	Load (7.5 g)	Load (10 g)	Load (15 g)
0.0	41.5	59.1	81.7	127.5
0.5	37.8	54.2	75.1	117.9
1.0	34.5	49.8	69.3	109.3
1.5	31.6	45.8	64.0	101.4
2.0	29.0	42.1	59.1	94.3
2.5	26.6	38.8	54.7	88.0
3.0	24.4	35.8	50.6	81.8
3.5	22.4	33.0	46.9	76.2
4.0	20.6	30.4	43.4	71.0
4.5	18.9	28.0	40.2	66.2
5.0	17.3	25.8	37.2	61.8
5.5	15.9	23.8	34.4	57.6
6.0	14.6	21.9	31.8	53.6
6.5	13.4	20.1	29.4	49.9
7.0	12.2	18.5	27.2	46.5
7.5	11.2	17.0	25.1	43.2
8.0	10.2	15.6	23.1	40.2
8.5	9.4	14.3	21.3	38.1
9.0	8.5	13.1	19.6	34.6
9.5	7.8	12.0	18.0	32.0
10.0	7.1	10.9	16.5	29.6
10.5	6.5	10.0	15.1	27.4
11.0	5.9	9.0	13.8	25.3
11.5	5.3	8.3	12.6	23.3
12.0	4.9	7.5	11.5	21.4
12.5	4.4	6.8	10.5	19.7
13.0	4.0	6.2	9.5	18.1
13.5	—	5.6	8.6	16.5
14.0	—	5.0	7.8	15.1
14.5	—	4.5	7.1	13.7

— = no information.
Note: This table has been approved by the Committee on Standardization of Tonometers of the American Academy of Ophthalmology and Otolaryngology. The table converts the scale reading obtained during Schiøtz tonometry to an intraocular pressure reading in mm Hg. Each column is specific for the given weight.
Source: R. O. Gulden & Co., Inc., 225 Cadwalader Ave., Elkins Park, PA 19117.

lower range (4–10 mm Hg). The Tono-pen lacks good correlation with Goldmann applanation tonometry when the IOP is higher than 30 mm Hg.[40–42]

Noncontact Tonometry

The noncontact tonometer (NCT) (Reichert, Buffalo, NY), introduced by Grolman in 1972,[43] distinguished itself by using a puff of air without direct eye contact to obtain an IOP reading. This air-puff design applies the same principle as the Goldmann applanation tonometer: calculating the amount of force necessary to flatten a fixed area of cornea.

The original NCT[44] consists of three operating systems. First, an optical alignment system allows for the proper positioning of the patient's cornea. Second, an opto-electronic applanation monitoring system projects collimated light at the corneal apex and detects parallel, coaxial rays reflected from the flattened cornea. Third, a pneumatic system creates the puff of air aimed at the cornea. When the cornea is aligned properly, a puff of air with increasing force is directed toward the cornea. At the instant when a 3.6-mm² area of the central cornea is flattened, the greatest amount of reflected light is transmitted to the electronic monitoring system, which converts the signal into an IOP reading that is digitally displaced.

The average NCT reading is measured over a time interval of approximately 1–3 ms, which represents $\frac{1}{500}$ of the cardiac cycle. The IOP measurement is therefore recorded randomly with respect to the ocular pulse, resulting in statistically significant variability. The probability that the pressure readings lie within a given IOP range increases as the number of readings, averaged together, increases. Consequently, it is recommended that a minimum of three readings within 3 mm Hg be averaged as the IOP.[45]

Perkins Tonometry

The Perkins tonometer (Clement Clarke Inc., Mason, OH) (Figure 3-22) is a handheld tonometer that makes use of the same biprism as the Goldmann applanation tonometer. It is portable and illuminated by a battery-powered light source. A counterbalance allows the Perkins tonometer to be used in any position, making it useful in the operating room, at a bedside, or with patients who are unable to maneuver into the slit lamp. Its portability makes it useful for patients in nursing homes.

Mackay-Marg Tonometry

The Mackay-Marg tonometer was designed to allow IOP measurements to be obtained through the sclera without anesthetic. However, the scleral IOP measurements were found to be inaccurate, and only readings taken on an anesthetized cornea were reliable. Although the original is no longer available, newer tonometers (e.g., the Tono-pen) apply similar principles. This tonometer measures the force required to keep the flat plate of a plunger flush with a surrounding sleeve against the pressure of the cornea. The force required to

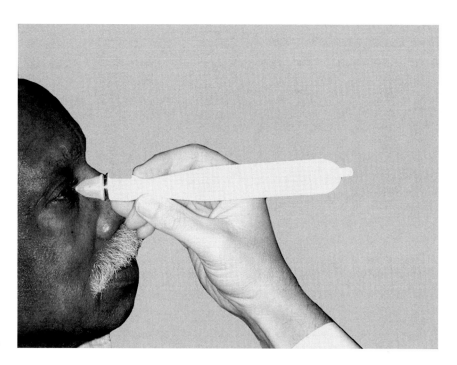

FIGURE 3-21. Tono-pen.

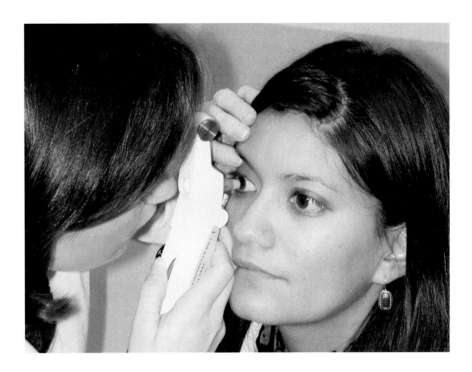

FIGURE 3-22. Technique of applanation tonometry with the Perkins tonometer.

deform the cornea (corneal rigidity) is transferred to the sleeve, allowing the plate to read only the IOP.[46]

Pneumotonometry

Similar to the Mackay-Marg tonometer, the pneumotonometer (Figure 3-23) uses a central sensor, which measures the IOP while the force required to bend the cornea is transferred to a surrounding structure. Air pressure works as the sensor in pneumotonometry,

replacing the flat electronic plate of the Mackay-Marg system. The instrument expresses a whistling sound when properly placed on the cornea.

The pneumatic tonometer is useful for measuring IOP in eyes with scarred, edematous, or irregular corneas. Additionally, the small tip makes this tonometer useful in animal studies. When compared with Goldmann tonometry readings, the pneumatic tonometer showed close correlation, but it tends to read slightly higher.[47,48]

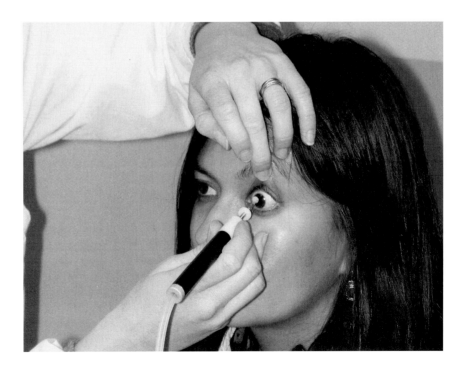

FIGURE 3-23. Technique of tonometry using the pneumotonometer.

CORNEAL THICKNESS AND IOP MEASUREMENT

IOP is an important parameter in the initial diagnosis and subsequent management of glaucoma. Although Goldmann applanation tonometry is currently the gold standard for measuring IOP, several factors, including corneal thickness, may affect its accuracy. A positive linear correlation has been reported between central corneal thickness (CCT) and IOP.[49,50] IOP obtained by applanation tonometry may be overestimated in thick corneas and underestimated in thin corneas. Ehlers and associates[51] reported that the Goldmann tonometer provided accurate readings when CCT was 520 μ. They calculated that applanation tonometry was overestimated or underestimated by approximately 5 mm Hg for every 70-μ deviation in corneal thickness.

Whitacre and coworkers[52] found that in eyes with thin corneas, IOP was underestimated by as much as 4.9 mm Hg, and in eyes with thick corneas, IOP was overestimated by as much as 6.8 mm Hg. The potential exists for patients with POAG who have thin corneas to be misdiagnosed with NTG.[53] Ehlers and Hansen[54] reported seven cases of NTG with an average CCT of 461 μ. A high incidence of NTG has been reported in one Japanese study.[55] It would be of interest to investigate the CCT of this population and re-evaluate the data. Similarly, normal patients with thick corneas may be misdiagnosed and treated for ocular hypertension. Johnson and coworkers[56] reported a case of a 17-year-old girl who consistently had IOPs of 30–40 mm Hg with normal visual fields and optic nerves. CCT was measured at 900 μ. Following unsuccessful medical treatment, the anterior chamber was cannulated with a pressure transducer and found to be 11 mm Hg. Central corneal pachymetry is therefore an important measurement that may be helpful in the accurate diagnosis and management of patients with glaucoma and patients in whom glaucoma is suspected.

With the surge in popularity of laser vision correction, an increasing body of evidence exists that CCT plays an integral role in the interpretation of applanation tonometry in eyes after refractive surgery. After laser refractive surgery, a reduction in IOP has been reported.[57] However, this reduction of IOP may be the result of the decreased CCT. It is important in the short- and long-term management of these patients to realize that the IOP is higher than the Goldmann applanation reading.

DIURNAL VARIATION OF IOP

Elevated IOP is one of the most significant risk factors for developing glaucoma. An IOP reading in the statistically normal range should not exclude diagnosing glaucoma. An IOP spike can never be ruled out. Tonometry is nonetheless complicated by the fact that, like many other biological parameters, the IOP demonstrates cyclic fluctuation. In normal eyes, the daily fluctuation can range from 3 to 6 mm Hg. In glaucomatous eyes, the diurnal pattern is an exaggeration of the slight variation seen in normal eyes. A fluctuation of 10 mm Hg is generally regarded as pathologic, and reports of glaucoma patients have yielded variations of more than 30 mm Hg.

The daily cycle of IOP variation generally follows a reproducible pattern, with the maximum pressure in the midmorning and the minimum pressure late at night. However, some individuals peak in the afternoon or evening, and others follow no consistent pattern.[58,59] Although many patterns of variation have been reported, it is believed that the diurnal fluctuation of IOP is, in part, due to changes in the rate of aqueous production.[60] Some reports, however, indicate that there may additionally be some small fluctuation in outflow facility accounting for diurnal changes. Further, reports of a small seasonal variation have been noted, with IOP slightly higher in the winter and lower in the summer.[61] The underlying mechanism of this has not been determined.

Brubaker and coworkers have established, through fluorophotometry (a technique that depicts aqueous production via diffusion of fluorescein into the anterior chamber and the dilution of that fluorescein concentration over time), that the rate of aqueous humor production is lowest during sleep and increases dramatically just before waking.[60] Brubaker suggests that circulating catecholamines, specifically epinephrine, may be responsible for the diurnal variation of aqueous production.

The clinical significance of diurnal IOP variation is the risk of missing a pressure elevation. The fact that IOP readings can vary dramatically during the day makes it unreasonable to assume that a single pressure reading represents a patient's average IOP. One study showed that one-half of IOP peaks occurred at times outside of normal office hours and that more elevated readings occurred in patients with suspected or documented progression of glaucomatous damage.[62] Various factors have been shown to increase or decrease IOP and should also be considered (Tables 3-7 and 3-8).

If the potential for IOP fluctuation is not accounted for, the effectiveness of medications can be misjudged. Target IOPs must also be based on diurnal fluctuations. It is recommended that before starting treatment in glaucoma patients, three IOP measurements should be obtained while the patient is off medications during different times of the day. Further, a modified diurnal curve measured in the office during

TABLE 3-7. Factors That May Lead to Increased
Intraocular Pressure

Age
>40 years
Gender
Female
Race
African American
Genetics
Family history of elevated intraocular pressure
Refractive error
Myopia
Seasonal
Higher intraocular pressure in winter months
Postural variation
Changing from sitting to supine
Exertional influences
Valsalva's maneuver
Electroshock therapy
Lid and eye movement
Blinking
Lid squeezing
Intraocular conditions
Secondary glaucomas
Increased corneal thickness
Systemic influences
Hypertension (especially systolic pressure)
Hyperthermia
Obesity
Pulse rate
Hemoglobin concentration
Diabetes
Hormonal influences
Adrenocorticotropic hormone
Glucocorticoids
Growth hormone
Hypothyroidism
Food and drugs
Caffeine
Tobacco
Corticosteroids

Source: Adapted from MB Shields (ed). Textbook of Glaucoma (3rd ed). Baltimore: Williams & Wilkins, 1992;70.

TABLE 3-8. Factors That May Lead to Lower
Intraocular Pressure

Exertional influences
Strenuous exercise lowers intraocular pressure transiently
Lid and eye movement
Decreased orbicularis tone
Horner's syndrome
Intraocular conditions
Uveitis
Retinal detachment
Decreased corneal thickness
Systemic influences
Myotonic dystrophy
Acute hypoglycemia
Hormonal influences
Progesterone
Estrogen
Chorionic gonadotropin
Relaxin
Hyperthyroidism
Food and drugs
Alcohol
Fat-free diet
Heroin
Marijuana
Nitroglycerin (administered by perfusion techniques)
Isosorbide dinitrate
Systemic digitalis
Beta-methyldigoxin
Prostaglandins
Beta blockers
Calcium channel blockers
Carbonic anhydrase inhibitors
Alpha agonists

Source: Adapted from MB Shields (ed). Textbook of Glaucoma (3rd ed). Baltimore: Williams & Wilkins, 1992;70.

the course of the day can often be helpful in identifying the extent of IOP variation.

SUMMARY

Each first-time patient in your office or clinic should be evaluated as a potential glaucoma suspect. The work-up includes a detailed history searching for risk factors associated with glaucoma development. The clinical examination follows the same protocol as the comprehensive eye evaluation. This includes best-corrected visual acuities, pupillary testing, confrontation fields, slit-lamp biomicroscopy, tonometry, and dilated fundus evaluation of the optic nerve and nerve fiber layer. If risk factors are present or clinical findings are suggestive of glaucoma, then additional testing of gonioscopy and visual fields is performed. The following four chapters cover gonioscopy, optic nerve, nerve fiber layer, and visual field examination.

REFERENCES

1. Asbell PA, Chang B, Amin A, Podos SM. Retinal acuity evaluation with the potential acuity meter in glaucoma patients. Ophthalmology 1985;92(6):764–767.

2. Pickett JE, Terry SA, O'Connor PS, O'Hara M. Early loss of central visual acuity in glaucoma. Ophthalmology 1985;92(7):891–896.

3. Anctil JL, Anderson DR. Early foveal involvement and generalized depression of the visual field in glaucoma. Arch Ophthalmol 1984; 102(3):363–370.

4. Levene RZ. Central visual field, visual acuity, and sudden visual loss after glaucoma surgery. Ophthal Surg 1992;23(6):388–394.

5. Lam BL, Thompson HS. A unilateral cataract produces a relative afferent pupillary defect in the contralateral eye. Ophthalmology 1989;97:334.

6. Shahinfar S, Johnson LN, Madsen RW. Confrontation visual field loss as a function of decibel sensitivity loss on automated static perimetry. Implications on the accuracy of confrontation visual field testing. Ophthalmology 1995;102:872–877.

7. Lakowski R, Drance SM. Acquired dyschromatopsias: the earliest functional losses in glaucoma. Doc Ophthalmol Proc Ser 1979;19:159–165.

8. Hart WM. Color Vision. In WM Hart (ed), Adler's Physiology of the Eye (9th ed). St. Louis: Mosby, 1992;722.

9. Drance SM, Lakowski R, Schulzer M, Douglas GR. Acquired color vision changes in glaucoma: use of 100-hue test and Pickford anomaloscope as predictors of glaucomatous field change. Arch Ophthalmol 1981;99:829–831.

10. Sample PA, Weinreb RN, Boynton RM. Acquired dyschromatopsia in glaucoma. Surv Ophthalmol 1986;31:54.

11. Korth M, Nguyen NX, Junemann A, et al. VEP test of the blue-sensitive pathway in glaucoma. Invest Ophthalmol Vis Sci 1994;35(5):2599–2610.

12. Hart WM Jr, Gordon MO. Color perimetry of glaucomatous visual field defects. Ophthalmology 1984;91:338.

13. Johnson CA, Adams AJ, Caasson EJ, Brandt JD. Blue-on-yellow perimetry can predict the development of glaucomatous visual field loss. Arch Ophthalmol 1993;111:645–650.

14. Jonas JB, Zach FM. Color vision defects in chronic open angle glaucoma. Fortschr Ophthalmol 1990;87(3):255–259.

15. Alpern M, Moeller J. The red and green cone visual pigments of deuteranomalous trichromacy. J Physiol (Lond) 1977;266:647.

16. Sample PA, Taylor JD, Martinez GA, et al. Short-wavelength color visual fields in glaucoma suspects at risk. Am J Ophthalmol 1993;115(2):225–233.

17. Johnson CA, Adams AJ, Casson EJ, Brandt JD. Progression of early glaucomatous visual field loss as detected by blue-on-yellow and standard white-on-white automated perimetry. Arch Ophthalmol 1993; 111:651–656.

18. Yamagami J, Koseki N, Araie M. Color vision deficit in normal-tension glaucoma eyes. Jpn J Ophthalmol 1995;39(4):384–389.

19. Skalka HW. Arden grating test in evaluating "early" posterior subcapsular cataracts. South Med J 1981;74:1368–1370.

20. Ghafour IM, Foulds WS, Allan D, et al. Contrast sensitivity in diabetic subjects with and without retinopathy. Br J Ophthalmol 1982;66:492–495.

21. Motolko MA, Phelps CD. Contrast sensitivity in asymmetric glaucoma. Int Ophthalmol 1984;7(1):45–49.

22. Ross JE. Clinical detection of abnormalities in central vision in chronic simple glaucoma using contrast sensitivity. Int Ophthalmol 1985;8(3):167–177.

23. Arden GB, Jacobson JJ. A simple grating test for contrast sensitivity: preliminary results indicate value in screening for glaucoma. Invest Ophthalmol Vis Sci 1978;17:23–32.

24. Arden GB. Testing contrast sensitivity in clinical practice. Clin Vis Sci 1988;2:213–244.

25. Marron JA, Bailey IL. Visual factors and orientation-mobility performance. Am J Optom Physiol Opt 1982;59:413–426.

26. Johnson CA, Samuels SJ. Screening for glaucomatous visual field loss with frequency-doubling perimetry. Invest Ophthalmol Vis Sci 1997;38(2):413–425.

27. Quigley HA. Identification of glaucoma-related visual field abnormality with the screening protocol of frequency doubling technology. Am J Ophthalmol 1998;125(6):819–829.

28. Kelly DH. Nonlinear visual responses to flickering sinusoidal gratings. J Optom Soc Am 1981;71:1051–1055.

29. Quigley HA, Dunkelberger GR, Green WR. Chronic human glaucoma causing selectively greater loss of large optic nerve fibers. Ophthalmology 1988;95:357–363.

30. Johnson CA. The Glenn Fry lecture: early losses of visual function in glaucoma. Optom Vis Sci 1995;72:359–370.

31. Shields MB. Glaucomas Associated with Intraocular Tumors. In MB Shields (ed), Textbook of Glaucoma (4th ed). Baltimore: Williams & Wilkins, 1998:302.

32. Weiss DI. Dual origin of glaucoma in encephalotrigeminal haemangiomatosis. Trans Ophthalmol Soc UK 1973;93:477.

33. Phelps CD. The pathogenesis of glaucoma in Sturge-Weber syndrome. Ophthalmology 1978;85:276.

34. Regenbogen LS, Naveh-Floman N. Glaucoma in Fuch's heterochromic cyclitis associated with congenital Horner's syndrome. Br J Ophthalmol 1987; 71(11):844–849.

35. Donaldson DD. Transillumination of the iris. Trans Am Ophthalmol Soc 1974;72:89.

36. Layden WE, Shaffer RN. Exfoliation syndrome. Am J Ophthalmol 1974;78:835.

37. Grant WM, Schuman JS. Tonometry and Tomography. In DL Epstein, RP Allingham, JS Schuman(eds). Chandler and Grant's Glaucoma (4th ed). Baltimore: Williams & Wilkins 1997;41.

38. Holladay JT, Allison ME, Prager TC. Goldmann applanation tonometry in patients with regular corneal astigmatism. Am J Ophthalmol 1983;96:90.

39. Mark HH. Corneal curvature in applanation tonometry. Am J Ophthalmol 76:223,1973.

40. Boothe WA, Lee DA, Panek WC, Pettit TH. The Tono-Pen. A manometric and clinical study. Arch Ophthalmol 1988;106:1214.

41. Frenkel REP, Hong YJ, Shin DH. Comparison of the Tono-Pen to the Goldmann applanation tonometer. Arch Ophthalmol 1988;106:750.

42. Hessemer V, Rossler R, Jacobi KW. Tono-Pen, a new hand-held tonometer: comparison with the Goldmann applanation tonometer. Klin Monatsb Augenheilkd 1988;193:420.

43. Grolman B. A new tonometer system. Am J Optom Arch Am Acad Optom 1972;49:646.

44. Shields MB (ed). Textbook of Glaucoma (3rd ed). Baltimore: Williams & Wilkins, 1992;70.

45. Moses RA, Arnzen RJ. Instantaneous tonometry. Arch Ophthalmol 1974;101:249.

46. Marg E, Mackay RS, Oechsli R. Trough height, pressure and flattening in tonometry. Vision Res 1962;1:379.

47. Quigley HA, Langham ME. Comparative intraocular pressure measurements with the pneumatonograph and Goldmann tonometer. Am J Ophthalmol 1975;80:266.

48. Jain MR, Marmion VJ. A clinical evaluation of the applanation pneumatonograph. Br J Ophthalmol 1976;60:107.

49. Kruse Hansen F. A clinical study of the normal human central corneal thickness. Acta Ophthalmol (Copenh) 1971;49:82–89.

50. Kruse Hansen F, Ehlers N. Elevated tonometer readings caused by a thick cornea. Acta Ophthalmol (Copenh) 1971;49:775–778.

51. Ehlers N, Bramsen T, Sperling S. Applanation tonometry and central corneal thickness. Acta Ophthalmol (Copenh) 1975;53:34–43.

52. Whitacre MM, Stein RA, Hassanein K. The effect of corneal thickness on applanation tonometry. Am J Ophthalmol 1993;115:592–596.

53. Copt RP, Thomas R, Mermoud A. Corneal thickness in ocular hypertension, primary open-angle glaucoma, and normal tension glaucoma. Arch Ophthalmol 1999;117:14–16.

54. Ehlers N, Hansen FK. Central corneal thickness in low-tension glaucoma. Acta Ophthalmol (Copenh) 1974;52:740–746.

55. Shiose Y, Kitazawa Y, Tsukahara S. Epidemiology of glaucoma in Japan: a nationwide glaucoma survey. Jpn J Ophthalmol 1991;35:133.

56. Johnson M, Kass MA, Moses RA, Grodzki WJ. Increased corneal thickness simulating elevated intraocular pressure. Arch Ophthalmol 1978;96:664–665.

57. Emara B, Probst LE, Tingey DP, et al. J Cataract Refract Surg 1998;24:1320–1325.

58. Kitazawa Y, Horie T. Diurnal variation of intraocular pressure in primary open angle glaucoma. Am J Ophthalmol 1975;79:557.

59. Costagliola C, Trapanese A, Pagano M. Intraocular pressure in a healthy population: a survey of 751 subjects. Optom Vis Sci 1990;67:204.

60. Brubaker RF. Flow of aqueous humor in humans: the Friedenwald lecture. Invest Ophthalmol Vis Sci 1991;32:3145–3166.

61. Epstein DL, Krug Jr JH, Hertzmark E, et al. A long-term clinical trial of timolol therapy versus no treatment in the management of glaucoma suspects. Ophthalmology 1989;96:1460–1767.

62. Wilensky JT, Gieser DK, Mori MT, et al. Self-tonometry to manage patients with glaucoma and apparently controlled intraocular pressure. Arch Ophthalmol 1987;105:1072.

4

Gonioscopy

Anthony B. Litwak

Gonioscopy is an essential diagnostic tool in the work-up of any patient diagnosed with or suspected of having glaucoma. Gonioscopy allows the clinician to view the anterior chamber angle anatomy, but more important, gonioscopy permits differential diagnosis of the glaucomas. Primary open-angle glaucoma includes more than 70% of the glaucomas, but it is a diagnosis of exclusion. It must be differentiated from primary and secondary angle-closure, as well as secondary open-angle glaucoma. The process of making this diagnosis begins with the patient history and includes evaluation of the anterior segment with slit lamp biomicroscopy. However, the pinnacle diagnostic test to differentiate the glaucomas is gonioscopy. This diagnosis is essential for proper management and treatment, as well as for medical-legal reasons. When glaucoma is diagnosed in any patient, the type of glaucoma must be specified in the patient's record. Any patient labeled as a *glaucoma patient*, *glaucoma suspect*, or *narrow-angle suspect* must have gonioscopy performed and recorded.

ANGLE ANATOMY

To document the gonioscopic findings, the clinician must have a basic knowledge of anterior chamber anatomy. The *anterior chamber angle* refers to the area between the peripheral anterior iris insertion and the peripheral posterior surface of the cornea (Schwalbe's line) (Figure 4-1). The primary function of the angle is to drain aqueous from the anterior chamber through the trabecular meshwork into Schlemm's canal (Figures 4-2 and 4-3).

Which angle structures are visible with gonioscopy depends on the concavity of the iris, the insertion point of the peripheral iris, and the depth of the angle chamber (see Figure 4-2D). The clinician should note the contour of the iris curvature as being flat, concave, or convex (Figure 4-4). A flat contour is the most common, whereas a concave contour may be an indicator of pigment dispersion syndrome (see Color Plates 1 and 3), and a convex contour may be seen in patients with anatomically narrow angles (Figure 4-5) who are at risk for angle-closure glaucoma. The insertion of the iris root is typically in the anterior face of the ciliary body. If the insertion is more anterior, then the ciliary body may not be visualized. The ciliary body is typically a brown-to-grey-colored band, and the width is typically the same as or smaller than the width of the trabecular meshwork band. If the ciliary body band is larger than the trabecular meshwork band, then an angle recession (splitting of the longitudinal and circular muscles of the ciliary body) may be present (see Color Plate 14). This finding represents previous trauma that may also affect trabecular meshwork function and increase the risk of secondary glaucoma. Occasionally, radially oriented physiologic blood vessels may be seen in the ciliary body. This should not be confused with angle neovascularization, which grows from the iris surface across the ciliary body and scleral spur and into the trabecular meshwork (see Color Plates 10 and 11).

The next anterior structure to the ciliary body is the scleral spur, which is a white band of collagen tissue representing the posterior lip of the scleral sulcus (see Figure 4-2A). The width of this band is usually approximately one-half of the trabecular meshwork band. The trabecular meshwork overlies the scleral sulcus and forms Schlemm's canal, which extends 360 degrees

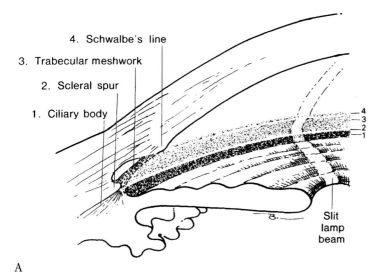

4. Schwalbe's line

3. Trabecular meshwork

2. Scleral spur

1. Ciliary body

Slit
lamp
beam

A

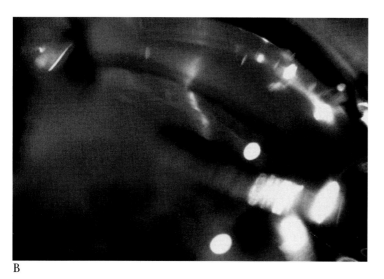

B

FIGURE 4-1. Normal anterior chamber anatomy. (A) Normal adult anterior chamber angle is shown in this artist's drawing of the gonioscopic appearance (*right*) and cross section of corresponding structures (*left*). (Reprinted with permission from MB Shields. Textbook of Glaucoma [2nd ed]. Baltimore: Williams & Wilkins, 1987;30.) (B) Gonioscopic view of a normal anterior chamber angle showing iris, ciliary body band, scleral spur, trabecular meshwork, and Schwalbe's line. By making a narrow beam and taking the slit lamp out of click stop, the clinician can observe reflections from the anterior and posterior surface of the cornea. These two reflections come to a point at Schwalbe's line. This patient has moderate pigmentation of the trabecular meshwork.

around the limbus (see Figure 4-2B). Aqueous exits the anterior chamber through the trabecular meshwork into Schlemm's canal. Intrascleral connecting channels drain the aqueous from Schlemm's canal into the episcleral veins.

The posterior two-thirds of the meshwork is the filtering portion for aqueous as it exits the anterior chamber into Schlemm's canal (see Figure 4-3). The filtering trabecular meshwork traps pigment and other debris from entering Schlemm's canal. Variable amounts of pigment can be trapped in the trabecular meshwork, resulting in a darkly pigmented band to a slightly beige band (see Color Plates 1 and 2). The anterior one-third of the trabecular meshwork is nonfiltering and usually has less or no visible pigmentation. Schlemm's canal is typically not visualized during gonioscopy, but when episcleral venous pressure is raised and is higher than the intraocular pressure (IOP), blood can reflux back into Schlemm's canal. The appearance is a red band beneath the trabecular meshwork (see Color Plate 16). Blood in Schlemm's

canal can be idiopathic or associated with Sturge-Weber syndrome, carotid-cavernous fistula, and obstruction of the superior vena cava.

The most anterior structure of the anterior chamber angle is Schwalbe's line, which represents the end of Descemet's membrane. Schwalbe's line is a slightly elevated ridge extending from the posterior surface of the cornea and may occasionally be pigmented. This is termed *Sampolesi's line*. Schwalbe's line is an important structure to identify, especially in patients with narrow angles. One clinical pearl for identifying Schwalbe's line is to take the slit beam out of click stop to approximately 15 degrees. Light from the narrow beam will reflect off the anterior and posterior surface of the cornea, and eventually the two lines will come to a point at Schwalbe's line (see Figure 4-1B). Once Schwalbe's line is identified, every structure posterior to it represents open angle. If the trabecular meshwork is visible, then the angle is open to the drainage of aqueous.

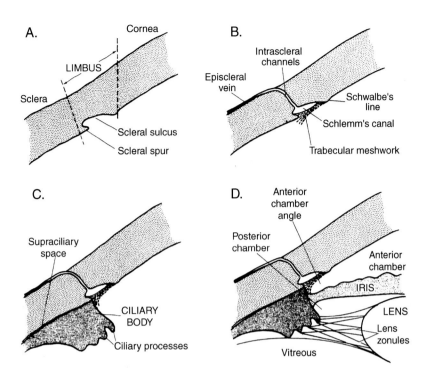

FIGURE 4-2. Construction of the anterior chamber angle. **(A)** The limbus is the transition area between the cornea and the sclera. The scleral sulcus is a recessed area in this tissue. The scleral spur is the posterior lip of the scleral sulcus. **(B)** Aqueous drains from the anterior chamber through the trabecular meshwork into Schlemm's canal and then into episcleral veins via intrascleral collecting channels. **(C)** The ciliary body is the site of aqueous production and attaches posterior to the scleral spur. **(D)** The iris inserts into the face of the ciliary body. (Reprinted with permission from MB Shields. Textbook of Glaucoma [2nd ed]. Baltimore: Williams & Wilkins, 1987;6.)

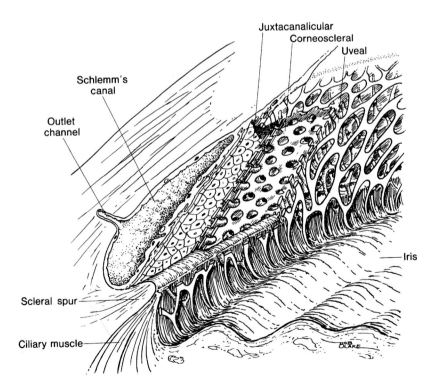

FIGURE 4-3. Three layers of trabecular meshwork (shown in cut-away views). The innermost layer is the uveal meshwork. The middle layer is the corneoscleral meshwork. The outer layer is the juxtacanalicular meshwork. (Reprinted with permission from MB Shields. Textbook of Glaucoma [2nd ed]. Baltimore: Williams & Wilkins, 1987;17.)

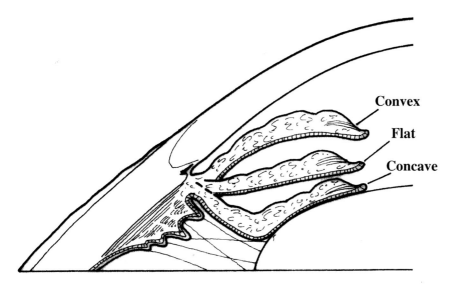

FIGURE 4-4. Iris contour. The iris may exhibit a convex, flat, or concave contour. Convex contour is associated with narrow angles and narrow-angle glaucoma, flat contours are the most common, and concave contours are found in patients with pigment dispersion syndrome and pigmentary glaucoma.

ZEISS FOUR-MIRROR GONIOSCOPY

Many types of lenses are available for performing gonioscopy. The gonioscopy lenses used most frequently in clinical practice are the indirect gonioscopy lenses. The two prototype lenses are the Zeiss four-mirror (Carl Zeiss, Thornwood, NY) and the Goldmann-style lenses (Haag-Strait, Berne, Switzerland). I have a strong personal bias for the Zeiss four-mirror lenses (Figure 4-6A). This lens is a four-mirror prism for angle evaluation with a central viewing portion for posterior pole fundus examination. The lens is mounted in an Unger holder. The Posner goniolens (Ocular Instruments, Bellevue, WA) (Figure 4-6B) is similar to the Zeiss lens, but the Posner lens is a lighter, one-piece

construction. The neck between the handle and lens can easily snap if the Posner lens is inadvertently dropped. The Sussman lens (Ocular Instruments, Bellevue, WA) (Figure 4-6C) is a hand-held version of the Zeiss four-mirror lens, which is held in a fashion similar to the Goldmann goniolens but has a footplate and posterior curvature comparable to the Zeiss goniolens.

The advantages of the Zeiss four-mirror lens over the Goldmann lens are as follows:

1. The footplate of the Zeiss lens (9 mm) is much smaller than that of the Goldmann lens (12 mm), which allows the clinician to insert the lens more easily onto the eye, especially useful for a noncooperative patient.

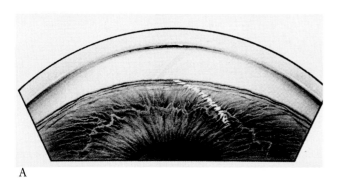

A

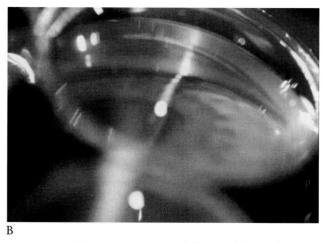

B

FIGURE 4-5. Narrow anterior chamber angle. (A) The drawing shows a convex iris contour without visibility of the angle structures. (Reprinted with permission from JJ Kanski, JA McAllister, JF Salmon [eds]. Glaucoma. A Color Manual of Diagnosis and Treatment [2nd ed]. London: Butterworth–Heinemann, 1996;61.) (B) This clinical gonioscopy photograph shows the eye of a patient with a convex iris contour and narrow anterior chamber angle. No angle structures are visible.

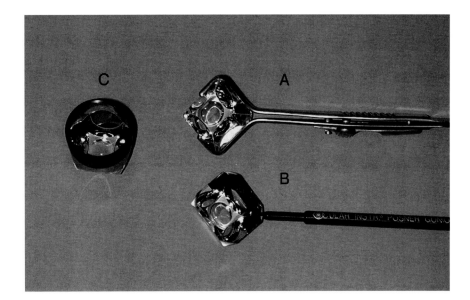

FIGURE 4-6. Four-mirror gonioscopy lenses. These lenses have posterior surfaces that mimic the anterior surface of the cornea. They do not require a coupling fluid and allow the clinician to perform pressure gonioscopy. (**A**) Zeiss four-mirror goniolens (Carl Zeiss, Thornwood, NY). (**B**) Posner goniolens (Ocular Instruments, Bellevue, WA). (**C**) Sussman lens (Ocular Instruments, Bellevue, WA).

2. The Zeiss lens has a flatter posterior curvature that mimics the anterior curvature of the cornea. This allows the clinician to avoid using a coupling fluid or gel. The flat posterior curvature also allows the clinician to perform pressure gonioscopy, which helps to determine whether patients with narrow angle have developed peripheral anterior synechiae (PAS).
3. The Zeiss goniolens has four mirrors, which allows the clinician to move the joystick of the slit lamp into the four mirrors to view 360 degrees of the anterior chamber angle without having to rotate the lens.

The main disadvantages of the Zeiss four-mirror lens over the Goldmann lens are as follows:

1. The Zeiss four mirror lens does not form a suction seal, so the patient may be able to blink the lens off of the eye. It is important not to inadvertently push the lens toward the eye (unintentional-pressure gonioscopy), because this may result in an artificially more opened angle and may mask a narrow-angle component.
2. Clinicians used to the Goldmann system may initially find the Zeiss technique more technically challenging; however, with a little experience, the speed of the procedure, the lack of need for a coupling gel, and the ability to perform pressure gonioscopy will convert most Goldmann users to Zeiss four-mirror gonioscopy.

PROCEDURE FOR ZEISS FOUR-MIRROR GONIOSCOPY

Before gonioscopy is performed, the patient should be instructed on the purpose and procedure of the test. I explain to the patient that I am going to examine the drainage portion of the eye and that the lens that I use might feel like an eyelash is in the eye, but it will not hurt. Topical anesthetic, such as proparacaine or Fluress, is applied to the cornea, and the patient is instructed to place his or her chin in the chin rest and forehead against the head rest of the slit lamp. Gonioscopy is typically performed after applanation tonometry. The outer canthus of the patient should be lined up with the notch mark on the columns of the slit lamp, so the chin rest will not have to be adjusted while the lens is on the eye. A fixation target should be given to the patient to keep the patient's eyes in primary gaze. The Zeiss lens is brought in from the side to rest on the edge of the lower lid (Figure 4-7A), the lens is then rotated onto the cornea, and the clinician focuses through the slit-lamp oculars. I prefer to position the lens in a diamond pattern (Figure 4-7B), rather than a square pattern (Figure 4-7C), so that I can keep the slit beam in a vertical position throughout the procedure. An elbow pad can be used to support your arm (Figure 4-7D).

I systematically start in the upper left-hand mirror and proceed to the upper right-hand mirror, followed by the inferior right and finally inferior left mirror. The angle being examined is 180 degrees from the mirror being viewed. Viewing just to the left of the center of the mirror corresponds to the angle directly opposite of, not diagonal to, the mirror. For

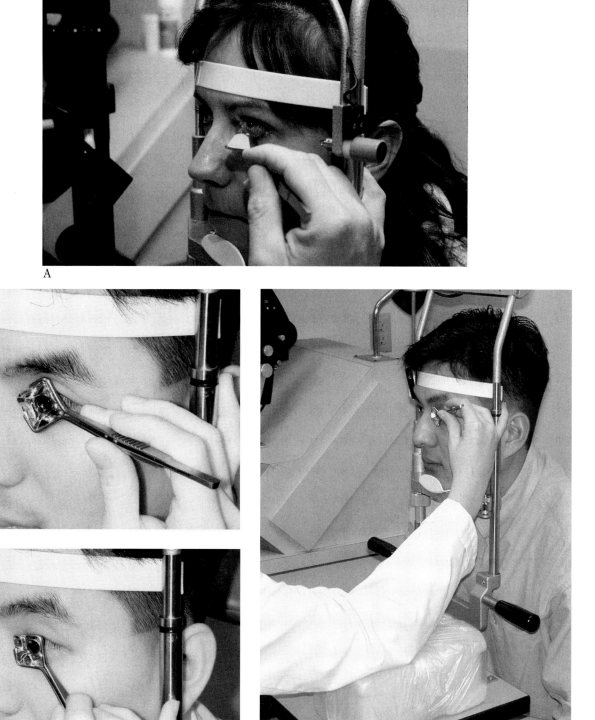

FIGURE 4-7. Insertion and holding positions of the Zeiss four-mirror goniolens. When the lens is being inserted, the patient is asked to look upward, and the lower lens is used to control the lower lid (**A**). The lens can be held in a diamond pattern (**B**) or square pattern (**C**). To help stabilize the lens, an elbow rest can be used, and the slit lamp can be hooked by the little finger (**D**).

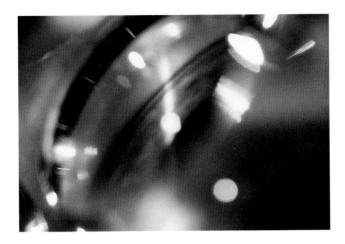

COLOR PLATE 1. Open anterior chamber angle to ciliary body with moderate to heavy pigmentation of the trabecular meshwork. Here the trabecular meshwork band is darker than the ciliary body band. Heavy pigmentation of the trabecular meshwork can be seen in patients with pigment dispersion syndrome and pseudoexfoliation of the lens.

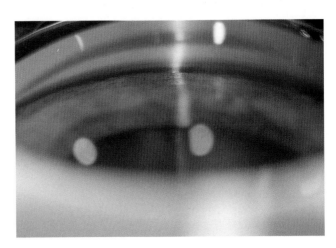

COLOR PLATE 2. Open anterior chamber angle to ciliary body with light pigmentation of the trabecular meshwork. Here the trabecular meshwork band is lighter than the ciliary body band. Little or no pigmentation of the trabecular meshwork may make it more difficult to identify other angle structures and grade the angle.

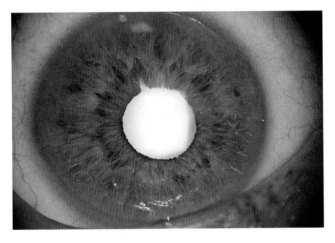

COLOR PLATE 3. Peripheral transillumination iris defects. Transillumination defects of the peripheral iris are typically seen in pigment dispersion syndrome. Pupillary transillumination defects are seen in pseudoexfoliation syndrome.

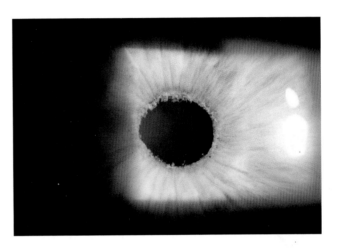

COLOR PLATE 4. Pseudoexfoliative (dandruff-like) deposits on the iris pupillary border.

COLOR PLATE 5. Pseudoexfoliation of the lens seen in retro-illumination. Note inner and outer ring of exfoliative material and middle ring absent of exfoliative material. This occurs because the iris brushes up against the lens as it dilates and constricts and pushes the exfoliative material from side to side.

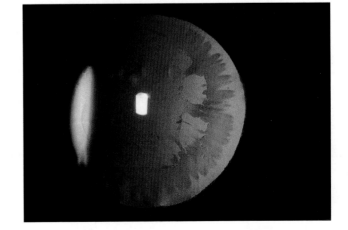

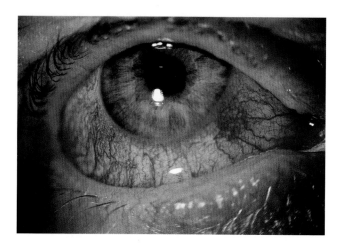

COLOR PLATE 6. Iritis. Note perilimbal injection of conjunctiva. Patient had 2+ cell and flare in the anterior chamber on slit-lamp biomicroscopy. Note also irregular pupil from posterior synechiae.

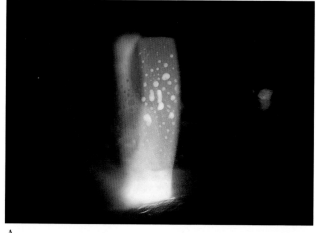

A

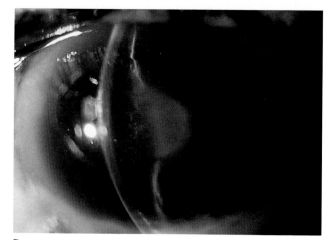

B

COLOR PLATE 7. Uveitis. (**A**) Keratic precipitates on the corneal endothelium in a patient with uveitis. This sign should alert the clinician to examine the angle for peripheral anterior synechiae. (**B**) Patient with severe uveitis. Note cell and flare in the anterior chamber.

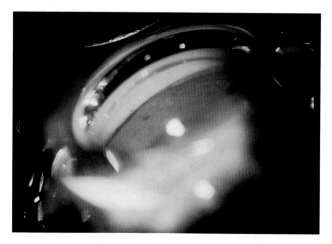

COLOR PLATE 8. Peripheral anterior synechiae. This patient had chronic angle closure with the development of peripheral anterior synechiae in the angle. After a peripheral iridotomy was performed, part of the angle (*right*) opens to ciliary body.

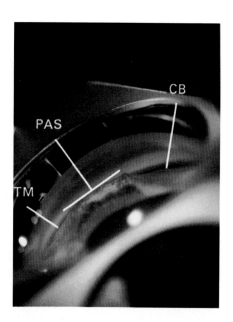

COLOR PLATE 9. Peripheral anterior synechiae (PAS). Iris adhesions are apparent above Schwalbe's line (high PAS). High PAS is typically seen in patients with penetrating injuries, flat anterior chambers after intraocular surgery, and in iridocorneal endothelial syndromes. This patient has iridocorneal endothelial syndrome. Note iris atrophy. (CB = ciliary body, TM = trabecular meshwork.) (Reprinted with permission from BM Fisch. Gonioscopy and the Glaucoma. Boston: Butterworth–Heinemann, 1993.)

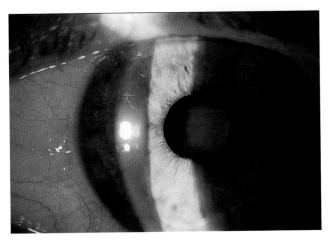

COLOR PLATE 10. Iris neovascularization. It typically appears at the pupillary border and can grow across the iris into the angle. The etiology of iris neovascularization is from ischemic retinal disease (e.g., diabetic retinopathy, central retinal vein occlusion).

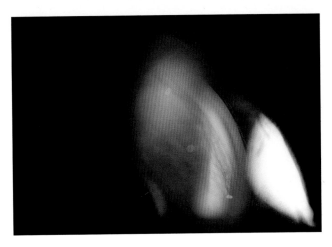

COLOR PLATE 11. Angle neovascularization. Neovascular vessels grow across the iris into the trabecular meshwork. Fibrovascular tissue forms and pulls the peripheral iris into the trabecular meshwork, leading to neovascular glaucoma. A minority of patients develop angle neovascularization without evidence of iris neovascularization.

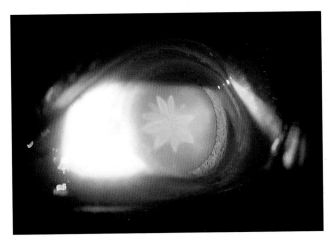

COLOR PLATE 12. Rosette cataract. This type of cataract is the result of previous trauma. Any trauma to the eye can lead to dysfunction of the trabecular meshwork, an increase in intraocular pressure, and traumatic glaucoma.

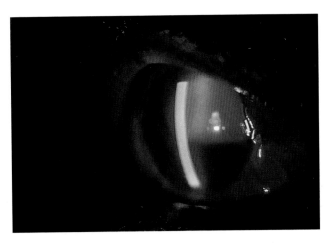

COLOR PLATE 13. Hyphema. Trauma to the iris or ciliary body can cause bleeding into the anterior chamber. This can result in an acute rise in intraocular pressure. After the hyphema resolves, patients are still at risk for developing traumatic glaucoma.

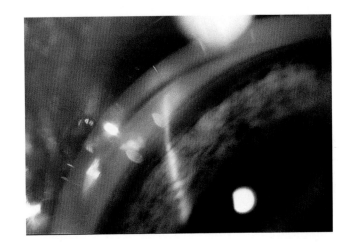

COLOR PLATE 14. Angle recession. With blunt trauma, the ciliary muscle can be separated, leading to a widening of the ciliary body band in the angle. Concurrent damage to the trabecular meshwork can lead to an increase in intraocular pressure and secondary glaucoma (traumatic).

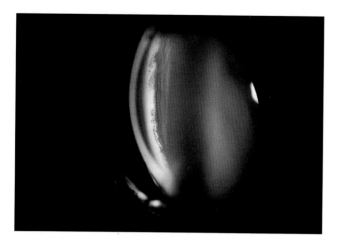

COLOR PLATE 15. Pigment clumping and scarring in the angle. Clumps of pigment in or above the trabecular meshwork can also be a sign of previous trauma, hyphema, or ocular surgery, and may be associated with the development of traumatic glaucoma.

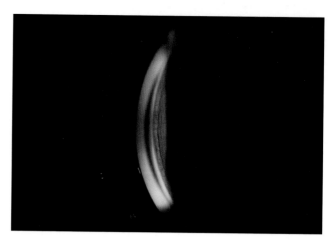

COLOR PLATE 16. Blood in Schlemm's canal. Blood in Schlemm's canal can be a sign of elevated episcleral venous pressure or may be an idiopathic finding. Elevated episcleral venous pressure is a risk factor for developing glaucoma.

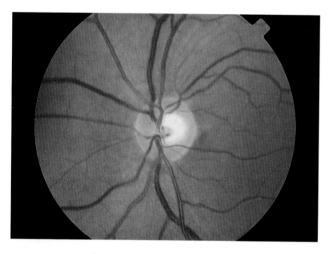

COLOR PLATE 17. Normal optic nerve. Neural-retinal rim tissue composed of ganglion cell axons and capillary beds has an orange-red appearance. Space in the center of the optic disc is devoid of axons and capillaries and is called the *optic cup*. Note visibility of the pores in the laminar cribrosa at the base of the cup. This patient has a medium-sized disc with a medium-sized cup. Note symmetric neuroretinal rim tissue between the superior and inferior poles, which is also greater than the temporal rim tissue.

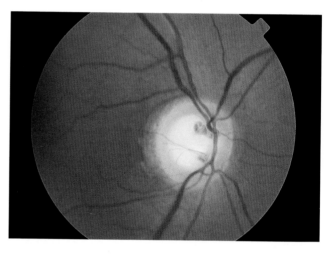

COLOR PLATE 18. Large physiologic cupping in a nonglaucoma patient. This patient has a large physiologic disc with large physiologic cupping. Note that the superior and inferior rim tissue is symmetric and greater than the temporal rim tissue.

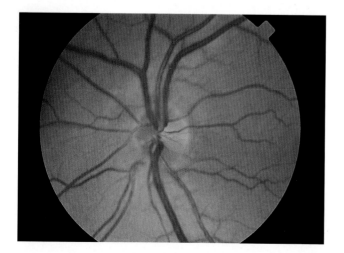

COLOR PLATE 19. Small physiologic disc with small cup. A small physiologic disc should have a small cup. Medium cups in a small disc should raise the suspicion of glaucoma, as should a large cup in a medium-sized disc.

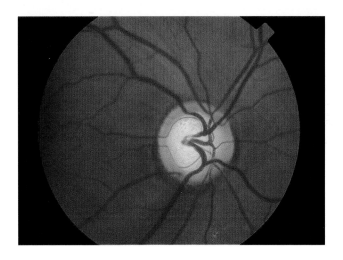

COLOR PLATE 20. Glaucoma in a large physiologic disc. Patient has a large cup and a large disc. However, the superior and inferior rim tissue are thin by comparison to the temporal rim tissue. In general, the superior and inferior rim tissue should be symmetric and approximately 1.5–2.0 times thicker than the temporal rim tissue. Glaucoma tends to affect the superior and inferior poles of the optic nerve, with relative sparing of the temporal pole. When the inferior or superior rim tissue is equal to or less than the temporal rim tissue, glaucoma damage should be suspected.

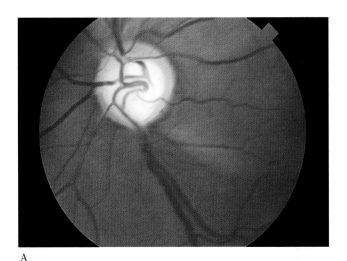

A

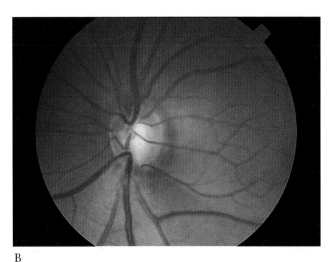

B

COLOR PLATE 21. Notch of the optic nerve. Notching in the optic cup represents a focal loss of ganglion cell axons, usually in the superior or inferior pole of the optic disc. It almost always corresponds to a visual field defect and nerve fiber layer loss. Notching is almost always a definitive sign of glaucoma damage. (A) Inferior notch in a large disc. (B) Inferior notch in a small disc. Note corresponding inferior nerve fiber layer loss.

COLOR PLATE 22. Endstage glaucoma damage to the optic nerve. Note complete cupping of the optic nerve, with undermining of the cup and bayonetting of the disc vessels. The optic disc appears pale because of exposure of the collagen tissue of the lamina cribrosa. Note also peripapillary atrophy.

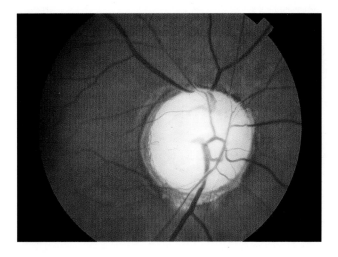

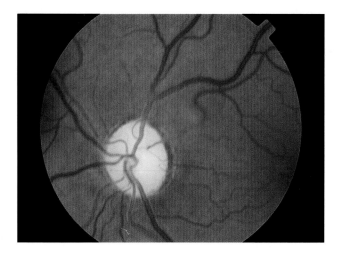

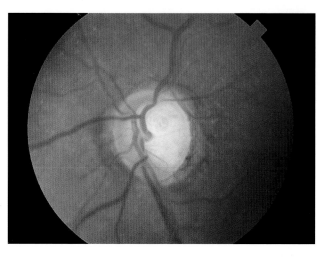

COLOR PLATE 23. Pallor of the optic nerve from nonglaucoma etiology. This patient displays moderate cupping, but the remaining rim tissue is pale. Pallor to the remaining neuroretinal rim tissue should alert the clinician to suspect an etiology (ischemia, compression, inflammation) other than glaucoma.

COLOR PLATE 24. Acquired pit of the optic nerve (APON) and peripapillary atrophy. APON is a focal depression within the lamina cribrosa that is an acquired sign of glaucoma damage. It tends to occur in the superior or inferior poles of the optic cup and is more frequently seen in normal-tension than high-tension glaucoma. This normal-tension glaucoma patient shows an APON in the superior part of the optic cup, which was associated with a inferior visual field defect just below fixation. Also note peripapillary atrophy, which tends to occur in an area of neuroretinal rim tissue thinning.

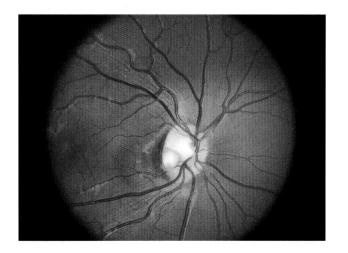

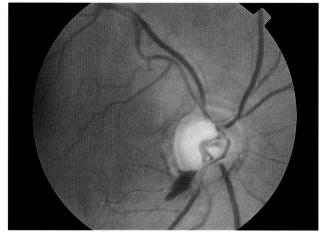

COLOR PLATE 25. Congenital optic pit. Note grayish-white lesion in the inferior temporal pole of the optic disc. Congenital optic pit represents a focal coloboma of the optic nerve and may result in a corresponding visual field defect. It can be differentiated from acquired pit of the optic nerve by its light grey appearance and lack of laminar dots.

COLOR PLATE 26. Drance hemorrhage. Disk hemorrhages (Drance hemorrhages) in the peripapillary retina or on the optic disc can also be a sign of glaucoma damage or progression. They tend to occur in the superior and inferior poles of the optic disc and are more common in normal-tension glaucoma than in high-tension glaucoma.

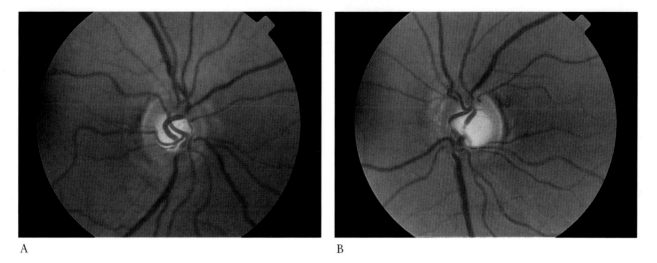

A   B

COLOR PLATE 27. Cup-to-disc asymmetry in a uveitic glaucoma patient. Note larger cupping in the left eye (**B**) compared with the right eye (**A**) in a patient with fairly symmetrically sized optic disks. Cup-to-disc asymmetry can be a sign of glaucoma damage, but it must be differentiated from asymmetric optic disc sizes.

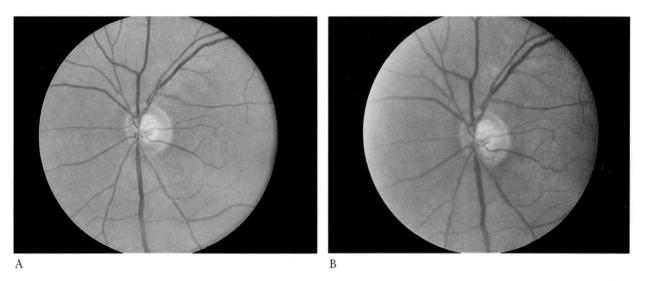

A   B

COLOR PLATE 28. Progressive cupping in glaucoma. Initial photograph (**A**) of a glaucoma suspect. Photograph (**B**) taken 2 years later documents progressive loss of neuroretinal rim tissue, especially in the inferior temporal pole. Note also nerve fiber layer loss inferior. Stereoscopic disc photographs should be taken on all glaucoma and glaucoma-suspect patients and used for serial comparisons.

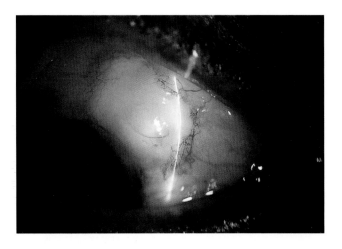

COLOR PLATE 29. Mitomycin C bleb. Mitomycin C filters have a distinct avascular, thin-walled, chalky-white appearance. They are less likely to scar down from fibrosis but are at a greater risk of developing a bleb leak.

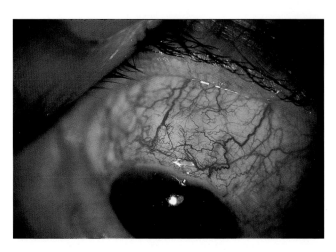

COLOR PLATE 30. Failing bleb. Signs of filtration failure include conjunctival injection, bleb vascularization, thickening of the bleb wall, lack of conjunctival elevation, and lack of conjunctival microcysts.

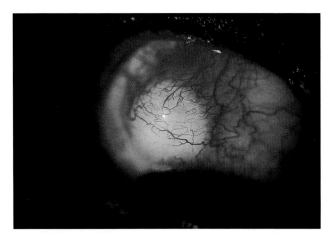

COLOR PLATE 31. Encapsulated bleb. Clinical signs of bleb encapsulation include a firm, opalescent localized bleb with a thick wall and progressive conjunctival hyperemia.

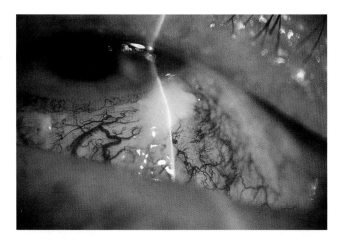

COLOR PLATE 32. Blebitis. Filtering blebs can become infected and lead to endophthalmitis. Note conjunctival injection and a mucous purulent discharge within an inferior temporal bleb.

example, viewing in the superior lens just to the right of the 12 o'clock position corresponds to the 5 o'clock angle (Figure 4-8), and viewing just to the left of 12 o'clock position corresponds to the 7 o'clock angle. The slit beam should be approximately 1–3 mm in width, and the light source should be on a low setting to reduce the amount of pupil constriction, which can alter the depth of the anterior chamber angle. The lens should be maintained perpendicular to the cornea; a tear-film seal provides clear, sharp views of the angle. If the film seal is disrupted by sliding of the lens or a change in eye movement, the view of the angle becomes distorted and the lens should be repositioned back onto the center of the cornea.

During the procedure, the iris contour and angle structures are evaluated (see Figure 4-1). The iris may exhibit a flat, convex, or concave contour (see Figure 4-4). Flat contours are typically seen in patients with deep anterior chambers and wide open angles. Concave contours are observed in patients with pigment dispersion syndrome (see Chapter 15). Concave iris contours should alert the clinician to examine the degree of pigment in the trabecular meshwork and look for peripheral iris transillumination defects and pigment on the corneal endothelium (see Color Plate 3). Convex iris contour is typically seen in patients with shallow anterior chambers and narrow anterior chamber angles (see Figure 4-5). These patients are more disposed to primary angle-closure glaucoma (see Chapter 16). It is important to tilt the goniolens to view the angle chamber angle in patients with convex iris contours (Figure 4-9). This is accomplished by tilting the lens towards the angle in view (if the inferior mirror is being viewed, the lens should be tilted towards 12 o'clock, which is the angle being examined). If the angle structures cannot be visualized with lens tilting, then the patient should be instructed to look in the direction of the mirror being viewed (e.g., if the clinician is looking at the 6 o'clock mirror and examining the superior angle, the patient should be instructed to look slightly down) (Figure 4-10).

The degree of lens tilt and change in patient gaze are incorporated into a grading system that helps to

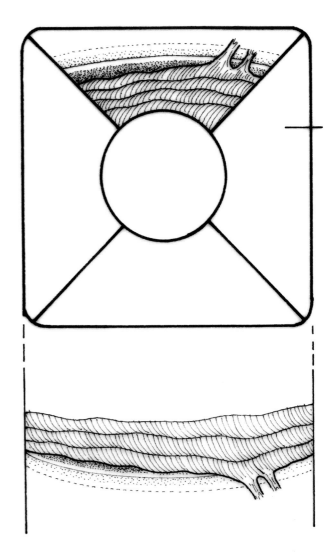

FIGURE 4-8. Corresponding angle with gonioscopy view. The gonioscopy mirror is viewing the anatomic angle 180 degrees away. In this case, the superior goniolens is viewing the inferior angle. However, angle structures viewed to the right of the 12 o'clock position (1 o'clock) in the goniolens correspond to the anatomic angle at 5 o'clock and not at 7 o'clock. In this drawing, peripheral anterior synechiae viewed at 1 o'clock in the goniolens correspond to the anatomic angle at 5 o'clock.

FIGURE 4-9. Dynamic gonioscopy: lens tilting diagram. With a convex iris contour, it may be necessary to tilt the gonioscopy mirror towards the angle being viewed to observe the angle structures. In this example, the clinician would view the inferior mirror and observe the superior angle. To view over the slightly convex iris contour, the goniolens is tilted slightly up. In this example, lens tilting reveals full trabecular meshwork. (SL = Schwalbe's line; TM = trabecular membrane.)

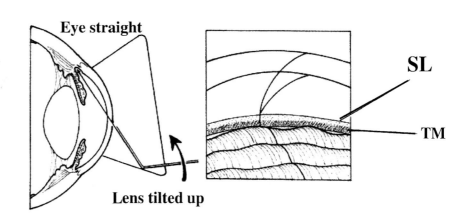

Eye straight

Lens tilted up

SL

TM

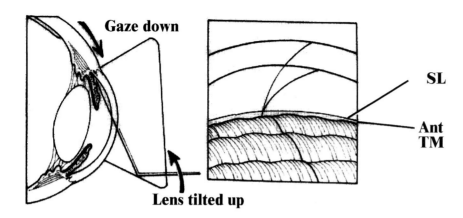

Gaze down

SL

Ant
TM

Lens tilted up

FIGURE 4-10. Dynamic gonioscopy with lens tilting and change in patient's gaze. If lens tilting does not reveal the anterior chamber angle due to a narrow angle, the patient should be asked to look slightly toward the angle mirror being viewed. In this case, the lens is tilted up, and the patient would be asked to look slightly down to view the angle structures in the superior angle. In this example, lens tilting and change in patient gaze reveal only anterior trabecular meshwork, indicating a very narrow angle. (SL = Schwalbe's line; Ant TM = anterior trabecular meshwork.)

classify angle grading and determine the risk for angle closure (Table 4-1 and Figure 4-11). For instance, an angle in which all structures including the ciliary body are visible without lens tilt or change in patient gaze is classified as a *grade 4 open angle* (see Figure 4-11A). If mild lens tilt is required to view the ciliary body, the angle is *grade 3* (see Figure 4-11B). If lens tilting only produces visibility of the full trabecular meshwork, the angle is *grade 2* (see Figure 4-11C). If lens tilting and a change in patient gaze allow visualization only of anterior trabecular meshwork, then the angle is *grade 1* (see Figure 4-11D). *Grade 1* angles should be considered for prophylactic laser peripheral iridotomy (see Chapter 16).

It is important to perform pressure gonioscopy to view the entire trabecular meshwork to uncover PAS. If PAS is present in conjunction with bilateral narrow anterior chamber angles, the patient is diagnosed with chronic primary angle-closure glaucoma and should be treated with a laser peripheral iridotomy. If no anterior chamber angle structures are visible with lens tilting and change in patient gaze, then the angle is closed (see Figure

4-11E), and pressure gonioscopy should be performed to determine whether PAS is present. Pressure gonioscopy is performed by gently pressing the gonioscopy lens against the cornea. This technique directs aqueous toward the peripheral anterior chamber and pushes the peripheral iris back to view the angle structure (Figure 4-12). When the iris is in appositional contact with the trabecular meshwork, adhesions may form between the iris tissue and meshwork, called *peripheral anterior synechiae* (Figure 4-13). PAS is not specific for primary angle-closure glaucoma, but it can occur in patients with chronic or severe iritis, neovascular glaucoma, and other causes of secondary angle-closure glaucomas. Thus, it is extremely important to differentiate primary angle-closure glaucoma, which is treated with a peripheral iridotomy, from secondary angle closures, which may have a much different treatment modality (see Chapter 17).

Patients with Grade 2 narrow angles without PAS should be re-evaluated with tonometry and gonioscopy after pharmacologic dilation. It is prudent to dilate one eye at a time with 0.5% tropicamide without phenylephrine and be prepared to manage an angle closure attack if it should occur. An increase in IOP of 6 or more millimeters of mercury in conjunction with narrowing of the anterior chamber angle is considered a positive mydriatic provocative test and an indication for prophylactic laser peripheral iridotomy. Acute angle-closure glaucoma, provocative narrow-angle testing, and the decision to prophylactically treat narrow angles with peripheral iridotomy are discussed in Chapter 16.

Clinical Pearl: When learning the technique of Zeiss gonioscopy, perform the procedure on all of your patients after applanation tonometry. This repetition allows improvement in technique and also allows the clinician to learn the physiologic variation of the anterior chamber angle.

TABLE 4-1. Dynamic Gonioscopy Angle Grading System

Grade 4: All angle structures can be seen (to ciliary body) without lens tilt or change in patient gaze.

Grade 3: All angle structures can be seen with minimal lens tilt (no change in patient gaze).

Grade 2: Full trabecular meshwork can be seen with lens tilt (no change in patient gaze).

Grade 1: Anterior trabecular meshwork can be seen with lens tilt and change in patient gaze.

Grade 0: Angle closed; no angle structures can be seen with lens tilt or change in patient gaze. Pressure gonioscopy should be performed to determine whether peripheral anterior synechiae are present.

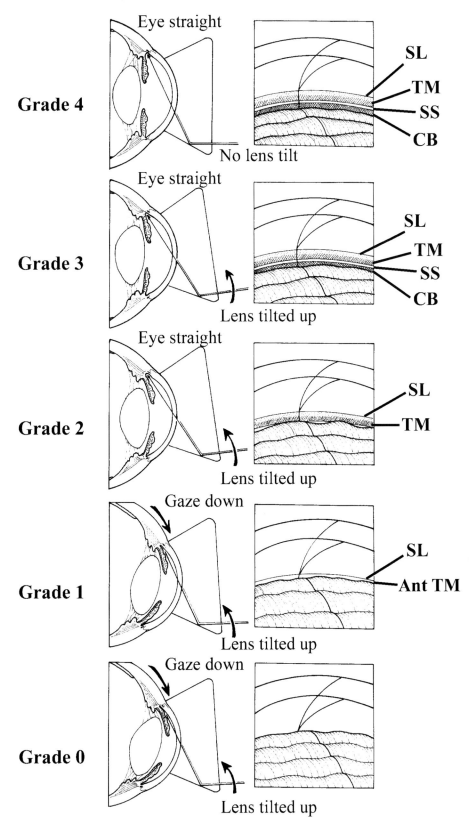

FIGURE 4-11. Litwak's dynamic gonioscopy grading system. Grade 4: All angle structures can be seen (to ciliary body) without lens tilt or change in patient gaze. Grade 3: All angle structures can be seen with minimal lens tilt (no change in patient gaze). Grade 2: Full trabecular meshwork can be seen with lens tilt (no change in patient gaze). Grade 1: Anterior trabecular meshwork can be seen with lens tilt and change in patient gaze. Grade 0: Angle is closed. No angle structures can be seen with lens tilt or change in patient gaze. Pressure gonioscopy should be performed to determine whether peripheral anterior synechiae are present. (Ant TM = anterior trabecular meshwork; CB = ciliary body; SL = Schwalbe's line; SS = scleral spur.)

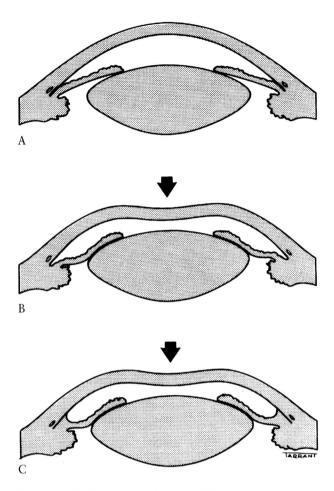

A

B

C

FIGURE 4-12. Pressure gonioscopy. When patients have narrow angles, making it difficult to view angle structures with lens tilting or change in patient gaze (**A**), the four-mirror gonioscopy lens can be pushed forward, toward the cornea. This directs aqueous into the peripheral anterior chamber and forces the iris to fall back from the angle (**B**). When peripheral anterior synechiae have formed in the angle, the iris stretches back with pressure gonioscopy, but the angle structures are not viewed (**C**). (Reprinted with permission from JJ Kanski, JA McAllister, JF Salmon [eds]. Glaucoma. A Color Manual of Diagnosis and Treatment [2nd ed]. London: Butterworth–Heinemann, 1996;15.)

GOLDMANN GONIOSCOPY

Another popular method of gonioscopy is performed with the Goldmann-type goniolens. Several varieties of this lens are available (Figure 4-14). Most popular is a three-mirror version that includes a central fundus lens for posterior pole examination and three peripheral lenses for angle, far fundus periphery, and midperiphery fundus evaluation. Single-, two-, and four-mirror versions are also used for gonioscopy. The single-mirror version must be rotated 360 degrees on the eye to view the entire anterior chamber angle. The two-mirror goniolens is rotated 180 degrees, alternating between the

two mirrors, and the four-mirror goniolens does not require rotation. The footplate of the Goldmann goniolens is larger and has a greater concave curvature than the Zeiss four-mirror goniolens. The larger footplate does not allow the clinician to perform pressure gonioscopy and is more difficult to insert onto the eye. The greater concave curvature requires the use of a coupling fluid to prevent air bubbles between the lens and the eye.

Traditional goniolens solutions like Goniosol are viscous and require lavage at the conclusion of the procedure, which may cause a superficial punctate keratitis. Superficial punctate keratitis can interfere with subsequent posterior pole examination and optic disc photodocumentation. Thicker artificial tear preparations, such as Ocucoat, AquaSite, and Celluvisc, can be substituted as a coupling fluid, which do not necessitate rinsing the eye out and reduces superficial punctate keratitis. The disadvantage to using tear preparations is the increased frequency of air bubbles underneath the lens if the lens is not inserted quickly onto the eye. The advantage of the Goldmann goniolens is the stability of the lens once it is inserted onto the eye. The suction seal that forms makes it very difficult for the patient to blink off the lens. The disadvantages are the requirement of a coupling fluid and the potential for air bubbles, longer examination time (if the lens needs to be rotated), and the inability to perform pressure gonioscopy.

PROCEDURE FOR GOLDMANN GONIOSCOPY

The initial set-up for Goldmann gonioscopy is similar to that for Zeiss four-mirror gonioscopy. The concave portion of the Goldmann lens should be filled with a viscous artificial tear solution, such as AquaSite, Ocucoat, or Celluvisc. Four-fifths of the concavity should be filled to help avoid bubble formation on insertion. The patient is asked to look up, and the lower lid is controlled with the edge of the goniolens (Figure 4-15A). The lens is then rotated quickly onto the cornea, and the patient is asked to look straight ahead at a fixation target (Figure 4-15B). The angle being examined is 180 degrees from the mirror being viewed. When the mirror is in the 12 o'clock position, examination of the inferior angle is possible. Viewing in the superior lens just to the right of the 12 o'clock position corresponds to the 5 o'clock angle (see Figure 4-8), and viewing just to the left of 12 o'clock corresponds to the 7 o'clock angle. Lens tilting or change in patient gaze should be used to allow visualization and grading of the anterior chamber angle (see Figure 4-11 and Table 4-1). Pressure gonioscopy is not possible with the Goldmann goniolens.

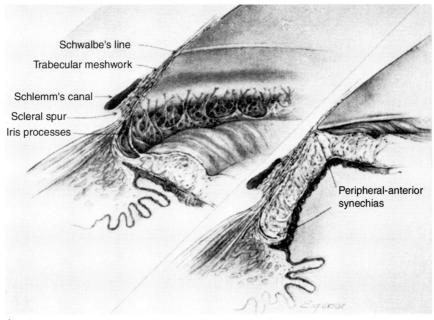

A

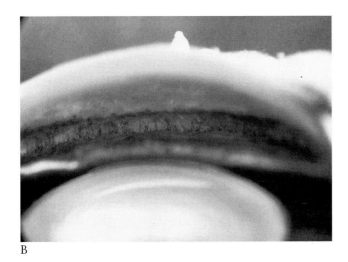

B

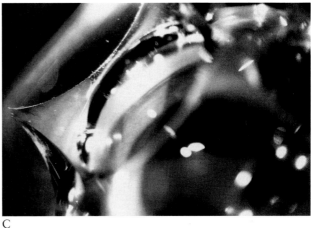

C

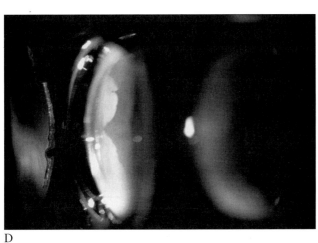

D

FIGURE 4-13. Peripheral anterior synechiae versus iris processes. (**A**) *Top left*: Iris processes represent thin strands of iris tissue that attach to the trabecular meshwork. They represent a physiologic variation of the normal angle. *Top right*: Peripheral anterior synechiae occur when broad bands of peripheral iris tissue adhere into the trabecular meshwork. This is an acquired finding and can occur from appositional angle closure, from chronic uveitis, and from angle neovascularization. (Reprinted with permission from HD Hoskins Jr, MA Kass. Becker-Schaffer's Diagnosis and Therapy of the Glaucomas [6th ed]. St. Louis: Mosby, 1989.) (**B**) Postmortem specimen of iris processes. (**C**) Clinical slide showing a band of low peripheral anterior synechiae in the angle. (**D**) Clinical slide of peripheral anterior synechiae extending above Schwalbe's line from a previously flat anterior chamber after filtering surgery (high peripheral anterior synechiae).

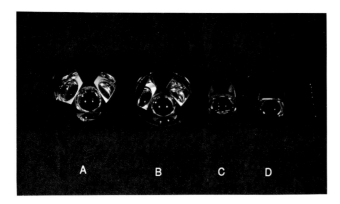

FIGURE 4-14. Goldmann gonioscopy. Goldmann-type gonios-copy lenses have a steeper posterior surface that requires the use of a coupling gel. Examples of different indirect Gold-mann-type lenses are shown here: (**A**) large three-mirror (one mirror for fundus periphery, one lens for midperipheral fundus examination, and one lens for gonioscopy); (**B**) small three-mirror; (**C**) two-mirror; and (**D**) one-mirror. (Reprinted with permission from BM Fisch. Gonioscopy and the Glaucomas. Boston: Butterworth–Heinemann, 1993;38.)

The Goldmann lens should be held with the thumb and middle finger, so that the index finger can be used to hold the face of the lens against the eye and the thumb and middle fingers can be repositioned to rotate the lens. A single-mirror Goldmann lens must be rotated 360 degrees to view the entire anterior chamber angle. After the entire angle has been examined, the lens suction seal is broken by gently pushing through the lid below the lens (see Figure 4-15C). Eye lavage is not necessary if an artificial tear solution is substituted for Goniosol.

ANGLE DOCUMENTATION AND ABNORMALITIES

Grading the anterior chamber and determining whether the patient is at risk for acute or chronic angle-closure glaucoma are important. The grading system that I use incorporates the structures of the angle viewed in addition to the amount of lens tilting or change in patient gaze required to view the angle anatomy (see Figure 4-11 and Table 4-1). The amount of pigmentation in the angle should also be graded. The majority of pigment will lie in the posterior two-thirds of the trabecular

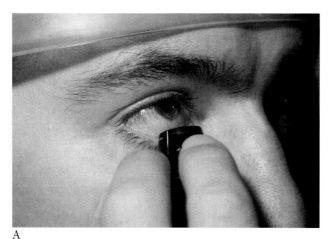

A

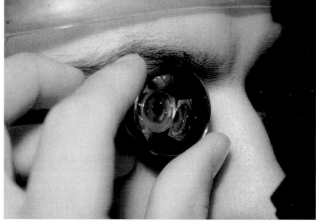

B

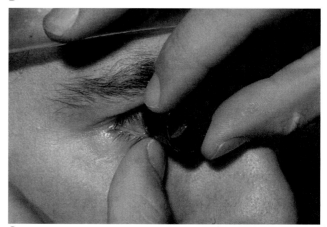

C

FIGURE 4-15. Goldmann gonioscopy procedure. (**A**) The patient is asked to look up, and the lens controls the lower lid. (**B**) The Goldmann three-mirror lens must be rotated 360 degrees to view the entire angle. (**C**) After the entire angle is viewed, gentle pressure is applied under the lower lid, and the suction seal is broken.

meshwork, which is the filtering portion of the meshwork, where aqueous drains into Schlemm's canal. Pigment may also be dispersed throughout the angle and is often present in greater quantities inferior in the angle because of gravitation. The pigment in the trabecular meshwork is graded from 0 to 4 (see Figure 4-1 and Color Plates 1 and 2). Zero or no pigmentation is a common finding and can make delineation of other angle structures more difficult. Any degree of trabecular meshwork pigmentation is helpful to establish other angle structures. Extensive pigmentation (grade 3 or 4) may be an indicator of pigment dispersion syndrome. The clinician should examine the iris for transillumination defects (see Color Plate 3) and the corneal endothelium for vertical deposition of pigment (Krukenberg's spindle). Pigment dispersion or excessive pigment in the trabecular meshwork is a risk factor for pigmentary glaucoma. Such patients who do not have glaucoma optic nerve damage should have their IOP routinely monitored every 6–12 months. IOP should also be checked after dilation and if the patient routinely participates in vigorous physical exercise, which may cause further pigment release and potential IOP spikes. Excessive pigmentation in the angle may also be a sign of exfoliation syndrome, previous trauma, or intraocular surgery.

Other angle abnormalities include adhesions of peripheral iris tissue into the trabecular meshwork (PAS). PAS must be differentiated from iris processes (see Figure 4-13). The latter are physiologic thin strands of iris tissue that extend from the iris surface into the trabecular meshwork. PAS are broader bands of iris adhesions and are usually acquired. They can be associated with chronic or recurrent iritis (see Color Plates 6 and 7), narrow angles, intraocular surgery, iris neovascularization, and other secondary angle-closure glaucomas (see Chapter 17). The location of PAS can be used to help determine the etiology. Superior PAS is commonly seen in patients with narrow angles because the superior angle is anatomically the narrowest. Superior PAS is frequently seen after cataract or filtering surgery if the incision was made at the 12 o'clock position. Inferior PAS is seen in patients with chronic or recurrent iritis. The inflammatory cells and released proteins gravitate and settle inferior to produce PAS. PAS above the trabecular meshwork is termed *high PAS* and is seen in patients with penetrating ocular injury and after flat anterior chamber in cataract or glaucoma filtering surgery (see Color Plates 8 and 9). High PAS is also observed in patients with iridocorneal endothelial syndrome (ICE) (see Chapter 17). PAS may also form in a patient who develops neovascularization of the anterior segment. In 90% of cases, the pupillary border is the initiation point for anterior segment neovascularization, which can grow across the iris surface, transverse the ciliary body and

scleral spur, and grow into the trabecular meshwork (see Color Plates 10 and 11). With the neovascular vessels grows fibrovascular tissue that can contract and pull the peripheral iris into the trabecular meshwork and form PAS.

It may take infiltration of one-half to three-fourths of the trabecular meshwork with angle vessels or PAS before an increase in IOP is detected. Furthermore, angle neovascularization without visible iris neovascular vessels may occur in 10% of cases of anterior segment neovascularization. Therefore, scrutiny of the angle with gonioscopy is required in all patients at risk for developing neovascular glaucoma, regardless of the iris status or tonometry reading. The etiology of anterior segment neovascularization is usually ischemic retinal disease (see Chapter 17). The most common causes are ischemic central retinal vein occlusion, proliferative diabetic retinopathy, and ocular ischemic syndrome (secondary to carotid artery disease). The treatment of iris or angle neovascularization is usually pan-retinal laser photocoagulation (PRP) of the ischemic retina. Aqueous suppressants may be used as adjunctive therapy to control IOP. Extensive PAS in the angle may require filtering surgery with antimetabolites or setons, or cycloablation procedures to the ciliary body to control elevated IOP.

One other angle abnormality to document is angle recession. This occurs from dehiscence of the longitudinal muscles from the circular muscles of the ciliary body. Angle recession may be localized or involve the entire 360 degrees of the angle (Figure 4-16). Comparing quadrants within the eye and between the two eyes is important. Anatomically, the inferior angle is larger than the superior angle, which tends to be the narrowest. Angle recession is evidence of prior trauma, but it does not necessarily mean that the patient will develop elevated IOP. Any sign or history of previous trauma (Table 4-2, and see Color Plates 12–14) may result in concurrent damage or dysfunction of the trabecular meshwork that may lead to a decrease in outflow and an increase in IOP. Clumps of pigment scattered throughout the angle are also a sign of prior trauma to the eye (see Color Plate 15). Elevated IOP can develop at any time after the traumatic event. Therefore, patients with evidence or history of previous trauma should be periodically monitored for IOP elevation and glaucoma development. Diagnosing traumatic glaucoma may also alter which medications or treatments are used. Pilocarpine and laser trabeculoplasty may be less effective in traumatic glaucoma (see Chapter 15). Blunt trauma may result in a separation of the ciliary body from the scleral spur (called a *cyclodialysis*), which may result in a drainage of aqueous into the suprachoroidal space with resultant hypotony (Figure 4-17).

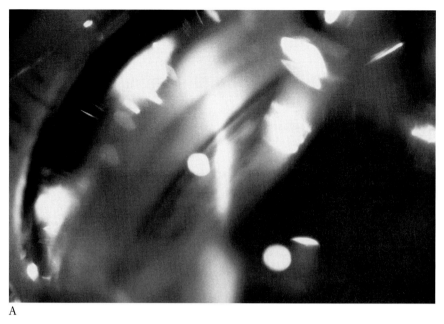

A

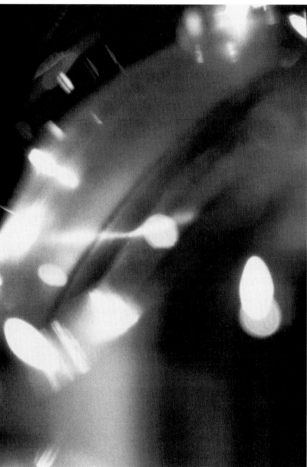

FIGURE 4-16. Three hundred sixty degrees of angle recession. Severe trauma can result in splitting of the ciliary muscle, causing an angle recession. It is often helpful to compare the degree of ciliary body band width between the two eyes. In this case, the patient's right eye has a normal ciliary body width (**A**) compared with the left eye, which has a much wider ciliary body band (**B**), indicating angle recession. Patients with angle recession have a greater risk of concurrent damage to the trabecular meshwork, resulting in an increase in intraocular pressure.

B

TABLE 4-2. Anterior Segment Signs of Trauma

Subconjunctival hemorrhage

Corneal scar or edema

Iritis

Hyphema

Iridodialysis

Sphincter tear of iris

Angle recession

Pigment clumping in the angle

Trabecular meshwork tear

Cyclodialysis

Asymmetric cataract or rosette cataract

Phakodonesis

Lens subluxation or dislocation

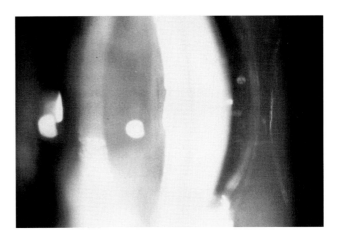

FIGURE 4-17. Cyclodialysis. Severe trauma can cause splitting of the ciliary body from the scleral spur, resulting in a cyclodialysis. Patients may exhibit hypotony because aqueous can drain into the suprachoroidal space.

SUMMARY

Gonioscopy is an essential test in the diagnostic work-up of any patient diagnosed with glaucoma, suspect for glaucoma, or having narrow anterior chamber angles. Gonioscopy allows the doctor to differentiate primary open-angle glaucoma from primary and secondary angle-closure glaucoma and secondary open-angle glaucoma. The type of glaucoma diagnosed should always be written in the patient's chart. The management and treatment plan should reflect the specific type of glaucoma diagnosed.

Clinicians should become adept at performing Zeiss four-mirror gonioscopy. The technique can be performed after applanation tonometry to improve technique and learn the physiologic variation of the anterior chamber angle. The angle structures that are visualized, the amount of lens tilting required to view the structures, and the contour of the iris help determine the angle grading system for gonioscopy. The amount of pigment in the trabecular meshwork should be graded. Angle abnormalities or negating abnormal findings (no PAS or angle recess) should also be recorded. Gonioscopy should be repeated once a year for all open-angle glaucoma patients and glaucoma suspects. It should be performed more frequently in patients with narrow angles or patients on chronic miotic therapy. Patients with chronic or recurrent iritis or patients at risk for anterior segment neovascularization should have gonioscopy performed at each follow-up visit.

Evaluation of the Optic Nerve

Anthony B. Litwak

Elevated intraocular pressure (IOP) is a risk factor for developing glaucomatous damage to the optic nerve. However, elevated IOP does not always cause glaucomatous damage, and some patients with a statistically normal IOP develop glaucoma. Thus, elevated IOP does not define glaucoma, and normal IOP does not exclude the diagnosis of glaucoma. Visual field loss should correlate with optic nerve damage, but 20–40% of the optic nerve's ganglion cell axons can be lost before reproducible visual field loss appears on automated white-on-white perimetry.[1] Thus, a normal visual field does not exclude the diagnosis of glaucoma. Glaucoma is a chronic progressive optic neuropathy, and therefore one of the most important tests to uncover glaucoma damage is the evaluation of the optic nerve.

The etiology of glaucomatous optic neuropathy is uncertain. Ganglion cell axons are dying at the level of the lamina cribrosa with retrograde atrophy back to their cell bodies in the retina. The laminar cribrosa is an important structure in the pathogenesis of glaucoma, because the axons must transverse the sieve-like openings to exit from the eye (Figures 5-1 and 5-2). Glaucomatous damage may be due to a variety or combination of inciting factors, including the following:

- Elevated IOP
- Ischemia or poor vascular perfusion pressure to the optic nerve
- Compression of ganglion cell axons
- Obstruction of axoplasmic flow within the ganglion cell axon
- Anatomic weakening of the lamina cribrosa

- Faulty connective tissue support in the lamina cribrosa
- Release of excitotoxins in the optic nerve
- Programmed cell death of the ganglion cell axons (apoptosis)[2,3]

Regardless of the etiology, glaucoma is a disease of the optic nerve. Glaucoma may be associated with certain risk factors (see Chapter 2), but none of these risk factors or combination of risk factors defines glaucoma.

ANATOMY

Ganglion cell axons make up 90% of the neuroretinal rim tissue of the optic disc. These axons come from receptor fields throughout the retina. They travel superficial in the retinal nerve fiber layer in a organized pattern (Figure 5-3). At the optic disc, they make a 90-degree turn and remain along the outer edge of the optic disc (Figure 5-4). The remaining constituents of the neuroretinal rim tissue include blood capillaries, glial cells, and astrocytes.[4] Capillary beds in the optic disc provide nutrition to the axons and give the neuroretinal rim tissue an orange-red appearance (Color Plate 17). Glial cells and astrocytes provide connective tissue support to the axons. The axons in the superior and inferior poles of the optic nerve have less structural support and may be more predisposed to glaucomatous damage (Figure 5-5).[5] These axons serve the nasal and arcuate visual fields, which are the site of initial visual field loss in most glaucoma patients.

The space in the center of the disc is often devoid of axons and capillaries and is called the *optic cup*.

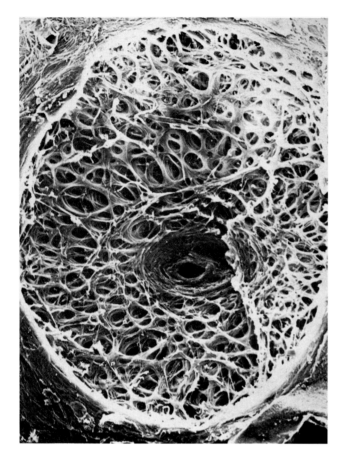

FIGURE 5-1. Photograph of the lamina cribrosa in which the ganglion cell axons have been dissolved away. Note the small pores where the ganglion cell axons transverse to exit the eye. One theory of glaucoma damage is poor structural support of the axons from faulty elastin structure of the lamina cribrosa. (Reprinted with permission from NR Miller. Walsh and Hoyt's Clinical Neuro-Ophthalmology [4th ed]. Baltimore: Williams & Wilkins, 1982;1:43.)

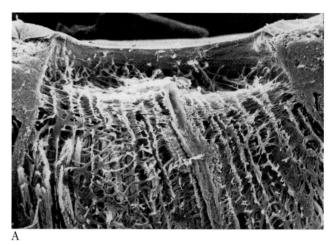

A

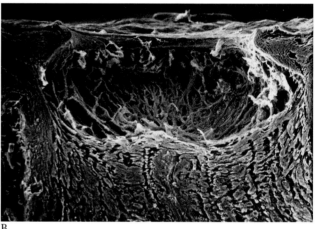

B

FIGURE 5-2. Cross section through the lamina cribrosa. (A) Normal patient without glaucoma. (B) Glaucoma patient showing bowing back of the lamina cribrosa. (Reprinted with permission from R Ritch, MB Shields, T Krupin. The Glaucomas [2nd ed]. St. Louis: Mosby, 1996;169.)

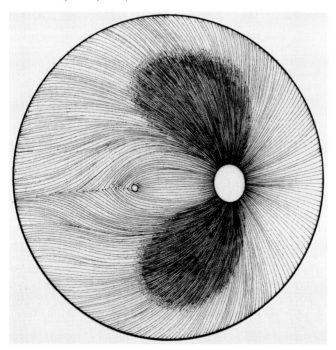

FIGURE 5-3. Pathway of the ganglion cell axons. Each ganglion cell body sends an axon across the retina to the optic nerve. These axon bundles (nerve fiber layer) travel in an organized arrangement. Axons from the temporal retina arc above and below the fovea to form the arcuate bundles. Axons from the macula travel in the papillomacular bundles. Axons in the nasal peripheral travel in the nasal bundles.

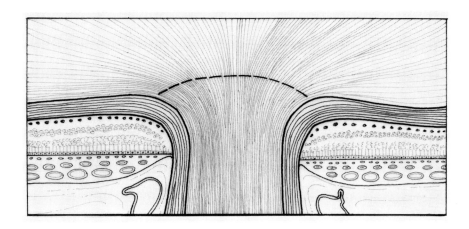

FIGURE 5-4. Neuroretinal rim tissue of the optic nerve. When the retinal ganglion cell axons reach the optic nerve, they make a 90-degree turn and remain along the outer edge of the optic disc to form the neuroretinal rim tissue. These axons must transverse the sieve-like lamina cribrosa to exit the eye. Glaucoma damage appears to occur at the level of the lamina cribrosa.

When present, the cup is pale in color because of visibility of the collagenous lamina cribrosa. Dots in the cup represent the fenestrations in the lamina cribrosa. These dots are not seen in all patients, but they may become more prominent with glaucoma damage. There is considerable physiologic variation in the size and appearance of the optic disc and cup that is often hereditary. The diameter of the scleral foramen can vary from approximately 1,000 to 3,000 μ.[6] A large scleral foramen results in a large physiologic disc that has more space to accommodate the ganglion cell axons and results in a large physiologic cup (Figure 5-6 and Color Plate 18). A smaller scleral foramen has a small disc and a small physiologic cup (Figure 5-7 and Color Plate 19). The number of ganglion cell axons can also vary in the normal optic nerve, with larger discs tending to have more axons than smaller discs.[6] These anatomic variations must be considered when the optic nerve is being evaluated.

In glaucoma, when ganglion cell axons are lost, there is a proportional loss of capillaries, thus maintaining an orange-red appearance in the remaining neuroretinal rim tissue. This is a feature unique to glaucoma. Other optic neuropathies, such as anterior ischemic optic neuropathy, optic neuritis, and compressive optic

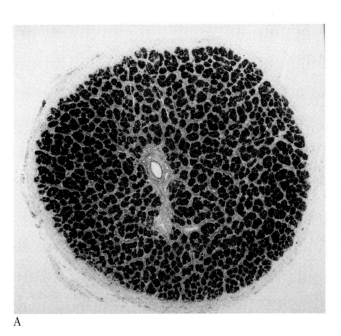

A

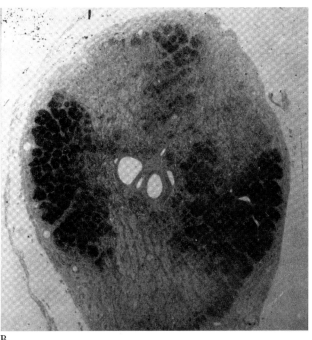

B

FIGURE 5-5. Cross section of the optic nerve in a healthy patient (**A**) and a patient with glaucoma (**B**). Healthy axons are staining dark. Note full complement of axons in healthy patient. In glaucoma, selective loss of axons occurs in the superior and inferior poles of the optic nerve with relative sparing of the temporal and nasal axons. (Reprinted with permission from NR Miller. Walsh and Hoyt's Clinical Neuro-Ophthalmology [4th ed]. Baltimore: Williams & Wilkins, 1982;1:330.)

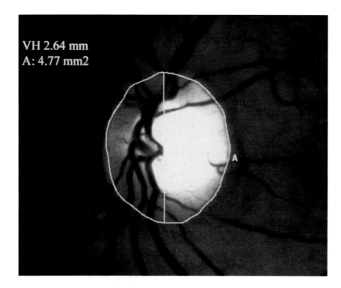

FIGURE 5-6. Large physiologic cup in large disc. When a Volk 60-D lens (Volk, Mentor, OH) was used at the slit lamp, the vertical height (VH) measured 2.9 mm in a patient with a cup-to-disc ratio of 0.8. Imagenet (Topcon, Paramus, NJ) showed a VH of 2.64 mm and a disc area (A) of 4.77 mm², which is more than 2 SD larger than the average-sized optic disc.

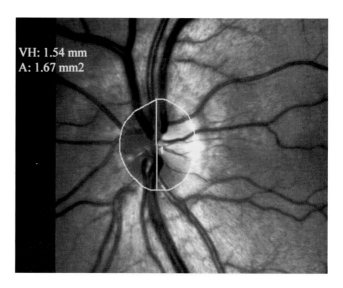

FIGURE 5-7. Small physiologic cup in a small disc. With a Volk 60-D lens (Volk, Mentor, OH) at the slit lamp, the vertical height (VH) measured 1.7 mm. Imagenet (Topcon, Paramus, NJ) showed a VH of 1.54 mm and a disc area (A) of 1.67 mm², which is 2 SD smaller than the average-sized optic disc.

neuropathies, usually cause pallor in the neuroretinal rim tissue. Pallor in the neuroretinal rim tissue should alert the clinician not to suspect glaucoma as the etiology of optic damage, even though the visual field loss may appear similar to that of glaucoma (Color Plate 23). One caveat: When the neuroretinal rim tissue becomes extremely thin in endstage glaucoma, the collagenous lamina cribrosa is more exposed, giving the appearance of rim pallor (Color Plate 22).

EXAMINATION TECHNIQUES

The most important step in the clinical optic nerve evaluation is to examine the optic disc in stereopsis through a dilated pupil. Monocular techniques, such as the direct ophthalmoscope, rely on color changes between the neuroretinal rim tissue and optic cup to estimate the cup-to-disc (C/D) ratio. This ratio represents fractional proportions of the optic cup size compared with the optic disc size. This method indirectly assesses the amount of neuroretinal rim tissue, which is mainly composed of ganglion cell axons. In glaucoma, saucerization of the optic disc can be present that extends beyond the color contour change of the optic cup. Observation of the color contour change rather than the topographic contour change results in erroneous underestimation of the optic cup (overestimation of the amount of neuroretinal rim tissue and underestimation of the degree of glaucoma damage) (Figure 5-8). Stereoscopic methods allow the examiner to evaluate the topographic contour of the

optic cup, which provides a more accurate assessment of the neuroretinal rim tissue. Careful inspection of the contour that the disc vessels transverse from the base of the cup to the edge of the disc also provides excellent topography clues to the remaining amount of rim tissue.

Several clinical techniques are available that provide stereoscopic examination of the optic nerve. Auxiliary lenses, such as a clear 78-, 66-, or 60-D lens, when used in conjunction with the biomicroscope, allow the clinician to obtain a magnified, stereoscopic view of the optic nerve (Figure 5-9). Patients tolerate the procedure very well because no direct eye contact is required; the condensing lens is held approximately 1–2 cm from the patient's eye. The only disadvantage to the technique is that the image viewed is reversed and inverted. The 78- and 66-D lenses also provide a wide enough field of view to allow the clinician to examine the entire posterior pole out to the equator. The 60-D lens provides more magnification but has the disadvantage of a smaller field of view. Depth of focusing is also more critical with the 60-D lens. A 90-D lens provides a wider field of view and is useful for posterior pole evaluation when pupillary dilation is poor. The lack of magnification makes it a less than optimal technique for optic disc evaluation. Most of the indirect biomicroscope condensing lenses come in either clear or yellow. Although the yellow-tinted lens may provide more patient comfort, the disadvantage of color artifact to the optic nerve (in judging disc pallor) and the inability to examine the retinal nerve fiber limits the usefulness of such lenses.

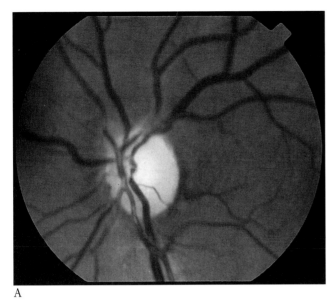
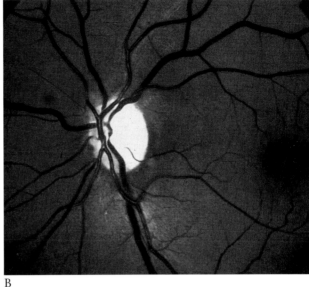

A   B

FIGURE 5-8. When monocular techniques, such as the direct ophthalmoscope, are used, it can be difficult to appreciate loss of neuroretinal rim tissue. In this patient, in two dimensions, there does not appear to be any significant cupping (**A**). However, close observation of the superior temporal rim tissue shows a deflection of the blood vessel right at the edge of the disc, indicating a notch. This is confirmed by the red-free photographs, which show severe nerve fiber layer loss in the superior arcades (**B**) and a dense inferior visual field defect (**C**) (*see next page*). This is one reason the optic nerve should always be evaluated in stereo.

Another technique for optic disc evaluation uses a Goldmann-type fundus contact lens (Haag-Streit, Berne, Switzerland) or the center of a Goldmann or Zeiss gonioscopy lens (Humphrey-Zeiss, Dublin, CA). This technique gives a true direct image of the optic nerve. The disadvantage of the Goldmann lenses is the use of a coupling gel and required direct eye contact. A viscous artificial tear preparation, such as Celluvisc or Ocucoat, used as a coupling medium reduces the incidence of corneal stippling when a Goldmann-type fundus contact lens or goniolens is used. The Hruby lens (–55 D) in conjunction with the biomicroscope also provides a direct, upright image of the optic nerve without direct eye contact. The disadvantages are a limited field of view and the requirement of good patient fixation.

HOW TO EVALUATE THE OPTIC NERVE

The purpose of the optic nerve evaluation is to assess the health of the ganglion cell axons. I recommend a systematic approach to examination of the optic nerve (Table 5-1).

Estimating the Physiologic Disc Size

There is considerable variation in the physiologic disc and cup size in the normal population.[6] African Americans have larger optic discs and larger optic cups than

whites.[7] The optic disc is also 2–3% larger in men than in women.[8] The first part of the optic nerve assessment is to evaluate the overall size of the disc to estimate the expected physiologic cup size. This can be accomplished by several techniques. One simple method estimates the number of arterial blood vessel widths that can be visualized across the horizontal surface of the optic disc. In a normal-sized disc, the number of blood vessel widths is approximately 10–12. A small physiologic disc will have

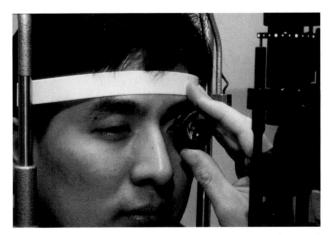

FIGURE 5-9. Using a 78-D lens at the slit lamp provides excellent magnification and stereoscopic viewing of the optic nerve. The procedure does not require direct eye contact. The image seen is inverted and reversed.

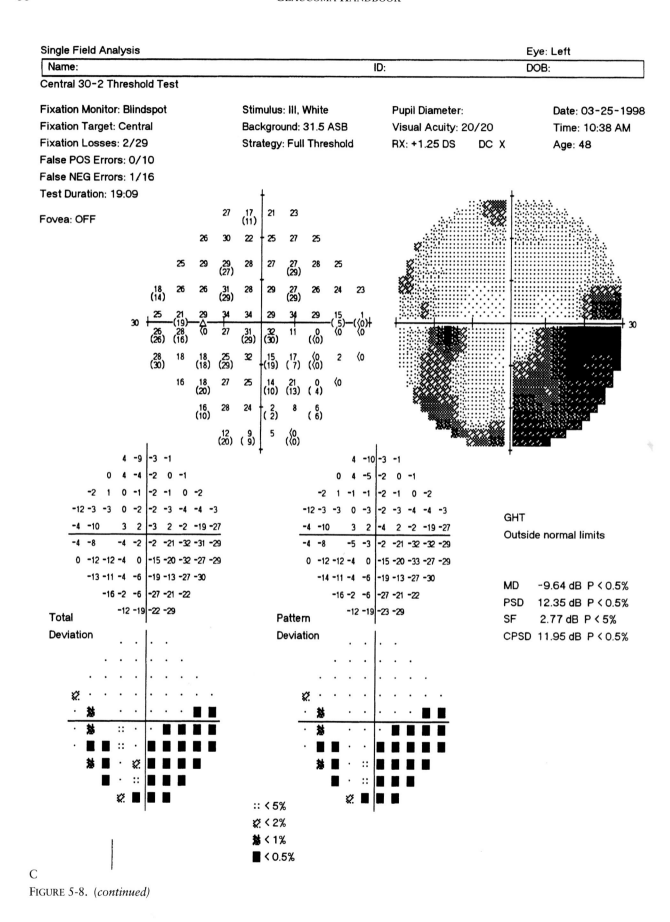

Single Field Analysis   Eye: Left

Name:	ID:	DOB:

Central 30-2 Threshold Test

Fixation Monitor: Blindspot   Stimulus: III, White   Pupil Diameter: Date: 03-25-1998
Fixation Target: Central   Background: 31.5 ASB   Visual Acuity: 20/20   Time: 10:38 AM
Fixation Losses: 2/29   Strategy: Full Threshold RX: +1.25 DS   DC X   Age: 48
False POS Errors: 0/10
False NEG Errors: 1/16
Test Duration: 19:09

Fovea: OFF

GHT
Outside normal limits

MD   -9.64 dB P < 0.5%
PSD   12.35 dB P < 0.5%
SF   2.77 dB P < 5%
CPSD 11.95 dB P < 0.5%

Total Deviation

Pattern Deviation

:: < 5%
✠ < 2%
▓ < 1%
■ < 0.5%

C

FIGURE 5-8. (continued)

TABLE 5-1. Optic Nerve Evaluation Checklist

Judge overall disc size (measure at the slit lamp with Volk 60-D lens [Volk, Mentor, OH])

Evaluate vertical cup-to-disc ratio in stereo (look at disc vessel topography rather than color changes)

  Compare with expected cup-to-disc ratio based on the vertical disc diameter (see Figure 5-10)

Evaluate for notches or thinning in the superior or inferior neural-retinal rim tissue

  Judge symmetry of neural rim tissue (superior versus inferior and between the two eyes)

  Compare rim tissue in the superior and inferior poles to the temporal rim tissue (should be greater in the superior and inferior poles than in the temporal pole) (see Figure 5-11)

Evaluate for acquired pits of the optic nerve within the cup

Evaluate for peripapillary atrophy

Evaluate for disc hemorrhage

Evaluate retinal nerve fiber layer (see Chapter 6)

---

fewer than 10, and a large disc will have more than 12. Another technique for estimating the overall disc size is to project a measuring target into the eye. This can be accomplished by using the circle target on the direct ophthalmoscope. The technique that I most frequently use requires a 60-D lens at the slit lamp. A thin vertical beam of light is directed at the optic nerve, and the vertical diameter length is adjusted at the slit lamp (Figure 5-10). After the beam length coincides with the superior and inferior edge of the optic disc, the measurement can be read from the slit lamp scale in millimeters. The values measured from the slit lamp do not represent the actual size of the optic disc, but they do approximate the relative size of the disc.[9] From these data, a normative database of relative physiologic disc sizes can be developed. In our patient population, using a Volk 60-D lens (Volk, Mentor, OH) with a Haag-Streit slit lamp, (Haag-Streit, Berne, Switzerland) the average vertical disc diameter is 2.0 mm. Ranges of 1 and 2 SD with the expected physiologic C/D ratios are listed in Figure 5-10B. It is important to remember that vertical height measurements vary depending on the manufacturer of the indirect lens, the power of the indirect lens, and the type of slit lamp used.

A large physiologic cup should be expected in a patient with a large disc (more than 1 SD from normal), and likewise a small physiologic cup should be expected in a small disc (less than 1 SD from normal) (see Color Plates 18 and 19). It should not be surprising to observe a C/D ratio of .7 or greater in a patient with a optic disc that is more than 2 SD from normal. A medium-sized cup in a small physiologic disc should arouse the same suspicion for glaucoma as a large cup in a normal-sized

disc (see Figure 5-10C and Table 5-2). A more sophisticated method of measuring physiologic disc size uses a digital imaging system (Imagenet Topcon, Paramus, NJ) (see Figures 5-6 and 5-7) or scanning laser ophthalmoscope (Topographic Scanning System [TOPSS]; Laser Diagnostic Technologies, San Diego, CA) and Heidelberg Retinal Tomograph (Heidelberg Engineering, Heidelberg, Germany), which allow both disc diameter and disc area measurements.

Judging Neuroretinal Rim Tissue and Cup-to-Disc Ratios

Next, using a stereoscopic technique (78- or 66-D lens at the slit lamp) with a dilated pupil, I assess the amount of neuroretinal rim tissue and judge the vertical C/D ratio. The grading of the C/D ratio suffers from poor interobserver variability,[10] which stems from different interpretations of where the neuroretinal rim tissue ends and where the optic cup begins and also from differences in the clinical instrumentation (monocular versus binocular) used. An experienced clinician using a stereoscopic technique greatly improves the intraobserver variability in assessing the C/D ratio. I judge the C/D ratio by looking at the first point of deflection of the disc vessels from the neural rim bending towards the optic cup. I record the vertical C/D ratio and compare it with the horizontal C/D ratio, because glaucoma preferentially damages ganglion cell axons in the superior and inferior poles of the optic nerve. I also record whether the slope of the optic cup is gentle or steep.

Loss of Rim Tissue and Notching of the Optic Nerve

Glaucoma damage typically causes a concentric enlargement of the C/D ratio from loss of ganglion cell axons in the neuroretinal rim tissue. However, there is a greater preference for damage to the axons in the superior and inferior poles of the optic nerve with relative sparing of the temporal and nasal axons. This results in a vertical elongation of the optic cup. Asymmetry of the neuroretinal rim tissue within the eye (comparison of superior to inferior rim tissue) and between the two eyes is one of the best clinical clues to diagnosing glaucoma damage.

When I examine the optic nerve, I evaluate the amount of neuroretinal rim tissue in the superior and inferior poles of the optic disc compared with the temporal pole (Figure 5-11). In general, the vertical poles of the disc should contain 1.5–2.0 times more neural rim tissue than the temporal pole (see Color Plates 17 and 18). The superior and inferior rim tissue should be symmetric, although slightly more ganglion cell axons are present in the inferior retina. In glaucoma, there is often selective damage to the ganglion cell axons in

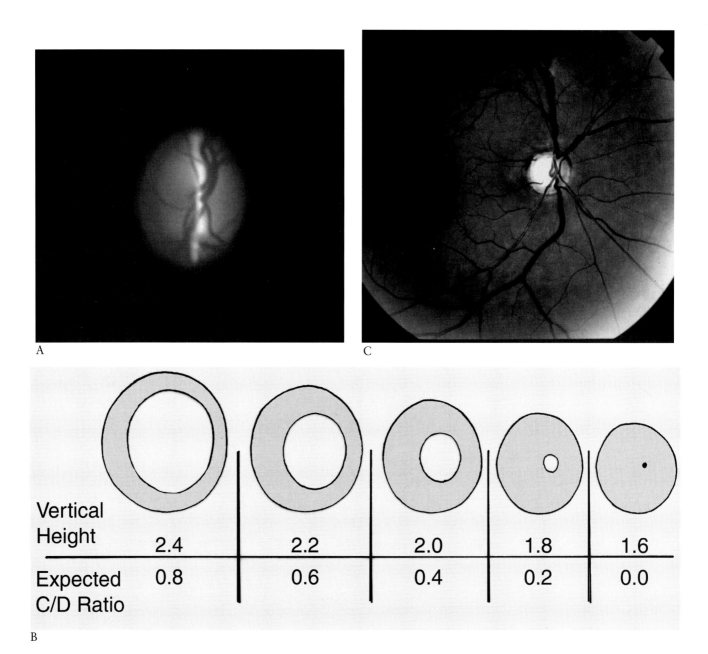

FIGURE 5-10. Measuring vertical height and estimating expected cup-to-disc (C/D) ratio. (A) Using a 60-D Volk lens (Volk, Mentor, OH) at the slit lamp, the clinician can estimate the vertical diameter of the optic disc by adjusting the length of the vertical streak with the superior and inferior borders of the disc and reading the number from the slit-lamp scale. (B) After estimating the vertical height, the clinician can predict the physiologic C/D ratio, because the size of the cup is related to the physiologic disc size. With a smaller disc, a small cup should be expected, and with a large disc, a large cup. (C) This patient has a C/D ratio of 0.7, but the vertical disc height is only 1.7 mm. A medium cup in a small disc should raise the suspicion for glaucoma. Note thinner rim tissue superior compared with inferior. This patient had glaucomatous visual field loss.

TABLE 5-2. Suspicion of Glaucoma Based on Cup and Disc Size

Cup size	Small disc	Medium disc	Large disc
Small	Expected	Normal	Normal
Medium	Abnormal	Expected	Normal
Large	Abnormal	Abnormal	Expected*

*Although a large cup should be expected in a patient with a large disc, glaucoma can be present in a large disc.

one or both vertical poles of the optic nerve, and relative preservation of the temporal and nasal axons. Therefore, when the amount of neuroretinal rim tissue in the temporal portion of the disc appears equal to or greater than that in the vertical poles, glaucoma damage should be suspected (see Figure 5-11B and Color Plate 20). With further focal damage, a notch of the neuroretinal rim tissue can be observed. Notches are defined as local areas of ganglion cell axons loss resulting in little or no remaining rim tissue in a focal area of the optic nerve (see Figure 5-11C and Color Plate 21). In glaucoma, notches are most typically observed in the superior temporal or inferior temporal neuroretinal rim tissue. An inferior notch is three times more common than a superior notch. Notches are usually pathognomonic of glaucoma damage and are associated with a corresponding visual field defect. They are a common sign of optic nerve damage and occur in approximately 30% of glaucoma patients.

With further glaucoma damage and loss of neuroretinal rim tissue, concurrent lateral and posterior disc excavation can occur. This results in bean potting of the optic nerve, in which retinal blood vessels disappear as they follow the lateral excavation of the optic cup and reappear at the base of the cup. This is a sign of endstage disease (see Color Plate 22).

Cup-to-Disc Asymmetry

Glaucoma may asymmetrically damage the inferior and superior poles of the optic nerve. Likewise, asymmetry in the C/D ratio or focal thinning of neuroretinal rim tissue between the two eyes can also be used to diagnose glaucoma damage (Color Plate 27). One caveat: Asymmetry in the C/D ratio may be the result of asymmetric optic nerve sizes (Figure 5-12). The best way to observe this phenomenon is to measure the vertical heights of the optic disc with a 60-D lens at the slit lamp. This measurement can be compared between the two eyes. Patients with asymmetric disc sizes will also probably have asymmetric physiologic cup sizes. If the patient has C/D asymmetry with similar disc sizes and the damage appears confined to one eye, the practitioner should investigate a secondary glaucoma (e.g., traumatic) as a possible etiology. However, many primary open-angle glaucoma patients exhibit asymmetric optic nerve damage. Typically, the eye with the greater damage shows a consistently higher IOP than the fellow

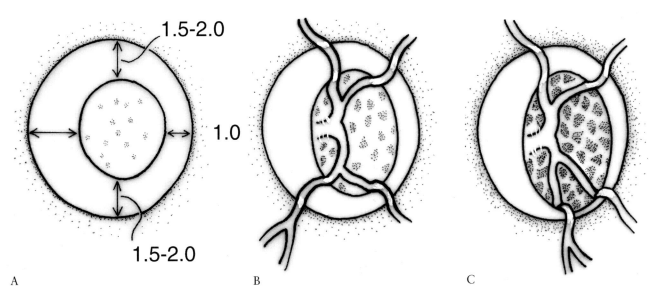

FIGURE 5-11. Patterns of optic nerve damage in glaucoma. (**A**) The amount of neuroretinal rim tissue in a normal optic nerve is generally 1.5–2.0 times greater in the superior and inferior poles of the optic disc than in the temporal pole. (**B**) In glaucoma, loss of neuroretinal rim tissue occurs, with a preference for the superior and inferior rim tissue. Here the inferior rim is slightly thinner than the superior rim. Also, the temporal rim tissue is now equal to or greater than the superior and inferior rim tissue, suggesting relative loss in the vertical poles from glaucoma damage. (**C**) With continued loss in one pole of the optic nerve, a notch of the neuroretinal rim tissue can occur. This example shows a notch in the inferior temporal portion of the optic nerve.

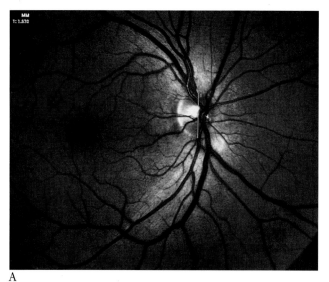
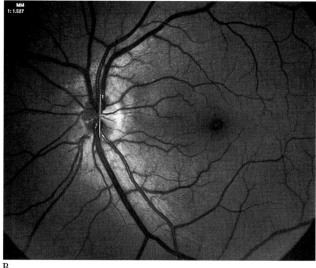

A   B

FIGURE 5-12. Asymmetric cup size secondary to asymmetric disc size. Patient is noted to have cup-to-disc asymmetry between the two eyes. However, measuring the vertical height of the optic nerve showed a larger physiologic disc in the right eye (**A**) than left (**B**). The right eye has a larger cup. In this case, the cup-to-disc asymmetry is physiologic and not secondary to glaucoma. Note intact nerve fiber layer in both eyes.

eye. When one eye has definite glaucoma, the fellow eye should be evaluated closely for subtle signs of glaucoma damage regardless of the IOP level.

Acquired Pits of the Optic Nerve

After assessing the neuroretinal rim tissue, I look carefully at the base of the optic cup. I judge the visibility of laminar dots and scrutinize for acquired pits of the optic nerve (APON). Laminar dots represent pores in the laminar cribrosa that allow the ganglion cell axons to exit the eye. They are not seen in all patients, but they can increase in size and number with progressive glaucoma damage. APON represent focal, discrete areas of depression or excavation within the lamina cribrosa. They signify focal areas of structural weakening of the lamina, usually in the superior or inferior poles of the optic cup[11] (Color Plate 24). The laminar dots are more pronounced in the area of the APON. APON is a subtle finding that is easily overlooked, but it is estimated to occur in approximately 20% of glaucoma patients.[12] The etiology may be ischemic, compressive, or genetic structural weakening of the laminar cribrosa. APON are often associated with focal visual field defects that are close to fixation or involve fixation and tend to be progressive.[13] They are more common in patients with normal-tension glaucoma than in those with high-tension glaucoma and tend to be unilateral.[13] APON should be differentiated from congenital optic pits, because the latter represents nonacquired focal coloboma of the optic nerve, which usually appears light to dark grey in color, and the absence of laminar dots (Color Plate 25). Congenital optic pits are not associated with glaucoma, although they may produce visual field defects typical of glaucoma damage. Congenital pits can be associated with serous macular detachment.

Peripapillary Atrophy

Next I evaluate the peripapillary area for evidence of atrophy or disc hemorrhages. Peripapillary atrophy is a nonspecific finding, but it has been associated with acquired damaged to the optic nerves from glaucoma.[14–16] The clinical appearance is a ratty or moth-eaten appearance to the retinal pigment epithelium, usually along the temporal aspect of the optic disc, and it corresponds to an area of neuroretinal rim thinning (Figure 5-13; see Color Plate 24). It also is seen more commonly in patients with normal-tension than high-tension glaucoma.[17–20] The exact etiology of this sign in glaucoma is unknown. The specificity for glaucoma is poor because this change is frequently observed as a physiologically aging change.

Disc Hemorrhage

Disc hemorrhage as an indicator of glaucoma damage (Drance hemorrhage) was first described by Stephen Drance in 1970.[21] These hemorrhages occur most frequently in the inferior pole of the optic nerve, followed by the superior pole and then the temporal pole. They are usually located on the optic disc or in the peripapillary area within 1 disc diameter of the optic nerve (Color

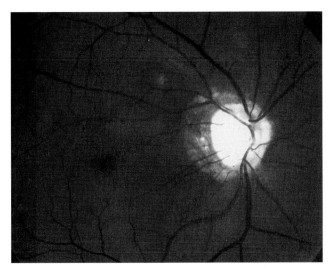

FIGURE 5-13. Peripapillary atrophy. Peripapillary atrophy can be an associated sign of glaucoma damage. It usually occurs along the edge of the disc, corresponding to thinning of the neuroretinal rim tissue. This glaucoma patient has extensive peripapillary atrophy along the entire temporal aspect of the disc. Note also the severe nerve fiber layer loss. Peripapillary atrophy is not specific for glaucoma and may be seen as a senile aging change.

months.[22] They are also more frequently observed in patients with normal-tension glaucoma. Disc hemorrhages can be an early sign of glaucoma damage and frequently precede visual field or nerve fiber layer loss (Figure 5-14). They can also indicate progressing glaucoma that is not adequately treated, or they may be an indication of poor compliance with medications. The appearance of a disc hemorrhage in a glaucoma suspect should give strong consideration for antiglaucoma therapy.[22] A disc hemorrhage in an established glaucoma patient warrants a re-evaluation of the treatment plan (lower target pressure) and suggests the possibility of patient noncompliance. Disc hemorrhages are not specific for glaucoma and can be seen after a posterior vitreous detachment in which a disc vessel was mechanically disrupted at the time of the posterior vitreous detachment and bled. It can be differentiated from retinal vasculopathies, such as diabetes or hypertension, because of the absence of retinopathy elsewhere in the posterior pole. Resolving hemorrhage after a venous occlusive event or peripapillary choroidal neovascular membrane can also mimic a Drance hemorrhage. When an isolated disc hemorrhage occurs in the superior temporal or inferior temporal peripapillary area without cause, then glaucoma diagnosis or progression should be considered as a possible etiology.

Stereoscopic Optic Nerve Photographs

Glaucoma is a chronic progressive disease of the ganglion cell axons. The best documentation of the optic nerve status is obtained by a set of stereoscopic disc photographs. It is extremely important to have baseline

Plate 26). They tend to be flame shaped when located superficial in the retinal nerve fiber layer. Disc hemorrhages located on the optic disc appear more blotlike. Disc hemorrhages occur in approximately 10% of glaucoma patients, but their number may be underestimated because they can resolve over a period of a few weeks or

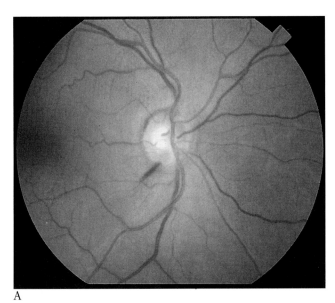

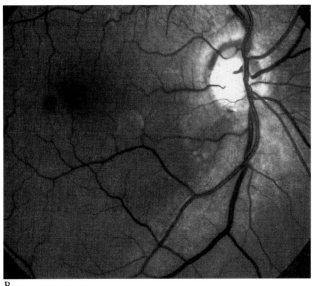

A   B

FIGURE 5-14. (A) Flame hemorrhage just inferior to the right optic nerve in a glaucoma suspect. (B) Six weeks later the hemorrhage is resolving, but the nerve fiber layer photograph shows an inferior wedge defect, and the patient developed a new corresponding visual field defect (C) (*see next page*).

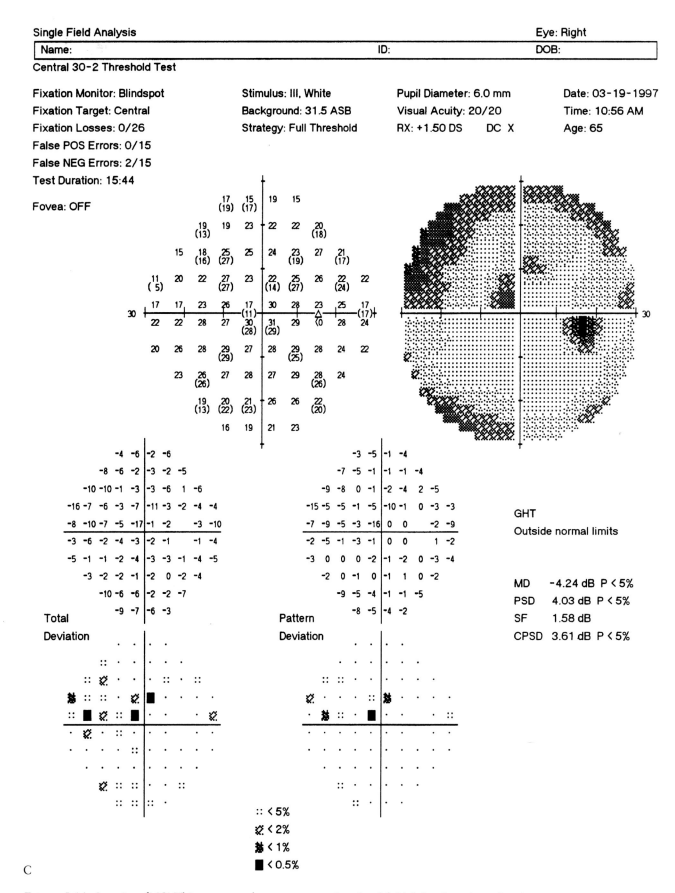

Single Field Analysis Eye: Right

| Name: | ID: | DOB: |

Central 30-2 Threshold Test

Fixation Monitor: Blindspot Stimulus: III, White Pupil Diameter: 6.0 mm Date: 03-19-1997
Fixation Target: Central Background: 31.5 ASB Visual Acuity: 20/20 Time: 10:56 AM
Fixation Losses: 0/26 Strategy: Full Threshold RX: +1.50 DS DC X Age: 65
False POS Errors: 0/15
False NEG Errors: 2/15
Test Duration: 15:44

Fovea: OFF

GHT
Outside normal limits

MD   -4.24 dB P < 5%
PSD   4.03 dB P < 5%
SF   1.58 dB
CPSD 3.61 dB P < 5%

Total Deviation

Pattern Deviation

:: < 5%
▨ < 2%
▩ < 1%
■ < 0.5%

C

FIGURE 5-14. (*continued*) (C) This corresponds to a new superior visual field defect just above fixation.

photographs for all glaucoma and glaucoma-suspect patients that can be used for future comparisons. When comparing disc photographs, looking for thinning of rim tissue and shifting of disc vessels as clues of glaucoma damage is important (Color Plate 28). These structural changes can often precede visual field loss in patients in whom a diagnosis of glaucoma is suspected. Progressive loss of neuroretinal rim tissue documented by serial photographs (increase in C/D ratio) is objective evidence of glaucoma damage. Established glaucoma patients can be followed with serial disc photographs in addition to serial visual fields to judge progression. Disc photographs are usually repeated every 2 years, sooner if progression is suspected.

REFERENCES

1. Quigley HA, Dunkelberger GR, Green WR. Retinal ganglion cell atrophy correlated with automated perimetry in human eyes with glaucoma. Am J Ophthalmol 1989;107:453–464.

2. Kerrigan LA, Zack DJ, Quigley HA, et al. TUNEL-positive ganglion cells in human primary open-angle glaucoma. Arch Ophthalmol 1997;115:1031–1035.

3. Quigley HA. Neuronal death in glaucoma. Prog Retin Eye Res Jan 1999;18:39–57.

4. Minckler DS. The organization of nerve fiber bundles in the primate optic nerve head. Arch Ophthalmol 1980;98:1630–1636.

5. Quigley HA, Addicks EM, Green WR, Maumenee AE. Optic nerve damage in human glaucoma. II. The site of injury and susceptibility to damage. Arch Ophthalmol 1981;99:635–649.

6. Jonas JB, Gusek GC, Guggenmoos-Holzmann I, Naumann GO. Variability of the real dimensions of normal human optic discs. Graefe's Arch Clin Exp Ophthalmol 1988;226:332–336.

7. Quigley HA, Brown AE, Morrison JD, Drance SM. The size and shape of the optic disc in normal human eyes. Arch Ophthalmol 1990;108:51–57.

8. Varma R, Tielsch JM, Quigley HA, et al. Race-, age-, gender-, and refractive error-related differences in the normal optic disc. Arch Ophthalmol 1994; 112:1068–1076.

9. Hancox MD. Optic disc size, an important consideration in the glaucoma evaluation. Clin Eye Vis Care 1999;11:59–62.

10. Varma R, Steinmann WC, Scott IU. Expert agreement in evaluating the optic disc for glaucoma. Ophthalmology 1992;99:215–221.

11. Stutman RS. Acquired pits of the optic nerve in glaucoma. Clin Eye Vis Care 1996;8:215–223.

12. Javitt JC, Spaeth GL, Katz J, et al. Acquired pits of the optic nerve. Increased prevalence in patients with low-tension glaucoma. Ophthalmology 1990;97: 1038–1044.

13. Cashwell LF, Ford JG. Central visual field changes associated with acquired pits of the optic nerve. Ophthalmology 1995;102:1270–1278.

14. Primrose J. Early signs of the glaucomatous disc. Br J Ophthalmol 1971;55:820–825.

15. Jonas JB, Nguyen XN, Gusek GC, Naumann GO. Parapapillary chorioretinal atrophy in normal and glaucoma eyes. I. Morphometric data. Invest Ophthalmol Vis Sci 1989;30:908–918.

16. Honrubia F, Calonge B. Evaluation of the nerve fiber layer and peripapillary atrophy in ocular hypertension. Int Ophthalmol 1989;13:57–62.

17. Primrose J. The incidence of the peripapillary halo glaucomatosus. Trans Ophthalmol Soc UK 1969;89:585–587.

18. Wilensky JT, Kolker AE. Peripapillary changes in glaucoma. Am J Ophthalmol 1976;81: 341–345.

19. Caprioli J, Spaeth GL. Comparison of visual field defects in low-tension glaucoma. Am J Ophthalmol 1984;97:730–737.

20. Buss DR, Anderson DR. Peripapillary crescents and halos in normal-tension glaucoma and ocular hypertension. Ophthalmology 1989;96:16–19.

21. Drance SM, Begg IS. Sector hemorrhage: a probable acute ischaemic disc change in chronic simple glaucoma. Can J Ophthalmol 1970;5:137–141.

22. Drance SM. Disc hemorrhages in the glaucomas. Surv Ophthalmol 1989;33:331–337.

Evaluation of the Retinal Nerve Fiber Layer

Anthony B. Litwak

Glaucoma is a chronic, progressive optic neuropathy. More specifically, glaucoma is a disease of the ganglion cell axons. The neuroretinal rim tissue of the optic nerve is primarily composed of ganglion cell axons. When ganglion cell axons die, a corresponding loss of neuroretinal rim tissue (or an increase in cup-to-disc ratio) eventually occurs. When more axons die, a corresponding visual field defect results. It is estimated that glaucoma patients lose 20–50% of their ganglion cell axons (because of the overlap of ganglion receptor fields) before they develop a reproducible visual field defect.[1,2] Automated perimetry is also a subjective test, and some patients are unable to reliably perform the test. Therefore, an objective diagnostic test that would uncover glaucoma damage at an earlier stage in the disease process (before visual field loss occurs) would be useful.

Evaluation of the retinal nerve fiber layer (NFL) is one method of assessing the health of the ganglion cell axons before they reach the optic nerve. Defects in the NFL may precede glaucomatous visual field loss and structural changes to the optic nerve.[3] The NFL evaluation can also be used to confirm visual field loss and can differentiate large physiologic cupping from glaucoma.[4] The technique is easy to learn and does not require expensive equipment. However, differentiating the physiologic variation of the normal NFL from early NFL loss does require some degree of experience.

ANATOMY OF THE NERVE FIBER LAYER

The retina contains approximately 1.0–1.5 million ganglion cell bodies. Each cell body sends an axon across the retina in the NFL toward the optic disc (Figure 6-1). The NFL lies superficial in the retina, just beneath the internal limiting membrane. The fibers travel in an organized pattern in which axons originating in the temporal periphery arc either above or below the macula in the retinal arcades and form the superior and inferior neuroretinal rim tissue of the optic nerve (Figure 6-2).[5] Fibers originating in the nasal retina insert into the nasal optic disc, and fibers originating in the macula insert into the temporal optic disc (papillomacular bundle). Because of this anatomic arrangement, the NFL is thickest and therefore clinically brightest in the superior and inferior arcades, and thinner or less bright in the papillomacular and nasal bundles.[6] This anatomic arrangement gives the normal NFL a characteristic bright-dimmer-bright pattern (Figure 6-3; see Figure 6-1).

CLINICAL NERVE FIBER LAYER EXAMINATION

The clinical examination of the NFL requires a bright light source and a red-free filter. The direct ophthalmoscope provides both, but it does not allow stereoscopic view of the optic nerve. I prefer to use the clear (non-yellow) 78-diopter (D) lens in conjunction with the biomicroscope, a technique that provides stereoscopic evaluation of the optic nerve head (see Chapter 5). After the optic nerve is examined, the light source on the biomicroscope should be turned up to the highest setting (this is very important), and the red-free filter should be flipped in to evaluate the NFL. The green light produced by the red-free filter is absorbed by the pigment in the retinal pigment epithelium and choroid, which will create a dark background to

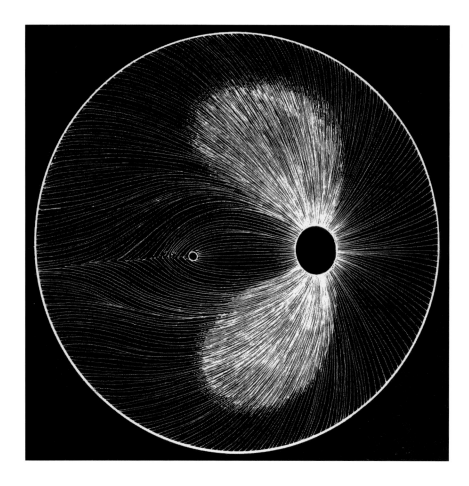

FIGURE 6-1. Pathway of the ganglion cell axons. Each ganglion cell body sends an axon across the retina to the optic nerve. These axon bundles (nerve fiber layer) travel in an organized arrangement. Axons from the temporal retina arc above and below the fovea to form the arcuate bundles. These axons become the superior and inferior neuroretinal rim tissue of the optic nerve. Axons from the macula travel in the papillomacular bundles and insert in the temporal optic nerve. Axons in the nasal peripheral travel in the nasal bundles and insert into the nasal optic nerve. Note that the nerve fiber layer is thicker and clinically brighter in the arcuate bundles than in the papillomacular and nasal bundles.

highlight the NFL. The NFL will reflect light and will be contrasted against the dark background from the pigmented posterior layers of the retina. Focus should be maintained on the superficial layers of the retina.

NORMAL NERVE FIBER LAYER

The normal NFL has a bright, linear, striated appearance with a course, fulminant texture. The NFL casts a white haze over the underlying retinal structures and obscures the smaller tertiary retinal blood vessels (Figure 6-4; see Figure 6-3). The brightness of the striations is dependent on the integrity of the NFL bundles (thickness), the amount of pigmentation in the retinal pigment epithelium and choroid, and the media clarity. The NFL is most prominent in the superior and inferior arcuate bundles and less bright in the papillomacular and nasal bundles. This gives the normal NFL a characteristic bright-dimmer-bright pattern corresponding to the superior arcuate–papillomacular–inferior arcuate

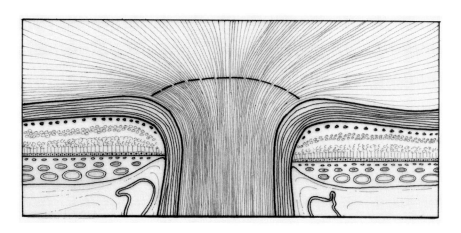

FIGURE 6-2. Neuroretinal rim tissue of the optic nerve. When the retinal ganglion cell axons reach the optic nerve, they make a 90-degree turn and remain along the outer edge of the optic disc to form the neuroretinal rim tissue.

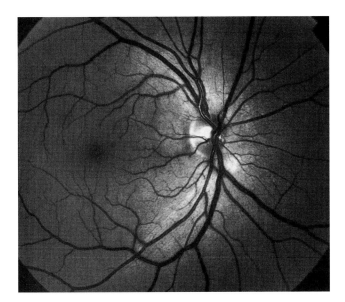

FIGURE 6-3. Normal clinical appearance of the nerve fiber layer. Note brighter silvery striations in the superior and inferior arcuate bundles and less brightness in the papillomacular and nasal bundles. This characteristic normal appearance of the nerve fiber layer occurs because more fibers travel in the arcuate bundles than in the papillomacular and nasal bundles. The thickness of the bundles is directly related to their brightness. Note also that the brightness diminishes farther from the optic nerve.

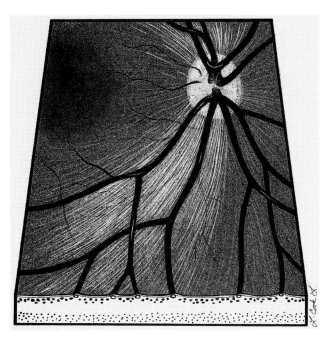

FIGURE 6-4. Artist's drawing of the normal nerve fiber layer. The normal nerve fiber layer consists of bright striations in the superficial layers of the retina that cast a white haze over the underlying retina, obscuring the smaller tertiary retinal blood vessels. The texture of the nerve fiber layer within a disc diameter of the optic nerve is more compact and fulminant because of the abundance of fibers plying up, one on top of each other.

bundles (see Figures 6-1 and 6-3). The brightness pattern should be fairly symmetric between the superior and inferior arcades and also between the two eyes. The NFL becomes dimmer farther away from the disc, and brighter approaching the disc. I recommend examining the NFL within 1–2 disc diameters from the optic nerve in the area between and including the arcuate bundles (5 o'clock to 1 o'clock in the right eye, and 11 o'clock to 7 o'clock in the left eye). It is not necessary to examine the NFL in the nasal bundles in glaucoma.

The first step in learning to evaluate the NFL is to become familiar with the normal physiologic appearance of the NFL in different age and ethnic groups. The NFL will be most prominent in young patients with clear media and heavy fundus pigmentation. Heavy pigmentation in the retinal pigment epithelium and choroid creates a dark background against which light reflected off the NFL is contrasted. In patients with a blonde fundus, the NFL will not be as bright, and it may not be visible at all if very little fundus pigmentation is present (Figure 6-5). Humans naturally lose approximately 2,500 ganglion cell axons per year, so over a lifetime each of us loses 10–20% of our allotted NFL. Thus, the NFL in an older patient will not be as bright as in a younger patient. Finally, media opacification, such as cataract, reduces the amount of reflected light off the NFL and blurs the clarity of the NFL striations. The clinician must take these factors into account when evaluating the NFL and

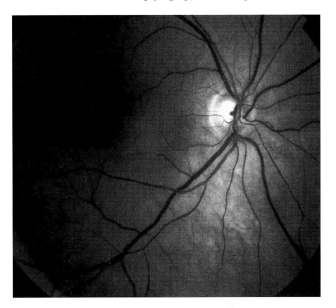

FIGURE 6-5. Poor visibility of the nerve fiber layer in a blonde fundus. This patient has less pigmentation in the retinal pigment epithelium and choroid, which allows for visibility of choroidal blood vessels, especially inferior to the optic nerve. The lack of pigmentation does not create a dark background to contrast with the reflections from the striations, resulting in poor visibility of the nerve fiber layer inferior compared with superior. This lack of visibility is the result of a blonde fundus and not caused by nerve fiber layer loss.

should examine the structure in all patients to become familiar with the presentations of the normal NFL.[7]

NERVE FIBER LAYER PHOTOGRAPHY

The NFL can also be evaluated by inspection of high-quality black-and-white photographs. Photographs are easier to evaluate than the clinical examination because they can be easily studied without eye movements or patient blinking. Comparisons between the superior and inferior arcades and between the two eyes are more assessable with high-quality photographs. Serial NFL photographs can also be taken to determine progressive NFL loss. However, proper equipment, film, and focus are required to produce photographs adequate for evaluation. The preferred photographic technique is to use 35-mm Technical Pan film (ASA 25) (Eastman Kodak, Rochester, NY), a short pass 560-nm cut-off filter (or red-free filter), and a high-quality 35-mm fundus camera.[8] Flash settings or the developing process may need to be bracketed, depending on media clarity, NFL brightness, and fundus pigmentation. For the Topcon TRC 50 V fundus camera (Imagenet Topcon, Paramus, NJ), I use a flash setting of 150 mW. The film is developed in an HC 110 developer dilution B for 8 minutes at 68°F. Contact printing or Kodalith film (Eastman Kodak, Rochester, NY) is used to convert the negative slide into a positive print or slide. I prefer a 35-degree field of view centered vertically at the optic nerve and just temporal to the optic nerve to highlight the arcuate bundles. Others prefer a 20-degree field focused each on the superior and inferior arcades just off the optic disc. This technique requires four photographs instead of just two.

Digital imaging systems are ideal for NFL documentation and provide instant images viewed on a monitor (without film) that can be reviewed for flash intensity and focus and stored and recalled from an optical disc or CD-ROM storage media. Inspection of high-quality photographs or images is the easiest way for novice observers to become familiar with the NFL evaluation; however, direct clinical evaluation is more convenient and avoids the time and cost of producing high-quality photographs. Quigley's manual, *Diagnosing Early Glaucoma with Nerve Fiber Layer Examination*, contains 100 test NFL photographs that can be graded and then compared with an experienced clinician's classification to improve interpretation skills.[9]

NERVE FIBER LAYER DEFECTS IN GLAUCOMA

In glaucoma, ganglion cell axons are damaged at the level of the lamina cribrosa with retrograde atrophy back to the ganglion cell body in the retina. There is selective damage to the superior and inferior arcuate bundles and relative sparing of the papillomacular and nasal bundles.[10] Defects in the NFL appear as darker zones in areas of expected brightness. Retinal blood vessels appear redder and darker, and smaller tertiary blood vessels become more visible. As more axons are lost, a grainy appearance may become apparent in the deep retina because of the visibility of the pigment in the retinal pigment epithelium and choroid. NFL loss in glaucoma has two main patterns: focal and diffuse atrophy.

Focal Nerve Fiber Layer Defects

There are two types of focal NFL loss in glaucoma: slit and wedge defects. Slit NFL defects represent focal damage to the ganglion cell axon at the level of the lamina cribrosa. Retrograde degeneration then reaches back to the ganglion cell body in the retina. Slit defects should be larger than one arteriole width in size and travel all the way to the optic disc (Figure 6-6A and B). If these two criteria are not met, the slit defect should not be considered a true NFL defect because this pattern (pseudoslit defect) is observed in approximately 10% of normal patients (Figure 6-6C). However, pseudoslits may be an early sign of glaucoma damage and should be observed for progression.

Wedge defects represent expanding focal damage to the optic nerve. The wedge becomes narrower closer to the optic nerve and broader farther from the disc, following an arcuate direction (Figure 6-7A and B). Wedge defects are associated with notching of the neuroretinal rim tissue and correspond to a visual field defect (Figure 6-7C). Because slit defects represent less ganglion cell axon loss than wedge defects, they may not produce white-on-white visual field loss. Often, focal slit or wedge defects can exhibit or develop adjacent diffuse NFL atrophy and eventually lead to diffuse overall thinning.

Focal defects can be graded according to whether the focal defect is relative (nerve fibers are still visible in the area of the focal loss) or absolute (no nerve fibers are visible in the area of focal loss) (Table 6-1).[9] Clinically, inferior focal defects occur more frequently than superior focal defects. Focal defects are the easiest type of NFL loss to identify in glaucoma, but they are not as common as the diffuse loss pattern.

Diffuse Nerve Fiber Layer Defects

Diffuse loss of the NFL in the superior and inferior arcuate zones is the most common pattern of NFL loss in glaucoma. The NFL looks thinned or raked, with the striations appearing less bright and having a less prominent texture. The amount of diffuse loss can be graded as mild, moderate, or severe (Figure 6-8 and Table 6-2).[9] In mild diffuse loss (D1), the striations are less bright and the texture is finer and less course. Medium-sized vessels are apparent, but small retinal

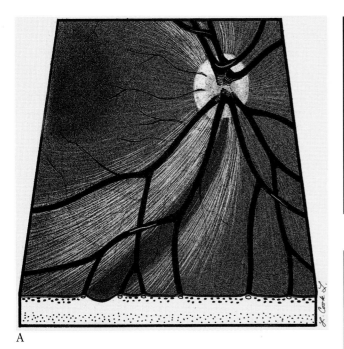

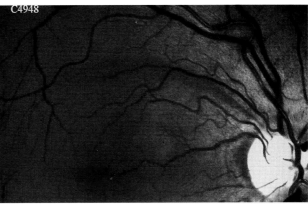

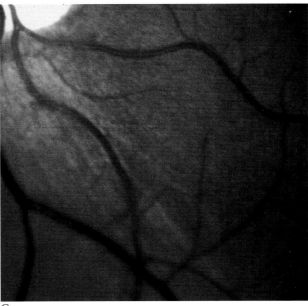

FIGURE 6-6. Slit defects and pseudoslits. Slit defect represents focal nerve fiber layer loss. (**A**) Slit defect is a dark focal band that should be larger than an arteriole width in size and travel all the way back to the optic nerve. (**B**) Clinical example of a slit defect in the superior arcade. Slit defects may or may not have damaged enough axons to cause an associated visual field defect. (**C**) Pseudoslits in the nerve fiber layer. As observation moves beyond 1 or 2 disc diameters from the optic nerve, the nerve fiber layer begins to thin out, and slit-type defects may be noted. They represent a variant of normal. Note that this slit defect in the inferior arcade does not go all the way back to the optic nerve.

blood vessels are not visible (see Figure 6-8B). In moderate diffuse loss (D2), the tertiary retinal blood vessels are more easily seen because the NFL striations are even less prominent (see Figure 6-8C). In severe diffuse loss (D3), few striations are visible, tertiary blood vessels are readily apparent, and the deep layers of the retina have a grainy appearance (see Figure 6-8D). With severe diffuse loss, the blood vessels may develop a pseudosheathing effect (see Figure 6-8D). This occurs because the blood vessels are made of collagen tissue, which is white (blood vessels appear red because of the red blood cells that flow through them). As the NFL is stripped away from the blood vessels, the outer collagen wall becomes more apparent.

Reproducible visual field loss appears at the stage of moderate NFL loss and becomes extensive with severe NFL loss. Visual field loss on white-on-white perimetry may not appear with mild NFL loss, but it may be detected with blue-yellow perimetry (see Case 6 in Chapter 18).

Diffuse loss in the early stages of glaucoma can be difficult to identify, and therefore comparison between the superior and inferior arcades in a single eye and between the arcades in both eyes is helpful in determining whether diffuse loss is present (Figures 6-9 and 6-10). Primary open-angle glaucoma is typically a bilateral disease, but glaucoma often asymmetrically damages one eye to a greater degree or damages asymmetrically between the superior and inferior poles. This asymmetry can give clues to the early diagnosis of glaucoma. Photograph inspection is especially useful in making NFL comparisons. NFL correlation to the amount of neuroretinal rim tissue is also a useful clinical pearl.

REVERSAL PATTERN

Glaucoma typically damages the superior and inferior arcuate bundles with relative preservation of the temporal and nasal bundles. As this pattern of damage continues,

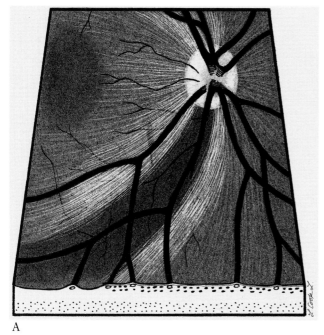
A

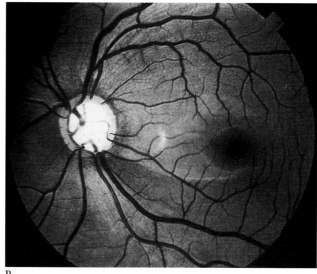
B

FIGURE 6-7. Wedge defect. Wedge defect represents expanding focal nerve fiber layer loss approximately one clock hour in size at the optic nerve (**A**). Clinical example of an inferior wedge defect associated with an inferior notch of the optic nerve (**B**) and corresponding visual field loss (**C**) (*see next page*).

patients with advanced disease may exhibit a reversal pattern to the retinal NFL (Figure 6-11). The papillomacular bundle will appear brighter than the superior or inferior arcuate bundles. This reversal pattern indicates significant NFL loss and will likely correspond with a double arcuate scotoma on visual field testing. Many glaucoma patients develop concurrent papillomacular and arcuate bundle damage, and the reversal pattern may not be observed. In endstage glaucoma, the NFL striations are not visible, and the retina appears dark, with prominent-appearing blood vessels, pseudosheathing of blood vessels near the optic disc, and a grainy appearance to the deep retina (see Figure 6-8D).

ADVANTAGES OF NERVE FIBER LAYER EXAMINATION

Evaluation of the NFL is a simple technique that does not require expensive equipment. Patients tolerate the procedure very well, and examining both eyes adds less than 1 minute of chair time. The primary advantage of examining the retinal NFL is to identify early glaucoma damage (see Figure 6-9). NFL defects can precede white-on-white field defects by up to 6 years.[3] In addition, the NFL examination can confirm the results of visual field testing. Confirmation of NFL loss corresponding to a subtle visual field defect can collaborate an early diagnosis of

TABLE 6-1. Grading Focal Nerve Fiber Layer Loss

Three questions to ask when evaluating for focal nerve fiber layer defects:

1. Are focal nerve fiber layer defects visible?

   No: normal

   Yes: proceed to Question 2

2. Are they less than one clock hour in size?

   No: wedge defect (W1 or W2)

   Yes: slit defect (S1 or S2)

3. Are striations visible in the area of the focal defect?

   Yes: relative focal defect (S1 or W1)

   No: absolute focal defect (S2 or W2)

TABLE 6-2. Grading Diffuse Nerve Fiber Layer Loss

Three questions to ask when evaluating the retinal nerve fiber layer for diffuse loss:

1. Are the nerve fiber layer striations bright, and is the texture course and fulminate in the arcuate bundles?

   Yes: normal

   No: proceed to Question 2

2. Are tertiary retinal blood vessels easily seen?

   Yes: proceed to Question 3

   No: mild diffuse loss (D1)

3. Are striations (although less bright) still fairly visible?

   Yes: moderate diffuse loss (D2)

   No: severe diffuse loss (D3)

Single Field Analysis

Eye: Left

Name:	ID:	DOB:

Central 30-2 Threshold Test

Fixation Monitor: Blindspot	Stimulus: III, White	Pupil Diameter:	Date: 06-11-1991
Fixation Target: Central	Background: 31.5 ASB	Visual Acuity: 20/20	Time: 2:27 PM
Fixation Losses: 1/26	Strategy: Full Threshold	RX: +1.00 DS DC X	Age: 37

False POS Errors: 1/18

False NEG Errors: 0/15

Test Duration: 14:18

Fovea: OFF

```
                27  19 | 29  29
            28  26  28 | 19  29  29
                       |(17)
        29  27  29  30 | 31  31  30  21
                (31)   |    (27)    (23)
    28  32  28  31  30 | 29  31  28  24  15
                (31)   |    (29)        (11)
30 --31--29--29--2--32-|--5--24--29--27--(0--
        Δ(0     ( 2)   |  ( 0)(24)      ( 8)
    30  26  <0  37  35 | 32  33  32  30  28
            (31)(33)   |(34)
    26  26  22  31  30 | 31  31  32  30  22
            (24)(29)   |    (33)        (26)
        28  30  29  29 | 30  31  30  29
            (30)       |        (32)
                28  30  32  25  28  31
                        (27)
                    25  31 | 29  26
```

```
        3  -6 | 4   4                          2  -6 | 3   3
     1  -1   1 |-10  1   2                   0  -2  0 |-11  0   1
  1  -2   1   1 | 1  -1   1  -6            0  -3   0  0 | 0  -2   0  -7
-1  2  -2  0  -1 |-3  -2  -2  -5 -14     -2  2  -3  0  -2 |-4  -3  -3  -6 -15
 1  -2     -30 -1 |-31 -8  -3  -3 -25     0  -3     -30 -2 |-32 -9  -3  -3 -26
```

GHT

Outside normal limits

```
-1  -5      2   1 | 0   0   0   0   0      -1  -6      1   0 |-1  -1  -1  -1  -1
-4  -5  -8  -2  -2 |-1   0   1   0  -4     -5  -6  -9  -3  -3 |-2  -1   0  -1  -5
   -2  -1  -2  -2 |-1   0   1   0           -3  -2  -3  -3 |-2  -1   0  -1
      -2   0   2 |-4  -1   2                   -3  -1   1 |-5  -2   1
         -4   2 | 1  -2                           -5   1 | 0  -3
```

MD   -2.70 dB

PSD   7.92 dB P < 0.5%

Total
Deviation

Pattern
Deviation

SF   1.46 dB

CPSD   7.75 dB P < 0.5%

```
::  < 5%
▨  < 2%
▩  < 1%
■  < 0.5%
```

C

FIGURE 6-7. (*continued*)

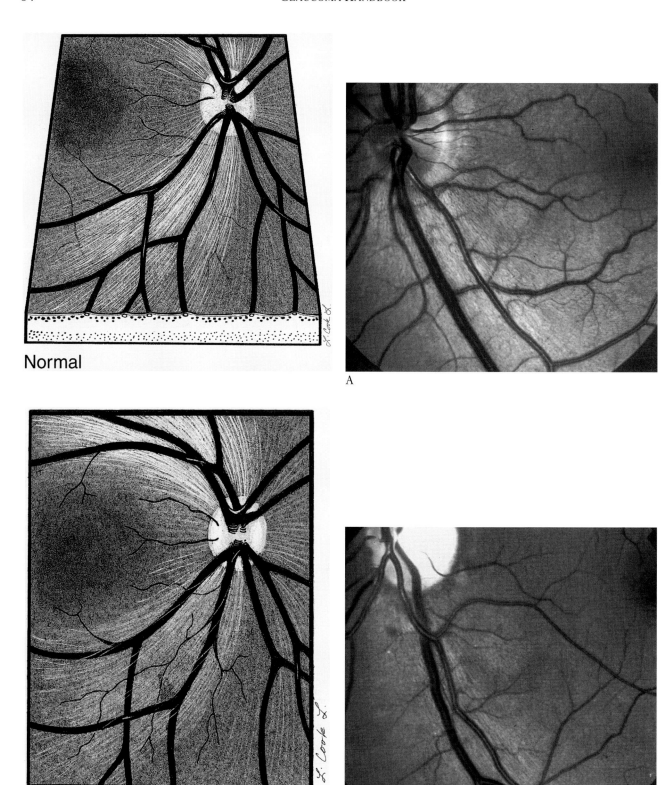

Normal

A

Mild

B

FIGURE 6-8. Normal nerve fiber layer and grading of progressive diffuse loss of the nerve fiber layer in glaucoma. (**A**) Normal nerve fiber layer with bright striations and fulminant texture. (**B**) Mild loss is represented by less bright striations and a thinner texture of the nerve fiber layer.

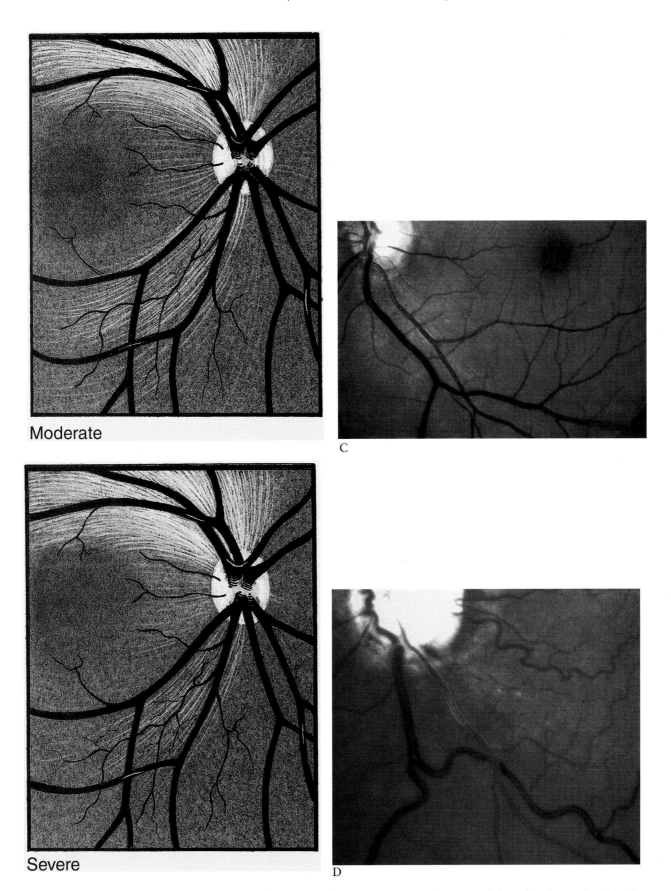

Moderate

Severe

C

D

FIGURE 6-8. (*continued*) (**C**) Moderate loss is defined by less distinct striations with more visibility of tertiary retinal blood vessels. (**D**) Severe loss shows very few visible striations. The blood vessels are dark and distinct. Note also pseudosheathing of the artery and disc hemorrhage.

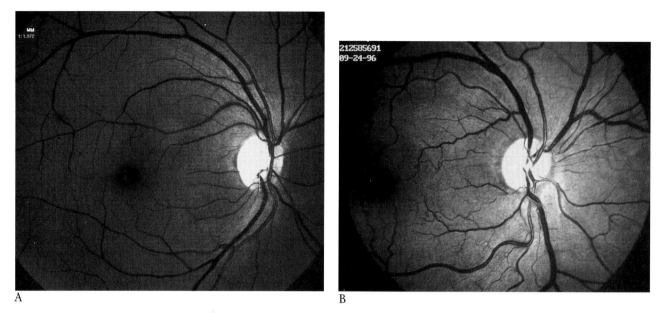

A   B

FIGURE 6-9. Nerve fiber layer comparison between superior and inferior arcades to detect glaucoma damage. (**A**) Note how the nerve fiber layer striations are less bright and fulminant in the inferior arcade (at 6 o'clock to 7 o'clock) compared with the superior arcade (at 11 o'clock to 12 o'clock). The smaller blood vessels are also darker and more easily seen at the 6 o'clock to 7 o'clock position. The nerve fiber layer defect would be classified as *mild diffuse loss in the inferior arcades*. The white-on-white visual field was normal. (**B**) Another example of mild diffuse loss in the superior arcades by comparison with its mirror image in the inferior arcades. Note also early slit defect in superior arcades.

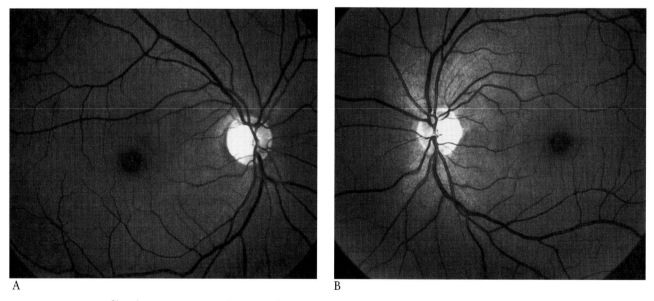

A   B

FIGURE 6-10. Nerve fiber layer comparison between the two eyes to detect glaucoma damage. Comparing the nerve fiber layer between the superior and inferior arcades or between the two eyes can be helpful to determine diffuse nerve fiber layer loss. Here the nerve fiber layer striations are less bright in the right eye (**A**) compared with the left eye (**B**), indicating mild to moderate diffuse loss both superior and inferior in the right eye.

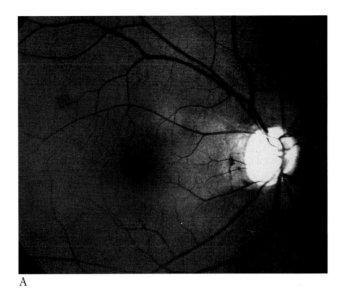

FIGURE 6-11. Nerve fiber layer reversal pattern in advanced glaucoma. Glaucoma typically damages the ganglion cell axons in the superior and inferior arcades with relative preservation of the axons in the papillomacular bundles. (**A**) This can lead to a pattern of nerve fiber layer loss in which the striations in the papillomacular bundle are brighter than the striations in the arcades. Note the complete lack of striations in the inferior and superior arcades and remaining striations in the papillomacular bundle. See visual field on next page (**B**).

A

glaucoma (Figure 6-12). The NFL examination can also help differentiate a large physiologic cup from glaucomatous cupping (Figure 6-13). Likewise, patients with anomalous optic nerves or who are unable to perform reliable visual field tests can be evaluated for glaucomatous damage. Serial photography of the NFL can be used to monitor for glaucoma progression (Figure 6-14).

DISADVANTAGES OF NERVE FIBER LAYER EXAMINATION

The NFL evaluation has potential pitfalls. Patients must have relatively clear media with good fundus pigmentation to evaluate the NFL (see Figure 6-5). It is important not to classify a pseudoslit NFL defect as a sign of glaucoma damage (see Figure 6-6C). Also, NFL loss is not specific for glaucoma—it can occur in any optic neuropathy or retinopathy. However, the pattern of NFL loss, the appearance of the optic nerves and visual fields, and patient symptomatology help differentiate glaucoma from other causes of NFL loss (Figure 6-15).

Finally, interpretation of the NFL takes time and experience, especially when the clinician is trying to differentiate a healthy eye from mild diffuse loss. The best way to learn the NFL technique is to examine the NFL in all healthy patients.[7] The physiologic variations that depend on age, race, media clarity, and fundus pigmentation should be learned. Next, the amount of NFL loss should be correlated with the degree of visual field loss in known glaucoma patients. The location and severity of the visual field defect can be predicted by the NFL evaluation (Figure 6-16). Comparisons of the NFL in the superior and inferior arcades and between the two eyes should be used to detect subtle loss (see Figures 6-9 and 6-10). After these steps have been achieved in hundreds of patients, the clinician can begin to use the NFL

to establish early optic nerve damage in glaucoma-suspect patients. Identification of NFL loss in patients in whom glaucoma is suspected confirms a diagnosis of glaucoma and may warrant therapeutic intervention. By establishing an early diagnosis of glaucoma, intervention with current therapies to lower intraocular pressure may help prevent or delay future visual field loss. NFL examination should not stand alone in treatment decisions but should be incorporated with other glaucoma risk factors and other clinical test results.

SCANNING LASER POLARIMETRY

Several instruments are commercially available that can give quantitative information about the NFL thickness, including a scanning laser ophthalmoscope (Heidelberg Retinal Tomograph [Heidelberg Engineering, Heidelberg, Germany] and TOPSS [Laser Diagnostic Technologies, San Diego, CA]) and an optical coherence tomographer (Zeiss Humphrey, Dublin, CA). A scanning laser polarimeter, GDx, (Laser Diagnostic Technologies, San Diego, CA) can measure the retardation of the NFL, which is directly related to NFL thickness (Figure 6-17). With software programs and normative databases, it may be possible to determine with probability values whether a patient's NFL thickness is statistically normal or abnormal. However, considerable overlap exists between the measurements in healthy patients and patients with early to moderate glaucoma. Looking at a combination of specific parameters may improve the sensitivity and specificity to detect glaucoma.[11] Quantitative NFL thickness with the GDx can also be measured over time to determine the stability or progression of glaucoma damage. However, at the present time, there are no long-term clinical trials to validate any of these instruments as a monitor for glaucoma progression, and the equipment is expensive.

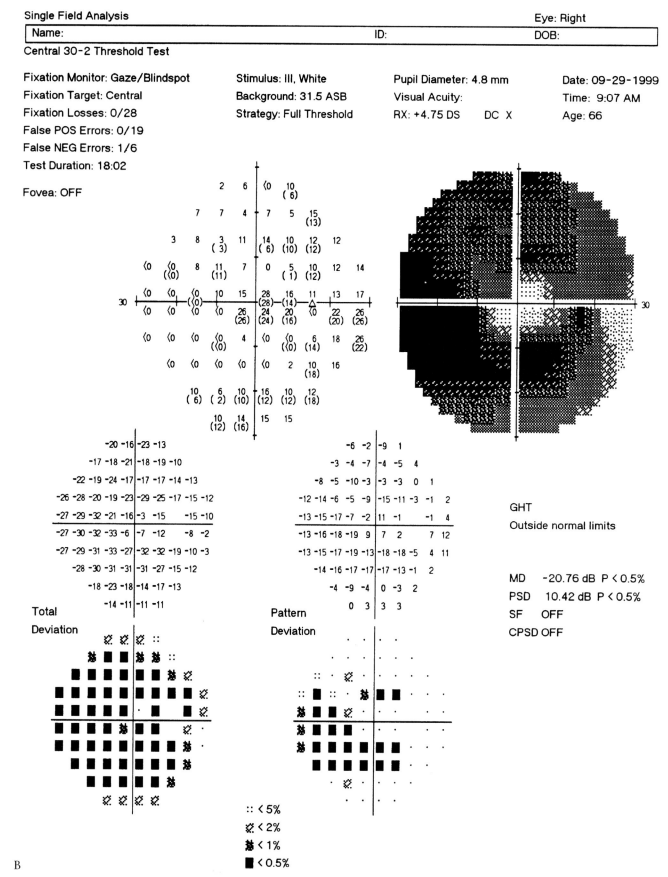

FIGURE 6-11. (*continued*) (**B**) This pattern of nerve fiber layer loss corresponds to a double arcuate visual field defect. Note how the central visual field is spared because of a relatively intact papillomacular bundle.

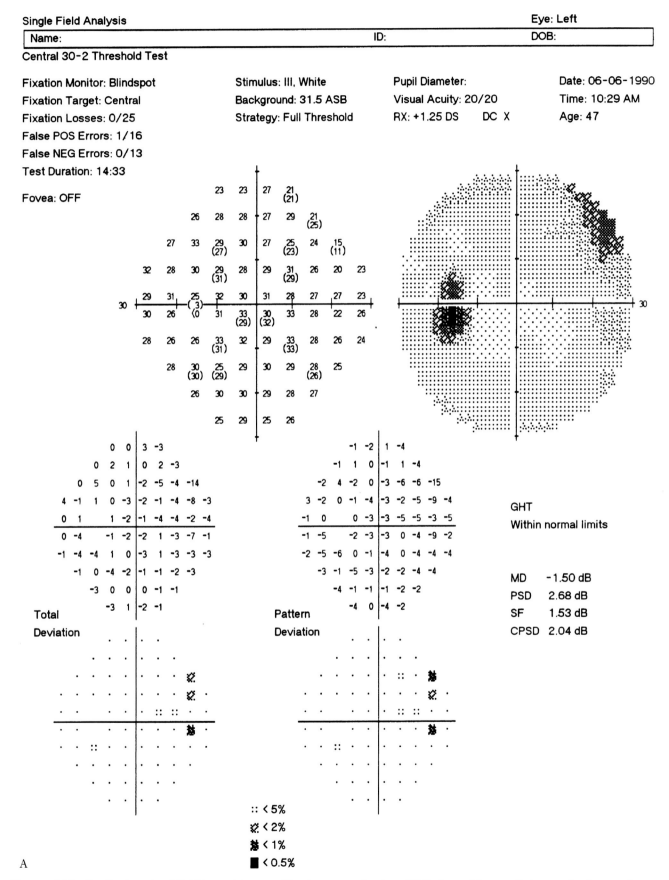

FIGURE 6-12. Confirming visual field loss with nerve fiber layer examination. (A) Patient with a small cluster of points on the pattern deviation plots in the superior nasal field. (B) Nerve fiber layer wedge defect in the inferior arcades confirms visual field defect (*see next page*).

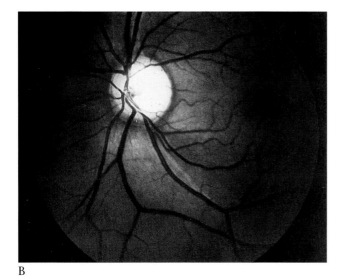

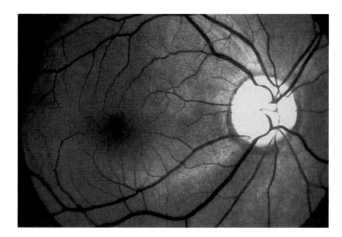

B

FIGURE 6-12. (*continued*). (**B**) Nerve fiber layer wedge defect in the inferior arcades confirms visual field defect.

FIGURE 6-13. Using nerve fiber layer examination to differentiate glaucoma cupping from large physiologic cupping. Patient has a large optic disc (vertical height, 2.4 mm) and a large cup. However, the color photograph of the optic nerve (Color Plate 20) shows thinning of the inferior rim tissue that is confirmed with an inferior wedge defect in the nerve fiber layer.

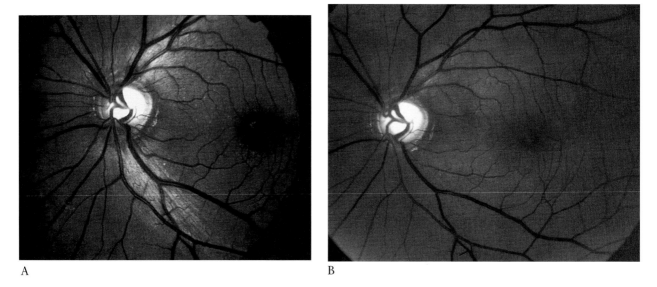

A   B

FIGURE 6-14. Progressive nerve fiber layer loss. This patient demonstrates progressive nerve fiber layer loss in the superior and inferior arcades (**B**) from his original nerve fiber layer photographs (**A**). This confirms glaucoma progression despite visual fields that appeared relatively stable (see Case 7 in Chapter 18).

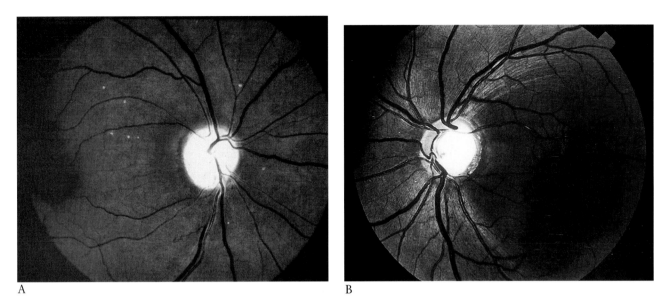

A B

FIGURE 6-15. Nerve fiber layer loss in nonglaucoma etiologies. (**A**) A 44-year-old African-American man with grade 4 hypertensive retinopathy and severe papilledema. Blood pressure was gradually controlled and disc swelling resolved, but disc pallor was present, indicating optic atrophy. Visual acuity was 20/60. Nerve fiber layer shows overall severe diffuse loss that is greatest in the superior arcades. (**B**) This patient had a history of alcohol abuse for 30 years and progressive visual acuity loss to 20/60 in both eyes. Optic nerves showed bilateral temporal pallor. Patient had toxic (alcohol-nutritional) optic neuropathy. Nerve fiber layer in the left eye shows marked dropout of the nerve fiber layer in the papillomacular bundle with sparing of the nerve fiber layer in the arcades. Any optic neuropathy can cause nerve fiber layer loss; however, the appearance of the optic nerve, the time frame of the vision loss, or the location of the nerve fiber layer defects help differentiate between glaucoma and other causes.

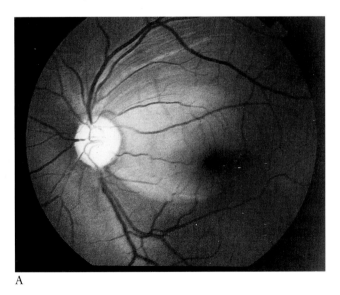

A

FIGURE 6-16. Correlating the nerve fiber layer examination to the visual field examination. When learning nerve fiber layer interpretation, it is helpful to predict the visual field loss based on the nerve fiber layer examination. (**A**) In this glaucoma patient, marked loss of the nerve fiber layer is visible in the inferior arcades, and moderate diffuse loss in the superior arcades. Note brighter papillomacular bundle (reversal pattern). (*See visual field on next page.*)

Single Field Analysis   Eye: Left

Name:	ID:	DOB:

Central 30-2 Threshold Test

Fixation Monitor: Blindspot   Stimulus: III, White   Pupil Diameter: Date: 08-23-1990
Fixation Target: Central   Background: 31.5 ASB   Visual Acuity: 20/20   Time: 12:04 PM
Fixation Losses: 0/25   Strategy: Full Threshold   RX: -0.25 DS +2.50 DC X 118 Age: 41.
False POS Errors: 1/9
False NEG Errors: 2/14
Test Duration: 14:47

Fovea: OFF

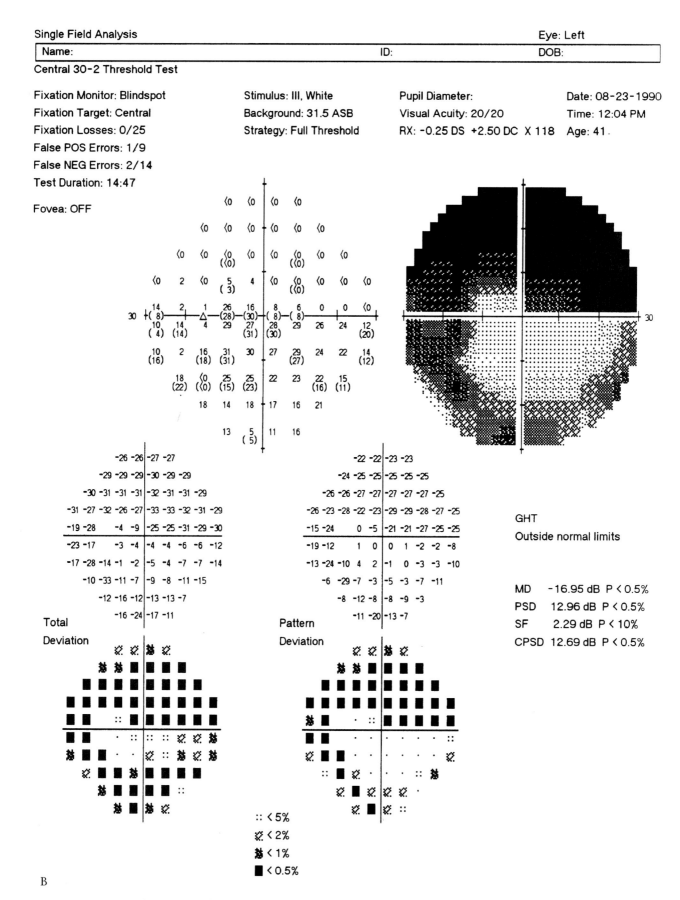

GHT
Outside normal limits

MD   -16.95 dB P < 0.5%
PSD   12.96 dB P < 0.5%
SF   2.29 dB P < 10%
CPSD   12.69 dB P < 0.5%

Total Deviation

Pattern Deviation

:: < 5%
▨ < 2%
▨ < 1%
■ < 0.5%

B

FIGURE 6-16. (*continued*) (**B**) Visual field can be predicted from nerve fiber layer loss. The patient has an almost complete superior altitudinal field defect and an early inferior arcuate defect. Note how the central visual field is spared due to a relatively intact papillomacular bundle.

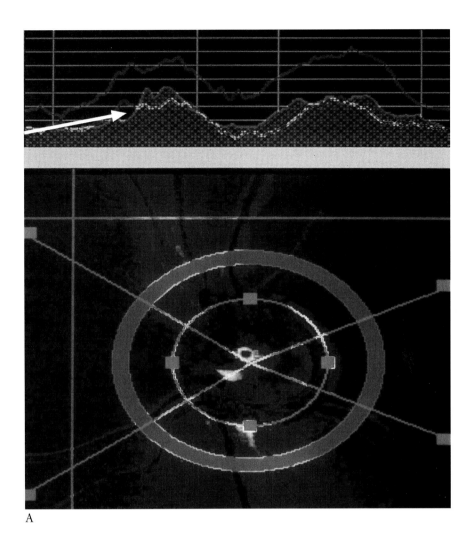

A

FIGURE 6-17. Scanning laser polarimetry: GDx (Laser Diagnostic Technologies, San Diego, CA) printout. The GDx measures retardation of the nerve fiber layer that is directly related to nerve fiber layer thickness. Here the GDx (**A**) shows less retardation (thickness), depicted by the depleted superior-temporal peak in the top graph (*arrow*) that corresponds to the superior nerve fiber layer loss in the clinical photograph (**B**), and an early inferior nasal step on the visual field (**C**). (*See next page.*)

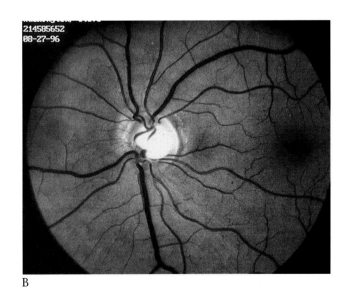

B

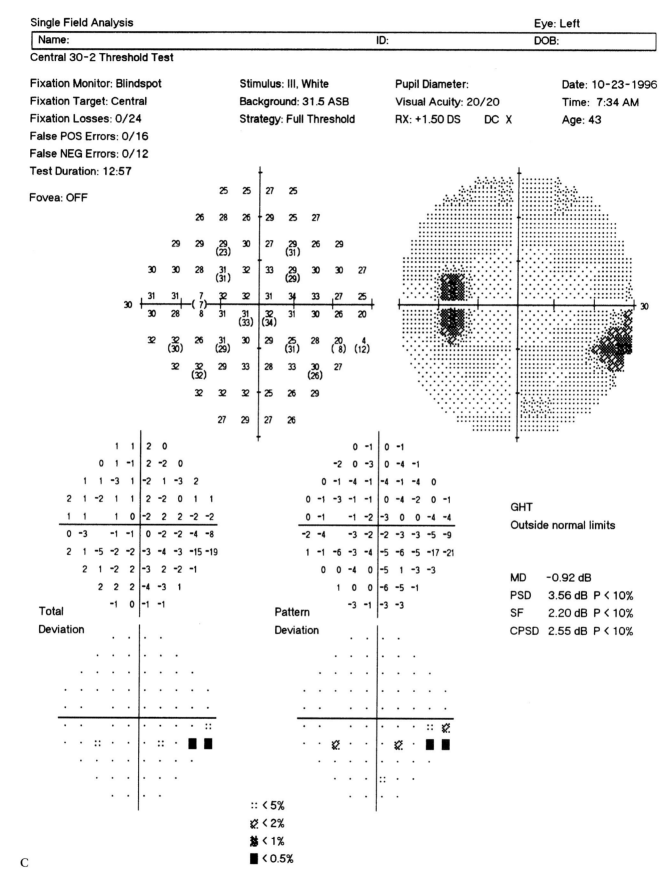

Single Field Analysis   Eye: Left

Name: ID: DOB:

Central 30-2 Threshold Test

Fixation Monitor: Blindspot   Stimulus: III, White   Pupil Diameter: Date: 10-23-1996
Fixation Target: Central   Background: 31.5 ASB   Visual Acuity: 20/20   Time: 7:34 AM
Fixation Losses: 0/24   Strategy: Full Threshold   RX: +1.50 DS   DC X   Age: 43
False POS Errors: 0/16
False NEG Errors: 0/12
Test Duration: 12:57

Fovea: OFF

GHT
Outside normal limits

MD   −0.92 dB
PSD   3.56 dB P < 10%
SF   2.20 dB P < 10%
CPSD   2.55 dB P < 10%

Total Deviation

Pattern Deviation

:: < 5%

▨ < 2%

▩ < 1%

■ < 0.5%

C

FIGURE 6-17. (continued)

REFERENCES

1. Quigley HA, Addicks EM, Green WR. Optic nerve damage in human glaucoma. III. Quantitative correlation of nerve fiber loss and visual field defect in glaucoma, ischemic neuropathy, papilledema and toxic neuropathy. Arch Ophthalmol 1982;100:135–146.

2. Quigley HA, Dunkelberger GR, Green WR. Retinal ganglion cell atrophy correlated with automated perimetry in human eyes with glaucoma. Am J Ophthalmol 1989;107:453–464.

3. Sommer A, Katz J, Quigley HA, et al. Clinically detectable nerve fiber atrophy precedes the onset of glaucomatous field loss. Arch Ophthalmol 1991;109: 77–83.

4. Jonas JB, Zach FM, Gusek GC, Naumann GO. Pseudoglaucomatous physiologic large cups. Am J Ophthalmol 1989;107:137–144.

5. Minckler DS. The organization of nerve fiber bundles in the primate optic nerve head. Arch Ophthalmol 1980;98:1630–1636.

6. Litwak A. Evaluation of the retinal nerve fiber layer in glaucoma. J Am Optom Assoc 1990;61:390–397.

7. Litwak AB. The retinal nerve fiber layer. Why some doctors just don't get it. Clin Eye Vis Care 1996;8:1–4.

8. Sommer A, D'Anna SA, Kues HA, et al. High-resolution photography of the retinal nerve fiber layer. Am J Ophthalmol 1983;96:535–539.

9. Quigley HA. Diagnosing Early Glaucoma with Nerve Fiber Layer Examination. New York: Igaku-Shoin, 1996.

10. Quigley HA, Sanchez RM, Dunkelberger GR, et al. Chronic glaucoma selectively damages large optic nerve fibers. Invest Ophthalmol Vis Sci 1987;28:913–920.

11. Weinreb RN, Zangwill L, Berry CC, et al. Detection of glaucoma with scanning laser polarimetry. Arch Ophthalmol 1998;116:1583–1589.

Evaluation of Automated Perimetry

Peter A. Lalle

The purpose of visual field examination is to aid in the diagnosis and management of glaucoma. Visual fields assist in determining the severity of damage so that an initial target pressure can be set and the effectiveness of treatment can be determined by following the patient's fields for glaucoma progression. For such an essential role in the management of this disease, it is critical that the visual field examination be reliable, accurate, and repeatable. Proper patient and test selection, as well as careful monitoring of the reliability indices, work toward this goal. Interpretation of the results requires recognition of artifacts that mimic glaucomatous defects. Application of basic algorithms provides initial guidance in the identification of defects and possible progression, although ultimately the interpretation of the test results rests with the clinician's knowledge of both the disease process and the individual patient's clinical presentation.

PATIENT SELECTION

Because of the key role visual field testing plays in the diagnosis and management of glaucoma, no patient should be prejudged to be incapable of performing visual field tests. Modifications to testing can be made to compensate for patients with physical or mental limitations.

Age is no limitation; patients from preteens to octogenarians are quite capable of giving reliable, consistent automated field results. However, several physical limitations may impede test taking. Adults without their dentures or young children may not be able to center their eyes when their chins are on the chin rest. In these cases,

a foam pad on the chin rest helps elevate and stabilize their heads. Patients with certain physical handicaps or who are wheelchair-bound may not be able to be positioned in the Humphrey Field Analyzer I (HFA I) perimeter (Zeiss Humphrey Systems, Dublin, CA). The new, smaller-bowl Humphrey Field Analyzer II (HFA II) is mounted on a special table that can be positioned to make perimetry possible for such individuals (Figure 7-1). Patients with physical ailments should be given frequent rests (at least 30 seconds of rest after every 5 minutes of testing) so that fatigue and discomfort do not interfere with their performance. The perimetrist should stay with the patient throughout the entire test to ensure that the patient remains centered, comfortable, and responding well. Test-shortening strategies may be useful for both physically challenged and neurologically impaired patients (see below). These patients are capable of giving reliable field results, and most benefit from a shortened test with frequent rests during the test.

TEST SELECTION

Proper test selection is the next step in obtaining reliable, interpretable visual field results. The following is a summary of tests:

Full Field 120 (F120): Suprathreshold test for glaucoma, useful as a "practice" test to lessen learning curve during threshold testing. Good sensitivity, fair specificity. Consider any field abnormal with 17 defects overall or 8 in any quadrant. Three-zone strategy gives additional qualitative information with minimal cost in time.

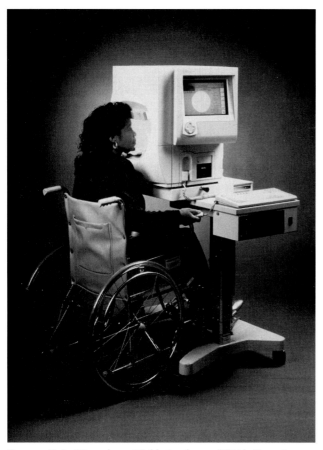

FIGURE 7-1. Humphrey Field Analyzer (HFA) II perimeter. The smaller bowl of the HFA II perimeter is mounted on a table that gives access to wheelchair patients. Swedish Interactive Thresholding Algorithm (SITA) and SITA Fast strategies are only available on the HFA II. (Photograph courtesy of Zeiss Humphrey Systems, Dublin, CA.)

Full Threshold 30-2: Gold standard by which all other tests are judged. Longest test, most susceptible to fatigue artifact. Tests 76 points in central 30 degrees.

Full Threshold 24-2: Eliminates all edge points from 30-2 except for two most nasal points along horizontal meridian, reduces test time by 10–20%. Comparable sensitivity and specificity to the 30-2 test. Eliminated edge points occasionally provide useful information. Tests 54 points in central 24 degrees.

Full Threshold 10-2: All test points are within 10 degrees of fixation, spaced 2 degrees apart (compared with 6 degrees with 24-2 and 30-2 tests). Preferred test in endstage glaucoma or when fixation is threatened to monitor central vision. Tests 68 points in central 10 degrees. Can be performed with either Full Threshold, FASTPAC, Swedish Interactive Thresholding Algorithm (SITA) Standard, or SITA Fast.

"Quick 24": Full Threshold 24-2 done with short-term fluctuation and fixation monitoring turned off. As sensitive as a standard threshold test, but quicker. Both glaucoma hemifield test and glaucoma change probability plots available.

"Turbo 24": Modified 24-2 with FASTPAC test strategy turned on, and short-term fluctuation and fixation monitoring turned off. Fastest threshold test on HFA I; not as sensitive as Full Threshold strategy, but may be useful for patients with profound fatigue artifact. Neither glaucoma hemifield test nor glaucoma change probability plots available. No validated cluster criteria available to confirm field defect. No criteria available to determine progression.

SITA Standard 30-2 or 24-2: Reduces test time by 33–50% compared with FASTPAC and Full Threshold strategies with similar sensitivities. Both glaucoma hemifield test and glaucoma change probability plots (planned) available.

SITA Fast 24-2 OR 30-2: Further reduces test time compared with standard SITA strategy. Approximately 75% faster than Full Threshold strategy. Like FASTPAC, some sacrifice is made in accuracy of threshold determination. Unlike FASTPAC, both glaucoma hemifield test and glaucoma change probability (planned) analysis are available.

Although the peripheral field outside 30 degrees was routinely tested in Goldmann kinetic bowl perimetry to find isolated nasal step defects, some practitioners question its continued usefulness in modern static perimetry.[1,2] For those who feel that testing of the peripheral field may supply useful information, the HFA provides a suprathreshold (screening) test of the entire visual field, the Full Field 120 (F120). It uses suprathreshold static targets to test the central field (inside 30 degrees) in the standard Armaly pattern, and a separate peripheral pattern that places the majority of its test points in the nasal field to maximize the detection of peripheral nasal field loss (Figure 7-2). When subsequent threshold field tests are performed, the additional information available from a previous F120 of the peripheral field may guide the practitioner in deciding whether a defect seen on threshold testing is a lens rim artifact (LRA) or a true defect. The F120's sensitivity and specificity have been validated through clinical studies, with good sensitivity and acceptable specificity. A positive test is defined by a total of 17 missed points or 8 missed points in any quadrant. It misses shallow scotoma and overcalls many normal patients, partly due to learning curve defects, because this test is only used for first fields.[3,4] Any positive finding on a screening test should be confirmed as soon as possible with a threshold test.

The HFA's central 30-degree field examination (30-2) remains the gold standard for testing glaucoma patients and is used in many glaucoma studies.[5,6] However, the edge points of the 30-2 are often depressed in normal patients and therefore have limited value in

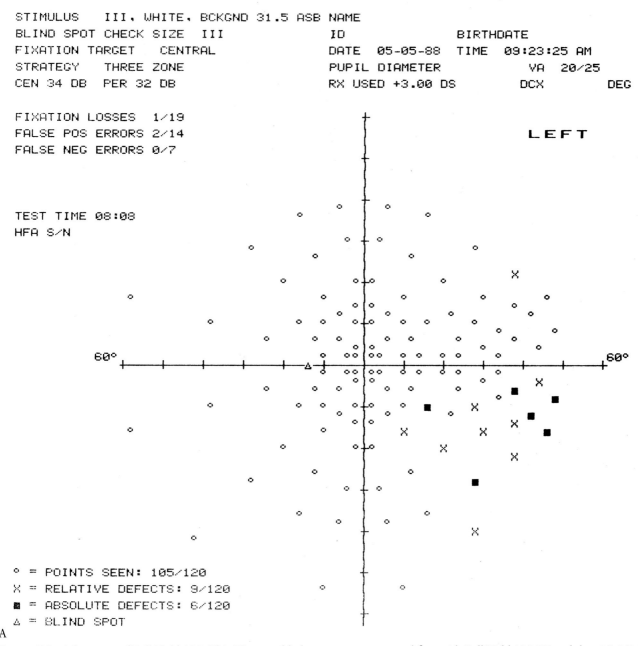

FULL FIELD 120 POINT SCREENING TEST

STIMULUS   III, WHITE, BCKGND 31.5 ASB NAME
BLIND SPOT CHECK SIZE   III   ID   BIRTHDATE
FIXATION TARGET   CENTRAL   DATE   05-05-88 TIME   09:23:25 AM
STRATEGY   THREE ZONE   PUPIL DIAMETER   VA   20/25
CEN 34 DB   PER 32 DB   RX USED +3.00 DS   DCX   DEG

FIXATION LOSSES   1/19
FALSE POS ERRORS 2/14   LEFT
FALSE NEG ERRORS 0/7

TEST TIME 08:08
HFA S/N

60°   60°

° = POINTS SEEN: 105/120
X = RELATIVE DEFECTS: 9/120
■ = ABSOLUTE DEFECTS: 6/120
△ = BLIND SPOT

A

FIGURE 7-2. Advantage of Full Field 120. This 73-year-old glaucoma suspect tested first with Full Field 120 (**A**) and then 30-2 Full Threshold (**B**) (*see next page*). Inspection of the 30-2 test raises the question of early inferior nasal step versus partial lens rim artifact. Inspection of the peripheral nasal field of the earlier F 120, which is tested without a trial lens, shows an obvious nasal step just encroaching on the central 30 degrees.

interpretation. In clinical practice, most clinicians choose the central 24-degree point pattern (24-2), which deletes most of these peripheral edge points, reducing the 76-point pattern to only 54 points.

Although the 30-2 and 24-2 may be considered equally useful in testing for glaucoma, they do not have an equal effect on the patient. The patient fatigues less with the shorter test, and hence higher sensitivities are often found (Figure 7-3). Thus, 30-2 and 24-2 tests should not be mixed when a patient is being monitored with sequential field tests. In addition to these considerations, all HFA 1 software revisions before revision 9.3 (including STATPAC for Windows Version 1.0 [Zeiss Humphrey Systems, Dublin, CA]) made errors in calculating the mean deviation (MD) index and the glaucoma change probability (GCP) plots when combining successive fields of 24-2 and 30-2. If the decision is made to change a patient from 30-2 to 24-2

Single Field Analysis   Eye: Left

| Name: | ID: | DOB: |

Central 30–2 Threshold Test

Fixation Monitor: Blindspot   Stimulus: III, White   Pupil Diameter: Date: 12-20-1989
Fixation Target: Central   Background: 31.5 ASB   Visual Acuity: 20/25   Time: 10:28 AM
Fixation Losses: 0/26   Strategy: Full Threshold   RX: +2.75 DS   DC X   Age: 73
False POS Errors: 0/20
False NEG Errors: 1/15
Test Duration: 16:17

Fovea: OFF

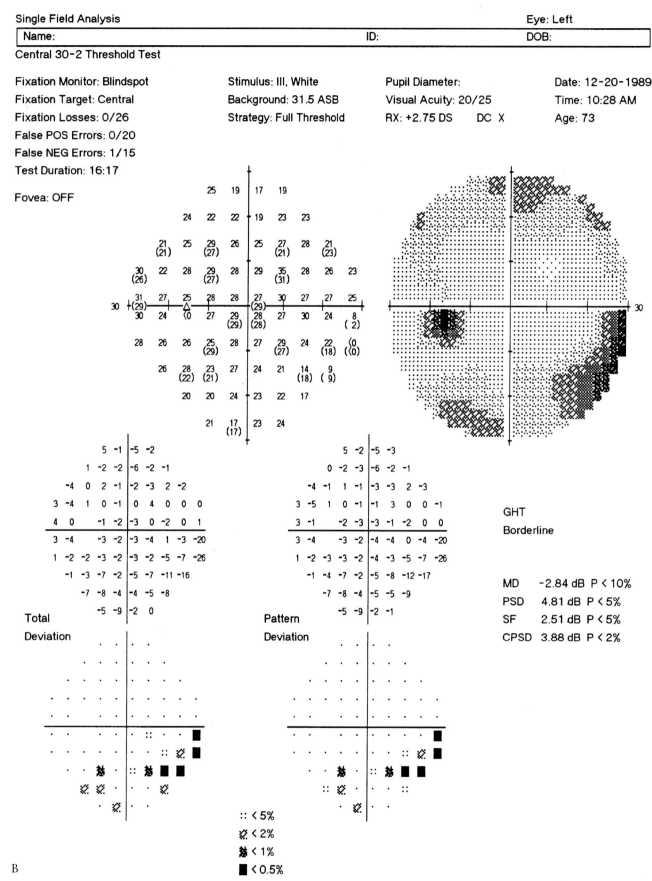

GHT
Borderline

MD   -2.84 dB P < 10%
PSD   4.81 dB P < 5%
SF   2.51 dB P < 5%
CPSD   3.88 dB P < 2%

Total Deviation

Pattern Deviation

:: < 5%
▨ < 2%
▦ < 1%
■ < 0.5%

B

FIGURE 7-2. (continued)

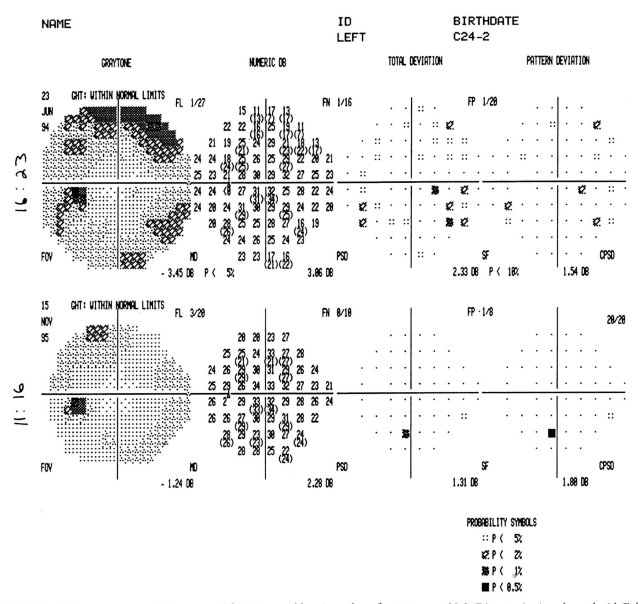

FIGURE 7-3. 30-2 strategy versus 24-2 strategy. This 66-year-old patient whose first test was a 30-2 (76 test points) performed with Full Threshold strategy, which took 16 minutes and 23 seconds. The patient was later tested with a 24-2 (54 test points) performed with Full Threshold strategy, which took only 11 minutes and 16 seconds. Visual fields improve with shorter testing strategies. It is important to keep the same testing strategy through subsequent tests. If a fatigue artifact is suspected, then a shorter testing strategy should be used.

testing, a new baseline should be established using only 24-2 tests.

The central 10 degrees of the visual field is critical because it monitors the status of fixation. Extinction of fixation occurs as successive hemifield involvement in which one-half of the central 10 degrees is lost (splitting fixation), followed by loss of the remaining half.[7,8] End-stage glaucoma patients should be tested with the central 10-2 to carefully monitor the remaining central isle of vision (Figure 7-4). The 6-degree spacing between test points of 24-2 and 30-2 is inadequate for monitoring the remaining visual field near fixation. In the 24-2 and 30-2 point patterns, the four points closest to fixation are 4.2 degrees away from fixation, which would allow a substantial drop in acuity before the scotoma was large enough to be detected. The 68 points of the 10-2 test are only 2 degrees apart, with the innermost four points only 1.4 degrees from fixation. This improved resolution allows detection of scotoma within the central 10 degrees missed by the larger spacing of the 24-2 or 30-2 tests and better monitoring of fixation.

THRESHOLD STRATEGIES

Determination of threshold values is made by one of four means. The HFA I is capable of only Full Thresh-

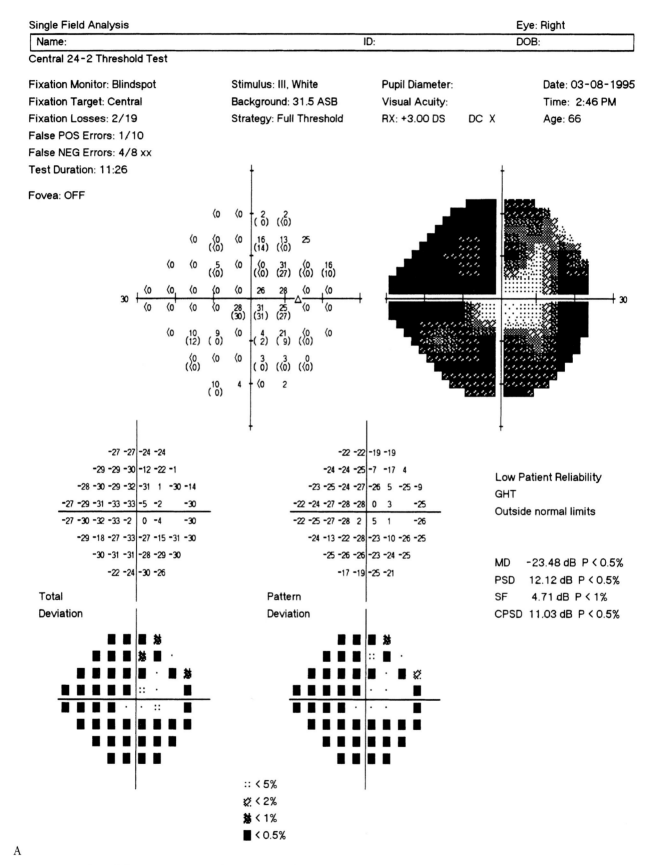

Single Field Analysis   Eye: Right

Name: ID: DOB:

Central 24-2 Threshold Test

Fixation Monitor: Blindspot   Stimulus: III, White   Pupil Diameter: Date: 03-08-1995

Fixation Target: Central   Background: 31.5 ASB   Visual Acuity: Time: 2:46 PM

Fixation Losses: 2/19   Strategy: Full Threshold   RX: +3.00 DS   DC X   Age: 66

False POS Errors: 1/10

False NEG Errors: 4/8 xx

Test Duration: 11:26

Fovea: OFF

Total Deviation

Pattern Deviation

Low Patient Reliability

GHT

Outside normal limits

MD   -23.48 dB   P < 0.5%

PSD   12.12 dB   P < 0.5%

SF   4.71 dB   P < 1%

CPSD   11.03 dB   P < 0.5%

:: < 5%

< 2%

< 1%

■ < 0.5%

A

FIGURE 7-4. Value of the 10-2 strategy. This patient with advanced glaucoma displayed severe visual field loss on the 24-2 (**A**). Fixation appears to be split from above on the 24-2 test, on which points are spaced 6 degrees apart, 3 degrees on either side of the horizontal.

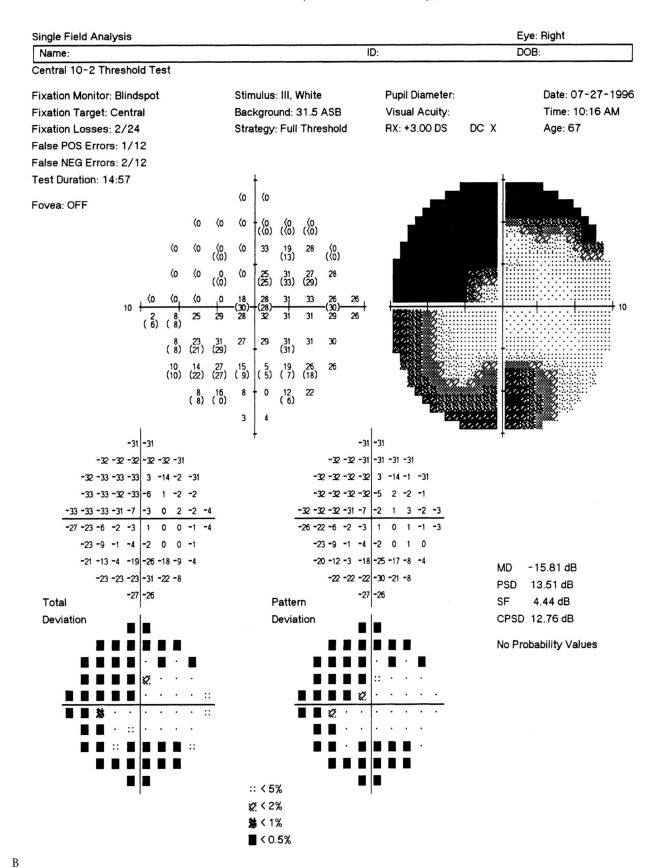

Single Field Analysis — Eye: Right

Name: — ID: — DOB:

Central 10-2 Threshold Test

Fixation Monitor: Blindspot | Stimulus: III, White | Pupil Diameter: | Date: 07-27-1996
Fixation Target: Central | Background: 31.5 ASB | Visual Acuity: | Time: 10:16 AM
Fixation Losses: 2/24 | Strategy: Full Threshold | RX: +3.00 DS   DC X | Age: 67
False POS Errors: 1/12
False NEG Errors: 2/12
Test Duration: 14:57

Fovea: OFF

MD   -15.81 dB
PSD   13.51 dB
SF   4.44 dB
CPSD 12.76 dB

No Probability Values

Total Deviation

Pattern Deviation

:: < 5%
✛ < 2%
✚ < 1%
■ < 0.5%

B

FIGURE 7-4. (*continued*) The 10-2 pattern shows a much higher sensitivity in the juxtafoveal points, 1.2 degrees from fixation (**B**). Serial 10-2 tests allow for better determination of progression of points near fixation than a 30-2 or 24-2.

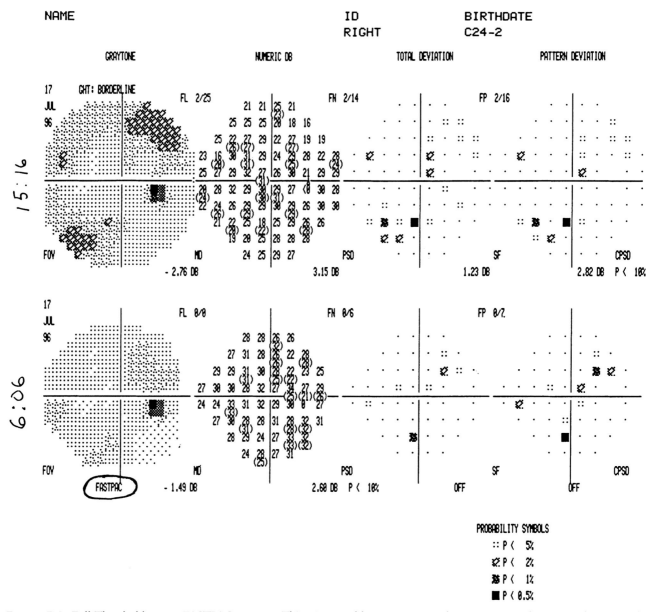

FIGURE 7-5. Full Threshold versus FASTPAC strategy. This 53-year-old patient required 15 minutes and 16 seconds to complete the first test using a 30-2 pattern with Full Threshold strategy. Patient was retested with a 24-2 pattern using FASTPAC; the resulting test time was 6 minutes and 6 seconds. FASTPAC strategy should be used when SITA strategy is not available and the patient has or is likely to show fatigue artifact on Full Threshold testing.

old and FASTPAC strategies, whereas the HFA II is capable of those plus two additional: SITA Standard and SITA Fast. The conventional staircase strategy used by the Full Threshold method crosses the threshold twice by changing the light in increments of 4 decibels (dB) until the light is not seen, and then increasing the light by 2 dB until it is seen again. FASTPAC is an alternative strategy that changes the intensity of the light by 3 dB and only crosses the threshold once. This strategy can reduce test time by as much as 40%, but the reduction is less in patients with extensive field loss (Figure 7-5).[9] The savings in time comes at the expense

of accuracy; FASTPAC's determination of threshold values is less precise than the Full Threshold strategy, and scotomas may be understated.[9] FASTPAC, in conjunction with the 24-2 pattern, is very useful for patients whose fatigue artifact with Full Threshold testing renders the field uninterpretable. The slight sacrifice in accuracy is outweighed by having meaningful test results. However, neither the glaucoma hemifield test (GHT), which analyzes the field for a defect, nor glaucoma change probability (GCP) analysis, which looks for significant progression, is available when FASTPAC is used.

Perimetrists have developed several strategies for reducing test time, both with and without FASTPAC. First, the 24-2 pattern is selected rather than the 30-2 pattern. Then, fixation loss (FL) catch trials (Heijl-Krakau) and short-term fluctuation (STF) are turned off. This strategy provides an easier test, saves approximately 5–8 minutes compared with an unmodified 30-2 test, yet still has all STATPAC data analysis (GHT and GCP) available. For patients still too taxed by the test, selecting the FASTPAC threshold strategy further minimizes overall test time. Five-minute threshold fields are possible with the addition of FASTPAC when only minimal visual field loss is present. As noted earlier, this technique has a drawback—neither GHT nor GCP is available. Further, because this shortened test causes less fatigue, dramatic improvement in sensitivity may occur in some patients that exceeds the change expected from the thresholding strategy alone.

SUMMARY OF TESTS

Testing patients who are undergoing perimetry for the first time presents a unique challenge. Regardless of testing strategy, a significant percentage of patients undergoing a visual field test for the first time exhibit a learning curve such that the initial field displays an overall depression, deeper in the periphery (Figure 7-6). In addition, spurious depressed points or a cluster of points that mimic scotoma are frequently found.[10]

The STATPAC database consists of the average of the second and third visual field tests of a group of normal patients. The first fields were too inconsistent compared with the results of the second and third to establish meaningful ranges of normal and consequently were excluded.[11,12] There is at least a theoretical consideration against using STATPAC to interpret the first field of a patient.

Testing first-time visual field patients with a suprathreshold F120 provides a useful warm-up examination before the patient undergoes Full Threshold testing, and it would validate the use of the STATPAC database on subsequent fields. Both the central and peripheral fields are examined with an average test time of 6–9 minutes per eye. If the F120 is normal, a threshold examination may be performed in 6 months. However, if the F120 is positive, a Full Threshold field should be performed at the earliest convenient time. The threshold test is then used to confirm visual field loss, and it becomes part of the baseline for follow-up care (see Figure 7-2).

Alternatively, the first visual field examination may be a threshold field using FASTPAC, and the standard Full Threshold may be used for subsequent testing or after a defect is identified with FASTPAC. However, starting the patient with either a suprathreshold test or

FASTPAC means that at some later date these fields will have to be discarded from the analysis after Full Threshold testing is performed.

Because of reluctance to discard tests, most practitioners still elect to test the first-time patient with a Full Threshold examination with the hope that the first field will not have to be discarded. Careful inspection of the result for evidence of learning effect is mandatory. All suspected defects should be confirmed by a second threshold test.

The HFA II provides two additional thresholding strategies: SITA Standard and SITA Fast (Figures 7-7 and 7-8). The SITA strategies have gathered a separate database of expected threshold values for normal patients. SITA uses this database, along with a more sophisticated knowledge of how different points influence the outcome at other points, to pick a starting testing stimulus that is close to the final value. As a result, the determination of threshold is reached with fewer questions asked, but with the same accuracy as a Full Threshold test. Unlike the Full Threshold strategy, SITA does not need to cross the threshold twice to determine the final value. SITA constantly monitors the test results of all points during a field examination and uses a complex statistical technique to assign a level of confidence for how close each test point is to its final value. When SITA believes that it is "confident" enough and knows what the final value for a point is, it stops testing that point. It does not have to double-cross the threshold to do this, and, hence, fewer questions are asked and test time is reduced. The reduction in test time results in a less-fatiguing examination, and, in general, SITA tests look better than Full Threshold tests, especially when evaluating the grayscales. However, because less variation in threshold values occurs with SITA, it accepts a narrower range of normal values for its STATPAC analysis. Although the SITA test grayscale may look better for a patient previously tested with Full Threshold, the probability plots of the SITA Standard and Full Threshold test will appear similar.

The principal difference between SITA Standard and SITA Fast is the level of confidence the program needs to stop testing at a given point. SITA Standard sets a higher level of certainty, requiring more trials at a given point. Thus, SITA Standard provides a more accurate assessment of the threshold value than SITA Fast, but SITA Fast takes less time.[13] In general, tests run with SITA Standard require approximately one-half the time of Full Threshold testing and approximately the same time as FASTPAC. SITA Fast takes approximately one-fourth of the time of Full Threshold and one-half the time of FASTPAC.[13] At present, the GHT is available for both SITA strategies. A new version of the GCP, not yet released, should be available soon for both SITA Standard and SITA Fast.

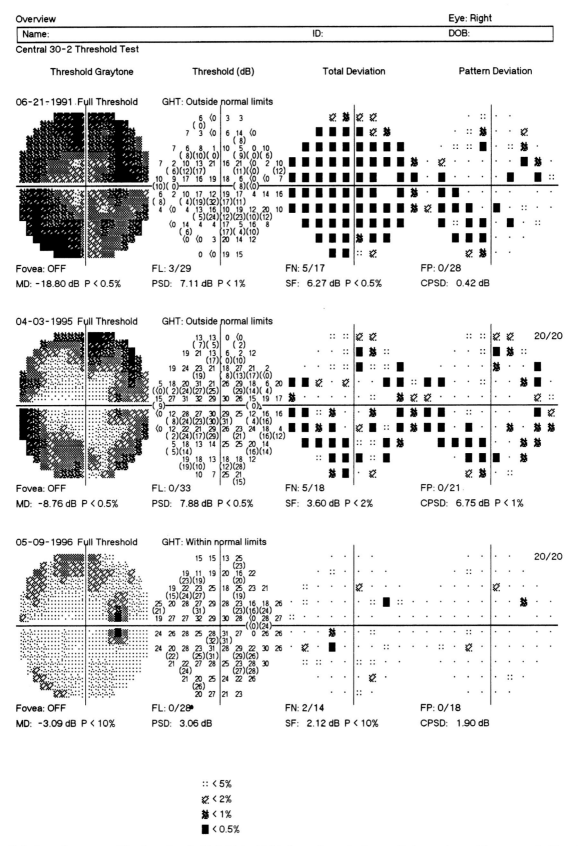

FIGURE 7-6. Learning curve. The first threshold field in 1991 showed marked overall depression with unremarkable reliability catch trials. The patient was not very responsive, and this type of behavior is often missed by standard catch trials. The second field shows somewhat better performance but still with marked fatigue artifact. By the third field, the test shows a mildly suspicious field with a normal glaucoma hemifield test message and no significant cluster in the pattern deviation plot.

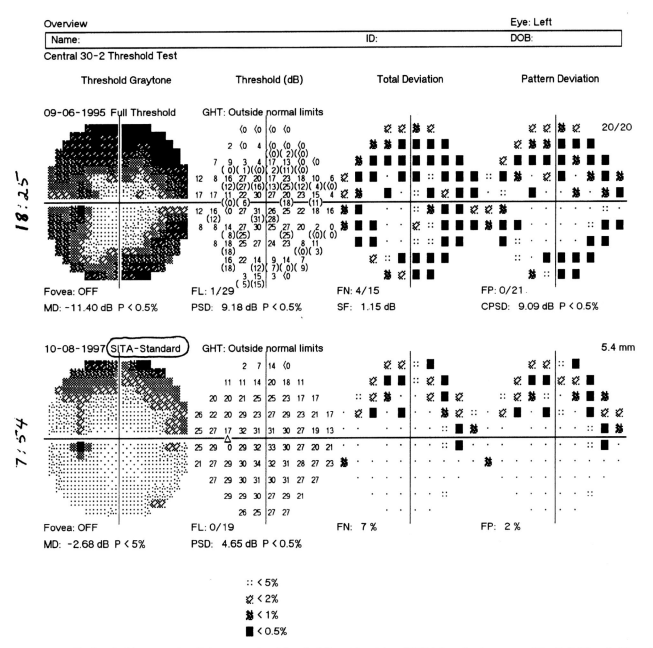

FIGURE 7-7. Full Threshold versus Swedish Interactive Thresholding Algorithm (SITA) Standard strategy. The Full Threshold took 18 minutes and 25 seconds for this patient and is marred by an overall constriction of the field representing a fatigue artifact. The field was repeated with SITA Standard, which took only 7 minutes and 54 seconds. With fatigue artifact removed, a superior arcuate defect is revealed that correlated to inferior rim tissue thinning of the optic nerve.

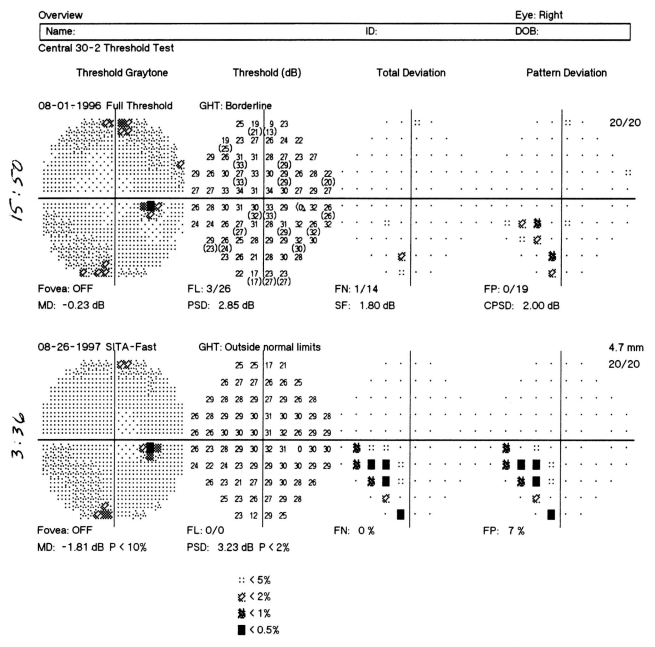

FIGURE 7-8. Full Threshold versus Swedish Interactive Thresholding Algorithm (SITA) Fast strategy. Test time was reduced from 15 minutes and 50 seconds to 3 minutes and 36 seconds by a shift from the Full Threshold to SITA Fast strategy. The Full Threshold field had no fatigue artifact despite the test time, and therefore the grayscale defect was similar in appearance in both fields.

Clinical Pearl:

There are, then, several options for patients undergoing field testing for the first time. For the HFA I, suprathreshold screening fields, threshold fields with FASTPAC, or threshold field testing with Full Threshold strategy can be used. Of these three, perhaps a suprathreshold test or FASTPAC threshold examination is the best field for patients without prior perimetric experience. Follow-up field tests should be performed with the Full Threshold strategy. If the patient fatigues with Full Threshold testing, the clinician should switch to the FASTPAC strategy. Users of the HFA II should select SITA Standard as the first field and use SITA Fast only for patients unable to perform SITA Standard without tiring.

After the initial field, follow-up fields should be kept as consistent as possible so that any change in the field is attributable to the disease process rather than a change in the testing condition. Keep the testing strategy the same, changing only to a faster strategy if patient fatigues with the initial strategy. Follow-up field testing should be carried out exclusively with either the 24-2 or 30-2 pattern, but it should not switch from one to the other. Whenever fixation is threatened (field loss extending within 5 degrees of fixation), a 10-2 test should also be used to follow the remaining central isle.

RELIABILITY INDICES

The next step in obtaining accurate, interpretable visual field results is ensuring that the test is reliable. The reliability indices serve as indicators of accuracy of fixation and consistency of the patient's responses. The following is a summary of reliability indices for the HFA I:

Increased FLs: Field is considered readable if false-negative and false-positive totals are acceptable. Monitor test stop examination, and plot blind spot if fixation losses occur in first 10 catch trials. Visual field tests with increased fixation losses may mask true defects.

Increased false-negatives: Consider field readable if fixation loss and false-positive totals are acceptable. Expect increase in false-negatives when visual field defect is large because of greater fluctuation of damaged receptor fields. If amount of damage is minimal or not expected, it probably represents patient fatigue or a patient who has changed his or her criteria for response during the test. Visual field tests with increased false-negatives look worse than expected from the optic nerve examination. These patients should be given frequent breaks during the test or switched to a shorter testing strategy.

Increased false-positives: No amount of false-positives is tolerable unless every threshold value is inspected (including repeated values) for points that are much greater in sensitivity compared with surrounding points. Regardless of fixation losses or false-negatives, any visual field test with unacceptable false-positives should be discarded, the patient reinstructed, and the test carried out again. Fields with increased false-positives mask defects and may show points of super sensitivity (white scotomas in grayscale, especially those with more than 38-dB threshold values).

Fixation Losses

Maintaining steady fixation on the central target is vital to accurate mapping of the field and for comparing follow-up test data. Often, a patient begins a test with steady fixation and gradually increases FLs by either tilting the head slightly during the test or losing attentiveness. The HFA I uses the Heijl-Krakau technique, which intentionally projects the target to an assumed location of the blind spot. If the patient's gaze is not on the fixation target, "seeing" retina is now in the predicted blind spot, and the patient responds to the light, which is recorded as an FL. The HFA I flags any FL score that equals or exceeds 20% of the total trials. However, the anatomic blind spot is not always where predicted, which can result in erroneous recordings of FLs. These may then lead the clinician to throw out the field as unreliable. To prevent this mistake, it has been recommended that if any FLs are recorded in the first 10 catch trials, the perimetrist should pause the test, have the instrument plot (find) the true blind spot, and then resume the test. This technique has been shown to greatly reduce the subsequently recorded FLs.[14] Alternatively, if the perimetrist constantly watches the patient, he or she can record a subjective interpretation in the patient's record without having to pause and lengthen the test. Constant monitoring of fixation by the perimetrist may negate the need to test fixation formally, and save time as well. When FLs are truly elevated, the resultant field is inconsistent with the rest of the clinical picture and usually looks better than the expected field (Figure 7-9).[15]

Gaze Tracking

The HFA II uses an entirely different technique to constantly monitor fixation wherein the alignment of corneal reflexes and the pupil are used. In the Heijl-Krakau technique, FL catch trials occur more frequently at the beginning of a test, so that a poorly fixating patient may be reinstructed and the test resumed. Very few catch trials occur at the end of the test, when the patient is likely to fatigue and lose fixation. Instead of intermittent catch trials dispersed throughout the test, the new technique records fixation at every stimulus presentation and displays a continuous bar graph in which the degree of fixation error is plotted over time as represented by the sequence of stimulus presentations (Figure 7-10). The newer technique provides a more accurate and representative assessment of the patient's fixation throughout the entire test. More importantly, no test time is devoted to FL catch trials. No agreed-on standard exists for indicating unreliable fixation using this technique, and the clinician is left to use subjective assessment of fixation. The clinician may choose to initially use both gaze tracking and blind-spot catch trials to serve as a reference until he or she becomes comfortable with interpreting gaze tracking.

False-Negatives

In Full Threshold and FASTPAC visual field testing, false-negative (FN) responses occur when a patient does not respond to a light that is 9 dB brighter than previously seen at the same location earlier in the examina-

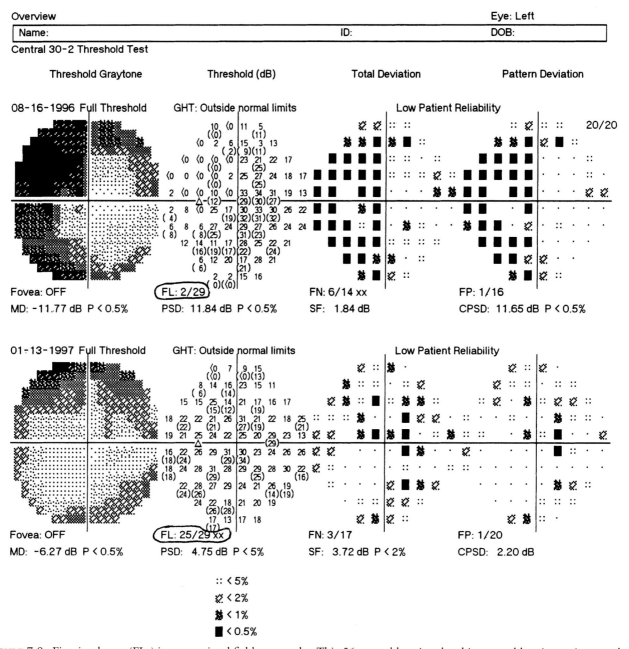

FIGURE 7-9. Fixation losses (FLs) improve visual field test results. This 56-year-old patient has bitemporal hemianopsia secondary to pituitary adenoma (only the left visual field is shown). In the second field, obtained just before surgery, the hemianopic defect "disappears" because of marked (25 out of 29) FLs. Patient "sees" in blind area because of constant searching.

tion. FNs are reported as a percentage of responses likely to be FNs (Figure 7-11A). Fatiguing, inattentive, or inconsistent patients have an increased number of FNs (Figure 7-11B). When FNs are elevated, the resultant field looks worse than the true field.[15] However, patients with glaucoma who are otherwise attentive and reliable, especially those with advanced disease, have been shown to have increased FNs compared with patients without glaucoma (Figure 7-11C).[16] Defective

areas vary more than normal areas in a glaucoma patient. The HFA flags any test with 33% or more FNs, but higher numbers have been suggested if the patient has advanced glaucoma damage to the optic nerve.

SITA threshold strategies take a different approach to FN testing. SITA looks at all the responses obtained at a given test point. It determines FNs by responses that occurred during threshold testing when a patient denied seeing a stimulus that was later found to be brighter

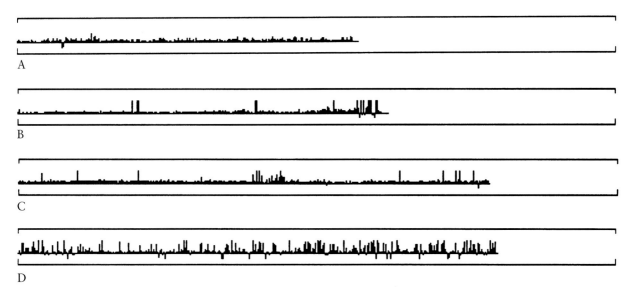

FIGURE 7-10. Gaze tracking interpretation. Gaze tracking provides constant rather than episodic monitoring. Upward deflections on graph represent gaze away from fixation, with the height of the bar representing the extent of the loss (up to 10 degrees). Downward deflections usually occur from either a blink or the loss by the gaze track on the edge of the pupil. (**A**) Normal gaze tracking: Patient maintained relatively steady gaze throughout the test. This gaze track display is representative of a compliant patient. There were no fixation losses recorded by the blind spot catch trial. (**B**) Late loss of fixation with fatigue: This patient maintained good fixation until the very end of test when his eyes began to wander. Of 16 fixation trials, only two losses were recorded. Fixation catch trials are more frequently tested in the beginning of the test than the end of the test. (**C**) Loss of fixation corrected with a pause in the test: Patient maintained good fixation until midway through the examination. The test was paused, and the patient rested. Patient then maintained good fixation until the very end of the test. The patient had no recorded fixation losses. (**D**) Poor fixation: Patient displayed erratic fixation throughout the test. Patient had more than 50% fixation losses with the blind spot monitor.

than the threshold found for that point. This is accomplished without having to spend time with a separate catch trial. When catch trials are performed, they occur only in normal areas of the field. FNs are reported as a percentage of responses likely to be FNs. Unlike FNs recorded by catch trials, FNs with SITA testing should not be elevated in glaucoma patients and should be assumed to be secondary to an inconsistent patient. Neither the manufacturer nor the literature has provided any suggested standards for abnormality.

False-Positives

In contrast to FNs, where patients deny seeing stimuli that are brighter than those previously seen for a point, false-positives (FPs) occur when patients claim to see a stimulus that wasn't presented (Figure 7-12). The instrument pauses during the testing routine without showing a stimulus, and if the patient responds, the response is recorded as an FP. These are typically recorded by patients who are anxious and afraid of doing poorly. The HFA flags the index when 33% of the trials are recorded as false-positive responses. However, Katz and Sommer have shown that even a 10% FP rate adversely affects the visual field examination.[15] Clinical experience has shown that even this figure may be too high. Any FP response should make the results suspect, and the field test should probably be discarded. Not only does the patient respond to lights that are not there, the patient responds to stimuli that are far too dim to have actually been seen. The grayscale of normal fields should also be searched for "white scotomas," or areas of hypersensitivity. The threshold values should likewise be inspected for values that are significantly better than surrounding values, especially if the obtained value is 38 dB or higher. When FPs are elevated, the resulting field test looks far better than the true field, masking defects.[15]

SITA eliminates catch trials for FPs and instead times a patient's response. If a patient responds to a stimulus faster than is known to be possible, that is considered an FP. SITA also measures the range of response times from a patient during a test, and if a particular response occurs significantly more quickly than the patient's previous responses, that response is considered an FP as well. SITA reports FPs as a percentage of responses that were likely to be FPs. Like FNs, there are no suggested criteria for abnormality for FP percentages determined with SITA testing.

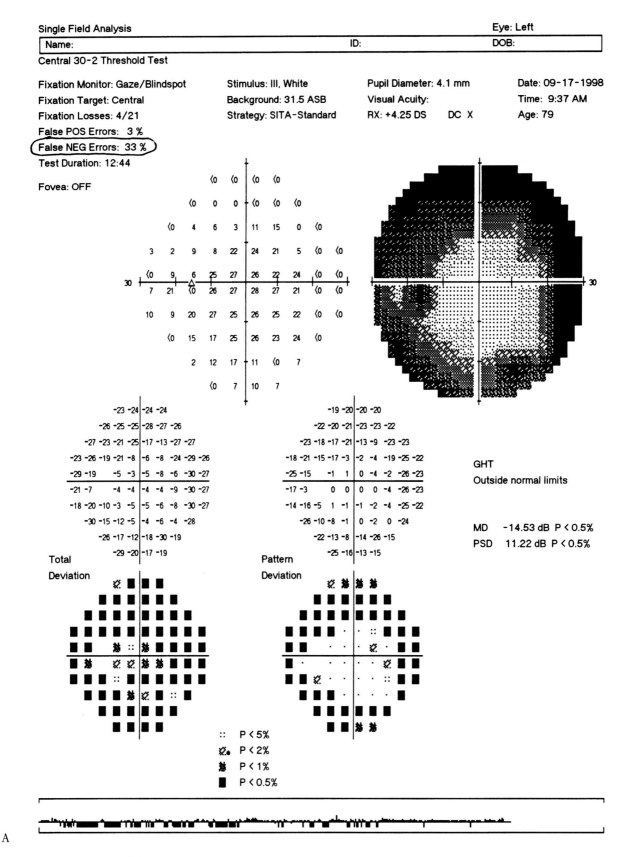

FIGURE 7-11. Increase in false negative (FN) errors. (A) Increased FN secondary to patient fatigue: With Swedish Interactive Thresholding Algorithm (SITA) testing, the FN errors are recorded at 33%. No set criteria are available for abnormal reliability indexes with SITA, but FNs greater than 10% should be viewed skeptically. In addition, the visual field looks much worse than would be expected from the appearance of the optic nerve. The generalized constriction of the visual field occurs because the far peripheral points are checked at the end of the test, when the patient is most tired.

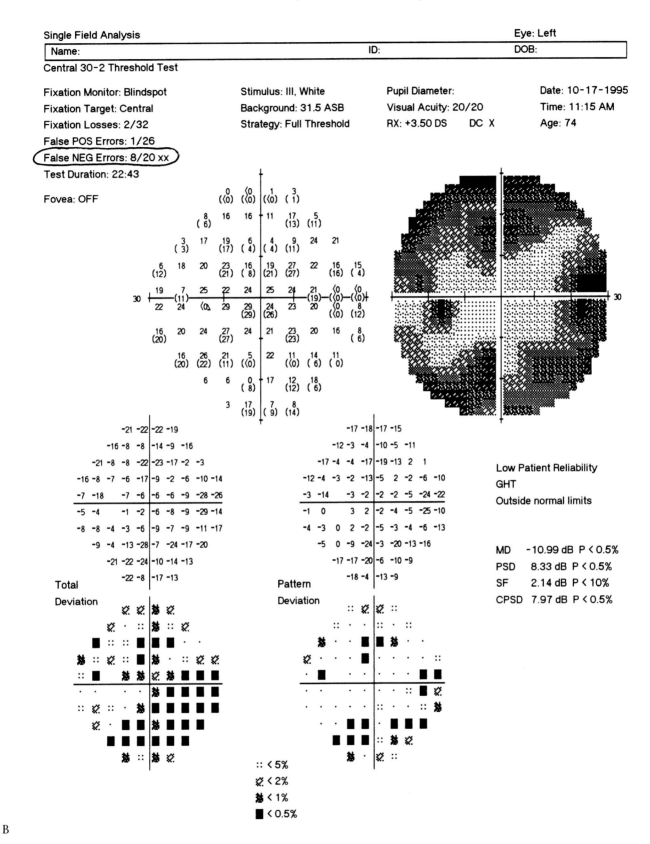

Name: ID: DOB:

Central 30-2 Threshold Test

Fixation Monitor: Blindspot   Stimulus: III, White   Pupil Diameter: Date: 10-17-1995
Fixation Target: Central   Background: 31.5 ASB   Visual Acuity: 20/20   Time: 11:15 AM
Fixation Losses: 2/32   Strategy: Full Threshold   RX: +3.50 DS   DC X   Age: 74
False POS Errors: 1/26
False NEG Errors: 8/20 xx
Test Duration: 22:43

Fovea: OFF

Low Patient Reliability
GHT
Outside normal limits

MD   -10.99 dB   P < 0.5%
PSD   8.33 dB   P < 0.5%
SF   2.14 dB   P < 10%
CPSD   7.97 dB   P < 0.5%

Total Deviation

Pattern Deviation

:: < 5%
⌀ < 2%
⊠ < 1%
■ < 0.5%

B

FIGURE 7-11. *(continued)* **(B)** Cloverleaf pattern: Increased FNs appear in a patient fatiguing during the test. The visual field looks much worse than would be expected from the appearance of the optic nerve. This cloverleaf pattern of visual field is a classic sign of patient fatigue. Four points in each quadrant just off fixation are tested during the beginning of the test. More peripheral points are tested at the end of the test. The cloverleaf pattern occurs because the patient is responding to the initially tested points but becomes unresponsive due to fatigue or lack of interest toward the end of the test. FNs were recorded as 8 out of 20.

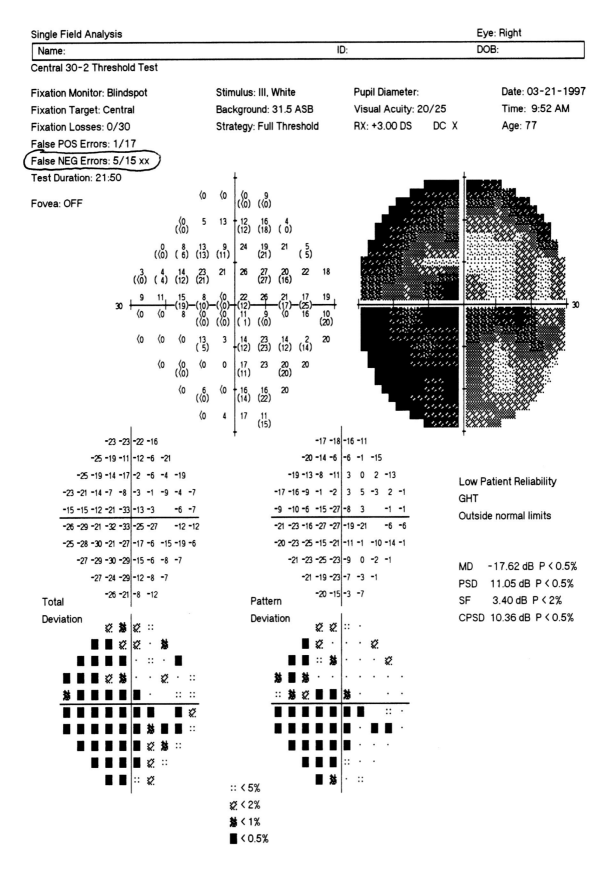

FIGURE 7-11. *(continued)* (C) Increased FNs in an advanced glaucoma patient: In a glaucoma patient with advanced visual field loss, an increase in FNs often occurs that is not necessarily a sign of inconsistency, but represents the high variability of ganglion receptor fields damaged by glaucoma. This endstage patient had otherwise reliable indices, but five FN responses out of 15 trials were recorded. In SITA testing, damaged areas of the visual field are not tested for FNs, theoretically improving its accuracy in determining patient fatigue.

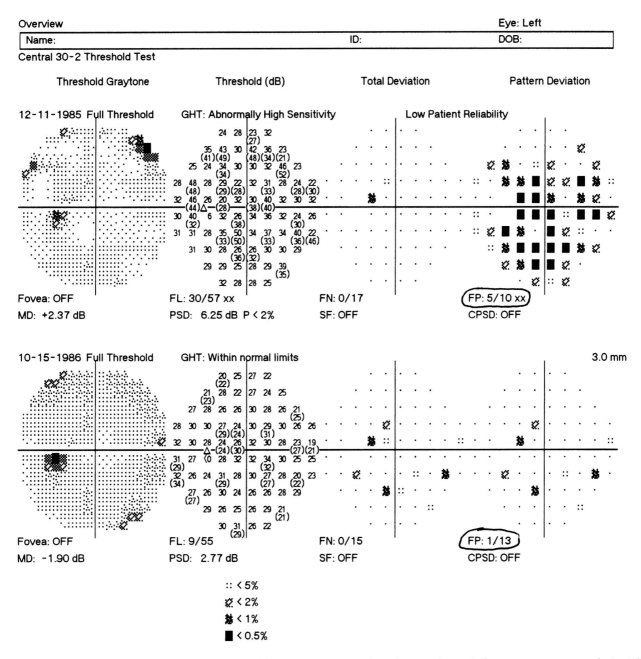

FIGURE 7-12. False positives (FPs), obvious and hidden. In 1985, FP catch trials were elevated (five FP responses out of 10 trials) with "white scotoma" present in the grayscale and threshold values exceeding 38 dBs. The total deviation plots are unremarkable. Because the point used to determine the general height indicator is much better than its expected value, the threshold values were markedly lowered and then appeared depressed in the pattern deviation plot, the opposite of pattern deviation reversal. Because of indiscriminate pushing of the response buttons, fixation losses (FLs) were also elevated. When the field was repeated in 1986, only 1 out of 13 FPs were recorded. However, inspection of the threshold values in the inferior temporal quadrant show values of 31, 32, and 34 dBs in the peripheral edge of the field, an unusually high sensitivity for this area. Inspection of other edge points show a sensitivity in the high 20s, more in line with what is expected. The patient is still showing a tendency to infrequent FPs that are not detected by the episodic catch trials. This could also be the result of wandering fixation.

Reliability Determination

The decision as to whether a visual field test should be discarded as unreliable is based on the assessment and integration of a number of factors. Visual field tests can first be classified as *reliable, unreliable,* or *readable*. In non-SITA visual field tests, if FL and FN are not flagged and there are no FP responses, and the field is consistent with the condition of the optic nerve, the test can be considered reliable. If both FL and FN are flagged, or more than one FP response is recorded, the field is unreliable. If a patient has increased FLs only and the perimetrist indicates that the patient fixated well despite the catch trial results, this field can be considered readable.[17] The results can be interpreted, bearing in mind that the field may look somewhat better than the true field. In a field tested with either Full Threshold or FASTPAC methods, if only FNs are flagged in a visual field with loss that was expected based on a damaged optic nerve, the field should also be considered readable, but it should be remembered that the field may look worse overall than the true field. Readable fields are kept but interpreted cautiously. For fields tested with SITA, it may be suggested that any field with more than 4% FPs or 12% FNs be viewed very skeptically. This is based solely on the author's opinion and initial experience with SITA. Formal studies have not been published to provide better guidance on this matter.

In non-SITA fields, even though there are no reliability indices flagged, the field may still be unreliable. Both FL and FP require the patient to press the button at an inappropriate time. Likewise, FN trials can only be performed at points that have at least 9 dB of sensitivity. A patient who is extremely unresponsive would therefore not be flagged, but the visual field result would be inconsistent with that predicted from the optic nerve. Also, during the course of serial follow-up fields, a normally reliable and responsive patient may experience a "bad day" where the reliability indices are unflagged but the field shows marked overall depression (Figure 7-13). On subsequent testing, the field returns to baseline.

ARTIFACTS, PSEUDODEFECTS, AND DEFECTS FROM OTHER DISEASES

Regardless of the testing strategy used, before a field can be interpreted for glaucomatous changes, it must first be assessed for artifacts (pseudodefects) and actual field defects that are the result of a disease other than glaucoma.

By far, the most common artifact is the learning curve, in which the initial field displays either an overall, concentric depression or focal defects that resolve on subsequent fields as the patient gains experience with the test (see Figure 7-6). For most patients, the learning curve flattens rather quickly, usually by the second field, although in some patients it may be longer than two fields. Caution should be exercised when interpreting a first field that shows defects because they may not be present on repeat testing.

Improper alignment of the trial lens holder results in a lens rim artifact (LRA) that may result in a dense concentric ring scotoma involving the edge points. If the trial lens holder is misaligned, only a

portion of the edge points may be depressed, mimicking a nasal step. A high refractive error can result in an LRA, with the trial lens thickness increasing the distance between the cornea and the lens edge, especially if a corrective cylindrical lens is also required. Any spherical prescription of more than 5 diopters should probably be corrected with a contact lens. Uncorrected refractive error causes an overall depression, and all patients should have a recent manifest refraction before field testing.[18,19]

The periorbital area and ocular media are common sources of visual field artifacts. The orbital rim can constrict the superior or supranasal fields beyond 30 degrees. Large noses with or without a head turn can cause defects that mimic inferior nasal steps. A palpebral fissure of 7 mm secondary to ptosis can cause a depression of at least 4 dB that extends inward to 24 degrees. It may extend all the way to fixation with a palpebral aperture of 5 mm, even though the pupil is not bisected by the lid (Figure 7-14).[20]

Clinically, media opacities, such as cataracts, have no effect other than an overall depression to all points, which is reflected in changes to the grayscale and total deviation plot (Figure 7-15).[21] The pattern deviation plot filters out the depression and is unaffected by overall depressions[22] (see the section Pattern Deviation Probability Plots). Pupils smaller than 2 mm may cause an overall depression, and most practitioners opt to dilate miotic pupils before testing. It is important that if pupils are dilated for one field, they should be dilated on all subsequent tests to maintain standard test conditions.

Retinal conditions, such as inflammatory and infectious diseases and vaso-occlusive events, which cause destruction of photoreceptors or axons, obviously lead to field defects (Figure 7-16). The defects are similar to those found in glaucoma.[23,24] Even diabetic retinopathy can cause relative and absolute defects secondary to areas of poorly perfused or nonperfused retina. Tilted discs, optic disc drusen, optic pits, anterior ischemic optic neuropathy, papillitis, chronic papilledema, and toxic optic neuropathy produce similar defects as well.[25]

Posterior chiasmal lesions, which are incongruous and incomplete, can produce defects that may be confused with anterior chiasmal lesions if care is not exercised when interpreting the visual field test results (Figure 7-17). Posterior chiasmal lesions generally respect the vertical midline and cause more temporal than nasal loss in one eye, and more nasal than temporal loss in the fellow eye. These visual field defects are most commonly misinterpreted when found in patients with an occult neurologic lesion. Patients with unexplained bilateral visual field defects that are greater temporally than nasal should be evaluated for a chiasmal lesion.

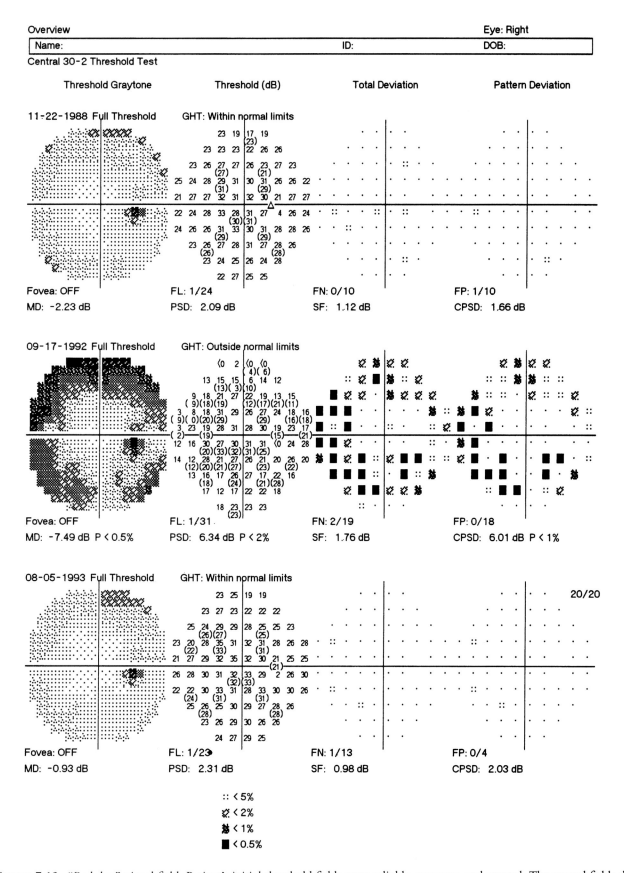

FIGURE 7-13. "Bad day" visual field. Patient's initial threshold fields were reliable, accurate, and normal. The second fields display a sudden worsening characterized by an overall depression, referred to as a *bad day field*, that was inconsistent with a stable clinical picture. The third field reverted back to the original status.

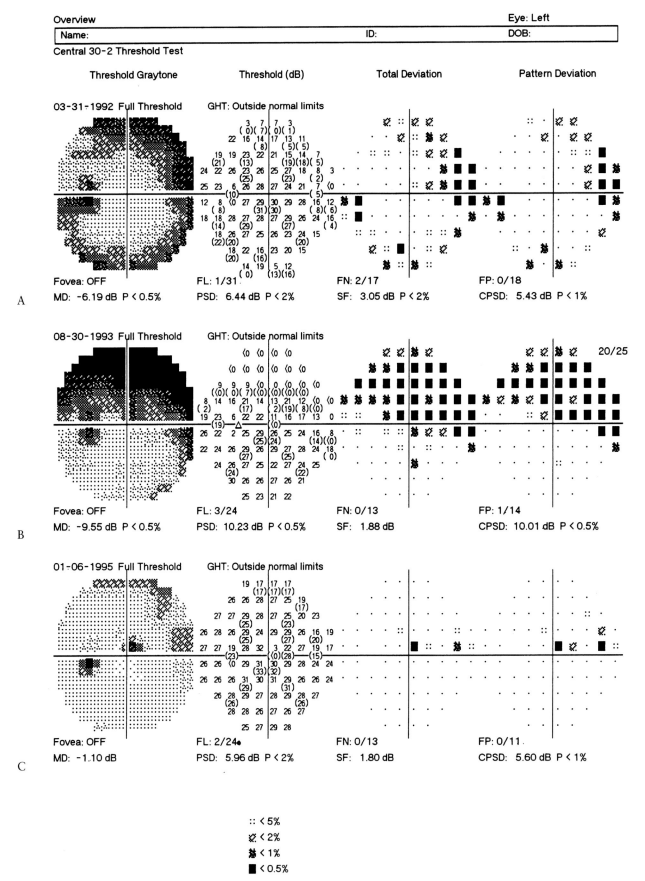

FIGURE 7-14. Upper lid artifact. This 80-year-old patient had progressive ptosis giving the false impression of rapid progression (**A** and **B**). In (**C**), the upper lid was taped, which removed the lid artifact and revealed the new central scotoma.

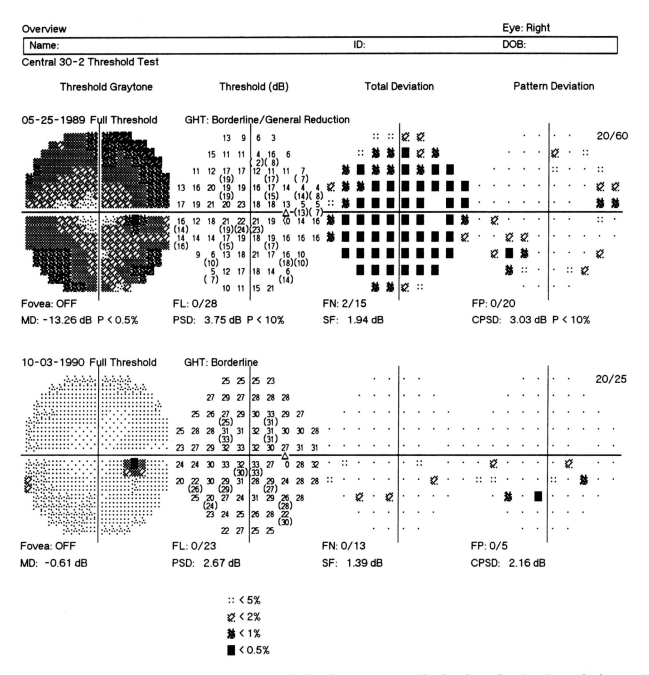

FIGURE 7-15. Cataract artifact. This glaucoma suspect had moderate cataract and reduced visual acuity. Grayscale shows uniform overall depression. The glaucoma hemifield test (GHT) shows borderline/general reduction of sensitivity. The total deviation plot shows uniformly abnormal *P* values. The pattern deviation plot corrects for overall depression from cataracts and miosis and shows an inferior nasal cluster. After cataract surgery, a marked overall improvement is seen in the grayscales and total deviation plots. Pattern deviation plots again suggest a mild abnormality in the inferior field, which correlates to superior nerve fiber layer and rim tissue thinning.

After visual field testing, the patient should be dilated and the field results reviewed with respect to the clinical examination. Close correlation of the visual field test with all other ocular findings is necessary to exclude nonglaucomatous field loss. Suspicion for nonglaucomatous etiology or poor visual field tester is high when the severity of field loss does not correlate to the extent or location of the optic nerve damage.

VISUAL FIELD INTERPRETATION

Field defects commonly found in early glaucoma are nasal steps, paracentral scotomas, and defects within

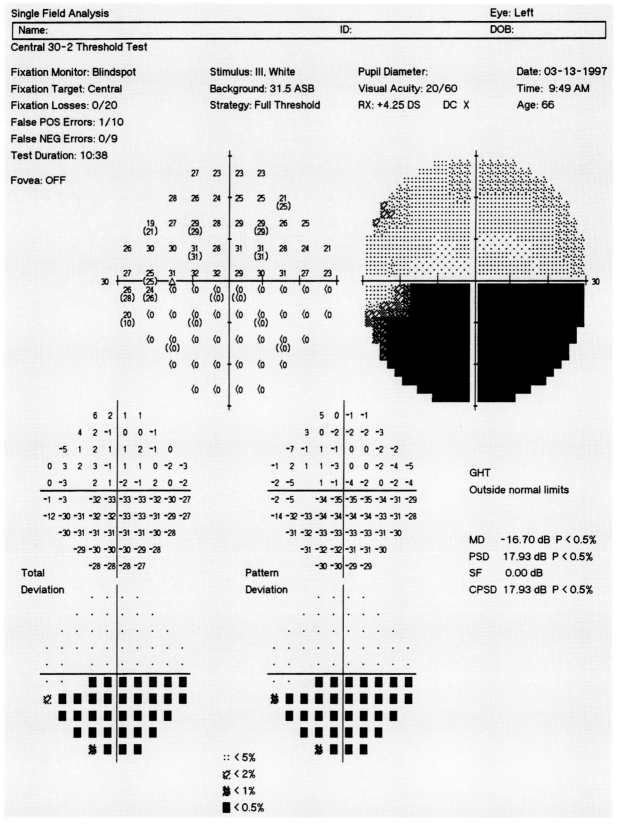

Single Field Analysis — Eye: Left

Central 30-2 Threshold Test

Fixation Monitor: Blindspot
Fixation Target: Central
Fixation Losses: 0/20
False POS Errors: 1/10
False NEG Errors: 0/9
Test Duration: 10:38

Fovea: OFF

Stimulus: III, White
Background: 31.5 ASB
Strategy: Full Threshold

Pupil Diameter:
Visual Acuity: 20/60
RX: +4.25 DS   DC X

Date: 03-13-1997
Time: 9:49 AM
Age: 66

GHT
Outside normal limits

MD   -16.70 dB P < 0.5%
PSD   17.93 dB P < 0.5%
SF   0.00 dB
CPSD 17.93 dB P < 0.5%

Total Deviation

Pattern Deviation

:: < 5%
⬚ < 2%
▦ < 1%
■ < 0.5%

A

FIGURE 7-16 (**A,B**). Glaucoma and branch retinal artery occlusion. Patient with normal tension glaucoma (both eyes) and a superior temporal retinal artery occlusion (left eye) (**A**). The right eye has a shallow, inferior arcuate defect that would be classified as *mild* (**B**). Note the inferior altitudinal field defect caused by superior artery occlusion in the left eye. There are several clues why the field defect in the left eye is caused by the artery occlusion. (*continued*)

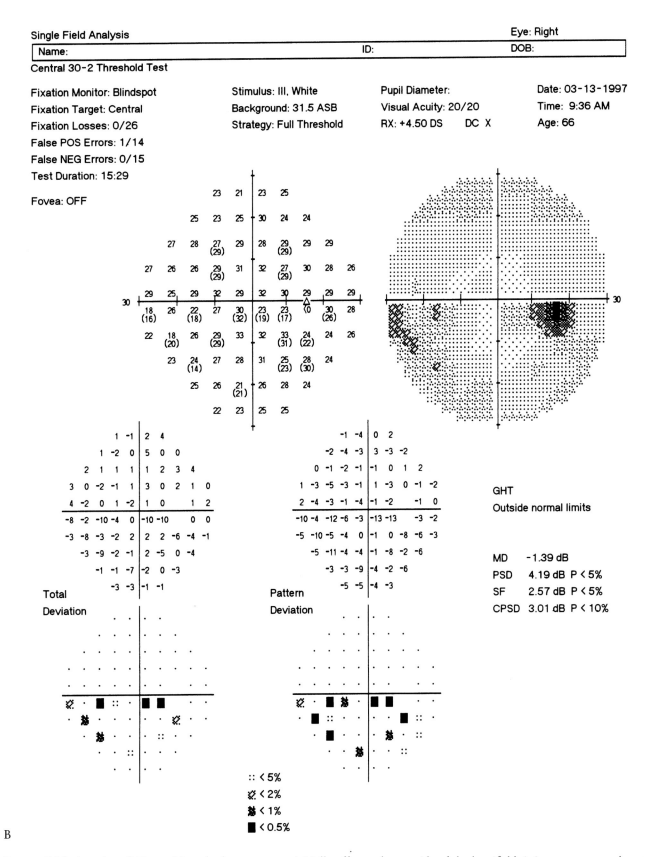

Name: ID: DOB:

Central 30-2 Threshold Test

Fixation Monitor: Blindspot   Stimulus: III, White   Pupil Diameter: Date: 03-13-1997
Fixation Target: Central   Background: 31.5 ASB   Visual Acuity: 20/20   Time: 9:36 AM
Fixation Losses: 0/26   Strategy: Full Threshold RX: +4.50 DS   DC X   Age: 66
False POS Errors: 1/14
False NEG Errors: 0/15
Test Duration: 15:29

Fovea: OFF

GHT
Outside normal limits

MD   -1.39 dB
PSD   4.19 dB P < 5%
SF   2.57 dB P < 5%
CPSD 3.01 dB P < 10%

Total Deviation

Pattern Deviation

:: < 5%
▨ < 2%
▩ < 1%
■ < 0.5%

B

FIGURE 7-16. *(continued)* First, although glaucoma may initially affect only one side of the hemifield, it is rare to see such total loss in one hemifield without the beginning of some defects in the other half. Second, even in endstage glaucoma, it is not common to see such total loss in the entire hemifield; usually one or two points within the defect still respond. And third, clinically the optic nerve cupping was similar in both eyes, and therefore the field loss was disproportionate to the status of the optic nerves.

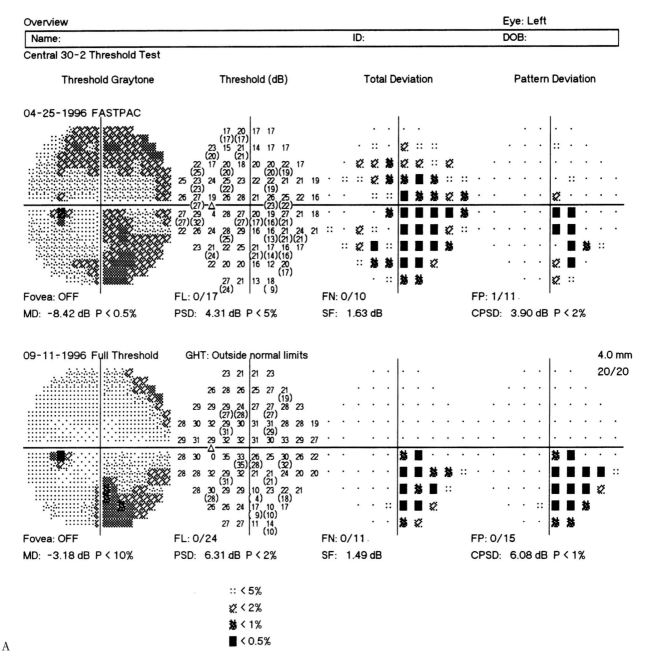

FIGURE 7-17. Posterior chiasmal defect mimicking glaucoma. This 50-year-old glaucoma suspect had a cup-to-disc ratio of 0.6–0.7. First field was done with FASTPAC. Total deviation plot in the left eye (**A**) shows an overall depression, especially in the nasal field, suggesting glaucoma damage. However, the pattern deviation plot shows a nasal defect that respects the vertical midline once the overall depression (part of the first field learning curve) is removed.

the arcuate bundles (Figure 7-18). With advanced disease, further axonal loss causes these defects to coalesce. Typically, one-half of the field is damaged extensively before the second half becomes equally involved. With endstage disease, only a central and/or temporal isle remains.

After ascertaining that the correct visual field was tested and that the test results are reliable, the field is inspected for these defects. The determination of

whether a defect exists is based on the comparison of the obtained data to an average value for normal. The critical issue is what value is used for "normal" and how it was determined. For Goldmann kinetic perimetry, commonly accepted definitions of a defect are available.[26] The definition for a paracentral defect (0.5 log unit or 5 dB below the expected value) became the de facto standard when the transition was made from kinetic to automated perimetry. Early software was

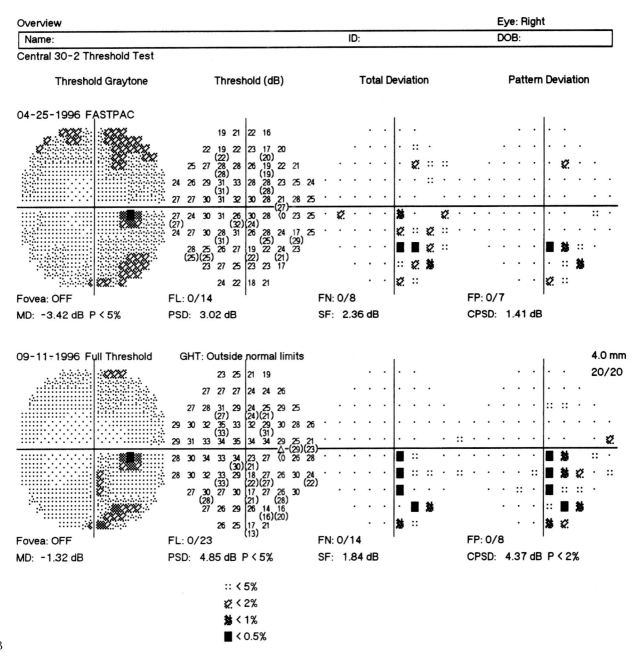

Overview   Eye: Right

| Name: | | ID: | DOB: |

Central 30-2 Threshold Test

Fovea: OFF

MD: −3.42 dB P < 5%   FL: 0/14   FN: 0/8   FP: 0/7

PSD: 3.02 dB   SF: 2.36 dB   CPSD: 1.41 dB

Fovea: OFF   GHT: Outside normal limits   4.0 mm   20/20

MD: −1.32 dB   FL: 0/23   FN: 0/14   FP: 0/8

PSD: 4.85 dB P < 5%   SF: 1.84 dB   CPSD: 4.37 dB P < 2%

:: < 5%
⊘ < 2%
▧ < 1%
■ < 0.5%

B

FIGURE 7-17. *(continued)* The right eye **(B)** deviation plots show an inferior temporal defect that also respects the vertical midline. The field was repeated, which confirmed the inferior quadrantanopsia. Magnetic resonance imaging revealed a left parietal lobe lesion thought to be secondary to either trauma or ischemia.

developed to show which points deviated from the expected value for normal by more than 4 dB. In these early versions of the HFA, the hill of vision was considered to have a fixed shape that did not change with age and was symmetric in all four quadrants.

As experience was gained, it became apparent that the hill of vision was not symmetric, nor did it remain the same shape throughout life.[10,12,27,28] More important, it was discovered that the proximity of a point to fixation determined how close a point would come to the average value. When a point around fixation is mea-

sured in a group of normal patients, a median value is determined that becomes the expected value. Because of normal variation, some patients may test at a value that is lower or higher than the median. The highest and lowest values in the normal group define the range of normal values. As long as the measured test value falls within this range of normal values, the point is considered normal. Points closer to fixation have a very small range (i.e., few points are greater or lesser than the expected value). Therefore, a point that is 5 dB less than the predicted value is highly unlikely to occur by chance

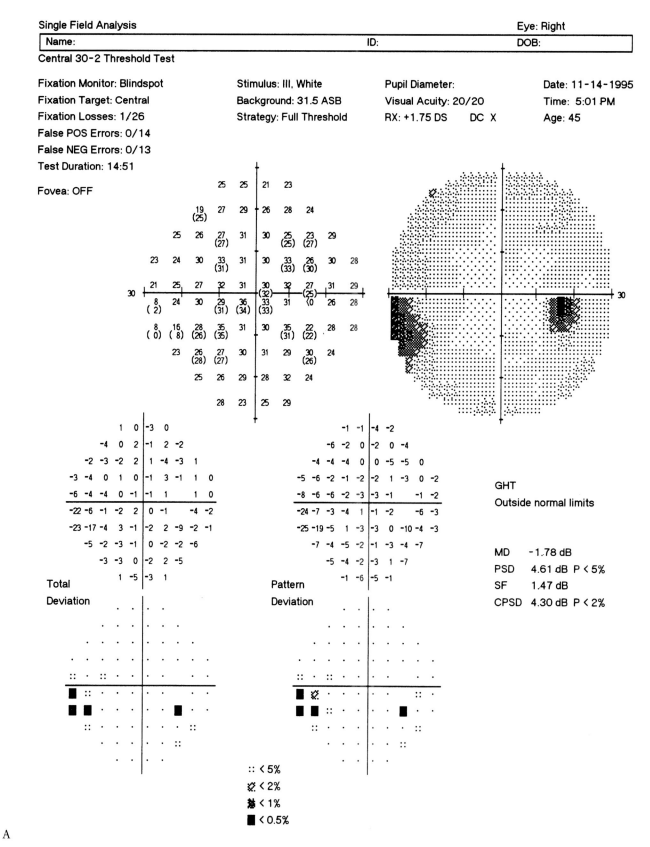

FIGURE 7-18. Common initial glaucoma visual field defects. (A) Nasal step.

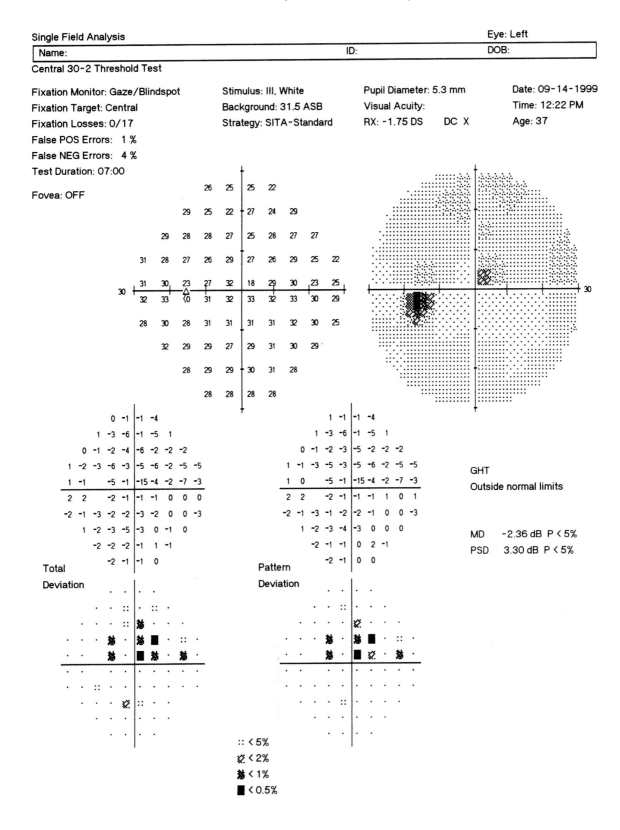

Single Field Analysis   Eye: Left

| Name: | ID: | DOB: |

Central 30-2 Threshold Test

Fixation Monitor: Gaze/Blindspot   Stimulus: III, White   Pupil Diameter: 5.3 mm   Date: 09-14-1999
Fixation Target: Central   Background: 31.5 ASB   Visual Acuity: Time: 12:22 PM
Fixation Losses: 0/17   Strategy: SITA-Standard RX: -1.75 DS   DC X   Age: 37
False POS Errors: 1 %
False NEG Errors: 4 %
Test Duration: 07:00

Fovea: OFF

```
            26  25   25  22
          29  25  22   27  24  29
        29  28  28  27   25  28  27  27
      31  28  27  26  29   27  26  29  25  22
      31  30  23  27  32   18  29  30  23  25
   30 ─ 32  33  0  31  32   33  32  33  30  29 ─ 30
      28  30  28  31  31   31  31  32  30  25
        32  29  29  27   29  31  30  29
          28  29  29   30  31  28
            28  28   28  28
```

```
Total                                   Pattern
Deviation                               Deviation

      0  -1 │-1  -4                          1  -1 │-1  -4
    1  -3  -6│-1  -5   1                   1  -3  -6│-1  -5   1
  0  -1  -2  -4│-6  -2  -2  -2           0  -1  -2  -3│-5  -2  -2  -2
1  -2  -3  -6  -3│-5  -6  -2  -5  -5   1  -1  -3  -5  -3│-5  -6  -2  -5  -5
1  -1     -5  -1│-15 -4  -2  -7  -3   1   0     -5  -1│-15 -4  -2  -7  -3
─────────────────────────────────    ─────────────────────────────────
2   2     -2  -1│-1  -1   0   0   0   2   2     -2  -1│-1  -1   1   0   1
-2 -1  -3  -2  -2│-3  -2   0   0  -3  -2 -1  -3  -1  -2│-2  -1   0   0  -3
  1  -2  -3  -5│-3   0  -1   0         1  -2  -3  -4│-3   0   0   0
    -2  -2  -2│-1   1  -1               -2  -1  -1│ 0   2  -1
      -2  -1│-1   0                        -2  -1│ 0   0
```

GHT
Outside normal limits

MD   -2.36 dB P < 5%
PSD   3.30 dB P < 5%

```
:: < 5%
▨ < 2%
▨ < 1%
■ < 0.5%
```

B

FIGURE 7-18. (B) Paracentral scotoma. (*continued*)

Single Field Analysis   Eye: Right

Name:	ID:	DOB:

Central 30-2 Threshold Test

Fixation Monitor: Gaze/Blindspot   Stimulus: III, White   Pupil Diameter: 6.1 mm   Date: 08-07-1997
Fixation Target: Central   Background: 31.5 ASB   Visual Acuity: 20/20   Time: 10:12 AM
Fixation Losses: 4/30   Strategy: Full Threshold   RX: +6.50 DS   DC X   Age: 66
False POS Errors: 1/21
False NEG Errors: 2/20
Test Duration: 18:41

Fovea: OFF

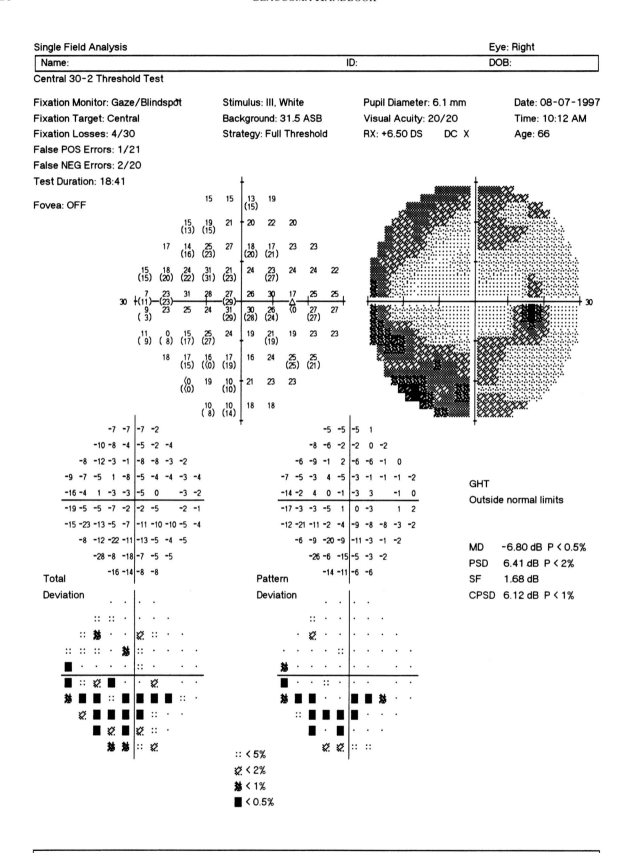

GHT
Outside normal limits

Total Deviation

Pattern Deviation

MD   -6.80 dB P < 0.5%
PSD   6.41 dB P < 2%
SF   1.68 dB
CPSD   6.12 dB P < 1%

:: < 5%
⌀ < 2%
⫶ < 1%
■ < 0.5%

C

FIGURE 7-18. (*continued*) (C) Defects in the arcuate bundles.

and represents a significant deviation from normal. However, the farther the point is from fixation, the larger the range of normal values. At 15 degrees superiorly from fixation, the range of normal values extends 5 dB on either side of the expected value. At 27 degrees superiorly from fixation, a value that is 20 dB lower than the age-matched expected value still falls within 95% of normal values.[12] Therefore, to determine whether a point is defective, knowledge of only the depth of the defect is insufficient.

Probability Values

Test points in early glaucoma are only mildly depressed, and the values for these abnormal points overlap the lowest values for normal. Threshold values within this overlapping area may represent early disease or the lower limit of normal and must, therefore, be viewed cautiously. STATPAC identifies where a point's obtained threshold value falls in a range of age-matched normal values stored in the on-board computer. The range of normal values is ranked from best to worst. *Normal* is defined as the values that range up to the 95th percentile. Statistical significance is assigned based on the percentile rank of a test value. When a test point's value is just above the 95th percentile, it is assigned a probability value of P <5%, meaning that only 4% of the age-matched normals have this value or worse. Probability values of P <2%, P <1%, and P <.5% are designated similarly.[29,30] It should be remembered that although these points are statistically significant, they are not necessarily abnormal. Probability values indicate the frequency at which the test results occur in normals.

Grayscale

A systematic review of the printout is the easiest approach to determining whether a field defect is present. The printout is similar for the Full Threshold, FASTPAC, and SITA field testing methods. First, the grayscale is inspected; most experienced clinicians view the grayscale with caution. The grayscale merely offers a shading of gray to represent the threshold values. It is easily influenced by artifact, and the interpreter of the results must remember that the areas between test points are interpolated, whereas the areas outside the test points are extrapolated. Further, because the hill of vision has a different shape for different ages and has an overall decline in sensitivity with age, the grayscale for a normal 20-year-old looks much different than one for a normal 70-year-old. Therefore, the grayscale should serve mostly as a first look, drawing attention to suspicious areas. The grayscale has a more useful role when evaluating a series of visual fields for progression.

Threshold Values

Included in the printout are the actual threshold values obtained during the test. Certain artifacts can be assessed by the threshold values, such as lid droop, which causes a horizontal row of threshold values of less than zero. In general, the probability plots are more useful than threshold values in the detection of defects. Threshold values are most useful in establishing the severity of the field loss and following the visual field tests for progression.

Total Deviation Probability Plots

Next is the inspection of the total deviation probability plots. The obtained value is compared with the stored range of age-matched normal values, assigned a probability of normal (see the section Probability Values), and displayed symbolically with a small dot for a point within the range of 95% of the normal values or with a shaded box (outside of 95% of normal values), indicating suspicion for abnormality (<5%, <2%, <1%, or <.5%). The darker the shade of gray in the box, the less frequently it occurs in normals. The total deviation probability plots will highlight shallow scotomas that are not noted by the grayscale. Because the probability plots do not interpolate between points like the grayscale, defects may not look exactly as they would with the grayscale or with isopter lines drawn with Goldmann kinetic perimetry.

Pattern Deviation Probability Plots

When the STATPAC database was being collected, patients with significant media opacities or miotic pupils were excluded because these conditions cause an overall depression. The total deviation plots assume the patient does not have a media opacity or miosis and that any depressed value is secondary to disease. However, in clinical practice, patients are far from the ideal. Many elderly patients have media opacities that depress the hill of vision. Other elderly patients have had cataract surgery, with media better than the database and point values that exceed the expected. Thus, these patients may exhibit either an overall depression or an elevation compared with the expected average values.

To compensate for this, a correction is made to the values of the test points. The deviation from expected value for each point (excluding edge points) is computed and then ranked. The value of the seventh-best point is then chosen to "correct" all the other values. This value is referred to as the *general height indicator*. If the point is better than expected, all values are lowered. If the point is worse than expected, all points are raised by the difference between the general height indicator and the obtained value. When the new value has been computed, it is again compared with a database, with the resultant analysis now displayed in the pattern deviation probability plots. When no significant overall depression is seen, the total and pattern deviation plots are similar. Conversely, overall depression causes the total and pattern deviation probability plots to differ. Studies have shown that the pattern deviation probability plot effectively filters out the depression from media opacities, highlighting focal defects, and pointing out the usefulness of this analysis (see Figure 7-15).[21,22]

Although some controversy exists as to whether mild overall depression can be seen as the earliest visual field loss,[31,32] it is well recognized to be present in later stages of glaucoma. The pattern deviation plots indiscriminately filter out depression caused by both artifact and real disease (Figure 7-19). When the pattern deviation plot looks better than the total deviation plot, the practitioner must decide whether significant media opacity or mitosis was present. If not, then the total deviation plot represents the true status of the field. If significant artifact from either media opacification or miosis is present, then the pattern deviation plot is the preferred analysis.

One final point should be made: When a 24-2 or 30-2 test is run on a patient with only a small central isle remaining, the seventh-best point might be severely depressed. This causes a very large correction to be added back to all points, so that severely depressed points now look normal (Figure 7-20). In this situation, the total deviation plots are all black boxes, whereas the pattern deviation plots reveal little, if any, defect. This has been termed *pattern deviation reversal*.[33]

Global Indices

Last, the global indices are inspected. In general, the global indices give a snapshot or quick overview of the field. The indices are computations with weighted points; that is, more value is given to points closer to fixation. But when the data from all the test points are combined into a single number, the spatial information from the test points is lost. For example, the MD index (see below) is the same value for a patient with a dense altitudinal defect as it is for a hemianopic loss. As in recording the probability plots, a probability value is assigned to each global index result that falls outside the range of 95% of normals.

MEAN DEVIATION

The MD index is the average deviation (difference) of each point from its expected value. It gives a quick assessment of the overall condition of the field. It has poor sensitivity in identifying a glaucomatous field because small, shallow defects are averaged out and overlooked.[17] The index is too easily influenced by cataracts and miosis, decreasing its specificity.

Short-Term Fluctuation

During the course of a Full Threshold or FASTPAC examination, 10 points are retested. The difference between the first and second value for each point is used for a weighted root mean square computation, the STF. The STF is an indicator of how consistent the patient's responses are. Historically, the STF index was thought to be an early indicator of glaucoma, but it did not prove useful in this respect. The index is also used as a quantitative measure of the consistency of responses. However, FN catch trials can provide a qualitative assessment that is just as useful, but less time consuming. Therefore, the STF global index is of limited use, and many practitioners elect to turn it off during testing. Without STF on, only four points are retested (part of the instrument initialization procedures), thus eliminating six points and shortening the test (see the section Test Selection).

Pattern Standard Deviation/ Corrected Pattern Standard Deviation

The pattern standard deviation (PSD) index measures the shape of the hill of vision and is elevated when focal defects are present. Next to the numeric value is a computed probability value, which only appears when the numeric value falls outside of the 95% range of normal. The corrected pattern standard deviation (CPSD) is similar to the PSD, but first "smoothes out" the hill of vision by using the STF index. When STF is off, CPSD is not computed. As is explained later, the PSD and CPSD are equally useful in assessing a visual field, and many practitioners elect to keep STF turned off.

So far in the initial analysis sequence, a visual field test is first appraised for being the correct test pattern and if the examination is reliable. Next, the grayscale, total deviation, and pattern deviation plots are inspected, in that order, for any discernible glaucomatous defect. Last, the global indices are quickly reviewed.

IDENTIFYING A GLAUCOMATOUS VISUAL FIELD LOSS

The presence of a nasal step or arcuate defect makes the diagnosis of a visual field loss straightforward, but most results with automated perimetry are not as clear-cut. Although threshold testing is more sensitive than manual perimetry in finding defects,[34] single points or even clusters of apparently defective points can be seen in normal visual fields.[10] The decision as to whether a defect is a paracentral scotoma or a statistical anomaly is challenging, especially in the presence of an overall depression.

As an aid to analysis, several algorithms are available, either on printout or computed by the practitioner

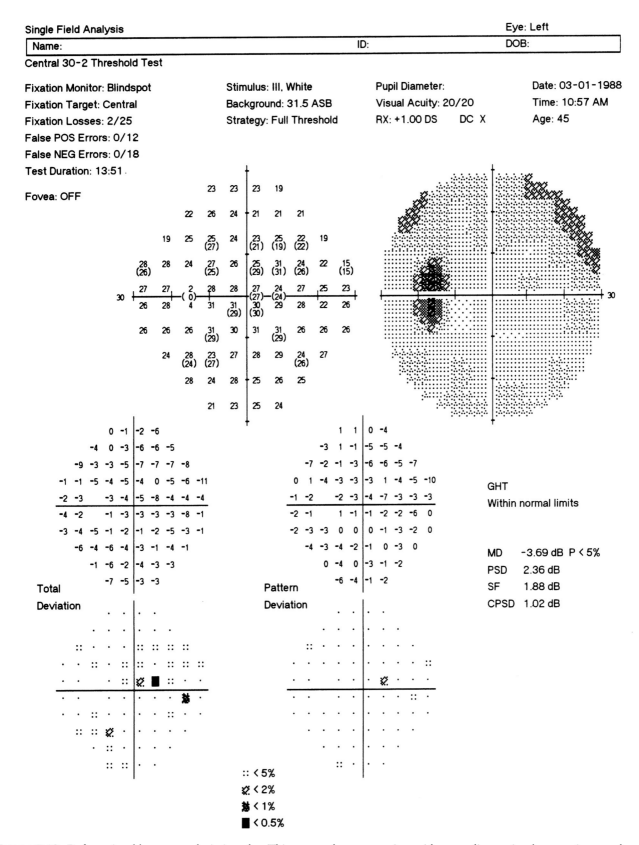

FIGURE 7-19. Defect missed by pattern deviation plot. This young glaucoma patient without media opacity shows an improved pattern deviation plot from the total deviation plot. In this patient, there is no media opacity and pupil size is normal. The overall depression "corrected" by the pattern deviation plot was caused by glaucoma, not media opacification. The nerve fiber layer shows an inferior wedge defect that corresponds to the superior nasal total pattern deviation plot. When no media opacity or miosis is present, the total deviation plot is the more accurate probability plot to interpret.

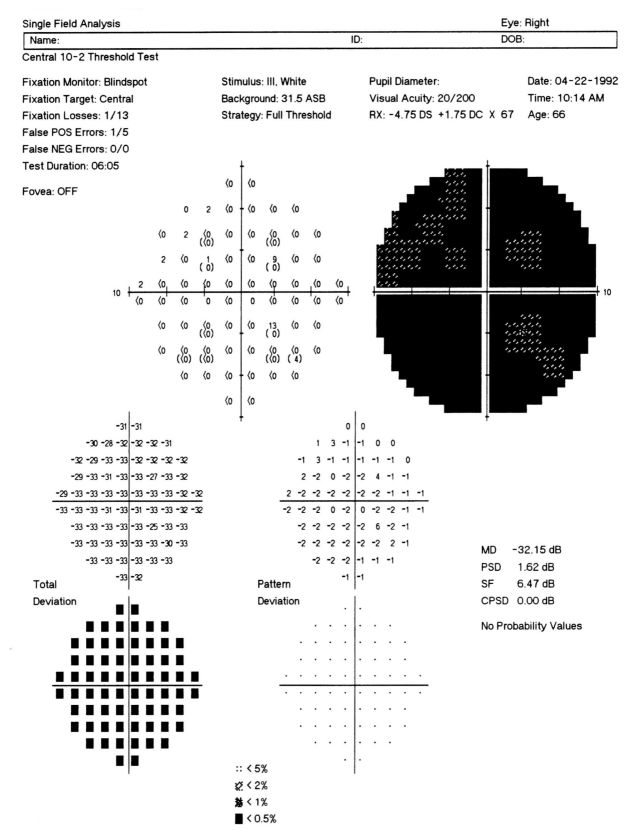

FIGURE 7-20. Pattern deviation reversal. Central 10-2 visual field shows an endstage field with very few points responsive to size III test target. Pattern deviation reversal has occurred in the pattern deviation probability plots, which falsely appear intact. With so few points responding to the size III stimulus, switching to the size V target is indicated (see Figure 7-31).

(Table 7-1). Three common analytic techniques take slightly different approaches to determining whether a field is abnormal. One approach assumes that although one or two points may be randomly abnormal, it is unlikely that a cluster of abnormal points exists by chance alone. A significant cluster of points is usually regarded as a defect. The definition of a *significant cluster* varies in the literature,[35–38] but it typically consists of three or more contiguous points on the same side of the horizontal meridian. (If the 30-2 pattern is used, no edge points are included except the two most nasal points straddling the horizontal meridian, whereas all points are considered in the 24-2 pattern.) Criteria differ in how they define which points are included in the cluster. Most criteria require that at least one of the three points be significantly depressed and the other two at least mildly depressed. For example, one point would have to be 10 dB lower than the expected value, whereas the other two would have to be at least 5 dB lower than expected.[36]

However, as mentioned in the Visual Field Interpretation section, it has been shown that in certain parts of the field, even 10-dB defects are not considered significant. Also, a normal hill of vision that has an overall depression secondary to cataracts or miosis has many depressed areas with false significant clusters. To compensate for these drawbacks, other cluster criteria have been proposed by Katz and colleagues.[17] In their cluster criterion, three contiguous abnormal points are searched for in the *pattern deviation* probability plots. If the 30-2 pattern is used, no edge points are included except the

two most nasal points next to the horizontal meridian, whereas all points are considered in the 24-2. At least one of the points has to be significant at the P <1% level. All points in the cluster must respect the horizontal meridian. By using the probability plots, the question of whether 10 dB is significant is answered. Overall depression from media opacities is compensated for by using the pattern deviation plots.

A similar approach to identifying a focal abnormality in the visual field is to evaluate the corrected standard pattern deviation (CPSD) from the global indices. The CPSD measures the shape of the hill of vision and is elevated when focal defects are present. If this value falls outside of the 90% of normal range, a probability value appears beside the number. If the probability value is less than 5%, then the visual field is considered abnormal.[17] If STF is not performed, then CPSD is not calculated. In this case, the PSD probability value can be used.

A third technique relies on the fact that one-half of the field is damaged first in glaucoma, progressing to moderate or severe loss before the other half becomes significantly involved. Therefore, one-half of the field can be used as the "normal" visual field and compared with the other half (superior versus inferior). The mirror-image analysis compares groups of points, or sectors, that correspond to areas of arcuate defects or nasal steps.[39] This technique requires the practitioner to add up the threshold values within one sector and compare the total to that in the mirror-image sector. If the difference between any two mirror-image sectors exceeds a predetermined amount, the field is considered abnormal. (Note: this technique has only been studied for glaucoma.) Overall depression is not a factor because it affects the entire field uniformly, and only a difference between halves is significant. However, to recognize visual fields that are severely depressed overall by disease, the analysis also adds all the sectors together and compares the total to a predetermined value. Use of the mirror-image analysis requires time-consuming manual calculations or a separate computer analysis[40] and is valid only for the 30-2 test pattern. The sensitivity and specificity are well established,[17,41] but the extensive calculations are not clinically practical.

Asman and Heijl further refined the cross-meridional strategy by developing the GHT.[42,43] Their analysis differs from the original mirror-image analysis in several ways. First, they used different paired sectors that they felt more closely matched the distribution of nerve fiber layer bundle defects (Figure 7-21). Second, instead of using raw threshold values, they computed differences between paired sectors based on probability values within the pattern deviation plots. Using probability plots eliminated overcalling 5-dB defects in the outer edge of the field. Using pattern deviation plots eliminated false identification of defects caused by overall

TABLE 7-1. Criteria for an Abnormal Field

If any one of the following three criteria is present on a repeatable visual field test, the visual field is considered abnormal.

1. Cluster criteria[17]

Three nonedge (but including on a 30-2 test the two most nasal points straddling the horizontal meridian and all points on the 24-2), contiguous (must be touching) points on the same side of horizontal median. On inspection of the pattern deviation probability plots, all three points must be identified as significant (P <5%), with at least one at the P <1% level.

2. Glaucoma hemifield test[17,42,43]

"Outside normal limits" message.

3. Corrected pattern deviation global index[17]

Corrected pattern standard deviation index significant at P <5% or more. (Note: If short-term fluctuation is turned off, use pattern standard deviation global index with the same criteria.)

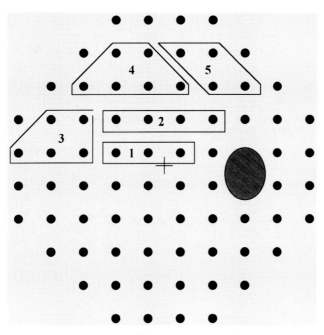

FIGURE 7-21. Diagram of the sectors used for the glaucoma hemifield test. Each of the five sectors in the superior field is compared with the mirror-image sector in the inferior field because glaucoma preferentially damages one-half of the optic nerve first.

depressions. Third, the analysis stratifies the field into "outside normal limits," "borderline," and "within normal limits" rather than "abnormal" versus "normal" classification of the mirror-image analysis. Fourth, the GHT attempts to find shallow, *symmetric* visual field loss between paired sectors by looking to see whether both sectors are depressed at a significant level. Finally, the general height indicator's value is analyzed and used to note whether the whole field has a statistically significant overall depression or is suspiciously overly sensitive. The GHT performs its analysis automatically and records it on the printout. The sensitivity and specificity of the GHT have been validated against patients with Goldmann visual field loss as the gold standard, and against patients with glaucomatous optic nerves regardless of visual field status. It has become the de facto standard for judging whether a visual field is normal.[5] The following is a list of glaucoma hemifield test messages and their definitions:

Outside normal limits: Either an upper zone differs from its corresponding lower zone at a P <1% level, or two corresponding zones are both depressed relative to normal at a P <.5% level.

Borderline: An upper zone differs from its corresponding lower zone at a P <3% level, but above the P <1% level.

General reduction sensitivity: The overall height of the hill of vision is reduced at a P <.5% level, but the

field does not satisfy the criteria for outside normal limits. The field may be borderline.

Abnormally high sensitivity: The overall height of the hill of vision is unusually high at a P <.5% level. With this occurrence, the upper and lower zones are not compared.

Within normal limits: None of the above criteria is met.

Clinical Pearl:
In clinical practice, a combination of techniques may be more useful than relying on a single technique for determining abnormality (Figure 7-22). Using a combination of techniques may help compensate for the individual deficiencies of a single analysis. After the initial analysis sequence has been completed the PSD index, the CPSD index, or both is checked; the GHT analysis is checked; and the PSD probability plots are inspected for a significant cluster defect. Despite the reasonable sensitivity and specificity of these algorithms, ultimately the clinician must be the final arbiter, integrating all other clinical information and using sound judgment in assessing the visual field. When a visual field defect is present, a second test should be performed to confirm the result and uncover any learning curve effect.[44] Visual field loss should be correlated to the optic nerve and nerve fiber before glaucoma is diagnosed as the cause of the defect.

CLASSIFYING THE SEVERITY OF FIELD LOSS

Once a visual field loss has been diagnosed, an assessment should be made to determine the severity of the defect. This information, combined with the assessment of optic nerve and nerve fiber layer damage and other risk factors, determines the initial target pressures for intraocular pressure (IOP) control. Hodapp and associates developed arbitrary, but useful, criteria classifying visual field loss into mild (Figure 7-23), moderate (Figure 7-24), or severe loss (Figure 7-25).[45] These criteria look at the MD index, the number and depth of depressed points on the pattern deviation probability plot, and the decibel value of the four points just off fixation. Table 7-2 is a modified version of this classification with greater significance placed on the points near fixation. Table 7-3 also provides classification of visual field loss using 24-2 Full Threshold and SITA Standard for both 30-2 and 24-2 tests. Visual field classification must be computed manually. Identifying the degree of glaucoma damage is essential for setting a target pressure (see Chapter 11). Because visual field loss is a continuum, not all fields fit neatly into a single category. More emphasis should be given to proximity of loss to fixation and defect depth of individual points when there is confusion in classifying the field.

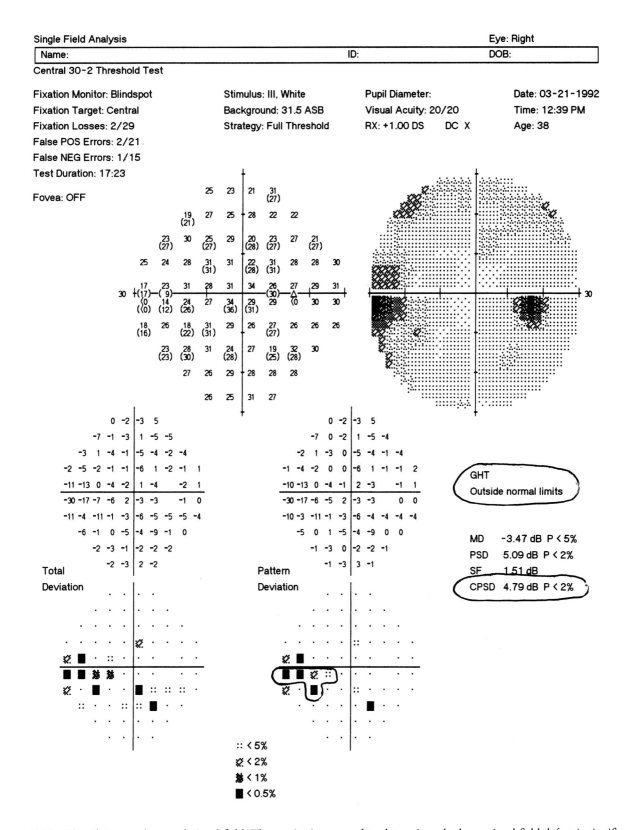

FIGURE 7-22. Classifying an abnormal visual field. Three criteria are used to determine whether a visual field defect is significant. One is an "outside normal limits" glaucoma hemifield test. Second is a cluster of three nonedge points (but including the two most nasal points on a 30-2 pattern that straddle the horizontal meridian and all points on a 24-2 pattern) that are contiguous (must be touching) and on the same side of the horizontal median. Two points must be significant at P <5% and one of the points must have a P value <1% or worse. Third is a corrected pattern deviation occurring with P <5%. A repeatable defect with *any* one of these criteria is considered a positive visual field defect. This patient exhibits all three criteria.

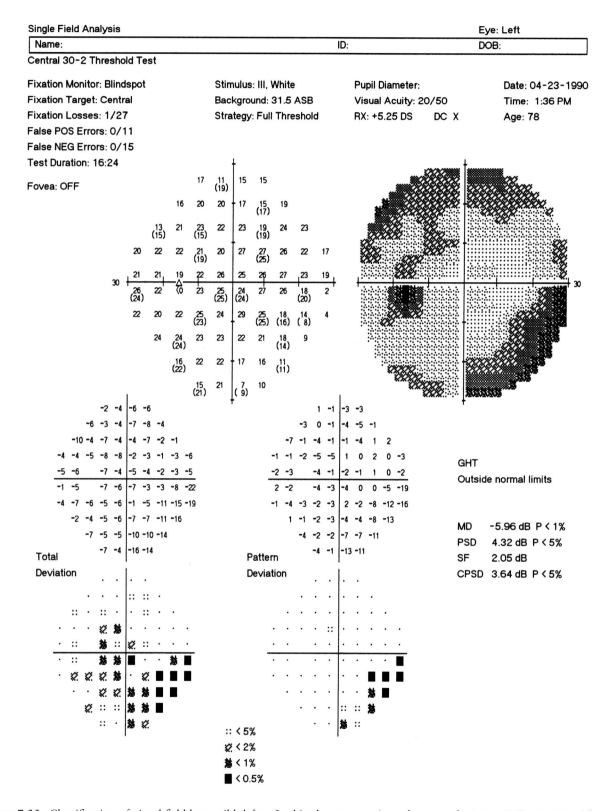

FIGURE 7-23. Classification of visual field loss: mild defect. In this glaucoma patient, the mean deviation (MD) is –5.96. There are 12 points with P values <5% and 8 points with P values <1% on pattern deviation plot, and the four central points are 26, 25, 25, and 24 dBs. Here the MD is better than –6; the number of points on the pattern deviation plots with P values <5% is less than 18, and with P values <1% is less than 10. None of the four points just off fixation has a value less than 20 dBs. It is also noteworthy that this patient has a moderate cataract that is lowering the MD and slightly reducing the four central values. In this case, the number of points on the pattern deviation plot gives the best estimate of the damage from glaucoma (see Table 7-4).

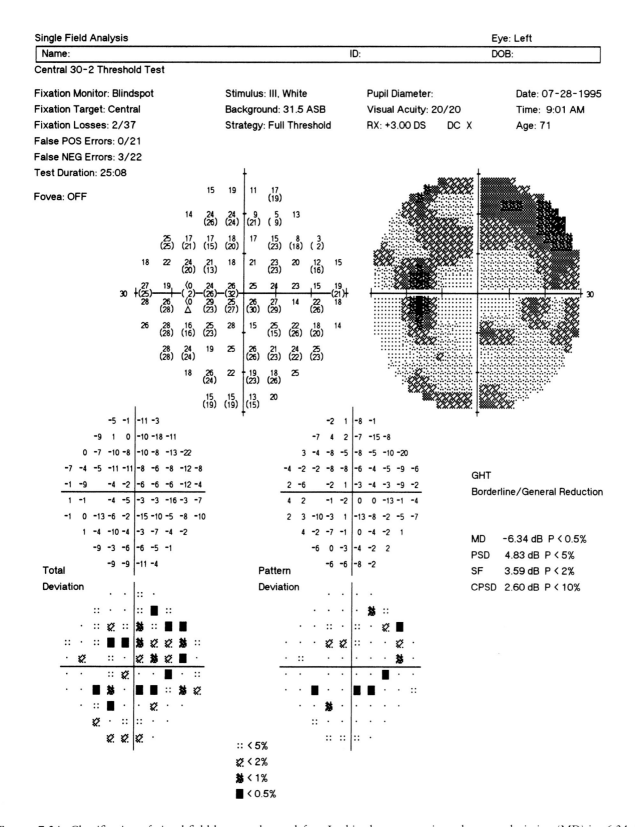

Single Field Analysis   Eye: Left

Name: ID: DOB:

Central 30-2 Threshold Test

Fixation Monitor: Blindspot   Stimulus: III, White   Pupil Diameter: Date: 07-28-1995
Fixation Target: Central   Background: 31.5 ASB   Visual Acuity: 20/20   Time: 9:01 AM
Fixation Losses: 2/37   Strategy: Full Threshold RX: +3.00 DS   DC X   Age: 71
False POS Errors: 0/21
False NEG Errors: 3/22
Test Duration: 25:08

Fovea: OFF

GHT
Borderline/General Reduction

MD   -6.34 dB P < 0.5%
PSD   4.83 dB   P < 5%
SF   3.59 dB   P < 2%
CPSD 2.60 dB   P < 10%

Total Deviation

Pattern Deviation

:: < 5%
☒ < 2%
☒ < 1%
■ < 0.5%

FIGURE 7-24. Classification of visual field loss: moderate defect. In this glaucoma patient, the mean deviation (MD) is –6.34; 22 points have P values <5%, and eight points have P values <1% on pattern deviation plot. The four central points are 29, 25, 26, and 28 dBs. (Also significant is the fact that both hemifields have significant cluster defects on the pattern deviation plots.) This patient is classified as having a moderate defect because the MD is better than –12 but worse than –6 dBs and the number of points on the pattern deviation plots with P values <5% is less than 36 but greater than 18 (see Table 7-4).

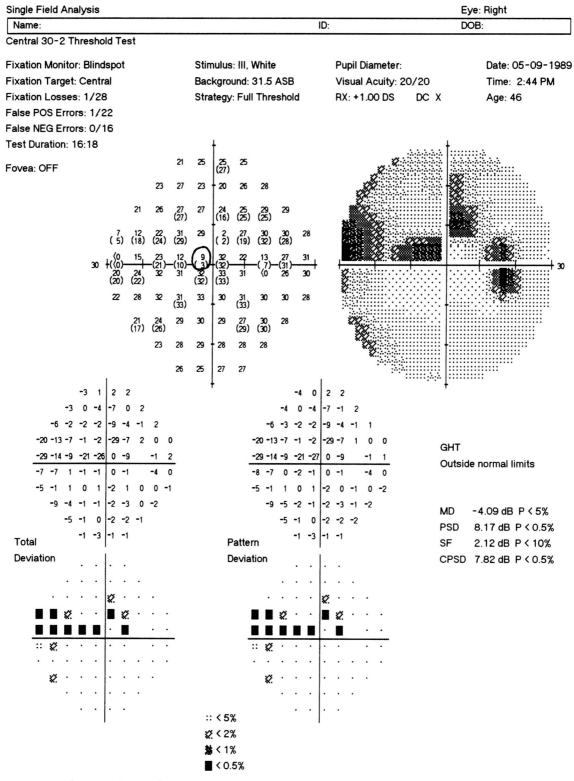

FIGURE 7-25. Classification of visual field loss: severe defect. In this glaucoma patient, the mean deviation (MD) is −4.09. There are 15 points with P values <5% and nine points with P value <1% on pattern deviation plot. The four central points are 6, 32, 32, and 33 dBs. In the severe classification, the MD is worse than −12 or the number of points on the pattern deviation plots with P values <5% is greater than 36—or the number with P values <1% is greater than 20 or any of the four points just off fixation have a value less than 10 dBs or less than 20 dBs in both hemifields. Note that the only reason this patient's visual field is classified as severe is because one of the central points has a dB value of 6 (average of 9 and 3 dBs). This is a cause for concern because the patient may be starting to split fixation and should be treated aggressively—hence the *severe* classification (see Table 7-4).

TABLE 7-2. Classification of Severity of Visual Field Loss Using Full Threshold 30-2 Test

Mild defect (all three conditions must be met):

1. Mean deviation index better than –6 dBs.

2. <18 points at P <5% and <10 points at P <1% on pattern deviation probability plot.

3. No point inside central 5 degrees (the four threshold points surrounding fixation) has threshold value <20 dB.

Moderate defect (all four conditions to be met):

1. Mean deviation index better than –12 dBs.

2. <37 points at P <5% and <20 points at P <1% on pattern deviation probability plot.

3. No point inside central 5 degrees has threshold value of <10 dBs.

4. One hemifield may have a point inside 5 degrees with threshold value <20 dBs, but not both hemifields.

Severe defect (any one of the four conditions is met):

1. Mean deviation index worse than –12 dBs.

2. More than 37 points at P <5% or more than 20 points at P <1% on pattern deviation probability plot.

3. Any point inside central 5 degrees of fixation has threshold value <10 dBs.

4. Both hemifields have defective points within central 5 degrees with threshold values <20 dBs.

P = probability.
Source: Modified from E Hodapp, R Parrish, D Anderson. Clinical Decisions in Glaucoma. St. Louis: Mosby, 1993;53–59.

IDENTIFYING PROGRESSIVE VISUAL FIELD LOSS

Perhaps the greatest challenge in automated perimetry is the recognition of progressive visual field loss. Rather than a static analysis that simply determines the presence of loss, detecting progression requires that the clinician recognize a glaucomatous change against a background of dynamic, physiologic artifact. Confounding variables that can masquerade as progressive loss are introduced that were not a factor in single-field analysis. Making matters worse, no commonly accepted algorithm or standard exists for defining progression with automated perimetry, despite years of clinical experience. This leads to differences of opinion even among expert observers in determining whether a visual field loss has worsened.[46,47]

Both Goldmann testing and automated visual field tests show progression in a similar fashion. Mikelberg established that Goldmann fields progress by either deepening of an existing defect, enlargement of an existing defect, or the appearance of a new defect in a previously normal area (Figure 7-26).[48] These may occur separately or in combination. The most frequently

occurring change was the deepening of an existing defect. These three possibilities occur in automated perimetry with progressive overall depression, as measured by a 2-db change in the MD index, suggested by Hodapp as a fourth means.[45] However, overall depression by itself is not universally accepted as an initial mean of progression.[32] Whether it occurs at all in early glaucoma is controversial, and its recognition is difficult in the presence of miosis or progressive change in the media. However, it is widely agreed that it is present in moderate to severe loss.

Maturing cataracts make the recognition of any type of progression difficult by creating an overall depression that can mask focal defects, as well as mimic the overall depression caused by advanced disease. Although cataracts may be present at the time of initial analysis for field loss, most algorithms can make the diagnosis in the presence of cataract-induced diffuse loss (see Figure 7-15). However, current software and algorithms do not factor out the development of cataracts during the course of follow-up, and clinicians must make this determination for themselves.

Even more vexing than cataracts is *long-term fluctuation* (LTF), which can be defined as the nonpathologic change in threshold values between tests. LTF is the greatest problem in determining progression. Several studies have determined that in stable glaucoma patients, the deeper the initial defect, the greater the fluctuation between tests.[49–51] Once a point has decreased to one-half its expected value, it may return to its expected value or not respond to the brightest stimulus at all on the next test. Therefore, the more extensive the initial field loss, the more the visual field fluctuates, even in stable glaucoma patients. In most clinical populations, patients display a combination of LTF and artifact, and true progression must be detected against this background of noise (Figure 7-27).

Overview

To rapidly review a series of fields for progression, it is recommended that the clinician first print out all the fields in an overview format that displays on a single row the grayscale, threshold values, total deviation plots, and pattern deviation plots (see Figure 7-26). The GHT analysis, reliability indices, and global indices are also listed for each field. Up to three fields can be displayed on a single page, which allows an easy scan of the elements of the display and ready assessment of trends. This display does not analyze the information or assign any statistical significance; it merely presents the available information in a convenient format.

The simplest technique for detecting progression is inspecting the grayscale for change (see Figure 7-26). Although fraught with artifact, the grayscale provides valuable information that is not available by

TABLE 7-3. Grading Glaucoma Damage and Setting Target Pressures Based on Different Visual Field Strategies

Damage level and suggested target pressures	30-2 Full Threshold	24-2 Full Threshold	30-2 SITA Standard	24-2 SITA Standard
Mild visual field loss: set target pressure 20–30% below baseline intraocular pressure	MD <–6 dB. AND <18 points below 5% level and <10 points below 1% level on pattern deviation plot. AND no central points* <20 dB.	MD <–6 dB. AND <14 points below 5% level and <8 points below 1% level on pattern deviation plot. AND no central points* <20 dB.	MD <–5 dB. AND <18 points below 5% level and <10 points below 1% level on pattern deviation plot. AND no central points* <20 dB.	MD <–5 dB. AND <14 points below 5% level and <8 points below 1% level on pattern deviation plot. AND no central points* <20 dB.
Moderate visual field loss: set target pressure 30–40% below baseline intraocular pressure	MD –6 to –12 dB. OR 18–36 points below 5% level or 10–20 points below 1% level on pattern deviation plot. OR central points* between 10–20 dB in one hemifield.	MD –6 to –12 dB. OR 14–28 points below 5% level or 8–16 points below 1% level on pattern deviation plot. OR central points* between 10–20 dB in one hemifield.	MD –5 to –10 dB. OR 18–36 points below 5% level or 10–20 points below 1% level on pattern deviation plot. OR central points* between 10–20 dB in one hemifield.	MD –5 to –10 dB. OR 14–28 points below 5% level or 8–16 points below 1% level on pattern deviation plot. OR central points* between 10–20 dB in one hemifield.
Severe visual field loss: set target pressure 40–50% below baseline intraocular pressure	MD >–12 dB. OR >36 points below 5% level or >20 points below 1% level on pattern deviation plot. OR <20 dB in both hemifields in central 5 degrees or any point in central 5 degrees has a value of <10 dB.	MD >–12 dB. OR >28 points below 5% level or >16 points below 1% level on pattern deviation plot. OR <20 dB in both hemifields in central 5 degrees OR any point in central 5 degrees has a value of <10 dB.	MD >–10 dB. OR >36 points below 5% level or > 20 points below 1% level on pattern deviation plot. OR <20 dB in both hemifields in central 5 degrees OR any point in central 5 degrees has a value of <10 dB.	MD >–10 dB. OR >28 points below 5% level or >16 points below 1% level on pattern deviation plot. OR <20 dB in both hemifields in central 5 degrees OR any point in central 5 degrees has a value of <10 dB.

MD = mean deviation; SITA = Swedish Interactive Thresholding Algorithm.
*Central points represent the four tested points within 5 degrees of fixation.

observation of changes in the total or pattern deviation probability plots. For example, a point near fixation that is depressed from an expected value of 32 to 26 dB would have a black box displayed in both the total and pattern deviation probability plots, signifying the greatest statistical likelihood of abnormality. If this same point now goes from 26 dB to 16 dB, the 10-dB change is not displayed by the probability plots that already received a black box at 26 dB. However, the change would be noticeable with the simple grayscale, which now displays a darker shade of gray. As the point continues to lose sensitivity over the course of several more visual field examinations, only the grayscale is capable of displaying any further change. But although change is detected, no determination of significance is made. In this example, whether the 10-dB decline is a significant change representing progression or is within the accepted range of LTF must be

determined. Therefore, although grayscale is good at displaying changes in sensitivity, it is left entirely up to the practitioner to decide whether the changes seen in the grayscale are LTF or progression (see Figure 7-27).

Next to the grayscale is the display of numbers representing the threshold values. Although manually comparing the changes in threshold values between one or two visual field tests is possible, it becomes a daunting task when all 76 points in each of four or five fields must be examined. It is better to concentrate only on the threshold values corresponding to suspicious points highlighted in either the grayscale or probability plots. But the practitioner is still left to decide how much the threshold values have to decline before the results can be considered true progression rather than LTF.

Next, both the total and pattern deviation probability plots can be examined for progression. Normal points or mildly defective points that worsen can be detected by

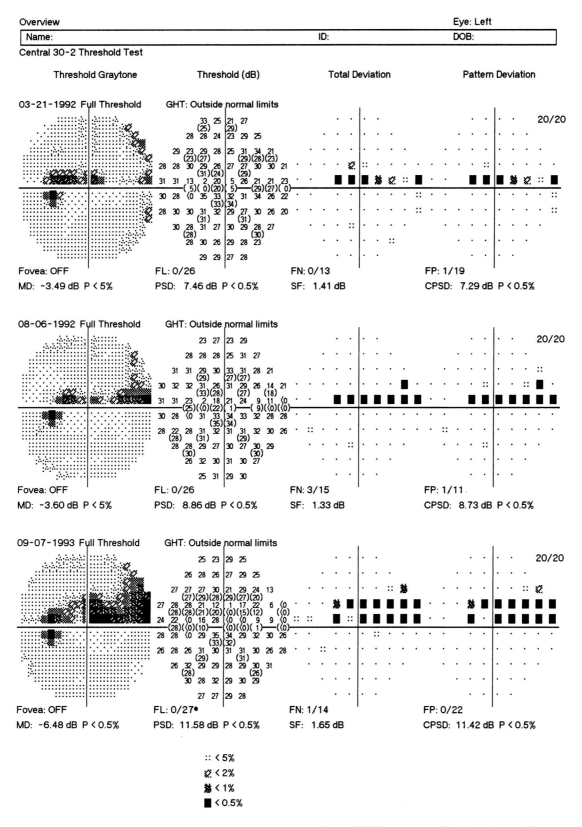

FIGURE 7-26. Overview printout of progressing defect. Progression of visual fields can occur by deepening, enlargement, or the appearance of a new defect in a previously normal location. This figure shows both deepening of the initial field defect (as seen by the darkening of the grayscale and decrease in the threshold dBs) and enlargement of the defect (as seen by enlargement of the defect in the grayscales and pattern deviation plots and decrease in the threshold dBs). Note that once the pattern deviation plots have reached a P value of <.5%, they no longer change, despite a further decrease in the threshold values. This change is, however, identified by a darkening of the grayscale.

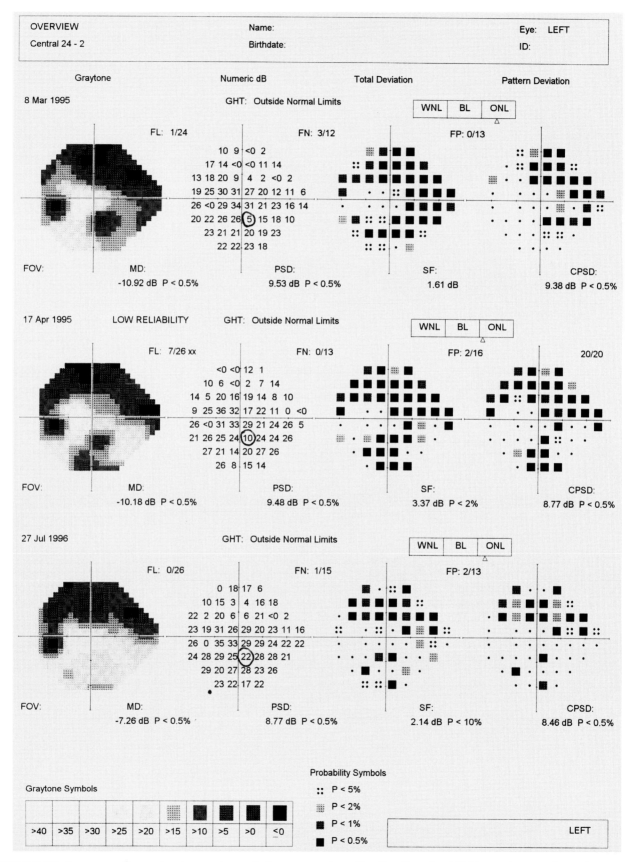

FIGURE 7-27. Long-term fluctuation in an advanced glaucoma patient. The first five visual fields on the overview printout were performed between March 1995 and June 1998. Note the change in the inferior paracentral scotoma depicted by the grayscales in the fields. Note that the threshold value in a point within this scotoma varied from 5, 10, 22, 6, and 25 dBs. This variation is called *long-term fluctuation* and is typically seen in a damaged area of the visual field.

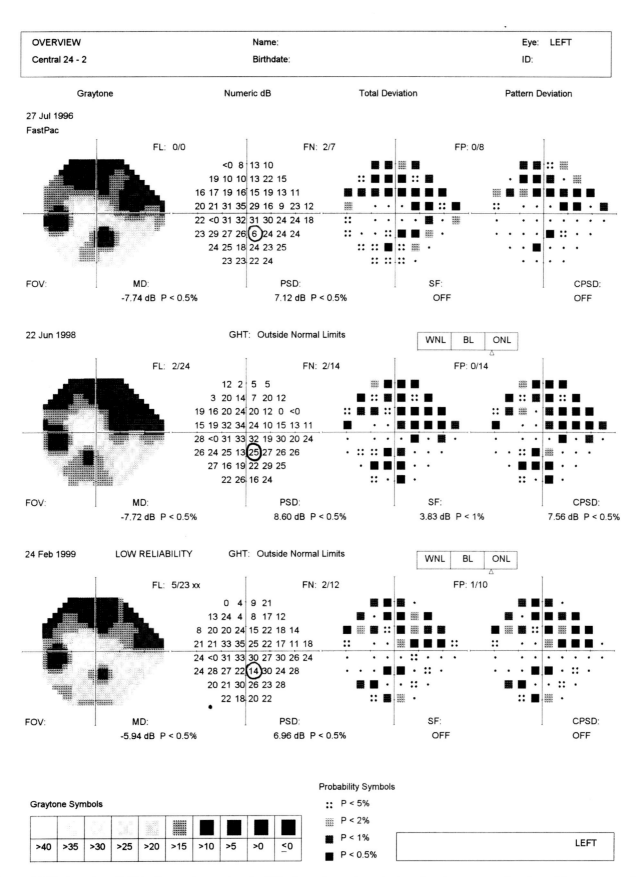

FIGURE 7-27. (*continued*) This fluctuation makes it difficult to determine whether the glaucoma patient is stable or progressing from the disease. The patient's latest visual field (February, 1999) shows a 14-dB value, and the surrounding points have remained unchanged. Through multiple visual field tests over time, the clinician can conclude that this patient has high long-term fluctuation, and the field is relatively stable.

TABLE 7-4. Criteria for Progression of Visual Field Loss

Establish a "baseline field":

- Average two or three representative visual fields.

- Record all values obtained in the baseline for each point.

In an area of field normal in baseline:

- Three contiguous points, same side of horizontal, must now be abnormal.

- One point by 10 dBs as found on the total deviation values.

- Two points by 5 dBs as found on the total deviation values.

In an area of field abnormal in baseline:

- Two contiguous points, same side of horizontal, must decrease from baseline by at least 10 dBs or three times the average short-term fluctuation in the baseline, whichever is higher.

- Suspected point's value must be lower than any value obtained for that point in the baseline tests.

To confirm visual field loss has progressed, change must be present in four out of five confirming visual field tests.

Source: Adapted from M Schulzer, Normal-Tension Glaucoma Study Group. Errors in the diagnosis of visual field progression in normal-tension glaucoma. Ophthalmol 1994;101:1589–1595; and Collaborative Normal-Tension Glaucoma Study Group. Comparison of glaucomatous progression between untreated patients with normal-tension glaucoma and patients with therapeutically reduced intraocular pressures. Am J Ophthalmol 1998;126:487–497.

the probability plots. In the absence of an overall depression, the change in the total deviation and pattern deviation is similar. In the presence of an overall depression, the total deviation plots appear worse than the pattern deviation plots. The challenge confronting the clinician is deciding whether the overall depression is secondary only to the disease process, in which case the total deviation plots are "correct," or whether the media has changed significantly and the pattern deviation plots are correct (see Figure 7-19). As mentioned earlier, the usefulness of the probability plots is limited by the fact that once a point is marked with the black box symbol corresponding to the highest P value of <.5%, no further worsening can be displayed. Although, the point may be only depressed less than 25% of its expected value. In general, the probability plots are useful for detecting progression in mild to moderate disease, but severely limited beyond this point.

Once an area of the field has been identified as possibly having progressed, the practitioner has to decide whether the change is significant enough to consider modifying current therapy. As discussed earlier in the section "Identifying Progressive Field Loss," no commonly accepted criteria exist for progression, and the criteria used for the Normal Tension Glaucoma (NTG) Study represent the best criteria presently available. Just as the use of a cluster of defects overcomes the probability of random points reaching significance when a determination is being made about whether a field is abnormal, a similar approach can be taken to

monitor for progression. Older criteria required that a point change by a predetermined amount.[35] This failed to account for the major influence of LTF.

The NTG Study has developed and subsequently modified criteria for change that have been partially validated against a statistical model and that attempt to account for an individual's LTF (Table 7-4).[36] The NTG criteria require the following:

- In areas that were *normal* in the baseline and now are suspected for having become abnormal, within a suspected cluster of three contiguous, nonedge points, one point must be at least 10 dB lower than its expected STATPAC value (as determined by the *total* deviation defect plot), whereas the other two must each be at least 5 dB lower than their expected STATPAC values. Judging progression in areas that were defective in the baseline (using the same cluster criteria) is more complex.

- A baseline is created by averaging three VF examinations. In areas that were *abnormal* in the baseline and are now suspected of worsening, *two or more points* within or adjacent to the defective area (at baseline) must decrease by an amount that exceeds three conditions. First, the change in threshold value in the suspected points must be at least 10 dB. Second, the change in threshold values must be greater than three times the average STF measured in the three baseline fields. Third, the value obtained on the follow-up field test must be worse than any value obtained for that point during the three baseline examinations. The second condition attempts to modify the strict 10-dB criterion to account for individual variation and requires that the STF be measured. Clinically, few reliable patients display STF over 3.33 dB, and it is probably more important to shorten the test than to measure the STF. The third criterion tries to correct for LTF by using all the values obtained in the three baseline examinations that serve on as a small, individual empirical database. Logically, a point should not be considered to have changed significantly if it was obtained in the baseline.

These criteria require a very time-consuming process of manually tabulating all the values obtained in the baseline visual fields for each point. This is best performed with a computer program, but none is commercially available.

Even using the strict NTG criteria that attempt to dampen the effect of LTF on visual field test results, statistical modeling and clinical experience showed a false-positive rate (overcalled stable fields as having progressed) of 57% that could be reduced to 2%, but only at the expense of performing four to six confirming field tests.[36,52] In a clinical setting, repeating a field examination four to six times is not a realistic practice. In general, two successive fields that show progression in the same area are probably the minimum to confirm progression if the clinical course is consistent (e.g., poor IOP control, disc hemorrhage, etc.). However, when invasive surgical intervention is contemplated, three confirming fields may be preferable if the first two are equivocal.

Glaucoma Change Probability

Rather than using the somewhat cumbersome criteria of the NTG Study to account for LTF, the GCP analysis uses a small, empirical database derived from stable glaucoma patients experienced in automated perimetry who underwent four visual field tests in 1 month. The range of expected fluctuation for individual points was determined based on the depth of the original defect and its location. By comparing a change in threshold values to this database of expected range of fluctuation, a statistical significance can be assigned to identify suspected progression (Figure 7-28). This greatly simplifies the identification of suspicious points.

The GCP averages the first two field tests to form a baseline. On the first page of the GCP, these two fields are shown with their grayscale and total deviation plots. A graph of the MD index for all the fields (both baseline and follow-up) is displayed to give a simple synopsis of the overall trend for that eye. If five fields are available, a regression analysis of the slope of the line drawn between the plotted MD indices is performed, and whether it is statistically significant for worsening is noted.

The printout of the follow-up fields displays four items. The grayscale and the total deviation probability plot are displayed and examined for new defects and enlarging and deepening defects. The grayscale displays worsening by darkening the area involved; this includes both normal and abnormal areas. However, whether this worsening is statistically significant is not determined. The total deviation plots readily display normal areas that are now defective, but, as previously discussed, these plots are limited in the ability to indicate abnormal points that have continued to worsen. The GCP has two other displays that are unique. First, the threshold value obtained in the follow-up field is subtracted from the averaged values in the two baseline fields and shown under the "Delta dB from Baseline" display. This allows the practitioner to quickly scan for defects that have worsened by 10 dB or more. The last display, "Delta Glaucoma Probability," notes the change from baseline and compares it to the GCP empirical database (see Figure 7-28B). If the change exceeds the LTF expected for 95% of the values in its database, a black delta (triangle) is displayed. Likewise, if the point is significantly improved, it is marked by an open delta. Stable points are represented by a black dot. A small "x" indicates that there were not enough points in the database to make a statistical assessment of the change in the value for that particular point. This usually occurs in baseline values that are very high (normal) or severely depressed (Figure 7-29). Differences between the somewhat rigid NTG criteria and the GCP are apparent. With the empirical delta glaucoma probability plots, it will be noted that some points can change less than 10 dB and be marked as exceeding the expected LTF, whereas other points change more than 10 dB and are noted as stable.

TABLE 7-5. Reviewing the Visual Field Test for Progression

1. Print out overview of all fields:

   - Inspect for reliability.
   - Determine when target pressure was reached and exclude earlier fields.
   - Select two or three fields to form baseline.
   - Inspect grayscales and probability plots of follow-up fields for worsening.
   - Correlate suspected areas with threshold values.

2. Print out glaucoma change probability analysis after selecting appropriate baseline tests:

   - Review grayscale and total deviation plots again.
   - Review difference in dBs from baseline and identify non-edge points (include two most nasal points) that have decreased by 10 dBs.
   - Correlate suspected points with change probability plot.
   - Two or three contiguous points are a significant cluster.

3. Suspected defect should be present on a minimum of two successive fields.

Both the NTG and the GCP are highly susceptible to overcalling progression caused by media worsening or increased miosis. Further, the small GCP database has limited information on patients with minimal defect or severe loss and has limited use for the analysis of these patients (see Figure 7-29). The NTG Study criteria were not developed for use on fields with severe loss either. Therefore, for those patients most prone to high LTF, little guidance exists in either the literature or the onboard analysis.

Both the NTG criteria and the GCP average several fields to cancel out or dampen the fluctuation while establishing the baseline. The selection of the fields to be included in the baseline is critical and should not be left entirely to onboard software, which routinely fails to detect the learning curve. (In the NTG Study, three fields are selected by the practitioner to represent the baseline and are averaged to form a master field.) Further, once progression has occurred, the old baseline has to be discarded and a new one established after the IOP has reached the new target IOP (Figure 7-30). A new baseline should not be established until the new target IOP has been reached because the field may continue to progress during this interval, and these field tests will not be representative of a stable baseline.

Miosis and cataracts are confounding variables, causing an overall depression. If the baseline was established before the addition of a miotic, subsequent fields should be performed while the eyes are dilated. No simple solution to progressive media opacification exists. At best, the overall depression induced by cataract could be determined by the clinician, and that amount

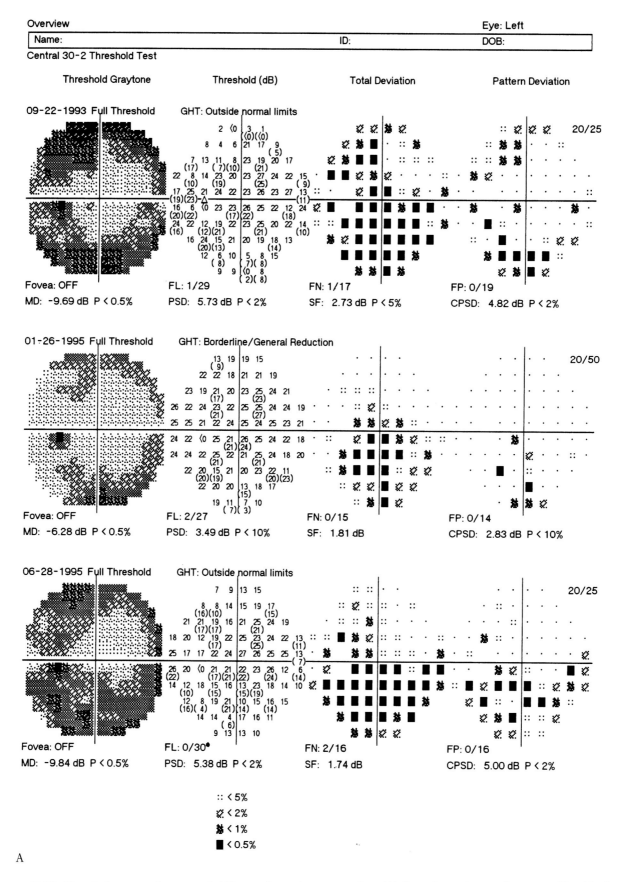

FIGURE 7-28. Use of glaucoma change probability to determine progression. (A) Overview printout shows considerable fluctuation in the patient's first three visual fields. It is difficult to judge with the grayscale and probability plots whether the field test of June 1995 represents progression or long-term fluctuation.

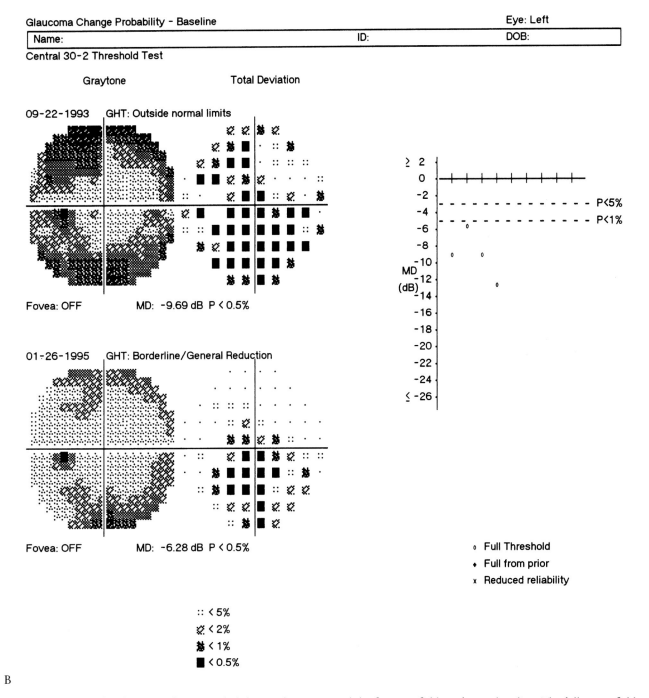

B

FIGURE 7-28. **(B)** The glaucoma change probability analysis averaged the first two fields to form a baseline. The follow-up fields of June 1995 and 1996 are compared with the baseline. (*continued*)

added to the values in the total deviation plot before the NTG Study criteria are applied. This might be accomplished by looking at the delta dB from baseline on the GCP, determining how much the stable areas of the field decreased, and assuming that this amount represents the overall depression. This would be valid only if the overall depression was exclusively caused by cataract, miosis, or both.

Just as the analysis of a single visual field test for abnormality uses several criteria, the analysis for change may require using several techniques to help diagnose progression. A suggested sequence for analyzing for progression is included in Table 7-5. Despite this analysis, it may not be clearly evident whether the field is stable or progressed. With any subjective analysis, a simple yes or no may not always be possible. In the final analysis, it is up to the practitioner's judgment to determine whether the field is stable. The practitioner's estimate of the probability that the field has progressed may be all that is possible.

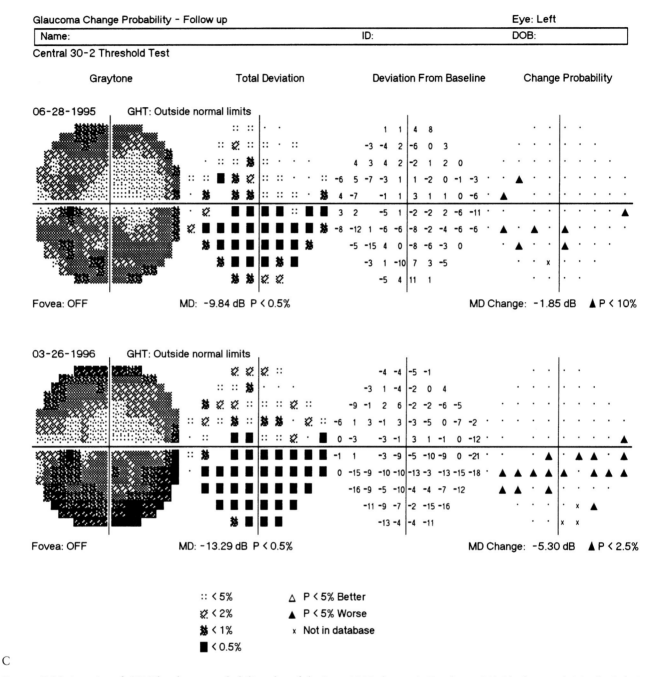

C

FIGURE 7-28. (*continued*) (C) The change probability plot of the June 1995 shows six P values <5% (*dark triangles*) in the inferior field. These dark triangles represent points that changed more than expected in the empirical database of stable glaucoma patients. The "deviation from baseline" plot also displays four points having dropped 10 dBs or more from the baseline. The 1996 field clearly shows progression in the inferior field by both the deviation from baseline and change probability plot.

IDENTIFYING PROGRESSION IN ENDSTAGE GLAUCOMA

As mentioned in the section, "Test Selection," not enough points respond to the size III stimulus in the 30-2 or 24-2 test pattern in endstage glaucoma to allow the visual field defect to be adequately monitored for progression. Although increasing the stimulus to size V increases the number of points that respond, the 30-2 pattern does not have sufficient spacing to carefully monitor fixation, a critical part of the care of an endstage glaucoma patient. Endstage glaucoma mandates a 10-2 pattern to monitor the central 10 degrees (fixation) (see Figure 7-4), and a 30-2 pattern with a size V stimulus can be used to follow the remainder of the field. When even a standard central 10-2 pattern fails to have enough responding points to

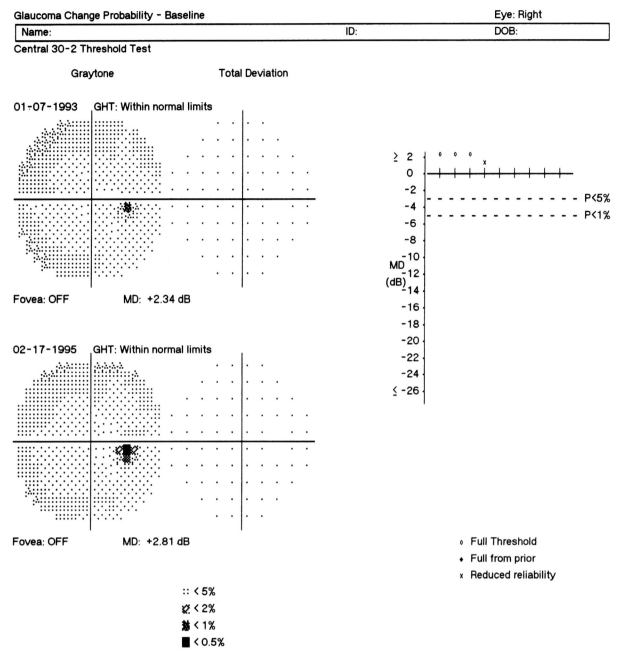

FIGURE 7-29 (A,B). (A) Small "x" in glaucoma change probability plot. In this glaucoma patient, the baseline threshold values are very high and normal. Because there are very few normal patients at baseline in the glaucoma change probability database, the program cannot make a statistical calculation for change in these points. Thus, there are numerous "x" signs in the glaucoma change probability plot, indicating the change at that particular point cannot be evaluated. (*continued*)

follow the patient's visual field for subsequent loss, the stimulus size should be changed from the standard size III to the nonstandard size V (Figure 7-31).

Identifying progression in endstage glaucoma is critical because loss of visual field in this area can lead to a precipitous drop in acuity. Many patients with only a small central isle note a subjective worsening of their "vision" with no change in acuity. This symptom proba-

bly represents a decay of the remaining visual field that does not yet impinge on fixation. The source of the patient's complaint may become apparent on a repeat 10-2 test. When analyzing the visual fields of a patient with endstage disease, all attention is directed toward preserving fixation. Typically, the superior nasal field progresses inward to split fixation, followed by loss in the inferior field that encroaches from the nasal field as well.[7,8]

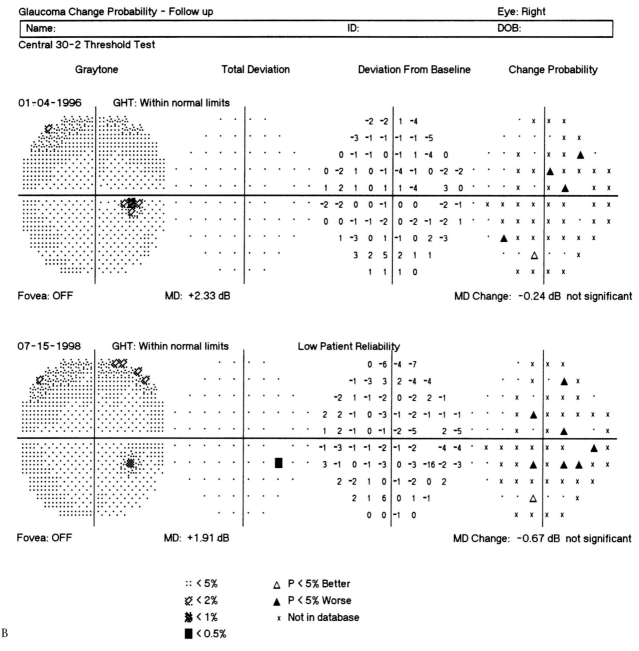

FIGURE 7-29. (*continued*) (**B**) Inspection of the deviation from baseline display shows that many of these points actually improved. Likewise, in patients with severe loss, the glaucoma change probability plot often shows the same x for points that have declined by more than 10 dBs. This, again, is secondary to the lack of patients with severe disease in the database. For patients with normal glaucoma hemifield test (GHT) results, it is best to follow the fields with an overview display until a defect is confirmed, and then use the glaucoma change probability plot. In severe disease, the glaucoma change probability plot can be used, but any point marked with an x should be inspected in the deviation from baseline display to determine the actual decline in dBs from baseline.

The GCP does not analyze central 10-2 fields, and endstage glaucoma patients followed with central 10-2 visual fields require manual analysis. Using the "average" function on the HFA I, two or three 10-2 field tests should be selected and averaged to form a baseline or *master* visual field. Follow-up fields can be subtracted from the master using the "compare" function on the

HFA. The HFA I is asked to compare the master with the most recent field, and the change in threshold values is displayed. The "average" and "compare" functions can also be used with the 10-2 fields taken with a size V stimulus. The HFA II can only perform the "compare" function, and a single field must be used as the baseline. No algorithms are recommended for use with the central

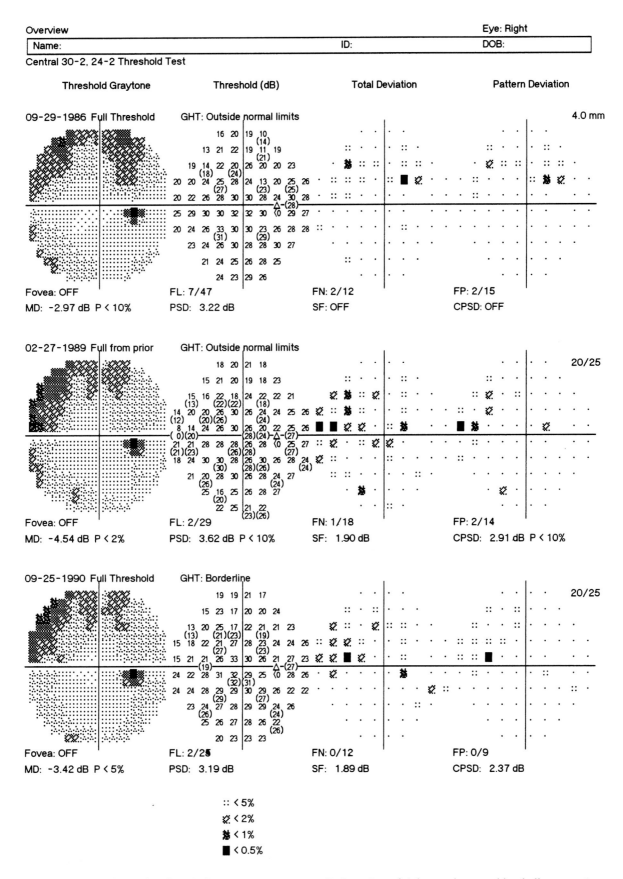

A

FIGURE 7-30. Need to change baseline to determine progression. (**A**) Overview of right eye shows stable, shallow superior arcuate defect from 1986 to 1990. (*continued*)

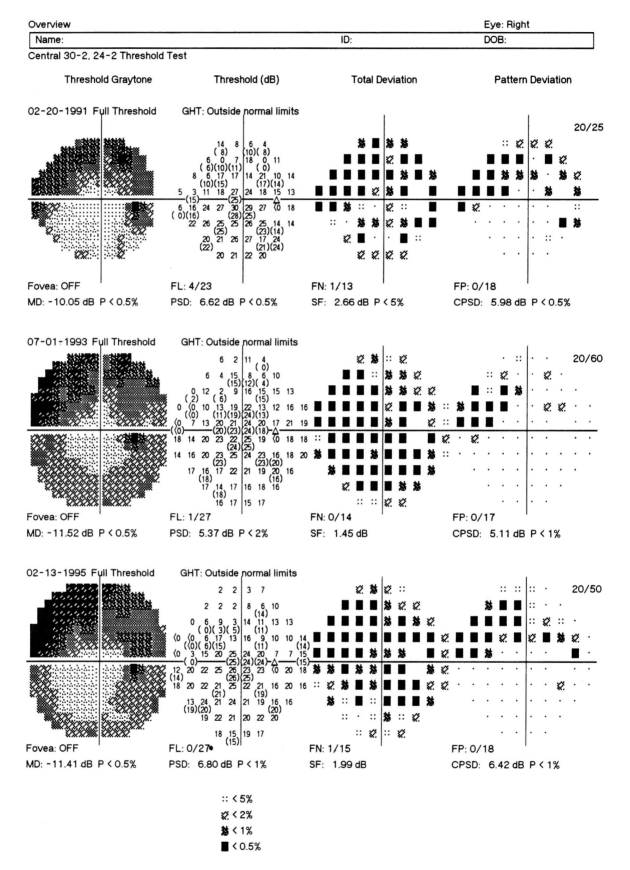

A

FIGURE 7-30A. (*continued*) Defect is classified as *mild* up to 1990, then changed suddenly to a moderate defect in 1991. The defect fluctuated somewhat between 1991 and 1995, but was a confirmed change from the prior three fields.

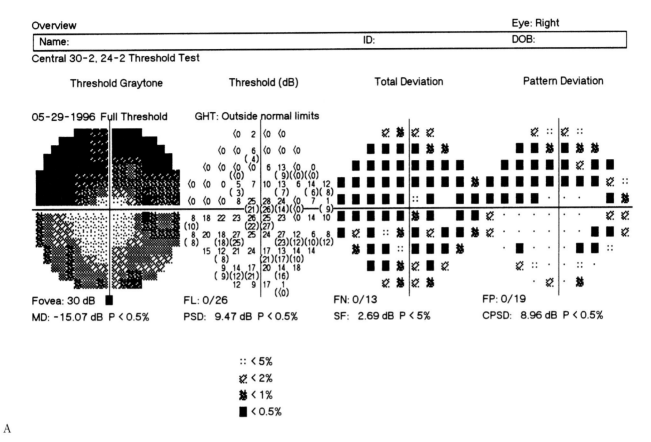

FIGURE 7-30A. *(continued)* From 1995 to 1996, the superior defect continued to deepen. From 1991 to 1996, the total deviation plots began to look worse than the pattern deviation plots. This was secondary to an overall depression from a maturing cataract. The pattern deviation plots showed the focal defects once the overall depression was removed. With most of the superior points significant at the P <.5%, worsening of the superior field is better appreciated with inspection of the grayscale and threshold values. *(continued on next page)*

10 degrees. The NTG Study criteria would seem to be a reasonable starting point in the analysis (see Table 7-4).

SHORT WAVELENGTH AUTOMATED PERIMETRY

Short wavelength automated perimetry (SWAP) was developed in the mid 1990s. Many patients with early glaucomatous nerve damage fail to show visual field loss on conventional white-on-white perimetry, whether kinetic or static. Histologic correlation by Quigley and colleagues suggested that up to 50% of the ganglion cell axons can be lost before kinetic perimetry detects a defect.[53] Automated static perimetry fares better, but up to 20–40% of the axons can be lost before a defect is apparent.[54] Attention has been directed toward developing a more sensitive visual field test.

SWAP uses a large blue stimulus (size V) against a bright yellow background. Several longitudinal clinical studies have shown that SWAP can identify a defect before it is detected by white-on-white perimetry, and that SWAP detects progression of the defect before it is found on white-on-white perimetry.[55-58] Visual field defects detected by SWAP may precede white-on-white defects by 5 years. It was proposed that a subset of the parvocellular visual pathway was selectively damaged in glaucoma to explain these results. However, other neural pathways also show damage earlier than with white-on-white perimetry.[59,60] The most likely explanation for the increased sensitivity of SWAP is reduced redundancy, which speculates that no selective loss occurs. Rather, because there are fewer axons in a normal eye that respond to a blue stimulus than axons that respond to a white stimulus, any diffuse loss preferentially affects the smaller subsystem.[61,62]

Although SWAP is more sensitive in detecting defects, its specificity needs to be closely watched. SWAP perimetry displays greater STF and LTF than does conventional white-on-white perimetry,[63] and cataracts introduce a greater artifact in SWAP.[64] The development of a normative database similar to STAPAC, termed *SWAPPAC*, has been critical for successful integration into clinical practice to minimize these confounding variables (Figure 7-32).[63]

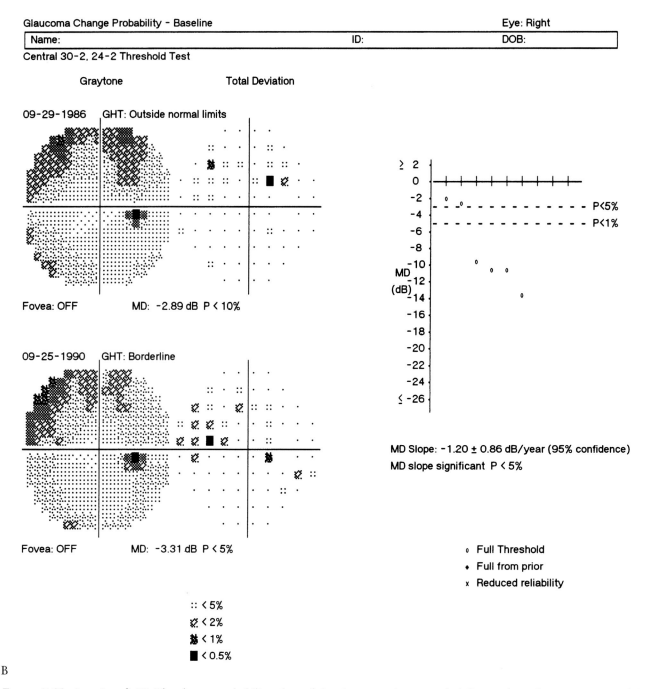

FIGURE 7-30. (*continued*) (**B**) The change probability plots of the glaucoma change probability analysis show worsening of the superior field in 1991 compared with the averaged baseline of the 1986 and 1989 fields.

Although the initial research indicated that SWAP might be capable of replacing conventional perimetry for many patients, its clinical use has been somewhat limited. First, even with the FASTPAC thresholding strategy, SWAP is a long and arduous test for most patients and has low patient acceptance. No version of SWAP is yet available for SITA testing, but if such a version becomes available, it may reduce testing time and improve patient acceptance. Second, patients with moderate to severe field loss on white-on-white perimetry have lost most of the axons responding to the blue stimulus and display an end-stage SWAP field, eliminating the test's usefulness in following these patients.[56] These patients should be followed with white-on-white perimetry instead of SWAP. Third, any significant cataract affecting the visual acuity may potentially induce a SWAP artifact. Therefore, cataract patients with vision of 20/40 or worse should not be tested with SWAP. Finally, in the original studies, a significant number of patients presented with defects on conventional white-on-white perimetry before blue-yellow.[55–57] A

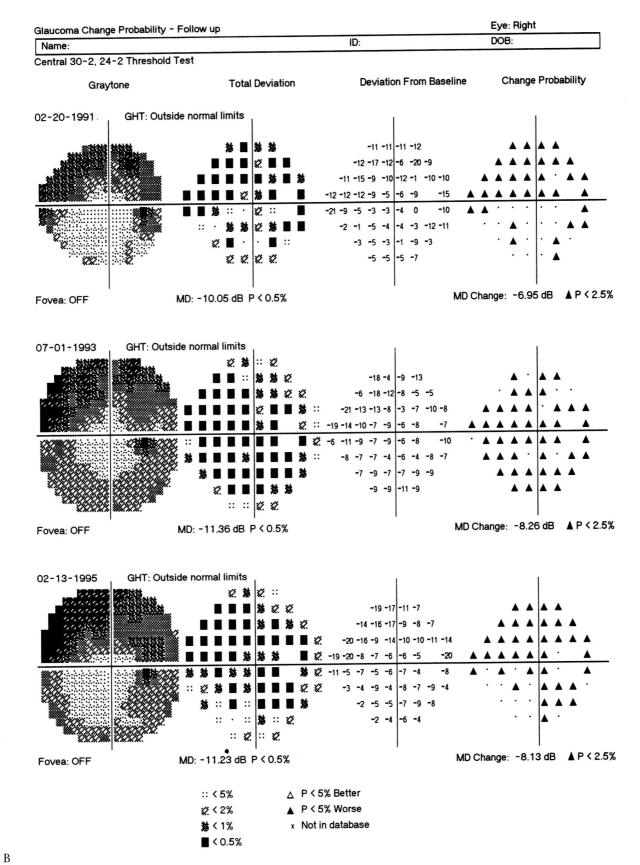

FIGURE 7-30B. However, subsequent worsening of the superior field in 1995 and 1996 could not be detected by the change probability plots, even though the deviation from baseline display showed continuing increase in loss in sensitivity. The later fields were still being compared with the baseline from 1986 and 1989. (*continued*)

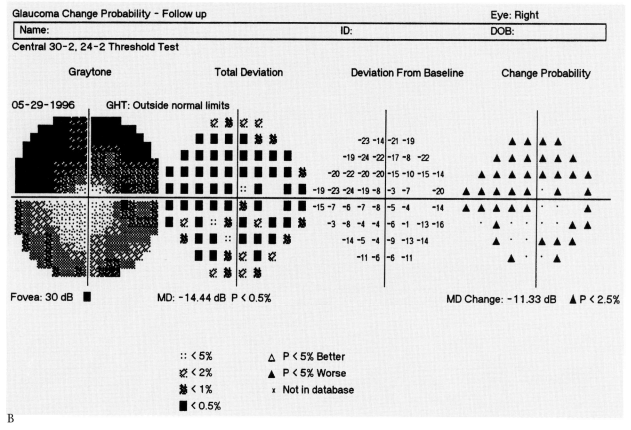

FIGURE 7-30B. (*continued*)

clinician cannot exclusively test glaucoma suspects with blue-yellow perimetry. It is suggested that for now SWAP be reserved for those high-risk glaucoma suspects who test normal with white-on-white perimetry (Table 7-6). A repeatable SWAP defect that correlates to the optic nerve and nerve fiber layer findings in a high-risk glaucoma suspect strongly supports the initiation of treatment (see Figure 7-32).

TABLE 7-6. Short-Wavelength Automated Perimetry Clinical Pearls

Use only for reliable visual field tester.

Use on high-risk glaucoma suspect.

Use when white-on-white visual field result is normal.

Use when minimal or no cataract is present.

Use 24-2 FASTPAC program.

Turn off short-term fluctuation.

If defect is present, repeat test to confirm.

Correlate with optic nerve and nerve fiber layer findings.

Some glaucoma defects may be present on conventional white-on-white perimetry before short-wavelength automated perimetry.

FREQUENCY-DOUBLING TECHNOLOGY PERIMETRY

Another new development in perimetry that attempts to detect visual field loss before it is evident on conventional white-on-white field testing is frequency-doubling technology (FDT). The FDT perimeter is a compact, lightweight, portable unit that does not require the special testing area of a conventional perimeter. The test can be performed with the patient's glasses in place in any ambient light setting. In the standard central 20-degree test, stimuli are presented at 17 locations: one central 5-degree target and four 10-degree peripheral targets per quadrant. The stimulus used in frequency doubling uses a grating of very low spatial frequency (0.25 cycles/degree) that is flickered at a high temporal frequency (25 Hz counterphase flicker). The dark bars become light and light bars become dark 25 times a second. At the right combination of spatial and temporal frequency and the proper contrast, only the total number of bars appears to double—hence the term *frequency doubling* (Figure 7-33). In the actual perimetric test, the contrast of the stimulus is varied, and the patient is asked to respond when they notice a dark, flickering stimulus.

Patients may experience a dimming of the background field when performing FDT or conventional

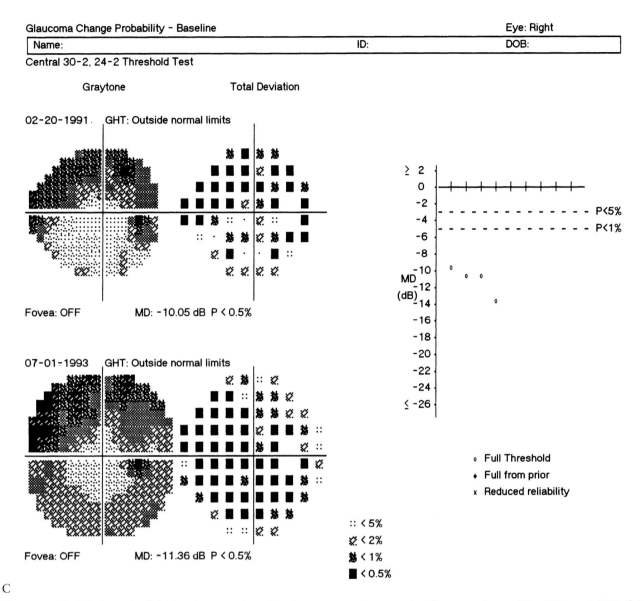

C

FIGURE 7-30. (C) Once the field has been confirmed to have worsened, a new baseline must be set. The 1991 and 1993 fields should be set as the baseline. (*continued*)

perimetry. This is called the *Troxler phenomenon*, and it occurs when a patient steadily fixates on a central target with a dim, uniform background.[65] Over time, the peripheral field may fade or disappear. Blinking or small eye movements eliminate the effect, and patients should be encouraged to blink normally during the test. Because the patient's eye is not observed during FDT perimetry, normal blinking should be encouraged. Clinically, this phenomenon may not be noticed during short-duration screening tests but is more likely during longer threshold examinations.

Frequency doubling is a phenomena mediated by the magnocellular pathway.[66] The magnocellular pathway is comprised of large-diameter axons that make up only 15% of the total number of axons. The subset of M-cells, the My, that respond to the frequency-doubling phenomena constitute less than 5% of the total number of axons. M-cells are thought to be affected preferentially in early glaucoma, and it is thought that by testing this specific group with minimal redundancy, defects will be seen on frequency doubling before they can be seen on white-on-white perimetry. Proof of that ability awaits the results of long-term studies. The available studies examining the ability of the frequency-doubling perimeter to detect defects that are already present on conventional white-on-white perimetry are very favorable (Figure 7-34).[67,68] Unlike conventional perimetry, in which screening fields play a secondary role in the perimeter's use, screening fields are an essential pur-

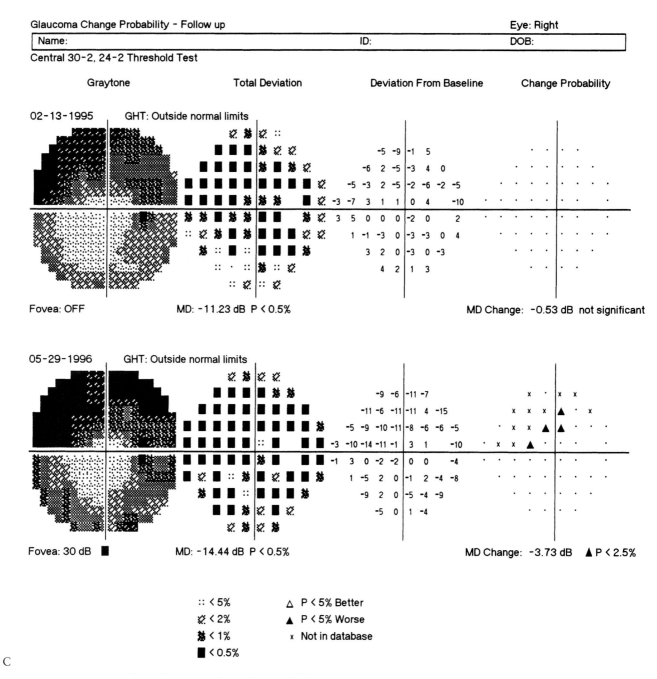

FIGURE 7-30C. (*continued*) In the new analysis, the 1995 field is stable, and only the superior half of the 1996 field shows progression. Several points are marked with an x, which denotes insufficient information in the limited glaucoma change probability database to generate a P value, and the point is left without analysis.

pose of this instrument. The excellent sensitivity and specificity obtained in the screening mode of the frequency doubling perimeter, which takes less than 1 minute per eye, offer practitioners a rapid field assessment with approximately the same diagnostic precision as formal visual field tests.

In conventional screening fields, the testing stimulus is an amount arbitrarily larger than the expected value for a particular point. The expected value is based on an unsophisticated version of the hill of vision, leading to many misclassified points. It assumes that all levels of severity of the disease present similarly. In reality, a broad spectrum of presentation is seen, ranging from mild defects that are barely distinguishable from normal visual fields to endstage disease with minimal remaining field. Recall that the purpose of a screening test is to provide rapid assessment if disease is present. Most screening strategies are designed to minimize overcalling normals, which may lead to patients with early disease being erroneously labeled *normal*. Clinically, the practitioner benefits from flexibility in the screening criteria to account for patients with known risk factors who are more likely to have the disease. Clearly the approach to screening a healthy, young white patient is vastly different from an elderly African-American patient with many times the risk for glaucoma.

The FDT perimeter offers two levels of screening based on an extensive database of normal visual fields. The screening tests evaluate the central 20 degrees of the visual field and allow the clinician to choose two levels of sensitivity and the corresponding specificity: the C-20-5 and C-20-1.

The C-20-5 screening test will first presents a stimulus known to be seen by 95% of people with normal visual fields. If missed, it then presents stimuli seen by 98% of people with normal visual fields, followed by 99% if the 98% stimulus is missed. This screening test offers the greater sensitivity but will overcall a number of normal patients as abnormal. The C-20-1 screening test first presents a stimulus known to be seen by 99% of stored tests with normal results for that patient's age group. If that stimulus is not seen, one seen by 99.5% is presented. If that stimulus is also missed, the instrument presents a stimulus of maximum contrast. Points missed only by the 99% stimulus are marked as mild defects. Points that are missed with the 99% and 99.5% stimuli but seen with the maximal contrast target are moderate defects. Severe defects are identified when no stimuli are seen at a particular point. The sensitivity of the C-20-1 is less than that of the C-20-5 and threshold FDT tests, because some early defects are missed with a stimulus seen by 99% of people with normal visual field test results flagged (Figure 7-35). Specificity is better with the C-20-1.

The availability of two levels for screening allows the practitioner to tailor the test to match the patient's risk factors for glaucoma and the setting in which the instrument is used. When screening a general population with minimal risk factors for glaucoma, the C-20-1 is the appropriate level. The C-20-1 may also be used for prescreening a first-time patient who is presenting to the office for a routine examination. Whenever a patient has been identified with risk factors for glaucoma (e.g., African American, elderly, strong family history), the appropriate level is the C-20-5. If prescreening is not routinely performed, a practitioner may elect to perform an FDT C-20-5 test after examination has revealed a suspicious finding. The results of the FDT perimetry can be used to judge if and when conventional static perimetry is necessary.

The literature provides some guidance for the interpretation of screening tests with the FDT perimeter (Table 7-7). Quigley has shown a sensitivity of 91% and specificity of 94% when two missed points, not necessarily adjacent, are used as a criterion for abnormality with the C-20-1 level.[68] The testing point corresponding to the area of the blind spot was excluded in the analysis. The subjects were drawn from a glaucoma specialty practice, and most were experienced Humphrey visual field testers. Johnson has presented data for the C-20-1 that use one significant point as the criterion for abnormality and reported a sensitivity of 84% in mild disease and 100% sensitivity with moderate to advanced disease.[69] His reported specificity was 100%. Using the C-20-5 screening test and two abnormal points, not necessarily adjacent, as the criterion, he reported a sensitivity of 92% for mild disease and sensitivity of 100% for moderate to advanced disease. Specificity was 93%.

With the C-20-1 screening test, the most reasonable approach is to use the one-point criterion to judge abnormality, with the additional requirement that the test be repeated and either the same point or an adjacent point be missed again. For the C-20-5 test, two points that do not have to be adjacent should be missed for the test results to be considered abnormal, and the results should be repeatable. Any patient failing either the C-20-1 or C-20-5 screening requires a conventional white-on-white static visual field test. If conventional white-on-white static perimetry is not available for a diagnostic, confirming test, then the FDT perimeter's threshold test may be performed. The FDT threshold test has been reported with acceptable sensitivity and specificity compared with conventional perimetry.[69]

For threshold examinations, FDT perimetry provides numerical threshold values, total and pattern deviation probability plots, and MD and PSD global indices similar to standard white-on-white perimetry. A central 20-degree program and 30-degree nasal program (tests two additional points in the nasal visual field) are available for the threshold test. Total test time per eye ranges from 2:30 minutes to 6:00 minutes depending on the severity of field loss. Although it takes a few more minutes, the threshold test provides substantially more information when defects are present. Such information is critical in following patients for changes in the visual field. If FDT perimetry proves capable of detecting defects before they are found on white-on-white perimetry, following patients with FDT visual field tests may become an accepted practice.

In general, the results of FDT perimetry and conventional static white-on-white perimetry seem to

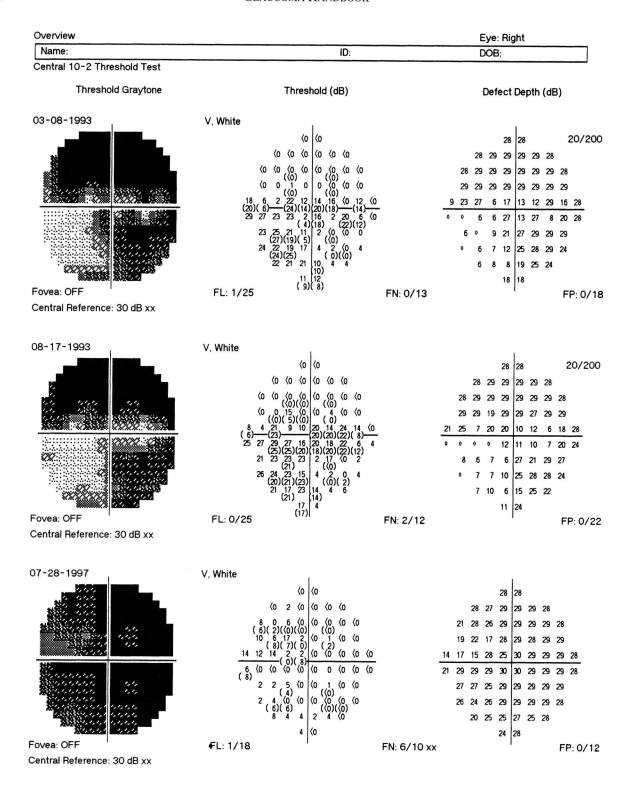

FIGURE 7-31. Progression with size V target. Central 10-2 pattern test showed an endstage field not responsive to the size III target (see Figure 7-20). The patient was switched to the size V target and subsequently followed with this stimulus. Inspection of gray-scale and threshold values show continued decline in the field. The defect depth display subtracts the obtained threshold from an expected hill of vision. The hill of vision used was not generated from an empirical database, and actual values have limited significance. However, the change in the values of the defect depth over time is significant and should be watched for further change.

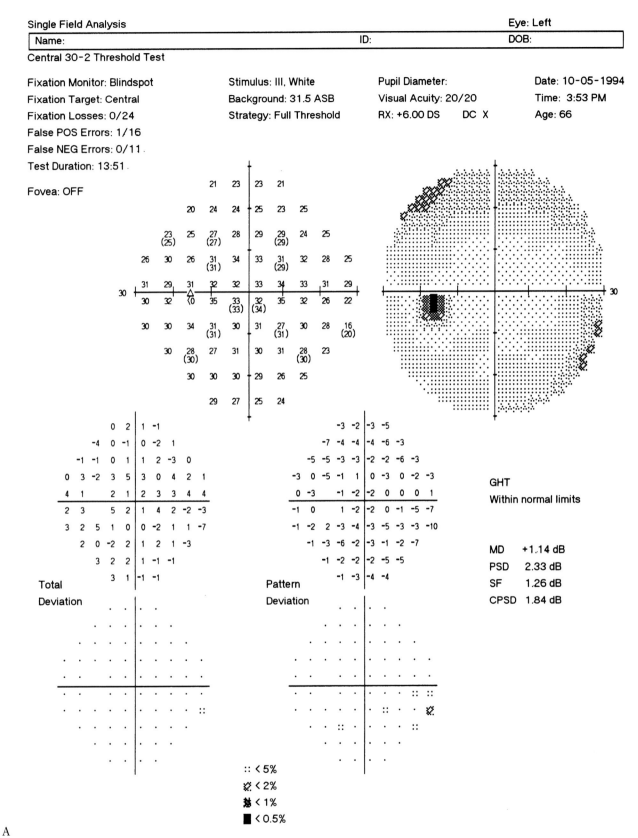

Single Field Analysis   Eye: Left

Name: ID: DOB:

Central 30-2 Threshold Test

Fixation Monitor: Blindspot   Stimulus: III, White   Pupil Diameter: Date: 10-05-1994
Fixation Target: Central   Background: 31.5 ASB   Visual Acuity: 20/20   Time: 3:53 PM
Fixation Losses: 0/24   Strategy: Full Threshold   RX: +6.00 DS   DC X   Age: 66
False POS Errors: 1/16
False NEG Errors: 0/11
Test Duration: 13:51

Fovea: OFF

GHT
Within normal limits

MD   +1.14 dB
PSD   2.33 dB
SF   1.26 dB
CPSD   1.84 dB

Total Deviation

Pattern Deviation

:: < 5%
⊗ < 2%
▨ < 1%
■ < 0.5%

A

FIGURE 7-32. Blue-yellow short-wavelength automated perimetry (SWAP). This glaucoma suspect showed a suspicious thinning of the superior rim tissue and retinal nerve fiber layer in the left eye. The white-on-white visual field was normal except for points with minimal significance in the inferior nasal pattern deviation plot. The cluster criteria, the glaucoma hemifield test (GHT), and corrected pattern standard deviation (CPSD) are normal (A). (continued)

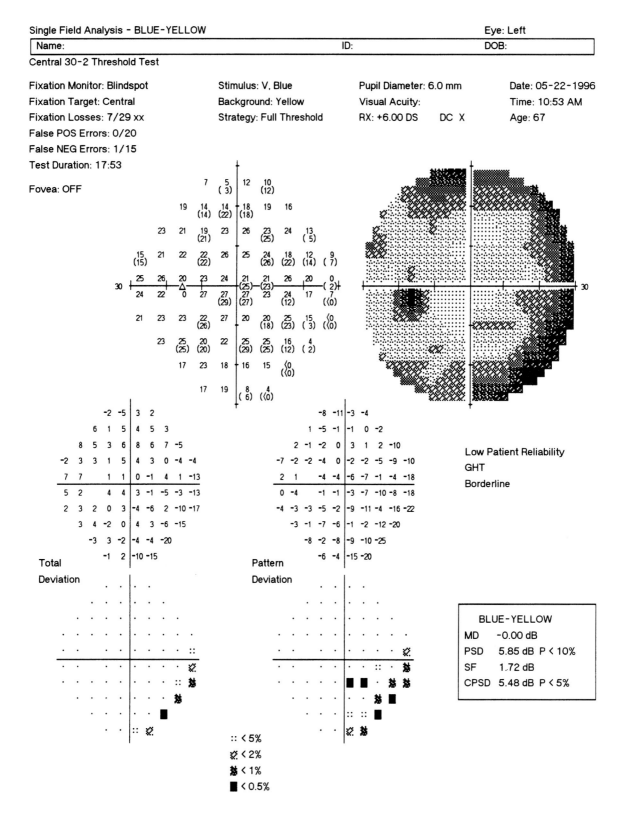

Single Field Analysis - BLUE-YELLOW   Eye: Left

| Name: | ID: | DOB: |

Central 30-2 Threshold Test

Fixation Monitor: Blindspot	Stimulus: V, Blue	Pupil Diameter: 6.0 mm	Date: 05-22-1996
Fixation Target: Central	Background: Yellow	Visual Acuity:	Time: 10:53 AM
Fixation Losses: 7/29 xx	Strategy: Full Threshold	RX: +6.00 DS DC X	Age: 67

False POS Errors: 0/20

False NEG Errors: 1/15

Test Duration: 17:53

Fovea: OFF

Low Patient Reliability
GHT
Borderline

Total
Deviation

Pattern
Deviation

BLUE-YELLOW	
MD	-0.00 dB
PSD	5.85 dB P < 10%
SF	1.72 dB
CPSD	5.48 dB P < 5%

:: < 5%
⊠ < 2%
▨ < 1%
■ < 0.5%

B

FIGURE 7-32. (*continued*) Testing with blue-yellow perimetry showed an inferior nasal defect on the pattern deviation plot with SWAPAC analysis (**B**). SWAP is able to identify defects earlier than white-on-white perimetry, but greater patient variability occurs with SWAP. At the time of this writing, SWAP should be used only on high-risk glaucoma suspects who test normal with white-on-white perimetry.

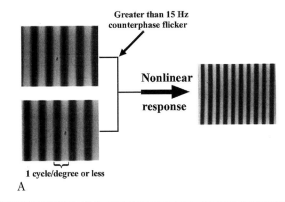

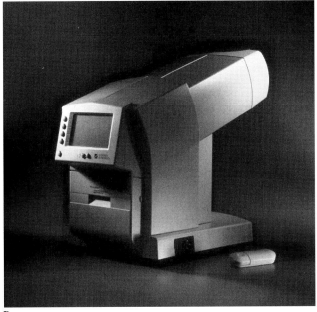

FIGURE 7-33. Frequency-doubling effect and technology. **(A)** Diagram shows frequency-doubling effect. Vertical light and dark bars are flickered back and forth so the light bars become dark and the dark bars become light. The patient appears to see twice the number of vertical bars, hence the term *frequency doubling*. It is proposed that a special subset of ganglion cell axons are sensitive to the frequency-doubling phenomenon. **(B)** Frequency-doubling technology instrument weighs approximately 19 lb, making it portable for screenings. (Photograph courtesy of Welch Allyn, Skaneateles Falls, NY.)

correlate fairly well (see Figure 7-34). It should be remembered that FDT perimetry and conventional white-on-white perimetry are two entirely different psychophysical tests, and some differences are expected. The screening programs of the FDT perimeter test out only to 20 degrees and may miss more peripheral nasal steps. The test target for FDT is larger than that used for conventional perimetry.

TABLE 7-7. Criterion for Abnormality with Frequency-Doubling Screening Perimetry

C-20-1 screening (use for low-risk glaucoma suspect):

One point missed, should be present at same or adjacent location on repeated test (area corresponding to blind spot excluded). If defect appears a second time, conventional test (Full Threshold or SITA [Swedish Interactive Thresholding Algorithm] 30-2 or 24-2) should be performed.

C-20-5 screening (use for higher risk glaucoma suspect, for example, African American, elderly, strong family history):

Two points missed that do not need to be adjacent and should be present at same or adjacent location on repeated test (area corresponding to blind spot excluded). If the defect appears a second time, conventional test (Full Threshold or SITA 30-2 or 24-2) should be performed.

Therefore, small scotomas may be missed with FDT, but broader diffuse loss may be uncovered early with FDT. The testing time is considerably shorter for FDT perimeter, which may reduce the incidence of fatigue artifacts.

At the time of this writing, it is recommended that the FDT perimeter be primarily used as a glaucoma screening device. The C-20-1 program should be used for low-risk glaucoma suspects and the C-20-5 program for high-risk glaucoma suspects. A positive defect on the FDT perimeter (see Table 7-7) should be confirmed and followed with conventional white-on-white perimetry. It may be possible that the threshold program on the FDT perimeter could be used to follow glaucoma patients for progression. However, the test offers fewer points to follow for progression than conventional perimetry (17 or 19 versus 54 or 76 points), and clinical studies are needed to prove its sensitivity and reliability before this becomes an accepted clinical practice.

CONCLUSION

Visual field testing plays an important role in the diagnosis of glaucoma. Visual field loss can also be classified by severity, playing a key role in the determination of the level of aggressiveness of therapy and setting a target pressure. Finally, visual fields are our primary indicator of the stability of glaucoma damage and the effectiveness of therapy. Although automated perimetry provides an invaluable tool, it requires a significant investment in resources and a firm commitment of time to master its intricacies.

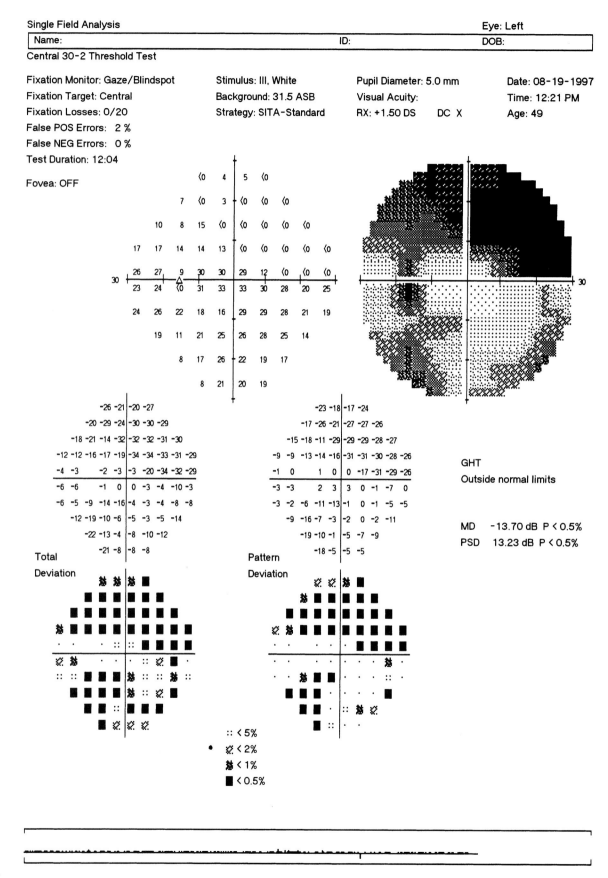

Single Field Analysis   Eye: Left

Name: ID: DOB:

Central 30-2 Threshold Test

Fixation Monitor: Gaze/Blindspot   Stimulus: III, White   Pupil Diameter: 5.0 mm   Date: 08-19-1997
Fixation Target: Central   Background: 31.5 ASB   Visual Acuity: Time: 12:21 PM
Fixation Losses: 0/20   Strategy: SITA-Standard   RX: +1.50 DS   DC X   Age: 49
False POS Errors: 2 %
False NEG Errors: 0 %
Test Duration: 12:04

Fovea: OFF

GHT
Outside normal limits

MD   -13.70 dB   P < 0.5%
PSD   13.23 dB   P < 0.5%

Total Deviation

Pattern Deviation

:: < 5%
✠ < 2%
⊠ < 1%
■ < 0.5%

A

FIGURE 7-34. Frequency-doubling technology (FDT) perimetry corresponding to static perimetry. This advanced glaucoma patient has a double arcuate visual field defect in the left eye that is greater above than below on Swedish Interactive Thresholding Algorithm (SITA) Standard perimetry (**A**). Test time was 12 minutes.

Full Threshold N-30

<u>LEFT EYE</u>

Test Duration 05:07 min

Threshold (dB)

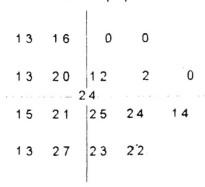

13	16	0	0	
13	20	12	2	0
15	21	25	24	14
13	27	23	22	

24

SCREENING C-20-1

<u>LEFT EYE</u>

Test Duration: 01:46 min

Deviation

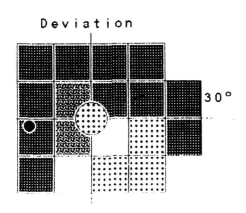

30°

Deviation

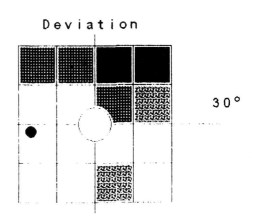

30°

```
MD    -9.84 dB   P  <  0.5%
PSD   +9.93 dB   P  <  1%

FIXATION    ERRS  :  0/6
FALSE  POS  ERRS  :  0/8
FALSE  NEG  ERRS  :  1/5
```

```
FIXATION   ERRS .  0/3
FALSE POS  ERRS. :  0/3
```

```
Probability Symbols
[       ]  P  > =  5%
[·······]  P  <   5%
[:::::::]  P  <   2%
[≈≈≈≈≈≈≈]  P  <   1%
[███████]  P  <   0.5%
```

```
[       ]  WITHIN NORMAL LIMITS
[≈≈≈≈≈≈≈]  MILD RELATIVE LOSS
[███████]  MODERATE RELATIVE LOSS
[███████]  SEVERE LOSS
```

B

C

FIGURE 7-34. (*continued*) FDT shows a similar deficit that is greater above than below. Note the better delineation of the vision loss on the N-30 (threshold) FDT (**B**) than the C-20-1 (screening) FDT (**C**). However, the testing times were 5 minutes and 7 seconds versus 1 minute and 46 seconds, respectively. Threshold FDT has better sensitivity than screening FDT, but the testing times are significantly longer.

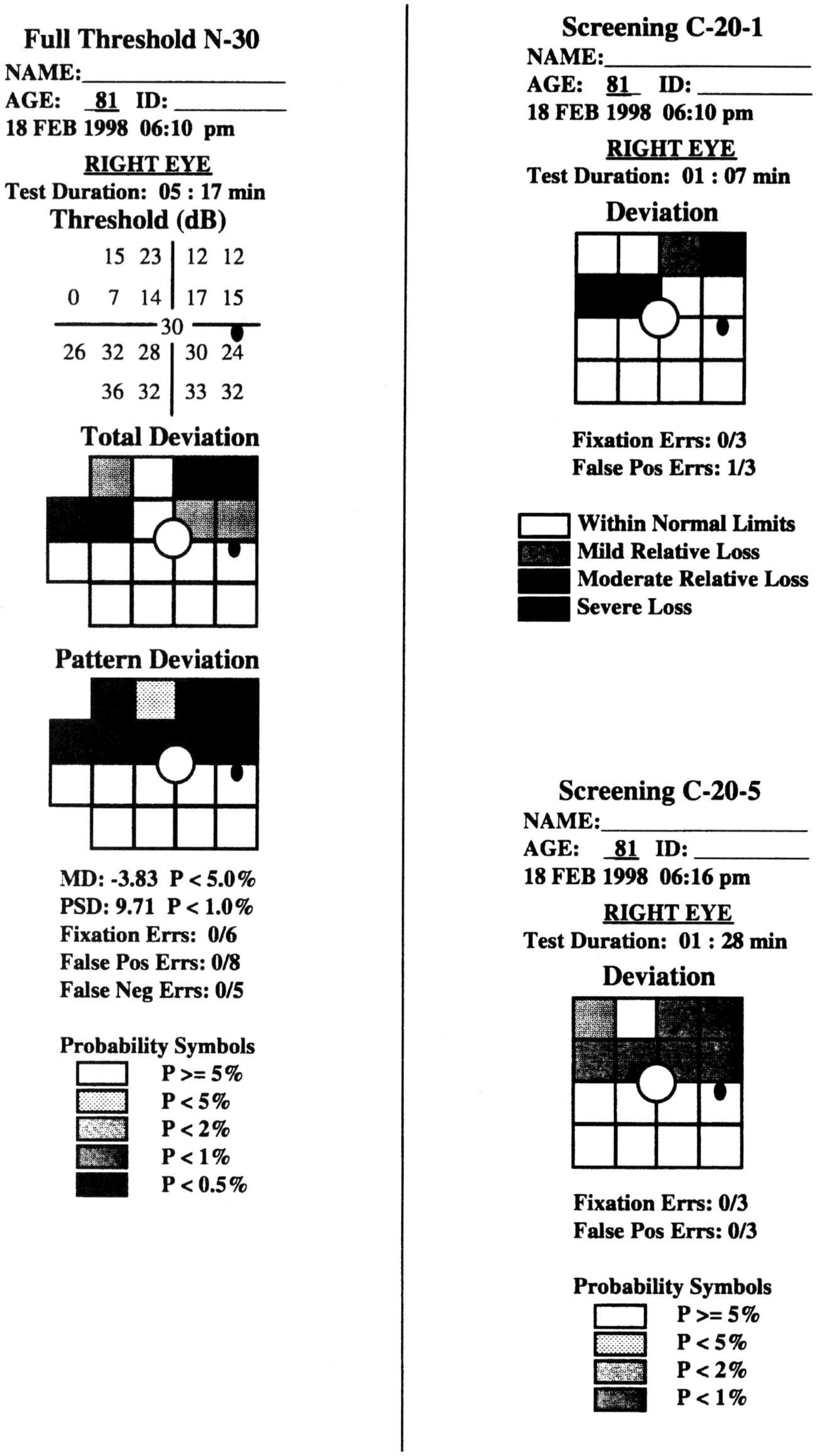

Full Threshold N-30

NAME:_____
AGE: __81__ ID: _____
18 FEB 1998 06:10 pm

<u>**RIGHT EYE**</u>
Test Duration: 05 : 17 min

Threshold (dB)

15	23	12	12	
0	7	14	17	15

———30———

| 26 | 32 | 28 | 30 | 24 |
| | 36 | 32 | 33 | 32 |

Total Deviation

Pattern Deviation

MD: -3.83 P < 5.0%
PSD: 9.71 P < 1.0%
Fixation Errs: 0/6
False Pos Errs: 0/8
False Neg Errs: 0/5

Probability Symbols

☐	P >= 5%
▒	P < 5%
▒	P < 2%
▓	P < 1%
■	P < 0.5%

Screening C-20-1

NAME:_____
AGE: __81__ ID: _____
18 FEB 1998 06:10 pm

<u>**RIGHT EYE**</u>
Test Duration: 01 : 07 min

Deviation

Fixation Errs: 0/3
False Pos Errs: 1/3

☐	**Within Normal Limits**
▒	**Mild Relative Loss**
▓	**Moderate Relative Loss**
■	**Severe Loss**

Screening C-20-5

NAME:_____
AGE: __81__ ID: _____
18 FEB 1998 06:16 pm

<u>**RIGHT EYE**</u>
Test Duration: 01 : 28 min

Deviation

Fixation Errs: 0/3
False Pos Errs: 0/3

Probability Symbols

☐	P >= 5%
▒	P < 5%
▒	P < 2%
▓	P < 1%

FIGURE 7-35. Frequency-doubling technology perimetry shows different sensitivities between screening C-20-1, C-20-5, and threshold N-30 testing strategies. The testing times are 5 minutes for the N-30 threshold test and less than 1.5 minutes for the two screening tests. The C-20-5 has better sensitivity for identifying defects than the C-20-1, but with slightly less specificity. It is recommended that high-risk glaucoma suspects be tested with the C-20-5 program and low-risk glaucoma suspects be tested with the C-20-1 program. (Courtesy of CA Johnson, M Wall, M Fingeret, et al. A Primer for Frequency Doubling Technology. Skaneateles Falls, NY: Welch Allyn; 1998;18.)

Acknowledgments

To Vincent Michael Patella, O.D., Zeiss Humphrey Systems, Dublin, CA, for all his patience and guidance in the preparation of this chapter.

REFERENCES

1. Seamone C, LeBlanc R, Rubillowics M, et al. The value of indices in the central and peripheral visual fields for the detection of glaucoma. Am J Ophthalmol 1988;106:180–185.

2. Caprioli J, Spaeth G. Static threshold examination of the peripheral nasal visual field in glaucoma. Arch Ophthalmol 1985;103:1150–1154.

3. Kosoko O, Sommer A, Auer C. Screening with automated perimetry using a threshold-related three level algorithm. Ophthalmology 1986;93(7):882–886.

4. Tielsch JM, Sommer A, Katz J, et al. Racial variations in the prevalence of primary open-angle glaucoma. The Baltimore Eye Survey. JAMA 1991;266(3):369–374.

5. Gordan MO, Kass MA. The Ocular Hypertension Study: design and baseline description of the participants. Arch Ophthalmol 1999;117(5):573–583.

6. Leske MC, Heijl A, Hyman L, et al. Early Manifest Glaucoma Trial: design and baseline data. Ophthalmology 1999;106:2144–2153.

7. Weber J, Schultz T, Ulrich H. The visual field in advanced glaucoma. Int Ophthalmol 1989;13:47–50.

8. Kolker A. Visual prognosis in advanced glaucoma: a comparison of medical and surgical therapy. Trans Am Ophthalmol Soc 1977;75:538–555.

9. Flanagan J, Wild JM, Trope GE. Evaluation of FASTPAC, a new strategy for threshold estimation with the Humphrey field analyser, in a glaucomatous population. Ophthalmology 1993;100:949–954.

10. Heijl A, Lindgen G. Normal variability of static threshold values across the central visual field. Arch Ophthalmol 1987;105(11):1154–1549.

11. Heijl A, Lindgen G, Olsson J. The effect of perimetric experience in normal subjects. Arch Ophthalmol 1989;107(1):81–86.

12. Heijl A, Lindgen G, Olsson J, Asman P. Visual field interpretation with perimetric probability maps. Arch Ophthalmol 1989;107(2):204–208.

13. Bentsson B, Olsson H, Heijl A, Rootzen H. A new generation of algorithms for computerized threshold perimetry, SITA. Acta Ophthalmol Scand 1997;75(4):368–375.

14. Sanabria O, Fuer WJ, Anderson DR. Pseudo-loss of fixation in automated perimetry. Ophthalmology 1991;98:76–78.

15. Katz J, Sommer A. Screening for glaucomatous visual field loss. The effect of patient reliability. Ophthalmology 1990;97:1032–1037.

16. Heijl A, Lindgen G, Olsson J. Reliability Parameters in Computerized Perimetry. In EL Greve, A Heijl (eds). Seventh International Visual Field Symposium, Amsterdam, Sept. 1986. Dordecht: Martinus Niijhoff/Dr. W Junk, 1987;593–600. (Doc Ophthalmol Proc Ser; 49).

17. Katz J, Sommer A, Gaasterland D, Anderson D. Comparison of analytic algorithms for detecting glaucomatous visual field loss. Arch Ophthalmol 1991;109:1684–1689.

18. Weinreb RN, Perlman JP. the effect of refractive correction on automated perimetric thresholds. Am J Ophthalmol 1986;101:706–709.

19. Goldstick B, Weinreb RN. The effect of refractive error on automated global analysis programs G-1. Am J Ophthalmol 1987;104:229–232.

20. Meyer DR, Stern JH, Jarvis JM, et al. Evaluating the visual field effects of blepharoptosis using automated static perimetry. Ophthalmology 1993;100:655–658.

21. Budenz DL, Fuer WJ, Anderson DR. The effect of simulated cataract on the glaucomatous visual field. Ophthalmology 1993;100(4):511–517.

22. Lam BL, Alward WL, Kolder HE. Effect of cataract on automated perimetry. Ophthalmology 1991;98(7):1066–1070.

23. Henricsson M, Heijl A. Visual fields at different stages of diabetic retinopathy. Acta Ophthalmol 1994;72:560–569.

24. Chee CK, Flanagan DW. Visual field loss with capillary non-perfusion in preproliferative and early proliferative diabetic retinopathy. Br J Ophthalmol 1993;77:726–730.

25. Burde RM, Savino PJ, Trobe JD. Clinical decisions in neuro-ophthalmology. St. Louis: Mosby, 1992:41–73.

26. Sommer A, Quigley H, Robin A, et al. Evaluation of nerve fiber layer assessment. Arch Ophthalmol 1984;102:1766–1771.

27. Katz J, Sommer A. Asymmetry and variation in the normal hill of vision. Arch Ophthalmol 1986;104(10): 65–68.

28. Young WO, Stewart WC, Hunt H, et al. Static threshold variability in the peripheral visual field in normal subjects. Graefes Arch Clin Exp Ophthalmol 1990;228:454–457.

29. Heijl A, Lindgren G, Olsson J. A package for the statistical analysis of visual fields. Doc Ophthalmol Pro Ser 1987;49:153–168.

30. Heijl A, Asman P. A clinical study of perimetric probability maps. Arch Ophthalmol 1989;07(2): 199–203.

31. Drance SM. Diffuse visual field loss in open-angle glaucoma. Ophthalmology 1991;98:1533–1538.

32. Asman P, Heijl A. Diffuse visual field loss and glaucoma. Acta Ophthalmol 1994;72:303–308.

33. Lalle PA. Visual Fields. In T Lewis, M Fingeret (eds). Primary Care of the Glaucomas. Norwalk, Conn.: Appleton & Lange, 1992;159–196.

34. Katz J, Tielsch J, Quigley H, Sommer A. Automated perimetry detects visual field loss before manual Goldmann perimetry. Ophthalmology 1995;102:21–26.

35. Glaucoma Laser Trial Research Group. The Glaucoma Laser Trial (GLT): 6. Treatment group differences in visual field changes. Am J Ophthalmol 1995; 120(1):10–22.

36. Schulzer M. Normal-Tension Glaucoma Study Group. Errors in the diagnosis of visual field progression in normal-tension glaucoma. Ophthalmology 1994;101:1589–1595.

37. Caprioli J. Automated perimetry in glaucoma. Am J Ophthalmol 1991;111(2):235–239.

38. Advanced Glaucoma Intervention Study Investigators. Advanced Glaucoma Intervention Study 2. Visual field test scoring and reliability. Ophthalmol 1994;101:1445–1455.

39. Duggan C, Sommer A, Auer C, Burkhard K. Automated differential threshold perimetry for detecting glaucomatous visual field loss. Am J Ophthalmol 1985;100:420–423.

40. Canner JK, Sommer A, Katz J, Enger C. ICE-PACK: a user friendly software package for processing Humphrey field analyzer diskettes. Invest Ophthalmol Vis Sci 1988;29(suppl):356.

41. Sommer A, Duggan C, Auer C, Abbey H. Analytic approaches to the interpretation of automated threshold perimetric data for the diagnosis of early glaucoma. Trans Am Ophthalmol Soc 1985;83:250–267.

42. Asman P, Heijl A. Glaucoma hemifield test. Automated visual field evaluation. Arch Ophthalmol 1992;110:812–819.

43. Asman P, Heijl A. Evaluation of methods for automated hemifield analysis in perimetry. Arch Ophthalmol 1992;110:820–826.

44. Katz J, Quigley H, Sommer A. Repeatability of the glaucoma hemifield test in automated perimetry. Invest Ophthalmol Sci 1995;36:1658–1664.

45. Hodapp E, Parrish R, Anderson D. Clinical Decisions in Glaucoma. St. Louis: Mosby, 1993;53–59, 99.

46. Werner E, Bishop K, Koelle J, et al. A comparison of experienced clinical observers and statistical tests in the detection of progressive visual field loss in glaucoma using automated perimetry. Arch Ophthalmol 1988;106:619–623.

47. Birch M, Wishart P, O'Donnell. Determining progressive visual field loss in serial Humphrey visual fields. Ophthalmol 1995;102:1227–1235.

48. Mikelberg F, Drance S. The mode of progression of visual field defects in glaucoma. Am J Ophthalmol 1984;98:443–445.

49. Heijl A, Lindgren A, Lindgren G. Test-retest variability in glaucomatous visual fields. Am J Ophthalmol 1989;108:130–135.

50. Werner EB, Petrig B, Krupin T, Bishop K. Variability of automated visual fields in clinically stable glaucoma patients. Invest Ophthalmol Vis Sci 1989;30:1083–1089.

51. Boeglin RJ, Zulauf M, Hoffman D, et al. Long-term fluctuation of the visual field in clinically stable glaucoma patients. Invest Ophthalmol Vis Sci 1991;32:1192–1198.

52. Collaborative Normal-Tension Glaucoma Study Group. Comparison of glaucomatous progression between untreated patients with normal-tension glaucoma and patients with therapeutically reduced intraocular pressures. Am J Ophthalmol 1998;126:487–497.

53. Quigley H, Addicks E, Green W. Optic nerve damage in human glaucoma. III. Quantitative correlation of nerve fiber loss and visual field defect in glaucoma, ischemic optic neuropathy, disk edema, and toxic neuropathy. Am J Ophthalmol 1983;673–679.

54. Quigley H, Dunkelgerger B, Green W. Retinal ganglion cell atrophy correlated with automated perimetry in human eyes with glaucoma. Am J Ophthalmol 1989;107(5):453–464.

55. Johnson CA, Adams AJ, Casson EJ, et al. Blue on yellow perimetry can predict the development of glaucomatous visual field loss. Arch Ophthalmol 111(15):645–650

56. Johnson CA, Adams AJ, Casson EJ, et al. Progression of early glaucomatous visual field loss as detected by blue-on-yellow perimetry and standard white-on-white automated perimetry. Arch Ophthalmol 1993;111(15):651–656.

57. Sample P, Martinez G, Weinreb R. Color visual fields: a 5 year prospective study in eyes with primary open angle glaucoma. In RP Mills (ed). Perimetry Update 1992/93. New York: Kugler Publications, 1993;467–473.

58. Sample P, Weinreb R. Progressive color visual field loss in glaucoma. Invest Ophthalmol Vis Sci 1992;33:240–243.

59. Casson E, Johnson C, Shapiro L. Longitudinal comparison of temporal-modulation perimetry with white-on-white and blue-on-yellow perimetry in ocular hypertension and glaucoma. J Opt Soc Am [A] 1993; 10(8):1792–1806.

60. Adams A, Rodic R, Husted R, Stamper R. Spectral sensitivity and color discrimination changes in glaucoma and glaucoma-suspect patients. Invest Ophthalmol Vis Sci 1982;23(4):516–524.

61. Lynch S, Demirel S, Johnson C. Are early losses of visual function in glaucoma selective or non-selective? Invest Ophthalmol Vis Sci 1996;37(3):S410 (abstract 1914).

62. Johnson CA. Selective versus nonselective losses in glaucoma. J Glaucoma 1994;3(suppl):S32–S44.

63. Wild JM, Moss ID, Whitaker D, O'Neill EC. The statistical interpretation of blue-on-yellow visual field loss. Invest Ophthalmol Vis Sci 1995;36:1398–1410.

64. Moss ID, Wild JM, Whitaker DJ. The influence of age-related cataract on blue on yellow perimetry. Invest Ophthalmol Vis Sci 1995;36:764–773.

65. Newman M. Visual Acuity. In R Moses (ed). Adler's Physiology of the Eye: Clinical Application. St. Louis: Mosby, 1970;581.

66. Maddess T, Henry GH. Performance of nonlinear visual units in ocular hypertension and glaucoma. Clin Vis Sci 1992;7:371–383.

67. Johnson CA, Samuels SJ. Screening for glaucomatous visual field loss with frequency doubling perimetry. Invest Ophthalmol Vis Sci 1997;38:413–425.

68. Quigley HA. Identification of glaucomatous visual field abnormality with the screening protocol of frequency doubling perimetry. Am J Ophthalmol 1998;6:819–829.

69. Johnson CA, Cioffi GA, Van Buskirk M. Evaluation of two screening tests for frequency doubling technology perimetry. Presented at International Perimetric Society meeting, Sept. 7, 1998. In Wall M, Wild J (eds). Proceedings of the XIIIth International Perimetric Society Meeting, Gardone Riviera (BS), Italy, September 6, 1998. Kruger Publications, The Hague/Netherlands, 103–109.

Glaucoma Treatment

8

Antiglaucoma Medications

Bruce E. Onofrey and Thomas R. Stelmack

ANATOMY OF AQUEOUS DYNAMICS

A brief review of the pertinent anatomy and physiology of aqueous humor production and flow is helpful in understanding the mechanisms of action of antiglaucoma drugs. Aqueous humor is produced by the ciliary body and flows into the posterior chamber at approximately 2–3 μl per minute.[1,2] There is a concurrent drainage of aqueous from the anterior chamber of the eye, so the complete turnover of aqueous in the eye occurs every 1–2 hours. Most of the aqueous comes from active secretion of the ciliary epithelium and, to a lesser extent, ultrafiltration (a passive pressure-driven process). Certain influences on secretion include local vasodilation or vasoconstriction of the ciliary body, the pH of the cell membrane, and the presence of carbonic anhydrase enzyme(s). Additionally, β-adrenergic agonist activity is thought to play a role in active secretion of aqueous. It is theorized that this happens at the level of the ciliary epithelium, but a vascular site has not been ruled out.[3] β Blockage of the ciliary body, mainly through a β_2 receptor, reduces the amount of aqueous production. α Receptors are also located on the ciliary body, and stimulation of the α_2 receptors causes a decrease in aqueous production.

After it is produced by the ciliary epithelium, the aqueous humor moves by bulk flow into the posterior chamber, across the anterior surface of the lens through the pupil into the anterior chamber. Aqueous provides metabolic and nutritional needs to the avascular lens and cornea. More than 80% of aqueous humor exits the eye through the trabecular meshwork (TM) into Schlemm's canal. There are three layers of TM (see Figure 4-3). The two innermost layers, the uveal- and corneoscleral meshwork, contain small pores that help filter and phagocytize debris from the aqueous. The outmost layer of the TM or inner layer of Schlemm's canal is the juxtacanalicular meshwork, which is the rate-controlling membrane that allows aqueous to drain from the anterior chamber into Schlemm's canal.

A resistance and a subsequent pressure decrease occur across the inner wall of Schlemm's canal[4-8] that thereby causes the pressure in the TM proximal to the canal (toward the anterior chamber side) to be higher than the pressure in the canal. TM outflow is pressure dependent. At elevated intraocular pressure (IOP), the TM distends and the inner wall moves toward the outer wall of the canal.[9,10] Cholinergic stimulation of the ciliary muscle causes the ciliary body to contract and stretch open the TM to increase aqueous outflow into Schlemm's canal. There may be β_2-adrenergic receptors on the TM that when stimulated also increase outflow. Once aqueous enters Schlemm's canal, it is drained into the episcleral venous plexus and episcleral veins via a series of intrascleral-collecting channels (see Figure 4-2B).

Up to 20% of the aqueous is drained through a separate route, the uveoscleral pathway. This pathway includes the absorption of aqueous by the ciliary body and iris, as well as the passage of aqueous through the longitudinal muscle fibers of the ciliary body to the suprachoroidal space, and exit via the vortex veins or through the sclera. Contraction of the ciliary muscle by cholinergic agonists may decrease uveoscleral outflow, whereas relaxing the ciliary muscle with a cycloplegic agent may enhance uveoscleral outflow facility.[11-13] Weak prostaglandin agents appear to alter the matrix of the ciliary body and increase uveoscleral outflow without inducing inflammation. Unlike trabecular outflow, which is limited by the pressure in the episcleral veins, uveoscleral outflow is independent of the IOP.[14,15]

The other important aspect of aqueous dynamics is diurnal variation. Brubaker[1] has shown that aqueous production has a range in healthy patients from 1.8 to 4.3 µl per minute; the rate is generally highest in morning hours, slightly lower during the afternoon hours, and approximately one-half of the morning rate during sleep. The hormonal basis is unknown, but it is symmetric in those with unilateral Horner's syndrome. This suggests a nonsympathetic mechanism. The rate declines by 3.2% per decade after the age of 10 years, and there is no gender difference.[16] Wilensky and Zeimer,[16] as well as Brown and colleagues,[17] have shown that IOP spikes on awakening, and that the increase lasts for approximately 30 minutes. Wide diurnal variations occur more frequently among glaucoma patients than nonglaucoma patients.[3,18,19] IOP spikes in glaucoma patients can be sporadic and not occur with any temporal pattern.

ANTIGLAUCOMA AGENTS

The pharmacologic agents used in the treatment of glaucoma are grouped by their pharmacologic or physiologic action (Table 8-1). This includes adrenergic agents (both antagonistic and agonistic), cholinergic agents (both direct and indirect [cholinesterase inhibiting] acting), carbonic anhydrase inhibitors (CAIs), prostaglandin agents, and hyperosmotics.

β-Adrenergic–Blocking Agents (Nonselective)

Timolol Maleate (Timoptic)

Timolol maleate (Merck, West Point, PA) was the first topical beta blocker to receive U.S. Food and Drug Administration (FDA) approval for the treatment of glaucoma. The oral drug was used before approval in the treatment of cardiac arrhythmias and hypertension. It is a nonselective blocking agent that has theoretically no preference for β_1- or β_2-receptor sites. It has no intrinsic sympathomimetic activity. Timolol's mode of action is to reduce aqueous production primarily via β_2 blockade of the ciliary body. Despite a small subgroup of patients who do not respond to timolol therapy,[20] most respond with a significant reduction in IOP. The average reduction reported is approximately 7 mm Hg (20–30%).[11] The drug's effectiveness can wane during the first 2 weeks by approximately 30–40% (short-term escape) with some additional loss during the first 3 months (long-term drift).[20] Because timolol has a remarkably constant effect on aqueous flow,[21] normalization of

inflow does not occur until 2–6 weeks after timolol has been discontinued.[22] For this reason, most clinicians use a 4-week period to "wash out" the medication before reassessing any change in IOP. Because the drug has significant systemic absorption, when one eye is treated, the fellow eye to a lesser degree can also exhibit a lowering of IOP. Data from the Glaucoma Laser Trial[23] suggested a 0.5-mm contralateral effect. However, information from the Ocular Hypertension Treatment Study indicates that the average contralateral effect of uniocular beta-blocker therapy is much higher (7% ± 12%).

Timolol is the most commonly prescribed beta-blocking agent. Beta blockers are the most frequently used first-line antiglaucoma drugs because of their cost effectiveness and because of the possibility of using a once- or twice-daily dosage, which improves compliance. Timolol is available in two concentrations: 0.25% and 0.5%. The 5-ml dropper bottle, with proper application, provides twice-daily treatment in both eyes for approximately 1 month. It is also available in 2.5-, 10.0-, and 15.0-ml dropper bottles. The 0.5% concentration is the most commonly prescribed, although the 0.25% concentration can demonstrate similar IOP lowering with fewer systemic side effects. Timoptic is available as a generic medication, as a gelrite formulation (Timoptic XE) (Merck, West Point, PA), and as pseudo-generic in the form of timolol hemihydrate (Betimol-R-Ciba) (CibaVision, Duluth, GA).

Timolol Maleate (Timoptic XE)

Timoptic XE (Merck, West Point, PA) is a thixotropic vehicle of timolol maleate that allows for once-daily dosing. It is available in 0.25% and 0.5% concentrations. The special vehicle changes from a liquid to a gel-like state when it is instilled. This sustained-release form has been shown to extend the effect of the drug for 24 hours. The gel formation can temporarily blur the patient's vision. The gel is also available as a generic.

Timolol Hemihydrate (Betimol)

Timolol hemihydrate (CibaVision, Duluth, GA) is a nonselective beta-blocking agent. It comes in a 0.25% and 0.5% concentration and is prescribed at a dosage of once or twice a day. The drug has the same IOP-lowering efficacy and systemic side effects as timolol maleate[24] but has been marketed at a much lower cost. Stewart showed that once-daily administration of Betimol 0.5% was equivalent to once-daily administration of Timoptic XE 0.5%.[25] It should be noted that even though timolol maleate and timolol hemihydrate drugs are pharmacologically similar and therapeutically equivalent, the pharmacist cannot automatically substitute them. Technically, prescriptions must specify Betimol or timolol hemihydrate.

TABLE 8-1. Pharmacologic Agents for Glaucoma

Drug	Concentration %/size	Dosage	Mechanism of action	Complications
Beta blockers				
Timolol maleate ophthalmic solution (Timoptic)	0.25, 0.5/2.5, 5.0, 10.0, 15.0 ml	qd–b.i.d.	Reduction of aqueous production via nonselective β-receptor blockade on ciliary body	Exacerbation of chronic obstructive pulmonary disease (asthma, emphysema, chronic bronchitis), congestive heart failure, cardiac arrhythmia, bradycardia, hypotension, headache, fatigue, depression, dizziness, impotence
Timolol maleate Ocudose dispenser (preservative-free unit dose container)	0.25, 0.5/0.45-ml	qd–b.i.d.	Same as above	Same as above
Timolol maleate ophthalmic gel-forming solution (Timoptic XE)	0.25, 0.5/2.5, 5.0 ml	qd	Reduction of aqueous production via nonselective β-receptor blockade via a thixotropic vehicle that turns from liquid to a gel-like state when instilled; allows for once-daily dose	Same as above
Timolol hemihydrate (Betimol)	0.25, 0.5/2.5, 5.0, 10.0, 15.0 ml	qd–b.i.d.	Same as timolol maleate	Same as timolol maleate
Metipranolol (Optipranolol)	0.3/5.0, 10.0 ml	b.i.d.	Same as timolol maleate	Same as timolol maleate with the addition of granulomatous uveitis
Levobunolol (Betagan)	0.25/5.0, 10.0 and 0.5/5.0, 10.0, 15.0 ml	qd–b.i.d.	Same as timolol maleate	Same as timolol maleate
Carteolol (Ocupress)	1.0/5.0, 10.0, 15.0 ml	b.i.d.	Same as timolol maleate with intrinsic sympathomimetic activity and less effect on serum lipoproteins	Same as timolol maleate with less risk of cardiac and central nervous system side effects because of intrinsic sympathomimetic activity
Betaxolol (Betoptic S)	0.25/2.5, 5.0, 10.0, 15.0 ml	b.i.d.	Reduction of aqueous production via β₁-selective-receptor blockade without intrinsic sympathomimetic activity; may have neuroprotectivity and increased perfusion to optic nerve via calcium channel–blocking properties	Fewer problems with pulmonary function than timolol maleate because of β₁ selectivity; ocular stinging
Adrenergic agonists				
Epinephrine (Glaucon, Epifrin)	0.5, 1.0, 2.0/15.0 ml	b.i.d.	Decreased aqueous production via α-receptor stimulation on ciliary body; increased outflow through the trabecular meshwork via stimulation of β₂ receptors	Pupil dilation, adrenochrome deposits, cystoid macular edema (20% of aphakes), follicular conjunctivitis, rebound hyperemia, hypertension, headache, systemic tachycardia, and palpitations

continued

TABLE 8-1. (*continued*)

Drug	Concentration %/size	Dosage	Mechanism of action	Complications
Dipivefrin (Propine)	0.1/5.0, 10.0, 15.0 ml	b.i.d.	Prodrug converted to epinephrine in the eye	Same as epinephrine, but fewer systemic side effects because lower concentration is used
Apraclonidine (Iopidine)	0.5/5.0, 10.0 ml	b.i.d.–t.i.d.	Decreased aqueous production via α_2 stimulation and increased uveoscleral outflow	Dry mouth, blanching of conjunctiva, mydriasis, lid retraction, allergic conjunctivitis, tachyphylaxis, minimal systemic cardiovascular effects
Brimonidine (Alphagan)	0.2/5.0, 10.0, 15.0 ml	b.i.d.–t.i.d.	Decreased aqueous production via α_2 stimulation and increased uveoscleral outflow with 1,000 times greater affinity for α_2 than α_1 receptors; possible neuroprotective properties	Ocular irritation, allergic conjunctivitis, blurring of vision, fatigue, reduction of systemic blood pressure, dry mouth
Cholinergics (miotics)				
Pilocarpine ophthalmic solution (Isopto carpine, Pilocar)	0.25, 0.5, 1.0, 2.0, 3.0, 4.0, 5.0, 6.0, 8.0, 10.0/15.0 ml	q.i.d.	Increased trabecular meshwork outflow via stimulation of ciliary muscle, which contracts and pulls the trabecular meshwork posteriorly; decreased uveoscleral outflow	Ocular stinging, headache, brow ache, accommodative spasm, retinal breaks, retinal detachment, gastrointestinal upset, potential heart block, rare bronchospasm; a high concentration may narrow the angle
Pilocarpine ophthalmic gel (Pilopine HS)	4.0/3.5-g tube	qhs	Same as above	Same as pilocarpine, corneal haze
Pilocarpine (Ocusert Pilo-20)	Pilo-20: 20 mg/h/8 systems per carton	q1w	Same as above	Same as pilocarpine, foreign body sensation
Pilocarpine (Ocusert Pilo-40)	Pilo-40: 40 mg/h/8 systems per carton	q1w	Same as above	Same as pilocarpine, foreign body sensation
Carbachol (Isopto Carbachol)	0.75, 1.5, 2.25, 3.0/15.0 ml	b.i.d.–q.i.d.	Increased trabecular meshwork outflow via stimulation of ciliary muscle, which contracts and pulls the trabecular meshwork posteriorly; decreases uveoscleral outflow; indirect- and direct-acting parasympathomimetic activity	Same as pilocarpine
Cholinesterase inhibitors				
Echothiophate iodide (Phospholine Iodine) (irreversible)	0.03, 0.06, 0.125, 0.25/5.0 ml	qd–b.i.d.	Prevents cholinesterase from removing acetylcholine from synapse between postganglionic/ciliary muscle receptor site resulting in continual stimulation of ciliary muscle	Same as pilocarpine ophthalmic solution with greater risk of central nervous system toxicity; also cataracts, iris cysts, posterior synechiae, and retinal detachment

TABLE 8-1. (*continued*)

Drug	Concentration %/size	Dosage	Mechanism of action	Complications
Physostigmine (Eserine Sulfate) ophthalmic ointment (reversible)	0.25/3.5-g tube	b.i.d.–q.i.d.	Same as echothiophate iodide	Same as echothiophate iodide
Demecarium bromide (Humorsol) (reversible)	0.125, .25/5.0 ml	b.i.d.	Same as echothiophate iodide	Same as echothiophate iodide
Topical carbonic anhydrase inhibitors				
Dorzolamide (Trusopt)	2.0/5.0, 10.0 ml	b.i.d.–t.i.d.	Decrease aqueous production via inhibition of carbonic anhydrase	Burning and mild hyperemia, sulfa sensitivities, bitter taste
Brinzolamide (Azopt) (suspension)	1.0/5.0, 10.0, 15.0 ml	b.i.d.–t.i.d.	Same as dorzolamide	Less ocular irritation than dorzolamide due to neutral pH; suspension may temporarily blur vision
Oral carbonic anhydrase inhibitors				
Acetazolamide (Diamox) (Diamox Sequels)	125-, 250-mg tablets; 500-mg extended-release capsules	q.i.d.–tablets, b.i.d.–sequels	Decrease aqueous production via inhibition of carbonic anhydrase	Paresthesias, malaise, gastrointestinal distress, polyuria, nephrolithiasis (renal stones), sulfa sensitivity, anorexia, urethral colic, metabolic acidosis, mental depression/confusion/psychosis, headaches, cardiac arrhythmias from potassium depletion, aplastic anemia
Methazolamide (Neptazane)	25-, 50-mg tablets	b.i.d.–t.i.d.	Same as acetazolamide	Same as acetazolamide
Dichlorphenamide (Daranide)	50-mg tablets	qd–t.i.d.	Same as acetazolamide	Same as acetazolamide
Prostaglandins				
Latanoprost (Xalatan)	0.005/2.5 ml	qhs	Increase uveoscleral outflow	Hyperemia, darkening of iris; cystoid macular edema; anterior uveitis; hypertrichosis, hyperpigmentation of lashes
Combination drugs				
Dorzolamide/Timolol maleate (Cosopt)	2.0/0.5 5.0, 10.0 ml	b.i.d.	Same as dorzolamide and timolol maleate	Same as dorzolamide and timolol maleate
Latanoprost/Timolol (Xalcom)	.005/0.5 2.5ml	qd	Same as timolol and latanoprost	Same as timolol and latanoprost
Hyperosmotics				
Oral route				
Isosorbide (Ismotic)	45%/220 ml	1.5 ml/lb of 45% solution	Reduces vitreal volume via an elevated plasma osmolarity gradient	Nausea, vomiting, headache, confusion, disorientation, gastrointestinal disturbances, dehydration, better tolerated by diabetics

continued

TABLE 8-1. (*continued*)

Drug	Concentration %/size	Dosage	Mechanism of action	Complications
Glycerin (Osmoglyn)	50/220 ml	2–3 ml/kg of 50% solution	Reduces vitreal volume via an elevated plasma osmolarity gradient	Nausea, vomiting, headache, confusion, disorientation, dehydration, cardiac arrhythmias, hyperosmolar nonketotic coma
Intravenous route				
Mannitol (various)	5.0, 10.0, 15.0, 20.0, 25.0 injection	7.5–10.0 ml/kg of 20% solution	Reduces vitreal volume via an elevated plasma osmolarity gradient	Nausea, vomiting, headache, dizziness, blurred vision, electrolyte imbalance, seizures, angina-like chest pain, dehydration, congestive heart failure
Urea (Ureaphil)	40 g/150 single-dose container	1.0–1.5 g/kg	Reduces vitreal volume via an elevated plasma osmolarity gradient	Nausea, vomiting, headache, disorientation, electrolyte imbalance, dehydration

Metipranolol (Optipranolol)

Like timolol, metipranolol hydrochlorate (Optipranolol 0.3%), manufactured by Bausch & Lomb in Rochester, New York is a nonselective beta-blocking agent that is usually prescribed as a twice-daily regimen. It lowers IOP that is higher than 24 mm Hg by 20–26%.[4,5] Optipranolol has no intrinsic sympathomimetic activity and produces weak local anesthesia.[6] It has the same cardiovascular side effects as timolol and slightly greater bronchospasm in asthmatics.[7] The most controversial adverse effect of metipranolol therapy was the development of granulomatous uveitis in two patients.[8] The use of the drug has been discontinued in England for this reason[9]; however, this effect may be associated with the method of sterilization and packaging in England. The major advantage of the drug has been its highly competitive pricing.

Carteolol (Ocupress)

Carteolol (Otsuka Pharmaceutical, Rockville, MD) is another nonspecific beta blocker, available as a 1% solution and prescribed twice daily. Most studies[10,26] comparing it to the other topical beta blockers indicate that it is probably equivalent, although one very short-term study[27] suggests that it is slightly less effective in lowering IOP than timolol. The manufacturer is promoting its intrinsic sympathomimetic activity as a safety advantage. The rationale is that beta blockers with intrinsic sympathomimetic activity have both antagonistic action (blocking) and partial agonistic action (stimulating) on some beta receptors.[26] Theoretically, these drugs may minimize systemic side effects, such as bradycardia and bronchial constriction. There is some evidence of less bradycardia and pulmonary effects with carteolol,[7] although the medication still should not be

used in patients with a history of bradycardia or restrictive airway disease. An additional benefit of carteolol is its relatively minimal effect on high-density lipoprotein (HDL) cholesterol.[28] In a comparison with timolol maleate, carteolol lowered beneficial HDL cholesterol by 3.3%, as compared with timolol's 8% decrease. This suggests that carteolol represents less of a risk to patients who have a significant history of coronary heart disease or unfavorable lipid profiles. An additional characteristic of carteolol is its lower lipid solubility. Decreased lipid solubility results in less drug crossing the blood-brain barrier and theoretically fewer central nervous system side effects.[29]

Levobunolol (Betagan)

Levobunolol (Allergan Pharmaceutical, Irvine, CA) is a nonselective beta blocker that has similar IOP-lowering effect and systemic side effects as timolol. It is available as 0.25% and 0.5% solutions. Pharmaceutical manufacturers are constantly striving to produce delivery systems or dosage regimens that improve patient compliance. When taken orally, levobunolol has a longer half-life than oral timolol: 6 hours versus 3 hours.[30] Dihydrolevobunolol, its major metabolite, is equipotent and equiactive with levobunolol and has a half-life of 7 hours.[30,31] When both chemicals are present, the theoretic functional half-life is therefore four times longer than that of timolol. The advantage of using levobunolol is, therefore, the ability to use it in a once-daily dosage that reduces costs, improves compliance, and lessens potential systemic side effects. Wandel et al.[32] have demonstrated greater IOP reductions with once a day dosage with levobunolol compared to once a day timolol. Derick and colleagues[33] showed once-daily equivalence to twice-daily dosing of levobunolol. Levobunolol is also available as a generic agent.

Side Effects and Contraindications to Nonselective Beta Blockers

Topical nonselective beta blockers are very effective antiglaucoma medications and are generally well tolerated both ocularly and systemically. However, beta blockers are not devoid of potentially serious systemic side effects. Outside of the eye, β_1 receptors are found primarily on the heart, and β_2 receptors on the bronchioles of the lungs. Side effects most frequently occur in patients who have some form of chronic obstructive pulmonary disease (COPD), such as emphysema, chronic bronchitis, or asthma. Beta blockers reduce the ability of the smooth bronchial muscle to dilate by blocking receptor sites and producing a narrowed lumen, causing difficulty with respiration. Patients with congestive heart failure, bradycardia (heart rate lower than 60 beats per minute), or heart block may suffer exacerbation of their condition with beta blockers. Patients using systemic beta-blocker or calcium channel blocker therapy should be closely monitored for additive toxicity (bradycardia or reduced cardiac output). When in doubt, consultation with the patient's cardiologist or treating physician is appropriate. Ocular side effects are relatively rare and include stinging, dry eye, hyperemia, and corneal anesthesia.

Some evidence suggests that beta-blocking agents may adversely affect insulin production, although this does not appear to occur with high frequency.[34] Of greater importance is the ability of beta-blocking agents to mask symptoms of hypoglycemia. Diabetic individuals should be warned of this potential effect and to carefully monitor their blood sugar when initialing beta-blocker therapy.

β-Adrenergic–Blocking Agents (β₁ Selective)

Betaxolol (Betoptic, Betoptic S)

Betaxolol (Alcon Pharmaceutical, Fort Worth, TX) is unique in that it is the only topical β_1 selective blocker available. It is one of the most potent of the cardioselective beta$_1$ blockers and exhibits no intrinsic sympathomimetic activity.[35] Betoptic lowers IOP by decreasing aqueous production.[36] It is available as a 0.5% solution (Betoptic) and a 0.25% suspension (Betoptic S) and is prescribed on a twice-daily schedule. The suspension vehicle contains an ionic exchange resin, which enhances corneal absorption. With this improved bioavailability, no difference is seen in IOP-lowering effectiveness between the 0.5% solution and the 0.25% suspension. Most clinicians prescribe Betoptic S over Betoptic

because of fewer systemic side effects and less stinging. The suspension should be shaken before instillation and may temporarily blur the patient's vision. The 0.5% solution is no longer available in the United States.

Side Effects and Contraindication of Betoptic

Because of its β_1 selectivity, Betoptic may have less of an adverse effect on pulmonary function than nonselective beta blockers.[11,15,37] However, patients with a history of COPD, asthma, or other breathing problems should avoid being prescribed any beta blocker, including betaxolol. There are reports of betaxolol exacerbating pulmonary function in patients with restrictive airway disease.[11] Furthermore, other categories of antiglaucoma medications exist (alpha agonists, CAIs, and prostaglandins) that are effective and do not affect pulmonary function.

Resting and nonresting bradycardia, seen with timolol, are reported to be negligible with betaxolol[12,13,38–40]; however, betaxolol should not be given to a patient with bradycardia, heart block, or congestive heart failure. Tear secretion and corneal sensitivity are reported to be unaffected with betaxolol.[38,41–43] Although the two drugs (timolol and betaxolol) demonstrate comparable efficacy, most studies show timolol to be slightly more effective in lowering IOP than betaxolol.[13,44,45]

Indications for Beta Blockers

The beta-blocking agents are very effective and are the initial glaucoma drug of choice for most clinicians, unless a contraindicating systemic condition, such as asthma, COPD, bradycardia, or heart failure, is present. It is advisable to initially prescribe the lowest concentration of a beta blocker at the lowest dosage (e.g., timolol 0.25% every day). The clinician should document that the patient is at the target pressure at the 24-hour postinstillation reading if once-daily therapy is prescribed. If the target IOP is not obtained, then a twice-daily dosage or a higher concentration can be tried. No clear standard has emerged regarding which of the beta-blocking agents to use first. The most commonly prescribed beta blocker has been Timoptic. However, some clinicians use Betoptic S or Ocupress because of their slightly better safety profiles. Betoptic may also have neuroprotective properties, although this is difficult to confirm. Ocupress may be a suitable choice among all the beta blockers for a patient with an elevated lipid profile. Timoptic XE, Betimol, and Betagan may have a longer duration of action and may be better choices for once-daily therapy. Betimol, Optipranolol, and generic timolol and levobunolol may have cost advantages over other trade-name beta blockers. The final cost of beta-blocker therapy is dependent on the manufacturer's retail price, the number of µls the manufacturer puts in the bottle, the size of the drop the bottle produces, and the ease of drop release from the bottle

(Table 8-2).[46] It is important to instruct the patient on proper drop instillation: Pressure should be placed on the bottom of the inverted bottle instead of on the sides.[47,48]

For medical-legal as well as clinical baseline, the patient's heart rate should be checked before initiating a beta blocker and during the course of treatment. Patients with bradycardia (resting pulse less than 60 beats per minute), heart arrhythmias, congestive heart failure, or second- or third-degree heart block should not be prescribed a beta blocker. Patients should also be questioned about pulmonary disease and shortness of breath before starting beta blockers. Any diagnosis of asthma, COPD, or shortness of breath is a contraindication for the use of beta blockers. Documentation of negative findings in the patient's chart is prudent (e.g., patient denies breathing problems or shortness of breath). Some internal medicine practitioners also evaluate respiratory function before and during systemic beta-blocker therapy. A simple peak-flow test can determine who is susceptible to compromise of the pulmonary function.

Adrenergic Agonists

Apraclonidine (Iopidine)

Clonidine was the first of the α_2 agonists to be investigated for its ability to lower IOP.[49] Due to high-lipid solubility, it easily crosses the blood-brain barrier. This results in significant reduction of systemic blood pressure via the central nervous system. The drug can also reduce perfusion of the optic nerve by the reduction of systemic blood pressure and reduction of local blood flow.[50,51] To capitalize on the IOP-lowering effects of clonidine and to minimize its side effects, the drug apraclonidine (Alcon, Fort Worth, TX) was developed. Apraclonidine exhibits much less lipid solubility than clonidine and therefore is unable to cross the blood-brain barrier. As a result, the systemic side effects are minimal.[52-55] Apraclonidine lowers IOP by decreasing aqueous production and may also increase uveoscleral outflow. It has demonstrated the ability to lower IOP within 1 hour of instillation, with a duration of at least 12 hours. A concentration of 1% was able to produce up to a 37% reduction in IOP, and the 0.5% concentration produced an average decrease in IOP of 27%.[53,56-59] It is available as a 1% concentration in a unit dose 0.5-ml ampule and as a 0.5% solution in a 5-ml bottle.

Side Effects and Contraindications of Apraclonidine

Although apraclonidine is devoid of significant cardiovascular and pulmonary side effects, it still can produce other systemic problems. The most common nonocular side effect of apraclonidine is dry mouth, which occurs in approximately 20–50% of patients. Sedation has been reported in fewer than 10% of patients.[56,60] Ocular side effects of apraclonidine are more common. Blanching of the conjunctiva, mydriasis, and lid retraction have all been reported. All are consistent with the α-agonist effect of the drug.[56,61] Of greater significance is the incidence of allergic reaction and tachyphylaxis associated with apraclonidine use. Allergic blepharoconjunctivitis occurs in 9% of patients within a 3-month period if a 0.5% concentration is used twice daily, and in up to 48% of individuals on longer-term therapy.[57,62,63] Another problem with the drug is its relatively short duration of efficacy. Tachyphylaxis can occur within several months of initiation of treatment.[64,65]

Indications for Apraclonidine

Apraclonidine was initially approved by the FDA in 1987 for its ability to prevent pressure spikes following anterior segment laser procedures. The 1% concentration was instilled 1 hour before surgery and immediately thereafter. The drug also was indicated for acute IOP lowering in patients with angle-closure glaucoma or another need to quickly lower IOP.[66] A study by Stewart and colleagues[62] illustrated that 0.5% apraclonidine could be used effectively in combination with timolol 0.5%. Furthermore, the study was able to show that apraclonidine had a much better IOP-lowering effect during sleep than that observed with timolol. As a result, in 1993, the FDA approved apraclonidine 0.5% three times daily for short-term use in the treatment of glaucoma in patients already on maximum medical therapy. Patients using the drug for longer-term therapy should be monitored for allergic response and tachyphylaxis. Most clinicians prescribe the drug on a twice-daily regimen as adjunctive therapy to reduce the incidence of allergic reaction.

Brimonidine (Alphagan)

Brimonidine (Allergan Pharmaceutical, Irvine, CA) was introduced in the United States in 1996. It comes in a 0.2% solution and is approved for initial glaucoma therapy on a thrice-daily dosage. It differs from apraclonidine in several ways. First, it is more lipophilic than apraclonidine and therefore exhibits better corneal penetration.[67,68] Second, it possesses greater specificity for the α_2 receptor, with 1,000 times the affinity for α_2 versus α_1 receptors.[69] Finally, brimonidine is less prone to oxidation than apraclonidine.[70] This is important because it is the oxidative products of clonidine compounds that are probably responsible for producing ocular allergy, which accounts for the much lower incidence of allergy with brimonidine when compared with apraclonidine. Brimonidine lowers IOP by decreasing aqueous production and by increasing uveoscleral outflow.[71]

Brimonidine 0.2% administered twice daily was found to be comparable to timolol 0.5% and superior to

TABLE 8-2. Drop Volume, Bottle Fill Volume, Days of Therapy, and Cost Per Month of Topical Beta Blockers

Drug	Percentage and nonproprietary name of medication	Manufacturer	Mean ± SD drop volume (ml)	Total volume (from density) (ml)	Used by patients (ml)	Wasted by patients (ml)	Percentage used correctly	Days of therapy per bottle	Cost per month ($)
Betagan	0.5 Levobunolol hydrochloride	Allergan Pharmaceuticals (Irvine, CA)	0.042 ± 0.002	10.10	4.22	3.62	54	32.3	40.50
AK-Beta	0.5 Levobunolol hydrochloride	Akorn Inc. (Abita Springs, LA)	0.045 ± 0.003	9.79	4.52	2.74	62	33.6	29.40
Ocupress	1.0 Carteolol hydrochloride	Otsuka America Pharmaceutical Inc. (Rockville, MD)	0.031 ± 0.005	9.88	3.11	1.17	73	58.0	20.40
Timoptic-XE	0.5 Timolol maleate gel-forming solution	Merck & Co. Inc. (West Point, PA)	0.049 ± 0.006	5.57*	4.86	2.96	62	35.3	27.30
Falcon generic	0.5 Timolol maleate	Alcon Laboratories (Fort Worth, TX)	0.032 ± 0.003	10.71	3.18	1.63	66	55.6	16.50
Schein generic	0.5 Levobunolol hydrochloride	Schein Pharmaceutical Inc. (Florham Park, NJ)	0.041 ± 0.003	9.83	4.08	2.10	66	39.7	23.70
Betoptic-S	0.25 Betaxolol hydrochloride	Alcon Laboratories (Fort Worth, TX)	0.040 ± 0.006	9.81	4.03	4.64	46	28.0	48.00
Bausch & Lomb generic	0.5 Levobunolol hydrochloride	Bausch & Lomb (Rochester, NY)	0.044 ± 0.003	9.85	4.42	3.68	55	30.6	30.90
OptiPranolol	0.3 Metipranolol	Bausch & Lomb (Rochester, NY)	0.040 ± 0.006	9.99	4.03	2.21	65	40.3	18.90
Betimol	0.5 Timolol hemihydrate	CibaVision Ophthalmics (Duluth, GA)	0.035 ± 0.006	10.44	3.52	2.12	61	45.3	18.30

*Average of two bottles.

Source: Modified from WC Stewart, C Sine, E Cate, et al. Daily cost of beta-adrenergic blocker therapy. Arch Ophthalmol 1997;115(7):855.

betaxolol.[72–74] The drug appears to be additive to other glaucoma therapeutic agents, although it should not be used with other epinephrine-like medications. Most clinicians prescribe brimonidine in a twice-daily regimen as adjunctive therapy. As primary therapy, the drug should be prescribed in a thrice-daily regimen because it has less trough IOP lowering than timolol.[73] If the drug is administered twice daily as initial therapy, then a 12-hour postinstillation IOP reading should be taken.

Animal studies are available that suggest that brimonidine exhibits neuroprotective properties. The first such study by Lair and colleagues demonstrated the drug's ability to protect rat neurons from kainic acid injury.[75] The second, by Mitchell and associates, used rabbit retinal ganglion cells. The drug inhibited glutamate-mediated injury.[76] These studies neither prove nor disprove brimonidine's ability as a neuroprotective agent in glaucoma. However, the safety and efficacy of brimonidine have made it one of the topical agents appropriate for initial therapy of glaucoma when beta blockers are contraindicated.

Side Effects and Contraindications of Brimonidine

The most common side effects of brimonidine are ocular irritation, allergy, and blurring of vision. Allergy occurs in as many as 10% of patients and is more frequent when a patient is kept on chronic therapy.[77] Brimonidine has not been shown to affect blood perfusion pressure to the optic nerve.[78] Fatigue, dry mouth, sedation, and reduction of systemic blood pressure are the most significant systemic side effects associated with brimonidine. Systemic side effects are more common with brimonidine than with apraclonidine because of brimonidine's greater lipid solubility and therefore greater penetration into the central nervous system.[79,80] Brimonidine should not be used in infants or children because of reported episodes of syncope, or in patients taking MAO inhibitors.

Epinephrine (Epifrin-Allergan, Irvine CA and Glaucon-Alcon, Fort Worth, TX)

Epinephrine is a nonselective direct-acting sympathomimetic agent. Reduction of IOP is mediated through α- and β-receptor stimulation. Stimulation of α receptors appears to be responsible for decreased aqueous production by reduction of blood flow to the ciliary processes. Increased outflow via the TM is enhanced by stimulation of β_2 receptors.[81–84] Schencker and associates have postulated that epinephrine also increases uveoscleral outflow.[85,86] Epinephrine has relatively poor corneal penetration. This requires the application of concentrations that range from 0.5% to 2.0%. Epinephrine is generally prescribed on a twice-daily regimen.

Side Effects and Contraindications of Epinephrine Drugs

Topical instillation of epinephrine drugs can result in significant systemic and local side effects. With 1% or 2% epinephrine, blood levels are produced through conjunctiva and nasal mucosal absorption sufficient to cause palpitations and tachycardia. Local side effects include adrenochrome deposits in the palpebral conjunctiva (oxidized epinephrine), follicular conjunctivitis, and rebound hyperemia. Cystoid macular edema (CME) in aphakic eyes increases in frequency (to 20%) with the use of epinephrine drugs.[20] Many of these cases are reversible[20] when epinephrine is discontinued, but if the CME persists or develops into a macular hole, the resultant visual acuity can fall to 20/200 or worse. No good data are available to indicate whether there is less frequent CME in pseudophakic patients on epinephrine drugs when compared with an aphakic group. Because of the risk of permanent vision loss from CME and the availability of other agents, topical epinephrine compounds should be avoided in all postoperative cataract patients. It is also important to note that all forms of epinephrine produce mydriasis. Therefore, any patient should be assessed for potentially occludable angles before initiation of therapy with these drugs. Patients may complain of blur and photosensitivity from the mydriatic nature of epinephrine and may require discontinuation of the drug.

Systemic side effects of epinephrine drugs include hypertension, tachycardia, cardiac arrhythmias, palpitations, and headaches. These agents can also potentiate the adrenergic effect of monoamine oxidase (MAO) inhibitors and tricyclic antidepressants.

Dipivefrin (Propine). Epinephrine in its divalent form (dipivalyl epinephrine; DPE) (Allergan, Irvine, CA) is a prodrug of epinephrine. As opposed to epinephrines in bitartrate or hydrochlorate forms, DPE is more lipophilic. This increase in lipid solubility improves corneal penetration by 17 times,[87,88] resulting in the lower concentration needed to achieve the same IOP reduction. Because DPE's equivalent concentration is only 0.1%, it produces systemic complications less frequently than topical epinephrine. Local ocular side effects, such as adrenochrome deposits, follicular conjunctivitis, and rebound hyperemia, can occur, although they seem to be less prevalent than with 2% epinephrine. CME in aphakes and pseudophakes should theoretically occur with the same frequency as 2% epinephrine because the same concentration is obtained inside of the eye. In summary, there is no good reason to use epinephrine drugs other than DPE because systemic side effects are significantly reduced with DPE. DPE is also available as a generic.

Indications for Dipivefrin. DPE and other epinephrine drugs are not frequently prescribed as first-line therapy because beta blockers are more effective and better tolerated. The clinical use of DPE is limited to younger patients who have contraindications to beta-blocking drugs and cannot afford other more expensive antiglaucoma medications. The dosing schedule is two times a day. Its effectiveness can approach that of betaxolol 0.5% as primary therapy.[89] DPE has little additive effect when combined with nonselective beta blockers, but may have a synergistic IOP-lowering effect when combined with betaxolol.[90–92] This is probably because epinephrine increases outflow by stimulating β_2 receptors that are not affected as greatly by the selective β_1 antagonism of betaxolol.[81–84]

Cholinergic Agents

The cholinergic or miotic agents include direct-acting and the indirect-acting (cholinesterase-inhibiting) drugs. It is important to note that miosis is not responsible for the IOP-lowering effect of the cholinergic drugs. These compounds reduce IOP by stimulation of the ciliary muscle, which pulls on the TM and increases the outflow of aqueous. Cholinergics are very effective in lowering IOP in most patients, with an average reduction of 25%. If the TM is abnormal or damaged, or if the mechanism of the glaucoma is other than TM dysfunction, cholinergics are less effective. They are additive to beta blockers, epinephrine drugs, CAIs, and α-adrenergic agonists. They are not additive to each other and may be less additive to prostaglandin agents because they inhibit uveoscleral outflow.

In primary angle-closure glaucoma, miotics can break the pupillary block component and allow aqueous to escape from the posterior chamber to the anterior chamber. In nonpupillary block angle-closure glaucoma (plateau iris syndrome), miotics help to pull the peripheral iris away from angle structures if peripheral anterior synechiae have not yet formed.

Pilocarpine (Isopto Carpine) and Carbachol (Isopto Carbachol)

The direct-acting cholinergic agents, pilocarpine and carbachol (Alcon Pharm, Fort Worth, TX), have equal potency for comparable concentrations. Pilocarpine is available as a 0.5%, 1%, 2%, 3%, 4%, 6%, 8%, and 10% solution and is usually administered four times a day. Carbachol is available as a 0.75%, 1.5%, 2.25%, and 3% solution and is prescribed three times a day. Pilocarpine and carbachol directly stimulate the cholinergic receptor sites (direct-acting). Carbachol has a longer duration of action because it directly stimulates the ciliary muscle, as well as being more resistant to cholinesterase hydrolysis (indirect-acting). Carbachol carries uniform charges on either end of its molecular structure, resulting in poor corneal penetration. The use

of benzalkonium chloride as a preservative enhances corneal penetration via a toxic effect on corneal epithelium. Carbachol is similar in IOP-lowering effect to pilocarpine, but can be prescribed three times a day instead of four.[20]

Pilocarpine concentrations of 1.0% and sometimes 2.0% are used for therapeutic miosis. They can be used while the patient is waiting for peripheral laser iridotomy for primary angle-closure glaucoma. They are used when pupil control is needed to prevent angle-closure in patients with plateau iris configuration (if laser iridoplasty cannot be performed). Another indication for chronic miosis is to prevent a dislocated lens from entering the anterior chamber and disrupting corneal endothelial integrity.

Lower concentrations of pilocarpine (.5% and 1%) are initially prescribed for primary open-angle glaucoma patients to reduce the common ocular side effects associated with cholinergic therapy. As the patient adapts to the ocular side effects, higher concentrations of pilocarpine can be used. A theoretical prediction that a 6% or higher concentration may offer better efficacy in darkly pigmented irides than 4% has not been adequately demonstrated.[93,94] In fact, due to the hyperosmotic nature of any solution more concentrated than 4%, concentrations this high induce tearing with subsequent dilution of the drug, and therefore should not be used. In general, for blue or light-colored irides, a maximum concentration of 2% is used, and in brown or dark irides, a maximum concentration of 4% should be used. If the IOP-lowering effect is not achieved or the patient has difficulty maintaining a four times a day schedule, the switch from 4% pilocarpine four times a day to 3% carbachol three times a day is made.

Pilocarpine is effective on ciliary muscle receptor sites for a limited time. The dose-response curve of pilocarpine peaks at approximately 4 hours after instillation. Hence, a more constant level of the drug's action on the ciliary muscle's receptor sites can be maintained if pilocarpine is used every 6 hours. Most clinicians prescribe one drop four times daily. The prescribed schedule[20] should be as close to every 6 hours as can accommodate the patient's lifestyle, or at least it should coincide with the diurnal (circadian) variation of the patient's IOP. With the advent of newer antiglaucoma agents with lower daily dosages and fewer ocular side effects, pilocarpine and other cholinergic agents are not as frequently prescribed. Cholinergic agents are better tolerated by patients older than 60 years and are less costly than the newer antiglaucoma agents.

Pilopine HS Gel. A gel form of pilocarpine, Pilopine HS (Alcon, Fort Worth, TX) is available in a 4% ointment. After penetrating the cornea, it resides in the aqueous in suspended droplets, which slowly dissolve into solution. Once in solution, the pilocarpine is available to act at the ciliary muscle receptors. This delivery system was originally designed to allow pilocarpine to be used once daily, preferably at bedtime. A 2-mm bead of this 4% gel is placed in the lower fornix. This delivery system was designed to improve patient compliance and reduce ocular side effects. Studies[94–100] indicate that at approximately 18 hours postinstillation of pilocarpine 4% gel, a rise in IOP occurs. This usually occurs in the late afternoon at approximately 5–6 PM. Frequently, the patient needs to add a drop of pilocarpine solution in the early evening for full 24-hour coverage. Corneal hazing and small gray opacities have also been reported with pilocarpine gel that are reversible on discontinuing the medication.

Ocusert. The Ocusert (Alza, Palo Alto, CA) delivery system for pilocarpine uses a rate-controlling membrane with a central reservoir of pilocarpine. It comes in a 20- and 40-μg concentration and is typically replaced once a week. The Ocusert is inserted into the lower fornix of the conjunctiva away from the cornea. It alleviates the necessity of multiple daily dosing, but the depo delivery system may cause local toxicity to the conjunctiva and reduce the success of filtration surgery. Extrusion and constant foreign body sensation have limited the use of the Ocusert system.

Echothiophate Iodide (Phospholine Iodine PI)

Echothiophate (Wyeth-Ayerst, Philadelphia, PA) iodide is the most commonly prescribed cholinesterase inhibitor. The cholinesterase inhibitors prevent the enzyme cholinesterase from removing acetylcholine at the postganglionic receptor site. Thus, acetylcholine accumulates and provides continual stimulation to the ciliary muscle. Echothiophate has a prolonged duration of action because it is an irreversible inhibitor of cholinesterase. The dosage of echothiophate is one drop once or twice daily of either a 0.03%, 0.06%, 0.125%, or 0.25% concentration. Shelf life is unstable, and the drug comes in a powder form, which needs to be mixed before the initial use. A 5-ml container with a rubber-stopped dropper is the standard packaging. Between dosing, the medication needs to be refrigerated. In addition to less frequent dosing than pilocarpine and carbachol, echothiophate is also more effective in IOP reduction.[101] Its use, however, is limited to pseudophakic and aphakic patient populations because it has cataractogenic properties. In younger patients, it may also produce iris cysts and can induce posterior synechiae formation and retinal detachment. These drugs are only administered once to twice daily in low concentrations due to their extremely long half-life and high potency. However, the benefit of infrequent dosing is generally overcome by the high incidence of systemic and ocular side effects.

Physostigmine (Eserine)

Physostigmine (Alcon, Fort Worth, TX) is a slightly less potent reversible anticholinesterase compound than echothiophate. It offers the advantage of not requiring refrigeration and is available as a 0.25% ointment. The dosage is generally twice daily.

Demecarium Bromide (Humersol)

Demecarium bromide (Merck, West Point, PA) is similar in potency, efficacy, and side effects to echothiophate. It differs in that it is stable in solution at room temperature and is a reversible cholinesterase inhibitor. It is available as a 0.125% and 0.25% solution and is usually administered one drop twice a day. Demecarium bromide is also used as a diagnostic and therapeutic agent in the management of accommodative esotropia.

Cholinergic Side Effects and Contraindications

Except for those who do not respond to miotics because of a totally occluded TM (peripheral anterior synechiae) or for whom traction on the corneal scleral cords will not open access to Schlemm's canal, few patients[20] do not respond to cholinergic therapy. Some evidence supports aging of the ciliary muscle as a factor that decreases the effectiveness of the cholinergics with age.[102] Cholinergic therapy is less effective in traumatic glaucoma and is contraindicated in uveitic, neovascular, and other secondary angle-closure glaucomas.

Cholinergics constrict the pupils and may limit peripheral and night vision. In a patient with a centrally positioned media opacity located at a nodal point, as in a posterior subcapsular cataract, miotics may profoundly affect visual acuity. This may prevent the patient from tolerating continued use of the miotic. One way to identify a potential problem is through an in-office trial with a 1% or 2% solution of pilocarpine. Conversely, some nuclear sclerotic cataract patients may experience a sharpening of vision due to the "pinhole effect" produced by constricting the pupil.

A second source of patient intolerance to miotics occurs from brow pain and accommodative spasm. The pain usually occurs within a few minutes after instillation and lasts on average 15–20 minutes. Pharmacologically induced pseudomyopia occurs in pre- and early presbyopic patients. If the induced myopia were stable, a new refractive correction would probably allow continued use of the cholinergic agent. However, the induced myopia is not constant—the greatest myopia immediately follows instillation of drops, with gradual reduction over the next 4 hours. For this reason, patients younger than 50 years poorly tolerate cholinergic drugs.

Other ocular side effects of cholinergic medications include posterior vitreous detachment, retinal break formation or retinal detachment. The high-risk group for retinal detachment primarily includes patients who have pre-existing peripheral retinal degenerations (i.e., lattice, retinal breaks), aphakia, pseudophakia, or high myopia. As the ciliary muscle contracts, it not only produces traction on the posterior margin of the TM, but also at the pars plana. Retinal traction in combination with pre-existing peripheral retinal degenerations can result in a retinal break.

Chronic miotic therapy can result in a pupil that becomes increasingly difficult to dilate. This can be troublesome for patients with peripheral retinal disease or diabetes who require adequate dilation to rule out retinopathy or perform laser treatment. The clinician needs to assess the benefit of using a miotic to achieve IOP control and weigh it against such side effects. With newer agents available that do not affect pupil size, cholinergics should probably be avoided in these patients.

Long-term use of stronger miotic agents (e.g., pilocarpine 4%) can narrow an anterior chamber angle. Gonioscopy should be repeated and monitored in all patients on miotic therapy. Two mechanisms[103] may be responsible for this effect: The peripheral iris becomes stretched and flaccid; "bunching" at its insertion. Also, the ciliary muscle, as it contracts, may shift anteriorly. This moves the iris-lens plane forward, narrowing the anterior chamber angle. This narrowing of the angle can block the TM and decrease aqueous outflow. When this occurs with concomitant gonioscopic evidence of anterior chamber angle narrowing, temporary discontinuance of the miotic is recommended.

Systemic side effects of cholinergic agents include gastrointestinal upset, salivation, abdominal cramping, and potential heart block.[104] These side effects usually occur with higher or more frequent dosages. Cholinesterase inhibitors were originally developed as insecticides and used in nerve gas. They therefore have the potential to produce systemic effects. This is enhanced by their high potency and long half-life. However, when used properly, even 0.25% echothiophate twice daily in one eye should not produce systemic problems in the average-sized adult. It is important to note that if the patient is exposed to other cholinesterase inhibitors, toxic systemic levels may be reached. Older forms of insecticides represent the most frequently encountered incidental exposure, which might produce central nervous system toxicity. Also, as with any antiglaucoma medication, the patient should be instructed not to exceed the prescribed dosage, with the explanation that no added benefit will result, but only additional side effects. A potentially fatal drug interaction is a risk in patients who undergo a surgical procedure that requires general anesthesia. Succinylcholine in combination with cholinesterase inhibitors can induce respiratory arrest.

It is important to educate patients and their physicians about this potential complication.

Oral Carbonic Anhydrase Inhibitors

Acetazolamide (Diamox)

CAIs decrease aqueous production by inhibiting the enzyme, carbonic anhydrase, that is part of the pathway of aqueous production. CAIs represent a very effective method of lowering IOP, with reductions of as much as 35% from baseline readings.[105] The most commonly prescribed oral CAIs are acetazolamide and methazolamide. Acetazolamide is available in 125-mg tablets, 250-mg (scored) tablets, and 500-mg time-release sequels. The standard dosage is 250-mg tablets four times a day or 500-mg sequels twice a day. Acetazolamide is the most effective of the oral CAIs and has the shortest onset of action. It should also be noted that, as opposed to the beta-blocking agents, acetazolamide continues to reduce aqueous flow during sleep.[1,106]

Methazolamide (Neptazane)

Methazolamide (Lederle, Wayne, NJ) is a CAI that has fewer systemic side effects than acetazolamide, although it is slightly less effective in lowering IOP. It is generally better tolerated for chronic use and therefore is often the initial oral CAI prescribed. Methazolamide has a longer onset of action and a longer duration of action than acetazolamide. It is commonly prescribed at a dosage of 50-mg three times daily, but thrice-daily 25-mg dosages, as well as twice-daily 50-mg dosages, can be effective. Methazolamide can also be tried if intolerable side effects occur from acetazolamide. However, if acute IOP lowering is needed, acetazolamide tablets are used because of their shorter onset of action.

Dichlorphenamide (Daranide)

Dichlorphenamide (Merck, West Point, PA) was developed to provide an oral CAI with greater efficacy than acetazolamide and fewer adverse effects. It is more potent than acetazolamide, requiring a dose of only 25–50 mg once to three times daily. It was hoped that this lowered dose would produce fewer side effects than acetazolamide; however, the side effects are similar to those accompanying acetazolamide use.[107]

Systemic Side Effects and Contraindications for Oral Carbonic Anhydrase Inhibitors

Systemic side effects are commonly encountered with chronic use of oral CAIs. The most notable side effects include paresthesias (tingling of the extremities), malaise, gastrointestinal distress, and polyuria. Because of its diuretic side effects and shifts in membrane permeability to electrolytes, kidney function can be severely affected over a long course of treatment. Nephrolithiasis (kidney stones) and some degenerative glomerular changes can occur. Methazolamide is metabolized mainly by the liver and is therefore a better choice for patients with compromised renal function. Potassium depletion is a significant problem with CAIs, especially in hypertensive patients using non K^+ sparing diuretics. Low K^+ levels can increase the risk of fatal cardiac arrhythmias. Low K^+ levels are particularly worrisome in patients using cardiac glycosides (digitalis, digoxin) because they increase the toxic effect of the drug by producing increased bradycardia.[108] Monitoring of K^+ levels, K^+ supplementation, or substitution of the diuretic should be considered before starting oral CAIs for treatment of glaucoma.

Other side effects of CAIs include sulfa allergy, anorexia, urethral colic, metabolic acidosis, and alterations in mental status. The latter include depression, mental confusion, and induced psychosis. With few exceptions, symptoms suggesting that these side effects have occurred come from family members. The clinician should therefore question family members at some time during the course of treatment. Impotency has also been reported with the use of CAIs.

Patients with a history of sulfa allergy should not be prescribed CAIs. Cases of erythema multiforme have been reported with acetazolamide as the precipitating agent. Aplastic anemia is a potentially fatal blood dyscrasia, where the bone marrow stops producing red blood cells, white blood cells, and platelets. It is a rare complication of oral CAIs, but it appears to be an idiosyncratic reaction, with no way to predict which patients are at risk.

CAIs are not well metabolized by the elderly. Therefore, it has been suggested that some reduction of dose should be made when CAIs are used in this population or in patients with reduced creatinine clearance.[109] The respiratory acidosis produced by oral CAIs can drop venous PCO_2 levels to 12 mm Hg or lower. Lastly, acetazolamide is contraindicated in pregnant women during the first trimester. Although it has never been shown to produce teratogenicity in humans, it has produced limb deformities in rats.[110]

Indications for Oral Carbonic Anhydrase Inhibitors

Oral CAIs have the potential to produce many side effects and patient intolerances, but their effectiveness commonly overrides the risks. With the advent of newer antiglaucoma medications and topical CAIs, oral CAIs are less frequently the choice for chronic use. They represent a significant part of the antiglaucoma armament for acute IOP lowering in patients with closed-angle

glaucoma or extremely elevated IOP. The standard treatment for these patients would be two 250-mg tablets of acetazolamide in conjunction with other topical therapy (see Chapter 16).

If CAIs are to be prescribed for chronic use, there are methods of reducing side effects. Methazolamide is generally prescribed before acetazolamide because it is better tolerated and less likely to cause kidney stones or metabolic acidosis. The clinician can start with a lower initial dosage of CAI and slowly increase it, such as 25 mg of methazolamide twice a day increased over time to 50 mg twice a day or three times a day. The use of sustained-release acetazolamide (Diamox Sequels) (Lederle, Wayne, NJ) can improve compliance because they are prescribed twice a day. They are also better tolerated than the tablet form of acetazolamide.[107]

Topical Carbonic Anhydrase Inhibitors

Dorzolamide (Trusopt)

Oral CAIs have great efficacy in lowering IOP, but have many adverse systemic side effects. Topical CAIs can alleviate many of the systemic sides effects, but they are generally less effective in IOP reduction as a result of poor corneal penetration. Dorzolamide (Merck, West Point, PA), a thienothiopyran-2-sulfonamide, was the first topical CAI approved by the FDA. It comes in a 2% solution and is prescribed in a thrice-daily regimen. Dorzolamide showed an IOP reduction of 21% in ocular hypertension.[111] Peak effect of the drug was seen at 2 hours, and average IOP reduction at 8 hours ranged from 17% to 24%. Dorzolamide is well tolerated and can be used in combination with other topical glaucoma agents, although it is only 13–19% additive to the beta blockers.[112] When prescribed as adjunctive therapy, the dosage is usually twice a day.

Side Effects and Contraindications of Dorzolamide

Side effects of dorzolamide include ocular stinging, mild hyperemia, and a bitter taste in the mouth. The stinging is due to the fact that the drug must be buffered at the acidic pH of 5.6. A single study that reports problems with increased corneal thickness due to reduced endothelial function[113] is not supported by other studies, which reported no alteration of endothelial function or increase in central corneal thickness.[114–116] However, topical CAIs should probably not be prescribed in patients with history of corneal dysfunction or dystrophy. Also, the drug should not be used in patients with sensitivity to sulfonamide drugs. The question of improved blood flow to the nerve using topical CAIs is unanswered, with one study showing no effect on optic nerve perfusion[117] and another suggesting improved perfusion.[118]

Brinzolamide (Azopt)

Brinzolamide (Alcon, Fort Worth, TX) is the newest of the topical CAIs. It comes as a topical 1% suspension and is prescribed for use three times a day as primary therapy and twice a day for adjunctive therapy. The use of a suspension form allows the drug to be buffered at physiologic pH. A study by Silver has shown that the drug is equivalent in IOP lowering effect (19–22%) to dorzolamide and produces less discomfort.[119] The most common side effect of brinzolamide is a temporary blur in vision from the suspension formulation. The contraindications for brinzolamide are similar to dorzolamide.

Timolol and Dorzolamide Combination (Cosopt)

Cosopt (Merck, West Point, PA) is a combination of 0.5% timolol and 2% dorzolamide. Studies show a similar IOP lowering with Cosopt prescribed bid with separate dosing of 0.5% timolol twice a day and 2% dorzolamide twice a day.[120] The convenience of taking a single drop versus two separate drops is weighed against the additional cost of Cosopt. Cosopt should not be prescribed as initial therapy. It is best as a substitute drug for a patient who did not reach the target pressure with timolol alone and showed an additive effect when dorzolamide was combined.

Prostaglandin Agents

In the body, prostaglandins are mediators in the inflammatory pathway. In the eye, the role of prostaglandins is much more complex than was first thought. These compounds significantly reduce IOP by increasing uveoscleral outflow. In this pathway, aqueous humor percolates through the iris and ciliary muscle to enter the supraciliary and suprachoroidal spaces. From these areas, the fluid passes through the sclera or out of the eye via the vortex veins.

Latanoprost (Xalatan)

Latanoprost (Pharmacia, Peapack, NJ) is prostaglandin PhXA41. The compound produces a reduction in IOP from 20% to 36% when administered once daily as a 0.005% solution.[121] The drug appears to be most effective when applied at night (35% reduction) rather than in the morning (31% reduction).[122,123] This exceeds the efficacy of the beta-blocking compounds. The drug is extremely potent and is generally well tolerated.

Side Effects and Contraindications for Latanoprost

Latanoprost has little effect on heart rate, blood pressure, or pulmonary function. Ocular side effects include stinging, tearing, and conjunctival hyperemia. Hyperemia tends to be mild but can be significant enough to discontinue the medication. Latanoprost may induce darkening of the iris by increasing melanin within the iris melanocytes. This effect only occurred in 10–16% of test subjects and was generally limited to blue-brown and green-brown eyes. Patients affected with the iris color change typically had light-colored irides in the periphery with a light brown pigmentation near the pupillary border. The effect does not cause an increase in pigment in the TM.[122,123] However, the iris change appears to be irreversible, and the long-term complications are unknown. Latanoprost also produces hypertrichosis and hyperpigmentation of the eyelashes.[124,125] Of greater significance are the cases of CME and anterior uveitis that occur in 6% of patients using the drug.[126–128] Aphakic and pseudophakic patients with posterior capsule breaks appear to be at greatest risk. Because of the potential exacerbating effect of prostaglandins on uveitis, they should be avoided in the presence of ocular inflammation.

Indications for Latanoprost

Latanoprost is a very effective IOP-lowering medication that is generally well tolerated both systemically and ocularly. Furthermore, the drug only has to be used once a day. However, the FDA recommends using latanoprost as a second-line therapy or as a primary agent if the patient has contraindications or has failed to achieve a target pressure with other primary antiglaucoma drugs. Latanoprost is additive to other antiglaucoma medications, including beta blockers. It may be less additive to pilocarpine due to the cholinergic reduction in uveoscleral outflow,[129] but an additive effect still occurs with cholinergic agents.[130] A combination drug of latanoprost and timolol is under investigation. Latanoprost also appears to be effective in lowering IOP in patients with normal-tension glaucoma and does not appear to affect perfusion pressure to the optic nerve.[131]

Latanoprost and Timolol Combination (Xalcom)

The U.S. Food and Drug Administration (FDA) has issued an approvable letter for the investigational fixed combination of latanoprost and timolol (Xalcom) (Pharmacia, Peapack, NJ) to treat glaucoma. The medication will be administered once a day and should be used for patients who have failed to achieve a target pressure on latanoprost or timolol alone.

Hyperosmotic Agents

Glycerin (Osmoglyn) and Isosorbide (Ismotic)

The oral hyperosmotic agents include glycerin 50% and isosorbide 45% (Alcon). Osmotic agents reduce IOP by reducing vitreal volume. The average shrinkage is 3–4%.[132] This can result in an IOP reduction of more than 30 mm Hg. Studies also suggest that the central mechanism of IOP reduction is poorly understood.[133] Because these agents cannot be used chronically and their effect is short term, they are usually reserved to treat a single event of highly elevated IOP found in either open- or narrow-angle glaucoma.

The osmotic agent should be ingested over a relatively short period of time and served over crushed ice. This keeps it close to room temperature on exposure to internal body temperature and preserves its osmotic function, which is directly proportional to viscosity. Serving the sweet-tasting drug on ice also improves its palatability and reduces the incidence of nausea seen with this group of agents. The recommended dosage for glycerin 50% solution is 2–3 ml/kg of body weight. For a 150 lb (68 kg) person, the calculation would be 3 ml × (150 lb/2.2kg) = 204 ml or slightly less than a full bottle of Osmoglyn (220 ml). The recommended dose for isosorbide 45% solution is 1.5 g/kg, which is equivalent to 1.5 ml/lb of body weight. Therefore, the dose for a 150-pound individual would be 150 lb × 1.5 ml/lb = 225 ml or approximately one full bottle of Ismotic (220 ml). Note that the glycerin calculation is in ml/kg and the isosorbide calculation is in ml/lb. Glycerin is broken down to free glucose, and extreme caution should be used when it is given to diabetic patients, especially those who are insulin dependent. Isosorbide is a better alternative for diabetic patients because it is not metabolized to glucose, although it has a slightly longer onset of action compared with glycerin.

Urea (Ureaphil) and Mannitol (Osmitrol)

Intravenous administration of hyperosmotic agents is less frequently used because of the availability of the laser peripheral iridotomy for primary angle-closure glaucoma, the effectiveness of topical antiglaucoma agents, improved understanding of malignant glaucoma, and the potential for significant complications with these agents (e.g., cardiac decompensation). Although the difference may not be clinically significant, intravenous administration produces a slightly faster action than oral glycerin does[20] and is useful if the patient's nausea and vomiting prevent oral drug use. The two agents administered by this route are urea (Abbott, Abbott Park, IL) and mannitol (various) 5%, 10%, 15%, 20%, and 25%. Mannitol is the drug of choice because it does not penetrate into the vitreous cavity. Penetration of the drug into the eye

and other body tissues reduces the hyperosmotic effect. The recommended dosage of mannitol is 7.5–10.0 ml/kg of a 20% solution.

Side Effects and Contraindications for Hyperosmotic Agents

Within 30 minutes after administration of the hyperosmotic agent, renal function increases and the patient experiences a full bladder. Thus, the tissue-fluid levels throughout the body are reduced. Dehydration can cause hyperthermia, especially in the elderly, as well as stressing the cardiovascular system as it increases output to compensate for a decreased blood and tissue volume. This additional stress could produce cardiac failure. Hyperosmotics may also produce nausea with occasional vomiting. Other side effects of hyperosmotics include headache, disorientation, dizziness, seizures, and chest pain.

REFERENCES

1. Brubaker RF. Flow of aqueous humor in humans (The Freidwald Lecture). Invest Ophthalmol Vis Sci 1991;32(13):3145.

2. Fink AI, Felix MD, Fletcher RC. The anatomic basic for glaucoma. Ann Ophthalmol 1978;10(4):397.

3. David R, Zangwill L, Briscoe D, et al. Diurnal intraocular pressure variations: an analysis of 690 diurnal curves. Br J Ophthalmol 1992;76(5):280.

4. VonDenffer H. Efficacy and Tolerance of Medipranolol. Results of a Multicenter Long Term Study. In H-J Mert (ed). Medipranolol: Pharmacology of Beta Blocking Agents and Use of Medipranolol in Ophthalmology, Vienna: Springer-Verlag, 1983;121–125.

5. Bausch D, Brew H, Edelhoff R. Medipranolol: Clinical Suitability in the Treatment of Chronic Open Angle Glaucoma. In: H-J Mert (ed). Medipranolol: Pharmacology of Beta Blocking Agents and Use of Medipranolol in Ophthalmology. Vienna: Springer-Verlag, 1983;132–147.

6. Bacon PJ, Brazier R, Smith SE. Cardiovascular responses in metipranolol and timolol eyedrops in healthy volunteers. Br J Clin Pharmacol 1989;27:1.

7. Jeunne CL, Hugues JL, Duffer Y, Munera LB. Bronchial and cardiovascular effects of ocular topical beta-antagonists in asthmatic subjects: comparison of timolol, carteolol and metipranolol. J Clin Pharmacol 1989;29:97.

8. Melles RB, Wong IG. Metipranolol-associated granulomatous iritis. Am J Ophthalmol 1994;118:712–715.

9. Schultz JS, Hoenig JA, Charles H. Possible bilateral anterior uveitis secondary to metapranolol therapy. Arch Ophthalmol 1993;111:1606–1607.

10. Duff GR, Graham PA. A double-crossover trial comparing the effects of topical carteolol and placebo on intraocular pressure. Br J Ophthalmol 1988;72:27.

11. Harris LS, Greenstein SH, Bloom AF. Respiratory difficulties with betaxolol. Am J Ophthalmol 1987;102(2):274.

12. DeSantis LM, Chandler M. Cardiac blockage after ocular instillation of beta adrenergic blockers in alert cynomolgus monkeys, safety profile for betaxolol. Invest Ophthalmol 1985;26(suppl):227.

13. Allen RC. Betaxolol in the treatment of glaucoma, multi-clinic trials. Ophthalmology 1984; 91(suppl):142.

14. Bill A. Conventional and uveo-scleral drainage of aqueous humor in the cyanomolgus monkey (Macaca irus) at normal and high intraocular pressures. Exp Eye Res 1966;5:45.

15. Timewell RM, Ward RL, Beasley CH. Betaxolol-timolol-placebo bronchospasm study in asthmatic bronchitis patients. Alcon Clinical Monitors Report. Ft. Worth, TX: Alcon Pharmaceuticals, 011-3432:0683, 1983.

16. Zeimer RC, Wilensky JT, Gieser DE. Presence and rapid decline of early morning intraocular pressure peaks in glaucoma patients. Ophthalmology 1990; 97(5):548.

17. Brown B, Burton P, Mann S, Parisi A. Fluctuations in intra-ocular pressure with sleep: II. Time course of IOP decrease after waking from sleep. Ophthalmic Physiol Opt 1988;8(3):249.

18. Wilensky JT. Diurnal variations in intraocular pressure. Trans Am Ophthalmol Soc 1991;89:757.

19. Henkind P, Walsh JB. Diurnal variations in intraocular pressure. Chronic open angle glaucoma: preliminary report. Aust J Ophthalmol 1981;9(3):219.

20. Kolker AE, Hetherington J. Becker-Schaffer's Diagnosis and Therapy of the Glaucomas (5th ed). St. Louis: Mosby, 1983.

21. Allen RC, Hertzmark MA, Alexander MW, Epstein MD. A double masked comparison of betaxolol vs timolol in the treatment of open angle glaucoma. Am J Ophthalmol 1986;101:537.

22. Schlect LP, Brubaker RF. The effects of withdrawal of timolol in chronically treated glaucoma patients. Ophthalmology 1988;95(9):1212.

23. The GLT Laser Trial Research Group. The Glaucoma Laser Trial (GLT): results of argon laser trabeculoplasty. Ophthalmology 1990;97(11):1403.

24. DuBiner HB, Hill R, Kaufman H, et al. Timolol hemihydrate vs timolol maleate to treat ocular hypertension and open-angle glaucoma. Am J Ophthalmol 1996;121(5):522–528.

25. Stewart WC, Leland TM, Cate EA, Stewart JA. Efficacy and safety of timolol solution once daily versus timolol gel in treating elevated intraocular pressure. J Glaucoma, 1998;7(60):402–407.

26. Rolando M, Muialdo U, Dolci A, et al. New beta blockers: comparison of efficacy versus timolol maleate. Glaucoma 1989;11:27.

27. Duff GR, Newcombe RG. The 12-hour control of intraocular pressure on carteolol 2% twice daily. Br J Ophthalmol 1988;72:890.

28. Freedman SF, Shields MB, Freedman NJ, et al. Topical beta blockers and plasma lipids-carteolol vs timolol. ARVO Annual Meeting Abstract, Tampa, May 2-6, 1993.

29. Gerber SL, Cantor LB, Brater DC. Systemic drug interactions with topical glaucoma medications. Surv Ophthalmol 1990;35:205–218.

30. DiCarlo FJ, Leinweber FJ, Szpiech JM, Davidson WF. Metabolisms of 1-bunolol. Clin Pharmacol Ther 1977;22:858.

31. Quast U, Vollmer KO. Binding of beta-adrenoreceptor antagonists to rat and rabbit lung. Special reference to levobunolol. Arzneimmittelforschung 1984;34:579.

32. Wandel T, Charap AD, Lewis RA, et al. Glaucoma treatment with once-daily levobunolol. Am J Ophthalmol 1986;101:298.

33. Derick RJ, Robin AL, Tielsch J, et al. Once-daily versus twice-daily levobunolol (0.5%) therapy. A crossover study. Ophthalmology 1992;99(3):424–429.

34. American Hospital Formulary Society Category. 52:36 Sterile Ophthalmic Solution Timoptic Package Insert 7115426 Endocrine, 1995.

35. Manoury P. Betaxolol, chemistry and biological profile in relation to its physiochemical properties. In Morelli, et al. (eds). Betaxolol and Other B1-Adrenoreceptor Antagonists, L.E.R.S. (vol 1). New York: Raven Press, 1983;13–19.

36. Reiss GR, Brubaker RF. The mechanism of betaxolol, a new ocular hypotensive agent. Ophthalmology 1983;90:1369.

37. Dunn TL, Gerber MJ, Shen AS, et al. Timolol induced bronchospasm; utility of betaxolol as an alternative ocular hypotensive agent in patients with asthma. Am Rev Respir Dis 1198;633(2): 264.

38. Musini A, Fabbri B, Bergamoschi M, et al. Comparison of the effects of propranolol, lidocaine and other drugs on normal and raised intraocular pressure in Man. Am J Ophthalmol 1971;72:773.

39. Atkins JM, Pugh BR, Timewell RM. Cardiovascular effects of topical beta blockers during exercise. Am J Ophthalmol 1985;99:173.

40. Berry DP Jr, Van Buskirk EM, Shields MB. Betaxolol and timolol. A comparison of efficacy and side effects. Arch Ophthalmol 1984;102:42–45.

41. Bonomi L, Zavarise G, Noya E, Michieletto S. Effects of timolol maleate on tear flow in human eyes. Graefe's Arch Clin Exp Ophthalmol 1980;213:19.

42. Nielson NV, Eriksen JS. Timolol transitory manifestations of dry eyes in long term treatment. Acta Ophthalmol 1979;56:418.

43. Van Buskirk EM. Corneal anesthesia after timolol maleate therapy. Am J Ophthalmol 1979;88:739.

44. Allen RC, Epstein DL. A double-masked clinical trial of betaxolol and timolol in glaucoma patients. Invest Ophthalmol 1982;22(suppl):40.

45. Levy NS, Boone L, Ellis E. A controlled comparison of betaxolol and timolol with long-term evaluation of safety and efficacy. Glaucoma 1985;7:54.

46. Stewart WC, Sine C, Cate E, et al. Daily cost of beta-adrenergic blocker therapy. Arch Ophthalmol 1997;115(7):853–856.

47. Merck, Sharp, and Dohme. Recommendations from the Manufacturer, Private correspondence from Associate Director of Professional Information, West Point, PA 1996.

48. Lederer CM, Harold RE. Drop size of commercial glaucoma medications. Am J Ophthalmol 1986;101:691.

49. DaHodapp E, Kolker A, Kass M, et al. The effect of topical clonidine on intraocular pressure. Arch Ophthalmol 1981;99:1208–1211.

50. Novak GD, Robin AL, Derrick RJ. New medical treatments for glaucoma. Int Ophthalmol Clin 1993;33:183–202.

51. Marquardt R, Pillunat LE, Stodtmeister R. Ocular hemodynamics following local application of clonidine. Klin Monatsbil Augenheikld 1988;193:637.

52. Robin AL. Short-term effects of unilateral 1% apraclonidine therapy. Arch Ophthalmol 1988;106:912.

53. Abrams, DA, Robin AL, Crandall AS, et al. A limited comparison of apraclonidine's dose response in subjects with normal or increased intraocular pressure. Am J Ophthalmol 1989;108:230.

54. Jampel HD, Robin AL, Quigley HA, Pollack IP. Apraclonidine, a one week dose-response study. Arch Ophthalmol 1988;106:1069.

55. Robin AL, Coleman AL. Apraclonidine hydrochloride: an evaluation of plasma concentrations and a comparison of its intraocular pressure lowering and cardiovascular effects to timolol maleate. Trans Am Ophthalmol Soc 1990;88:149–162.

56. Abrams DA, Robin AL, Pollack IP, et al. The safety and efficacy of topical 1% ALO 2145 (p-aminoclonidine hydrochloride) in normal volunteers. Arch Ophthalmol 1987;105:1205–1207.

57. Nagasubramanian S, Hitchings RA, Demailly P, et al. Comparison of apraclonidine and timolol in chronic open-angle glaucoma. A three month study. Ophthalmology 1993;100:1318.

58. Lee DA, Topper JE, Brubaker RF. Effect of clonidine on aqueous humor flow in normal human eyes. Exp Eye Res 1984;38:239–246.

59. Butler P, Mannschreck M, Lin S, et al. Clinical experience with the long-term use of 1% apraclonidine. Arch Ophthalmol 1995;113:293.

60. Morrison JC, Robin AL. Adjunctive glaucoma therapy: a comparison of apraclonidine to dipivefrin when added to timolol maleate. Ophthalmology 1989;96:3–7.

61. Jampel HD, Pollack IP, Quigley HA, et al. Apraclonidine. A one-week dose-response study. Arch Ophthalmol 1988;106:1069–1073.

62. Stewart WC, Ritch R, Shin DH, et al. The efficacy of apraclonadine as an adjunct to timolol therapy. Arch Ophthalmol 1995;113:287–292.

63. Butler PJ, Jones B. Incidence of characteristics of allergic reaction to apraclonidine 0.5%. Invest Ophthalmol Vis Sci 1996;37(3):S201. Abstract 936.

64. Cardakli F, Smythe B, Eisele J, et al. Effect of chronic apraclonidine treatment on intraocular pressure in advanced glaucoma. J Glaucoma 1992;1:271–278.

65. Lish A, Camras C, Podos S. Effect of apraclonidine on intraocular pressure in glaucoma patients receiving maximally tolerated medication. J Glaucoma 1992;1:19–22.

66. Krawitz PL, Podos SM. Use of apraclonidine in the treatment of acute angle-closure glaucoma. Arch Ophthalmol 1990;108:1208.

67. Yaldo MK, Shin DH, Parrow KA, et al. Additive effect of 1% apraclonidine hydrochloride to non-selective beta blockers. Ophthalmology 1991;98:1075–1078.

68. Chien DS, Homsy JJ, Gluchowski C, Tang-Liu DD. Corneal and conjunctival/scleral penetration of p-aminoclonidine, AGN 190342 and clonidine in rabbit eyes. Curr Eye Res 1990;9:1051–1059.

69. Burke J, Manlapaz C, Kharlamb A, et al. Therapeutic Use of Alpha-2 Adrenoreceptor Agonists in Glaucoma. In S Lanier, L Limbird (eds). Alpha-2-Adrenergic Receptors: Structure, Function and Therapeutic Implications. Reading, U.K.: Harwood Academic Publishers, 1996;179–187.

70. Toris CB, Tafoya ME, Cambras CB, et al. Effects of aproclonidine on aqueous humor dynamics in human eyes. Ophthalmology 1995;102(3):456–461.

71. Toris CB, Cambras CB, Yablonski ME. Effects of brimonidine on aqueous humor dynamics in human eyes. Arch Ophthalmol 1995;113:1514–1517.

72. Schuman JS. Clinical experience with brimonidine 0.2% and timolol 0.5% in glaucoma and ocular hypertension. Surv Ophthalmol 1996;41:S27–S37.

73. Schuman JS, Horwitz B, Choplin NT, et al. A one year study of brimonidine twice daily in glaucoma and ocular hypertension. A controlled, randomized, multicenter clinical trial. Arch Ophthalmol 1997;115:847–852.

74. Javitt J, for the Brimonidine Outcome Study Group. The clinical success rate and quality of life assessment of brimonidine tartrate 0.2% compared with timolol 0.5% administered twice-daily, in patients with previously untreated open-angle glau-

coma or ocular hypertension. Invest Ophthalmol Vis Sci 1997;38(4):S729. Abstract 3363.

75. Lai R, Hasson D, Chun T, Wheeler L. Neuroprotective effect of ocular hypotensive agent brimonidine. XIth Congress of the European Society of Ophthalmology Proceedings 439–444, 1997.

76. Mitchell CK, Nguyen CK, Felman RM. Neuroprotection of retinal ganglion cells. Invest Ophthalmol Vis Sci 1998;39(4):S261. Abstract 1187.

77. Serle JB. A comparison of the safety and efficacy of twice daily brimonidine 0.2% versus betaxolol 0.25% in subjects with elevated intraocular pressure. Surv Ophthalmol 1996;41(suppl):S39–S47.

78. Katz BA, Pillunat LE, Bohm AG, Hammard P, Richard G. Effect of brimonidine on optic nerve head blood flow. Invest Ophthalmol Vis Sci 1998;39(4):S270. Abstract 1230.

79. Sneddon JM, Turner P. The interactions of local guanethidine and sympathomimetic amines in the human eye. Arch Ophthalmol 1969;81:622.

80. Bonomi L, DiComite P. Outflow facility after guanethidine sulfate administration. Arch Ophthalmol 1967;78:337.

81. Neufeld AH, Jampol LM, Sears ML. Cyclic-AMP in the aqueous humor: the effects of adrenergic agents. Exp Eye Res 1972;14:242.

82. Neufeld AH, Sears ML. Adenosine 3'-5'-monophosphate analogue increases the outflow facility of the primate eye. Invest Ophthalmol Vis Sci 1975;14:688.

83. Robinson JC, Kaufman PL. Effects and interactions of epinephrine, norepinephrine, timolol and betaxolol on outflow facility in the cynomolgus monkey. Am J Ophthalmol 1990;109:189.

84. Sears M, Caprioli J, Kondo K, Bauscher L. A Mechanism for the Control of Aqueous Humor Formation. In SM Drance, AH Neufeld (eds). Glaucoma: Applied Pharmacology in Medical Treatment. New York: Grune and Stratton, 1984;303–324.

85. Miyake K, Miyake Y, Kuratomi R. Long term effects of topically applied epinephrine on the blood-ocular barrier in humans. Arch Ophthalmol 1984;105:1360.

86. Schenker HE, Yablonski ME, Podos SM, Kinder L. Fluorophotometric study of epinephrine and timolol in human subjects. Arch Ophthalmol 1981;99:1212.

87. Mandell AL, Stenz F, Kitabachi AE. Dipivalyl epinephrine: a new pro-drug in the treatment of glaucoma. Ophthalmology 1978;85:268.

88. Wei CP, Anderson JA, Leopold I. Ocular absorption and metabolism of topically applied epinephrine and a dipivalyl ester of epinephrine. Invest Ophthalmol Vis Sci 1978;17:315.

89. Albracht DC, LeBlanc RP, Cruz AM, et al. A double masked comparison of betaxolol and dipivefrin for the treatment of increased intraocular pressure. Am J Ophthalmol 1993;116:307.

90. Tsoy EA, Bettina BM, Shields MD. Comparison of two treatment schedules for combined timolol and dipivefrin therapy. Am J Ophthalmol 1986; 102:322.

91. Allen RC, Epstein DL. Additive effect of epinephrine to betaxolol and timolol in primary open angle glaucoma. Arch Ophthalmol 1986;104:1178.

92. Knupp JA, Shields MB, Mandell AI, et al. Combined timolol and epinephrine therapy for open angle glaucoma. Surv Ophthalmol 1983;28(suppl):280.

93. Ritch R, Shields MB, Krupin T. The Glaucomas: Pharmacology. New York: Mosby, 1989.

94. Sherman SE. Clinical comparison of pilocarpine preparations in heavily pigmented eyes: an evaluation of the influence of polymer vehicles on corneal penetration, drug availability, and duration of hypotensive activity. Ann Ophthalmol 1977; 9(10):1231.

95. Johnson DH, Epstein DL, Allen RC, et al. A one-year multi-center clinical trial of pilocarpine gel. Am J Ophthalmol 1984;97:723.

96. Goldberg I, Ashburn FS, Kass MA, Becker B. Efficacy and patient acceptance of pilocarpine gel. Am J Ophthalmol 1979;88:843.

97. Stewart RH, Kimbrought RL, Smith JP, Ward RL. Long-acting pilocarpine gel: a dose-response in ocular hypertensive subjects. Glaucoma 1984;6:182.

98. March WF, Stewart RM, Mandell AI, Bruce LA. Duration of effect of pilocarpine gel. Arch Ophthalmol 1982;100:1270.

99. Aldrette J, McDonald TO, DeSouse B. Comparative evaluation of pilocarpine gel and timolol in patients with glaucoma. Glaucoma 1983;5(5):236.

100. Weintraub M, Evans P. Pilocarpine: the method is the message. Hosp Form 1985;20:177.

101. Harris LS. Comparison of pilocarpine and echothiophate in open angle glaucoma. Ann Ophthalmol 1972;4(7):736.

102. Crawford K, Gabelt BT, Kaufman PL. Age-related decline in outflow facility and facility response to pilocarpine in rhesus monkeys. ARVO abstract 1672, poster 18, 1990.

103. Rieser JC, Schwartz B. Miotic-induced malignant glaucoma. Arch Ophthalmol 1972;87:706.

104. Littman L, Kempler P, Rhola M, et al. Severe symptomatic AV block induced by pilocarpine eye drops. Arch Intern Med 1987;147:586.

105. Friedland BR, Mallonnee J, Anderson DR. Short-term dose response characteristics of acetazolamide in man. Arch Ophthalmol 1977;95:1809–1812.

106. McCannel CA, Heinrich SR, Brubaker RF. Acetazolamide but not timolol lowers aqueous humor flow in sleeping humans. Graefes Arch Clin Exp Ophthalmol 1992;230(6):518.

107. Lichter PR, Newman LP, Wheeler NC, Beall OV. Patient tolerance to carbonic anhydrase inhibitors. Am J Ophthalmol 1978;85:495–502.

108. Epstein DL, Grant WM. Carbonic anhydrase inhibitor side-effects: serum chemical analysis. Arch Ophthalmol 1977;95:1378–1382.

109. Chapron DJ, Sweeney KR, Feig PU, Kramer PA. Influence of advanced age on the disposition of acetazolamide. Br J Clin Pharmacol 1985;19(3):363.

110. Layton WM, Hallesy DM. Deformity of forelimb in rats: association with high doses of acetazolamide. Science 1965;149:306–308.

111. True-Gabelt B, Kaufman PL, Polanski JR. Ciliary muscle muscarinic binding sites, choline acetyltransferase and acetylcholinesterase in aging rhesus monkeys. Invest Ophthalmol Vis Sci 1990;31:24–31.

112. Strahlman ER, Vogel R, Tipping R, Clineschmidt CM. The use of dorzolamide and pilocarpine as adjunctive therapy to timolol in patients with elevated intraocular pressure. The Dorzolamide Additivity Study Group. Ophthalmology 1996;103:1283–1293.

113. Herndon LW, Choudri SA, Cox T, et al. Central corneal thickness in normal, glaucomatous and ocular hypertensive eyes. Arch Ophthalmol 1997;115(9):1137–1141.

114. Kaminski S, Hommer A, Koyuncu D, et al. Influences of dorzolamide on corneal thickness, endothelial cell count and corneal sensibility. Acta Ophthalmol Scand 1998;76(1):78–79.

115. Lass JH, Khosrof SA, Laurence JK, et al. A double-masked, randomized, 1 year study comparing the corneal effects of dorzolamide, timolol and betaxolol. Arch Ophthalmol 1998;116(8):1003–1010.

116. Egan CA, Hodge DO, McClaren JW, Bourne WM. Effect of dorzolamide on corneal endothelial function in normal human eyes. Invest Ophthalmol Vis Sci 1998;39(1):23–29.

117. Grunwald JE, Mathur S, Dupont J. Effects of dorzolamide hydrochloride 2% on the retinal circulation. Acta Ophthalmol Scan 1997;75(3):236–238.

118. Harris A, Arend O, Arend S, Martin B. Effects of topical dorzolamide on retinal and retrobulbar hemodynamics. Acta Ophthalmol Scand 1996;74(6):569–572.

119. Silver LH. Clinical efficacy and safety of brinzolamide, a new topical carbonic anhydrase inhibitor for primary open-angle glaucoma and ocular hypertension. Am J Ophthalmol 1998;126(3):400–408.

120. Hutzelmann J, Owens S, Shedden A, et al. Comparison of the safety and efficacy of the fixed combination of dorzolamide/timolol and the concomitant administration of dorzolamide and timolol: a clinical equivalence study. International Clinical Equivalence Study Group. Br J Ophthalmol 1998;82:1249–1253.

121. Alm A, Camras CB, Watson PG. Phase III latanoprost studies in Scandinavia, the United Kingdom and the United States. Surv Ophthalmol 1997;41(2):S105–S110.

122. Wistrand PJ, Stjernschantz J, Olsson K. The incidence and time course of latanoprost-induced radial pigmentation as a function of eye color. Surv Ophthalmol 1997;41(S2):S129–S138.

123. Camras CB, Alm A. Initial clinical studies with prostaglandins and their analogues. Surv Ophthalmol 1997;41(2):S61–S75.

124. Wand M. Latanoprost and hyperpigmentation of eyelashes (letter). Arch Ophthalmol 1997;115(9):1206–1208.

125. Johnstone MA. Hypertrichosis and increased pigmentation of eyelashes and adjacent hair in the region of the ipsilateral eyelids of patients treated with unilateral topical latanoprost. Am J Ophthalmol 1997;124:544–547.

126. Warwar RE, Bullock JD, Ballal D. Cystoid macular edema and anterior uveitis associated with latanoprost use. Ophthalmology 1998;105(2):263–268.

127. Gaddie IB, Bennett DW. Cystoid macular edema associated with the use of latanoprost. J Am Optom Assoc 1998;69(2):122–128.

128. Rowe JA, Hattenhauer MG, Herman DC. Adverse side-effects associated with latanoprost. Am J Ophthalmol 1997;124(5):683–685.

129. Bill A, Phillips CI. Uveoscleral drainage of aqueous humor in human eyes. Exp Eye Res 1971;12:275.

130. Linden C, Alm A. Latanoprost and physostigmine have mostly additive ocular hypotensive effects in human eyes. Arch Ophthalmol 1997;115:857–861.

131. Drance SM, Crichton A, Mills RP. Comparison of the effect of latanoprost 0.005% and timolol 0.5% on the calculated ocular perfusion pressure in patients with normal tension glaucoma. Am J Ophthalmol 1998;125(5):585–592.

132. Robbins R, Galin MA. Effect of osmotic agents on the vitreous body. Arch Ophthalmol 1969;82:694.

133. Podos SM, Krupin T, Becker B. Effect of small-dose hyperosmotic injections on intraocular pressure of small animals and man when optic nerves are transected and intact. Am J Ophthalmol 1971; 71:898.

CHAPTER 9

Laser Trabeculoplasty

J. James Thimons

Laser trabeculoplasty (LTP) or argon laser trabeculoplasty (ALT) is a procedure that has been used since the early 1980s as an adjunct therapy in the management of open-angle glaucoma. The first procedures to use laser application in the treatment of glaucoma were attempted by Krasnov in 1973.[1] Krasnov performed laser puncture of the trabeculum with direct access to Schlemm's canal to increase aqueous drainage and reduce intraocular pressure (IOP). This procedure was initially successful, but it did not demonstrate good long-term IOP control because of scarring and closure of the trabecular openings.[1,2] In the late 1970s, a variation of this technique was applied by Wise and Witter in which small, less intense, focal burns of the trabecular surface were used to lower IOP.[3] This form of the procedure, named *argon laser trabeculoplasty*, showed significantly greater success with fewer complications. The role that this procedure plays in glaucoma management has evolved significantly since the 1980s from a last-resort procedure before filtering surgery to one commonly used during all stages of glaucoma management, including first-line therapy. Although it has not replaced medical or incisional surgical therapy, ALT clearly has established itself as a valuable element in the treatment armamentarium.

MECHANISM OF ACTION

The mechanism by which ALT lowers IOP is thought to be related to a mechanical transformation of the tissue in the trabecular meshwork. Focal argon laser application produces an absorption of heat/energy and a localized contraction of the trabecular beams in the immediate area of application. The surrounding trabecular beams are widened, which increases spacing and creates greater outflow of the trabecular region.[4–6] This is due to the direct anatomic relationship between trabeculum and the scleral tissue immediately posterior that serves as a fixed ring of attachment for the trabecular meshwork. The evidence of this mechanical effect is best demonstrated in patients with pigmentary deposition in the trabecular meshwork. In these individuals, treatment of a portion of the angle demonstrates a marked decrease in the level of pigmentary deposits at approximately 4–6 weeks after the procedure, indicating that the flow of debris through the trabecular meshwork is increased.[7,8]

In addition to the mechanical theory, there is demonstrated histopathologic evidence that endothelial cellular activity is increased and this relative change is responsible for an increase in phagocytosis of trabecular meshwork debris. Cellular activity of this type may be related to a direct stimulation by the argon laser energy or may be an indirect response to some form of biochemical substance that is liberated by the laser at the time of the treatment.[9–11] In either event, the net effect of the procedure is a lowering of IOP of approximately 20–30%. This is approximately equivalent to 5–8 mm in the average glaucoma patient. ALT has also been shown to reduce diurnal pressure elevation in glaucoma patients by 25%.[12]

PATIENT SELECTION

Patient selection is an important aspect of successful treatment with ALT. Certain types of glaucoma are more

TABLE 9-1. Indication for Argon Laser Trabeculoplasty (ALT) Based on Type of Glaucoma

Favorable response to ALT	Variable response to ALT	Poor response to ALT
Primary open-angle glaucoma	Uveitic glaucoma	Juvenile glaucoma
Pseudoexfoliative glaucoma	Aphakic glaucoma	Iridocorneal endothelial syndromes
Pigmentary glaucoma	Angle-recession/traumatic glaucoma	Steroid-induced glaucoma
Primary open-angle glaucoma with uncomplicated pseudophakia		Neovascular glaucoma

responsive and some forms of glaucoma are relatively refractile to ALT or in their presence may provoke an increase in IOP (Table 9-1). Typically, primary open-angle glaucoma patients respond favorably and with consistency to ALT.[13,14] Patients with pseudoexfoliation or pigmentary glaucoma can also be dramatically responsive to ALT.[15–17] Patients with primary open-angle glaucoma who have undergone uncomplicated cataract extraction are generally good candidates for ALT, although the response is less predictable.

Other secondary forms of glaucoma, such as uveitic and traumatic/angle-recession glaucoma, are often less responsive to ALT and can have significant complications, such as IOP spikes and iritis. Juvenile glaucoma, steroid-induced glaucoma, individuals with iridocorneal endothelial syndromes, and other forms of secondary angle-closure glaucoma are generally not indicated for this procedure because of the poor response.[7] Additionally, in every patient who is considered for ALT, the potential benefits must be weighed against the relatively infrequent but real risk of a postoperative rise in IOP. Although the vast majority of patients do not experience postoperative IOP spikes when treated with apraclonidine, IOP may become elevated and relatively refractile to additional ocular antihypertensive therapy. It is therefore appropriate to select patients based not only on the type of glaucoma but the severity of the disease, judging by optic nerve head damage and visual field loss. For this reason, the procedure is best implemented in the early to moderate stages of glaucoma. Use in the endstage glaucoma patient is still considered, but postoperative IOP spikes can be damaging to remaining ganglion cell axons.

CLINICAL APPLICATIONS OF LASER TREATMENT

The success of ALT depends on the accurate placement of the laser energy into the trabecular meshwork (Figure 9-1). The appropriate location of the laser burns is at the junction of the pigmented and nonpigmented trabecular meshwork. This is best accomplished through the use of moderate slit-lamp magnification and adjunctive gonioscopy lenses, such as the Goldmann three-mirror or Ritch lens (Ocular Instruments, Bellevue, WA). The selection

of the energy levels for treatment is variable, depending on the level of pigmentation of the trabecular meshwork and the patient's individual response. Generally, treatment for ALT is instituted with a 50-μm spot size at 0.1-second duration with a power setting of approximately 600–800 mW. In patients with significant pigmentation of the trabecular meshwork, the absorption of laser energy is more efficient, and a reduction in the power setting may be necessary for the appropriate treatment level. In patients with a relatively pale trabecular meshwork, the power may need to be increased up to 1,000 mW to achieve the appropriate level of tissue interaction. The desired end point of the laser therapy is a mild blanching or whitening of the trabecular meshwork tissue (see Figure 9-1). The production of a vesicular response should be avoided; it usually represents an excess of laser energy and can produce subsequent inflammation and potential scarring of the trabecular meshwork, resulting in an increase in IOP.[18] The selection of the laser type is generally one of convenience. Both argon and diode lasers have demonstrated efficacy in this procedure.[19]

Therapy can be performed over 180 degrees or 360 degrees of angle surface at the initial treatment.[20] Both treatment options have advantages and disadvantages (Table 9-2). The number of spots placed in a typical 180-degree session is approximately 40–60, and they are spaced two spot widths apart from each other. If the entire 360 degrees of the trabecular meshwork is to be treated, 80–100 spots are usually applied. When treating 180 degrees, it is typical for the clinician to initiate therapy inferiorly between the 3 o'clock and 9 o'clock positions. This area is selected because in most patients the level of pigmentation is greatest in the inferior angle, which aids in laser energy absorption.[21,22] The remaining superior 180 degrees can be treated 6 weeks later. If the initial 180-degree treatment achieves the desired IOP lowering, then the remaining 180 degrees of treatment can be deferred until it is needed.

Several steps must be taken to prepare the patient for the ALT procedure (Table 9-3). As in all laser procedures, informed consent should be obtained before treatment. The patient is instructed to take all glaucoma medications as prescribed on the day of the procedure. α Agonists, such as apraclonidine or brimonidine, are

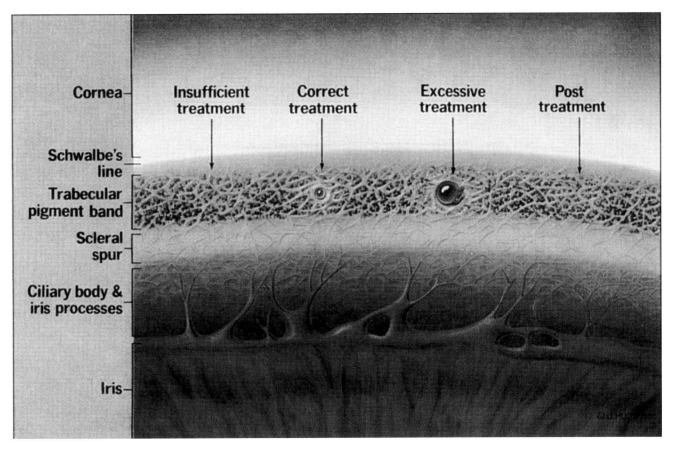

FIGURE 9-1. The laser burns for argon laser trabeculoplasty should be directed at the junction of the pigmented and nonpigmented trabecular meshwork. The intensity of the burn should be adjusted to create a mild blanching of the trabecular meshwork. (Reprinted with permission from Reiss GR, Wilensky JT, Higginbotham EJ. Laser trabeculoplasty. Surv Ophthalmol 1991;35:407–416.)

used to prevent a potential post-treatment IOP rise that is associated with ALT in some patients. Although 1% apraclonidine had been the preferred agent, studies have demonstrated that 0.5% is equal to 1% in preventing IOP spikes.[23] One drop is applied approximately 1 hour before the procedure. In patients who are using α agonists as chronic glaucoma agents, the IOP-decreasing effect of apraclonidine after ALT may be significantly diminished.[24]

Individuals who have a relatively convex iris surface or a narrow approach to the anterior chamber angle that either obscures or makes the view of the trabecular meshwork difficult may need to be treated with low-dose pilocarpine before the procedure to achieve better visibility of the trabecular meshwork. Pilocarpine is applied approximately 1 hour before the procedure. The preferred concentration of pilocarpine is 1–2%, depending on iris pigmentation. In a small subset of patients who demonstrate significant optic nerve head damage and significant visual field loss, it may be necessary to further protect the potential for IOP rise through the use of an oral carbonic anhydrase inhibitor. The appropriate

TABLE 9-2. Advantages of 180-Degree versus 360-Degree Treatment with Argon Laser Trabeculoplasty (ALT)

180 degrees	*360 degrees*
Less severity in postoperative iritis	Better initial intraocular pressure lowering
Less risk of postoperative intraocular pressure spikes	Longer duration of effectiveness
Remaining 180 degrees can be treated at a later date if ALT fails to control intraocular pressure or if the effects of ALT diminish	Less delay in moving to more aggressive therapy (filtering surgery) if ALT is not effective

TABLE 9-3. Pre- and Post-Treatment Regimens

Preprocedure treatment	Postprocedure treatment
Maintain current antiglaucoma regimen	Apraclonidine 0.5% 1 gtt immediately after the procedure
Apraclonidine 0.5% 1 gtt 1 hr before the procedure	Assessment of anterior chamber reaction at 1 hr postprocedure
Pilocarpine 1–2% (depending on iris pigmentation) 1 gtt if view of trabeculum is compromised because of a convex iris contour	Intraocular pressure measurement at 1 hr postprocedure
	If intraocular pressure is at or below pretreatment level, patient should be discharged on all glaucoma medications, with the addition of prednisolone acetate (Pred Forte) q4hr, tapering one drop per day until the medication is discontinued after 1 wk
Oral carbonic anhydrase inhibitors (250 mg × 2) 1 hr before procedure, if optic nerve damage is severe and pressure spike could produce further injury	Follow-up scheduled 1 wk after procedure, if no complications occur

application of this agent is two 250-mg acetazolamide tablets approximately 1 hour before the procedure.

At the time of ALT therapy, the patient undergoes topical anesthesia with proparacaine. Numerous lenses are available to deliver the laser treatment, but the two most commonly used are the Goldmann three-mirror lens and the Ritch lens, which are specifically designed for anterior segment treatment. These lenses must be kept in optimum condition, and the surface of the lens and its coatings must be maintained to maximize the delivery of the laser energy. Additionally, the use of a coupling solution, such as Celluvisc (Allergan Pharmaceuticals, Irvine, CA) or Goniosol (Ciba Vision, Atlanta, GA), is appropriate to maintain the cornea-goniolens contact and to allow for an undistorted view of the anterior chamber angle. Visualization of the anterior chamber angle is crucial, and, to this end, patients who have significant corneal surface abnormalities should be treated appropriately for those conditions to the point of best resolution before ALT therapy. Corneal edema or significant disturbance of the corneal epithelial surface can produce a diffusion of the laser beam, minimizing its effectiveness, and can potentially be absorbed into the cornea and produce tissue injury. Treatment in patients such as this should be deferred until the corneal integrity has been restored and good visualization of the anterior chamber is possible.

POST-TREATMENT CARE

After the ALT procedure is completed, the patient is retreated with one drop of 0.5% apraclonidine and subsequently monitored for approximately 1–2 hours to assess the degree of anterior chamber inflammation and the potential elevation of IOP.[25] A mild anterior chamber reaction is common. Once it has been established that the IOP is being maintained at a safe level, then the patient can be discharged. This typically means IOP is equal to or less than pretreatment levels. In individuals in whom the pressure elevates after ALT, appropriate

measures for reducing IOP should be undertaken. This includes the application of further ocular antihypertensive agents, such as beta blockers, α agonists, and oral carbonic anhydrase inhibitors, when appropriate. The cholinergic agents should be avoided because they can provoke a worsening of the inflammatory response.[26] Latanoprost (Xalatan) may be a potential IOP-lowering agent in this situation, but the possibility of exacerbation of the inflammation must be weighed against the potential for IOP reduction. In severe IOP rises unresponsive to topical therapy or oral carbonic anhydrase inhibitors, oral hyperosmotic agents should be instituted. Such a patient should be maintained in the clinic or the office until the IOP shows a definite response to the additional medical therapy. A 1-day follow-up visit may be appropriate for a patient who develops a significant IOP spike after the ALT procedure.

Post-treatment medications in uncomplicated cases include all of the patient's pretreatment glaucoma therapy and the addition of a topical anti-inflammatory agent, such as prednisolone acetate (Pred Forte), on a tapering dose over several days. This anti-inflammatory dose can be varied depending on the severity of the patient's postoperative inflammatory response. In most instances, a first-day schedule of q4h (six times per day) tapering down one drop per day over 1 week is an adequate treatment. Cycloplegic agents are not necessary in this treatment regimen. Typically, patients who have had an uneventful course are seen again in 1 week, an assessment of the status of the cornea and anterior chamber is undertaken, and IOP is measured. Iritis should be significantly diminished, and the prednisolone acetate should be discontinued and taken from the patient so the medication is not confused with a glaucoma drop. If the inflammation has not subsided or is worse, the prednisolone acetate should be increased and the patient followed closely until the inflammation is controlled. Patients taking pilocarpine or latanoprost with persistent iritis should temporarily discontinue these medications because they may exacerbate the inflammatory component. It is not unusual for the IOP to be relatively unchanged at the 1-week visit, but some individuals may demonstrate an IOP lowering. If the patient's IOP and anterior chamber status are acceptable, then a 4- to 6-week follow-up visit is routinely scheduled, anticipating that the full effect of the laser treatment will be apparent. It can take up to 6–8 weeks after the procedure to achieve the total IOP-lowering capacity of ALT. If the desired target pressure has not been reached 6 weeks after ALT, the remaining 180 degrees can be treated (if the patient's initial treatment was 180 degrees). If 360 degrees was initially treated and the target pressure is not achieved, then additional therapy or filtering surgery should be considered.

RETREATMENT

Once 360 degrees of the trabecular meshwork has been treated with ALT, retreatments are typically not attempted. Retreatments tend to be less successful in IOP lowering and may induce greater anterior chamber inflammation and trabecular scarring. Grayson and associates demonstrated that in individuals with initial successful therapeutic response to ALT, retreatment can be accomplished,[27] but this is usually reserved for individuals who have had a good initial response and over time have demonstrated a "leakage" of the IOP back towards retreatment levels. In these patients, an additional 60–70 spots can be placed on the full 360-degree circumference of the trabecular meshwork. The IOP reduction does not typically achieve the same percentage of IOP lowering of the initial procedure.[28,29] Obviously the risk for inflammation and potential IOP spikes must be considered, and patients who developed complications or had a poor initial response to ALT should not be retreated. The pretreatment and post-treatment care is the same for the second session as it is for the original ALT procedure.

ROLE OF ARGON LASER TRABECULO-PLASTY IN GLAUCOMA THERAPY

ALT plays an important role in the overall management of the glaucoma patient. The Glaucoma Laser Trial (GLT) provides the most direct evidence of the effectiveness of the therapy and its capacity to be integrated into medical management of the glaucoma patient.[30] The design of the GLT was to evaluate the initial therapy of topical medications versus ALT. As initial glaucoma treatment, the initial success of IOP control is excellent in ALT patients, approaching 95% at the 3-month follow-up. But the procedure shows declining effectiveness to only 44% successful IOP control without medication after 24 months. After 5 years, only one out of five patients continues to demonstrate IOP control without medical therapy. Notably, in the GLT study, the nonlaser

group used a stepwise medical therapy that was successful in approximately one-half of the patients with a single medication and two-thirds successful with up to two medications at the 2-year follow-up. A combination of laser and topical medical therapy was successful in 89% of the patients. It is reasonable to conclude that ALT can be used in conjunction with topical medical therapy to achieve a desired target pressure.[31]

The GLT has shown that the laser can be an effective tool in IOP management, and its use has moved forward significantly in the overall scheme of glaucoma therapy. Although it is still most common for initial therapy to be medically directed, it is important that practitioners give consideration to ALT in individuals who have contraindications to medications, have demonstrated inadequate response to topical therapy, have compliance problems with medical treatment, or to whom cost of medication becomes a hardship. The GLT showed that patients who had undergone ALT used less medication to achieve successful IOP management than individuals who were on medical therapy alone. This has the potential to have several positive effects on the overall management of the glaucoma patient. The first of these effects is the decrease in potential side effects from using less topical medical therapy to control the disease. The second effect is the potential for increased compliance by simplification of the glaucoma management process, and the third is the decrease in the financial cost. Cost-effectiveness is a significant consideration in choosing ALT. If the procedure is effective, medication use can be significantly decreased in many patients, with a concurrent decrease in the cost per month to the patient of their glaucoma care. For most individuals, if only one medication is removed due to ALT success for 1 year, the cost of the procedure is negated. The improved quality of life that is offered to patients when ALT is successful is also a significant factor.

COMPLICATIONS

Although ALT is a well-established and generally safe procedure, the potential exists for complications. These include increased IOP, ocular inflammation, peripheral anterior synechiae, loss of vision/visual field, corneal damage, and failure of the procedure.[32–34] One of the more common complications is post-treatment IOP rise. This increase in IOP is relatively unpredictable and can be both acute in its onset and severe in its intensity in a small subset of patients (especially in patients with a history of uveitis or trauma). The obvious risk that this creates is the potential for loss of vision in an eye that already demonstrates a compromised optic nerve. Apraclonidine has been demonstrated to be significantly effective in the prophylaxis of this complication. Before its introduction, from 20% to 50% of patients experienced a postoperative IOP spike. Pretreatment medication with apraclonidine significantly reduces the incidence of postoperative IOP elevation to 20% or less, and significant increases in IOP are relatively rare.[35,36] Additionally, a small number of patients (less than 5%) have a long-term increase in IOP after the procedure, even with medical therapy.

Post-treatment inflammation is another common sequela with ALT. It is present in almost 100% of patients after therapy, but with appropriate anti-inflammatory regimens, the rate of significant complications is rare. Inflammation of the trabecular meshwork with inflammatory precipitates (trabeculitis) can occur but may be difficult to identify with gonioscopy. The development of these precipitates is appropriately treated with anti-inflammatory agents with aggressive pulse therapy.[37] Some individuals demonstrate persistent post-ALT inflammatory response, and, in these individuals, appropriate use of topical steroidal and nonsteroidal agents can be very helpful in extinguishing the inflammatory reaction. Persistent inflammation should be treated to prevent the onset of broad peripheral anterior synechiae and posterior synechiae. The mechanisms for the inflammation and the subsequent IOP elevation are most likely related.[38] It has been postulated that a biochemical response (prostaglandin activity) may be one of the causes, and the development of inflammatory material, as well as pigment and other debris, could well serve to mechanically obstruct the trabecular meshwork. Topical prostaglandin agents, such as latanoprost, may need to be temporarily discontinued if severe or persistent iritis is present after ALT.

Studies have shown that the ideal location for laser application is the anterior third of the pigmented trabecular meshwork. Placement of burns more posteriorly toward the ciliary body can incite local inflammatory response with the potential for small, tuft-like peripheral anterior synechiae formation.[39] These generally do not interfere with IOP control over the long-term management of the patient, but if they are severe, they can serve as an initiating point for future compromise of the angle. Peripheral anterior synechiae extending high into the trabecular meshwork, although not a common sequela of ALT, can occur if excessive laser energy is used.

CONCLUSION

ALT can be considered as another effective "medication" in our armamentarium against glaucoma. It may be used as initial therapy in patients who are noncompliant, have contraindications to topical medications, are unable to instill eye drops, or cannot afford the cost of medications. ALT is most commonly used as an adjunctive therapy and should be considered in a patient's treatment after two or three topical medications have been prescribed and the target pressure has not been met or the patient is showing progression of the disease.

Even though most patients achieve an initial IOP lowering with ALT, the effect of the procedure diminishes over time with a failure rate of approximately 10% or more per year. Which patients will lose IOP control is unpredictable, as is the time frame in which the loss of IOP control will be exhibited. Glaucoma patients must be monitored with serial IOP, optic nerve evaluation, and visual field testing to determine whether more aggressive therapy is required.

ALT has varying rates of success, depending on the nature of the glaucoma being treated. Patients with secondary glaucoma presentations such as steroid-induced glaucoma, iridocorneal endothelial syndromes, neovascular glaucoma, and other angle-closure glaucomas, as well as congenital or juvenile glaucoma, are not good candidates for ALT. Patients with traumatic angle recession or uveitic glaucoma are generally much less successful ALT candidates. The risks and benefits of the procedure must be weighed for each individual. In patients with chronic open-angle, pigmentary, or pseudoexfoliative glaucoma, the benefits of ALT outweigh the potential risks in most patients.

REFERENCES

1. Krasnov NM. Laser-puncture of anterior chamber angle in glaucoma. Am J Ophthalmol 1973;75:674–678.

2. Worthen DM, Wickham MG. Argon laser trabeculotomy. Trans Am Acad Ophthalmol Otolaryngol 1974;78:371–375.

3. Wise JB, Witter SL. Argon laser therapy for open-angle glaucoma: a pilot study. Arch Ophthalmol 1979;97:319–322.

4. Bylsma SS, Samples JR, Acott TS, Van Buskirk EM. Trabecular cell division after argon laser trabeculoplasty. Arch Ophthalmol 1988;106:544–547.

5. Melamed S, Pei J, Epstein DL. Short-term effect of argon laser trabeculoplasty in monkeys. Arch Ophthalmol 1985;103:1546–1552.

6. Van Buskirk EM, Pond V, Rosenquist RC, Acott TS. Argon laser trabeculoplasty: studies of mechanism of action. Ophthalmology 1984;91:1005–1010.

7. Robin AL, Pollack IP. Argon laser trabeculoplasty in secondary forms of open-angle glaucoma. Arch Ophthalmol 1983;101:382–384.

8. Ritch R, Liebmann J, Robin A, et al. Argon laser trabeculoplasty in pigmentary glaucoma. Ophthalmology 1993;100(6):909–913.

9. Melamed S, Pei J, Epstein DL. Delayed response to argon laser trabeculoplasty in monkeys: morphological and morphometric analysis. Arch Ophthalmol 1986;104:1078–1083.

10. Van Buskirk EM. Pathophysiology of laser trabeculoplasty. Surv Ophthalmol 1989;33(4):264–272.

11. Alexander RA, Grierson I. Morphological effects of argon laser trabeculoplasty upon the glaucomatous human meshwork. Eye 1989;3(6):719–726.

12. Greenidge KC, Spaeth GL, Fiol-Silva Z. Effect of argon laser trabeculoplasty on the glaucomatous diurnal curve. Ophthalmology 1983;90:800–804.

13. Bergea B, Bodin L, Svedbergh B. Primary argon laser trabeculoplasty vs pilocarpine. II. Long-term effects on intraocular pressure and facility of outflow. Study design and additional therapy. Acta Ophthalmol 1994;72(2):145–154.

14. Gillies WE, Dallison IW, Brooks AM. Long-term results with argon laser trabeculoplasty. Aust N Z J Ophthalmol 1994;22(1):39–43.

15. Higginbotham EJ, Richardson TM. Response of exfoliation glaucoma to laser trabeculoplasty. Br J Ophthalmol 1986;70(11):837–839.

16. Sherwood MB, Svedbergh B. Argon laser trabeculoplasty in exfoliation syndrome. Br J Ophthalmol 1985;69(12):886–890.

17. Lehto I. Long-term follow up of argon laser trabeculoplasty in pigmentary glaucoma. Ophthalmol Surg 1992;23(9):614–617.

18. Wilensky JT, Jampol LM. Laser therapy for open-angle glaucoma. Ophthalmology 1981;88:213–217.

19. Chung PY, Schoman JS, Netland PA, et al. Five-year results of a randomized, prospective, clinical trial of diode versus argon laser trabeculoplasty for open angle glaucoma. Am J Ophthalmol 1998;126:185–190.

20. Honrubia FM, Ferrer EJ, Lecinena J, et al. Long-term follow up of the argon laser trabeculoplasty in eyes treated 180 degrees and 360 degrees of the trabeculum. Int Ophthalmol 1992;16(4–5):375–379.

21. Grayson D, Chi T, Liebmann J, Ritch R. Initial argon laser trabeculoplasty to the inferior vs superior of trabecular meshwork (letter). Arch Ophthalmol 1994;112(4):446–447.

22. Takenaka Y, Yamamoto T, Shirato S. One-quadrant argon laser trabeculoplasty and its indication. Jpn J Ophthalmol 1987;31(3):483–488.

23. Threlkeld AB. Apraclonidine 0.5% versus 1% for controlling intraocular pressure elevation after argon laser trabeculoplasty. Ophthalmic Surg Lasers Aug ,1996.

24. Chung HS, Shin DH, Birt CM, et al. Chronic use of apraclonidine decreases its moderation of post-laser intraocular pressure spikes. Ophthalmology 1997;104:1921–1925.

25. Dapling RB, Cunliffe IA, Longstaff S. Influence of apraclonidine and pilocarpine alone and in combination on post laser trabeculoplasty pressure rise. Br J Ophthalmol 1994;78(1)30–32.

26. Ofner S, Samples JR, Van Buskirk EM. Pilocarpine and increase in intraocular pressure after trabeculoplasty. Am J Ophthalmol 1984;97:647–649.

27. Grayson DK, Camras CB, Podos SM, Lustgarten JS. Long-term reduction of intraocular pressure after repeat argon laser trabeculoplasty. Am J Ophthalmol 1988;106(3):312–321.

28. Brown SV, Thomas JV, Simmons RJ. Laser trabeculoplasty re-treatment. Am J Ophthalmol 1985;99(1):8–10.

29. Richter CU, Shingleton BJ, Bellows AR, et al. Re-treatment with argon laser trabeculoplasty. Ophthalmology 1987;94(9):1085–1089.

30. Glaucoma Laser Trial Research Group. Glaucoma Laser Trial (GLT) and Glaucoma Laser Trial Follow Up Study. 7. Results. Am J Ophthalmol 1995;120(6):718–731.

31. Glaucoma Laser Trial Research Group. Glaucoma Laser Trial (GLT). 2. Results of argon laser trabeculoplasty versus topical medicines. Ophthalmology 1990;97(11):1403–1413.

32. Keightley SJ, Khaw PT, Elkington AR. The prediction of intraocular pressure rise following argon laser trabeculoplasty. Eye 1987;1(5):577–580.

33. Mermoud A, Pittet N, Herbort CP. Inflammation patterns after laser trabeculoplasty measured with the laser flare meter. Arch Ophthalmol 1992;110(3):368–370.

34. Thoming C, Van Buskirk EM, Samples JR. The corneal endothelium after laser therapy for glaucoma. Am J Ophthalmol 1987;103(4):518–522.

35. Dapling RB, Cunliffe IA, Longstaff S. Influence of apraclonidine and pilocarpine alone and in combination on post laser trabeculoplasty pressure rise. Br J Ophthalmol 1994;78(1):30–32.

36. Holmwood PC, Chase RD, Krupin T, et al. Apraclonidine and argon laser trabeculoplasty. Am J Ophthalmol 1992;114(1):19–22.

37. Fiore PM, Melamed S, Epstein DL. Trabecular precipitates and elevated intraocular pressure following argon laser trabeculoplasty. Ophthalmic Surg 1989;20(10):697–701.

38. West RH. The effect of topical corticosteroids on laser-induced peripheral anterior synechiae. Aust N Z J Ophthalmol 1992;20(4):305–309.

39. Traverso CE, Greenidge KC, Spaeth GL. Formation of peripheral anterior synechiae following argon laser trabeculoplasty. A prospective study to determine relationship to position of laser burns. Arch Ophthalmol 1984;102(6):861–863.

10

Glaucoma Filtering Surgery

Judith E. Goldstein

Glaucoma filtration surgery, better known as *trabeculectomy*, has undergone significant technical advances since the procedure was first performed in the nineteenth century. Glaucoma surgery is no longer a treatment of last resort, but is instead an intervention that may be considered at any time during the management of the patient. The risk-benefit ratio must be weighed for each patient with an emphasis on the potential impact on an individual's quality of life. Some of the quality of life indices to consider include reduction in side effects from glaucoma medication, cost of medication, and inconvenience of instilling eye drops.

INDICATIONS FOR SURGICAL INTERVENTION

The decision to recommend and perform glaucoma filtration surgery is based on many factors, including, but not limited to[1,2]:

1. Magnitude and duration of intraocular pressure (IOP) elevation
2. Extent and progression of visual field defects
3. Extent of damage to the optic nerve head
4. Patient's own sense of visual function
5. Course of the contralateral eye with or without treatment
6. General health and life expectancy of the patient
7. Relative risk of surgical complications in a specific eye

In traditional glaucoma management, filtration surgery is indicated when medical and laser therapy is insufficient to control the disease. Medical therapy is

thus deemed insufficient and surgical intervention is indicated if:

- The IOP cannot be lowered enough to prevent further damage.
- The medication cannot be tolerated.
- Compliance cannot be achieved.

It is important to mention that studies within the last decade suggest that some forms of glaucoma therapy, including chronic topical beta-blocker therapy and argon laser trabeculoplasty, may have an adverse effect on the success rate of trabeculectomy.[3] Chronic pilocarpine use[4–7] may induce changes in the conjunctival tissue that reduce the surgical success rate compared with the success rate of surgery used as the primary intervention.[8–13] Potential changes in the conjunctival tissue include an increase in the number of macrophages, lymphocytes, mast cells, and fibroblasts and a decrease in the number of epithelial goblet cells.[3] This increase in the number of inflammatory cells as a result of chronic medical therapy suggests a greater likelihood of external bleb scarring and ultimate filtration surgery failure, raising the question of whether surgery or medications should be the initial therapy for primary open-angle glaucoma.[10,11,14] The Collaborative Initial Glaucoma Treatment Study (CIGTS) is an ongoing clinical trial designed to determine whether medications or filtering surgery should be first line therapy for newly diagnosed glaucoma patients.

PATIENT EDUCATION

Glaucoma filtration surgery, like any other medical or surgical intervention, must be explained to the patient to

TABLE 10-1. Complications of Filtration Surgery

Decrease visual acuity "snuffing of vision"

Irregular astigmatism

Photophobia

Ptosis

Foreign body sensation and tearing

Corneal dellen and possible decompensation

Cataract formation

Shallow or flat anterior chamber

Persistent intraocular inflammation

Bleb leak

Chronic hypotony

Hyphema

Choroidal detachment

Macular edema or hypotony maculopathy

Failure of filtration procedure

Suprachoroidal hemorrhage

Malignant glaucoma

Endophthalmitis

Phthisis bulbi

TABLE 10-2. Factors Affecting the Success Rate of Glaucoma Filtering Surgery

Favorable factors for surgical success

Older patients (>60 years of age)

Surgical success in fellow eye

Virgin eye (no previous surgical procedures)

No ocular inflammation

Experienced surgeon

Unfavorable factors for surgical success

Younger patients (<60 years of age)

African-American race

Aphakic or pseudophakic eyes

History of ocular inflammation (uveitic glaucoma)

Neovascular glaucoma

Conjunctival cicatrizing diseases

Previous ocular surgery

Prior failed filtering surgery

establish appropriate consent and, more important, realistic expectations. The risks and benefits must be carefully conveyed, with an emphasis on the possibilities of ocular discomfort, corneal decompensation, infection, vision loss, and cataract formation (Table 10-1). The patient must understand that the goal of surgery is stabilization of glaucomatous visual field loss rather than reversal of damage that has already occurred.

SURGICAL SUCCESS

The definitions of surgical success used in the literature are ambiguous. The definitions offered in studies vary anywhere from IOP control (which itself is poorly defined) without medications, to preservation of visual field, to IOP control with the use of additional medications. With this said, studies point to trabeculectomy success rates between 65% and 90%.[14,15] These rates depend on a variety of factors (Table 10-2), including the type of glaucoma, age of the patient, previous failure of glaucoma surgery in that eye or the fellow eye, use of antimetabolites, conjunctival scarring from a previous surgery, and aphakia or pseudophakia.

TYPES OF SURGICAL PROCEDURES

The goal of surgical intervention for glaucoma is to create an additional outflow channel for aqueous to escape from the anterior chamber, resulting in lowered IOP. The two types of procedures currently in use are the partial-thickness (guarded) procedure and the full-thickness (unguarded) procedure (Figure 10-1). These procedures are differentiated according to whether a scleral flap is present to regulate the flow of aqueous. The partial-thickness trabeculectomy is favored because of the reduced rate of complications.

Partial-Thickness (Guarded) Trabeculectomy

In the partial-thickness procedure (Figure 10-2), once the eye is anesthetized and the patient's individual surgical anatomy inspected, a conjunctival flap is created (see Figure 10-2A). The operation site is typically at the superonasal corneoscleral junction. This location provides the easiest surgical access and leaves room temporally for future cataract surgery, and the resultant bleb will be covered by the upper eyelid. This prevents diplopia caused by surgical iridectomy and assists in maintaining a normal cosmetic ocular appearance. An additional advantage of creating a superior surgical site is a possible decrease in the rate of infection as compared with an inferior filter site.[16] In cases of reoperation, an alternate site may be chosen because of the difficulty in dissecting scarred conjunctiva.

Before creating any incision, the surgeon must decide whether the conjunctival flap will be limbal-based or fornix-based. The terms *limbal-based* and *fornix-based* describe where the flap is anchored. Most surgeons perform one type more than the other, according to individual preference. With a limbal-based flap, a curved circumferential incision is made at least 8 mm posterior to the limbus, and the conjunctiva is dissected anteriorly;

FIGURE 10-1. **(A)** Full-thickness procedure with direct flow of aqueous from the anterior chamber into the subconjunctival space. **(B)** Guarded procedure (trabeculectomy). A sutured scleral flap provides resistance to aqueous drainage from the anterior chamber to the subconjunctival space. (Reprinted with permission from EJ Higginbotham, DA Lee. Management of Difficult Glaucoma. Cambridge: Blackwell Scientific, 1994;326.)

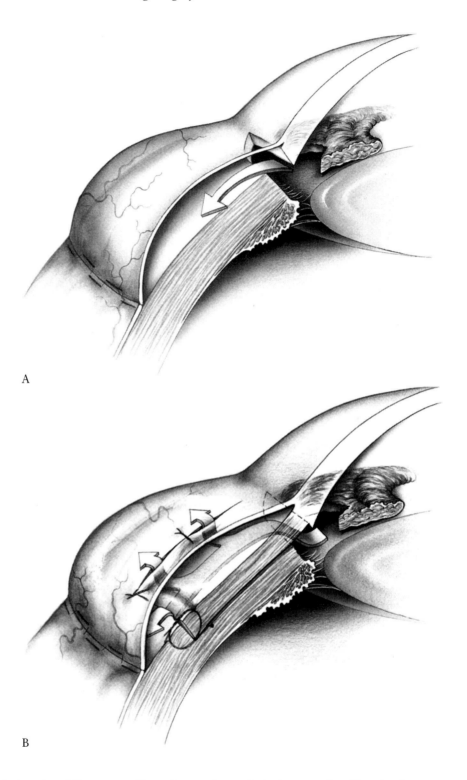

A

B

therefore, the flap is based at the limbal region (Figure 10-2A). In contrast, with a fornix-based flap, the incision is made anteriorly at the limbus, and the conjunctiva is dissected posteriorly. Neither flap is clearly superior in reducing IOP or in its long-term success rate.[17,18]

While creating the conjunctival flap, the surgeon must contend with two distinct external tissue layers. Most external is the conjunctival mucous membrane. Below the conjunctiva and the subconjunctival space is

Tenon's capsule, a relatively avascular, fibroelastic structure. The first operational incision is the creation of the conjunctival flap. Both the conjunctiva and Tenon's capsule must be dissected either anteriorly or posteriorly (based on the flap type), away from the sclera.

Once the conjunctival flap is created and cautery is applied to bleeding scleral vessels, the surgeon demarcates the outline of the scleral flap (see Figure 10-2A). Scleral flaps can be triangular, square, rectangular, trapezoidal,

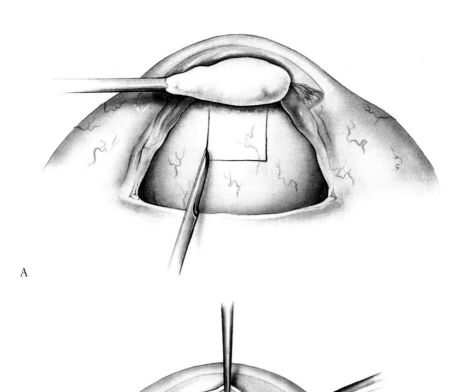

FIGURE 10-2. Anatomic drawings of elements of a guarded trabeculectomy procedure. (**A**) Once the limbal-based conjunctival flap has been created, the outline of the scleral flap is incised to approximately one-half scleral depth. (**B**) The scleral flap is dissected and then elevated with forceps while the inner scleral flap is outlined and then excised.

or semicircular in shape, depending on the surgeon's preference. The size of the flap is also variable and may depend on the shape chosen. Flaps usually vary from 3 to 5 mm circumferentially and 2 to 4 mm radially. In partial-thickness or guarded procedures, the outline of the flap is incised so that the flap created is approximately one- to two-thirds of the total scleral thickness. The flap is then dissected anteriorly toward clear cornea. It is important to carry the scleral flap far enough anteriorly to avoid incising the ciliary body, which may lead to excessive bleeding. Good surgical technique is also critical in incising the scleral flap, partially because accidental perforation may create an undesired full-thickness flap and, in turn, full-thickness drainage.

After a paracentesis track is made (later used to reform the anterior chamber), a sclerostomy (hole in the sclera) is created. An inner sclerotrabecular block of tissue, smaller than the scleral flap (e.g., 2 mm × 2 mm), is removed (see Figure 10-2B). This can be done by incising

with a knife, scissors, or a Kelly Descemet's punch. This hole through the sclera is called the *sclerostomy site*. The sclerostomy site is an important anatomic feature for postoperative evaluation should the clinician suspect filter failure. Blockage of the sclerostomy site, as determined through gonioscopic evaluation, prevents aqueous flow out of the anterior chamber. Once the sclerostomy is made, the surgeon creates a peripheral iridectomy to prevent the underlying iris from prolapsing through the sclerostomy site and ultimately blocking the flow of aqueous (see Figure 10-2C).

Before closure of the scleral flap, the eye is carefully inspected for any bleeding at the iris root or ciliary body that may have occurred while the iridectomy was being created. The scleral flap is then sutured to the scleral bed using one to four sutures (see Figure 10-2D). The amount of scleral flap tightening significantly affects the titration of aqueous outflow. The goal is to tie the sutures loosely enough to permit adequate filtration, but tightly enough to

FIGURE 10-2. (*continued*) (**C**) A peripheral iridectomy is performed through the sclerostomy site. (**D**) Scleral flap is closed, followed by Tenon's capsule and conjunctival closure. (Reprinted with permission from EJ Higginbotham, DA Lee. Management of Difficult Glaucoma. Cambridge: Blackwell Scientific, 1994;350–357.)

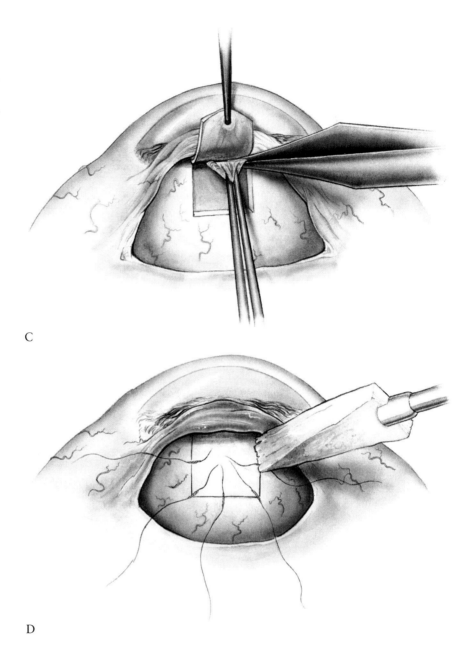

C

D

prevent overfiltration and hypotony. A popular technique is to tie the sutures tight to avoid excessive postoperative hypotony and then selectively cut or release sutures as needed in the early postoperative period.

The anterior chamber can then be reformed through the paracentesis track using a 30-gauge cannula and balanced salt solution. By applying cellulose sponges around the edges of the scleral flap, visualization of the amount of aqueous humor leaking out can be determined. Suture tension may then be adjusted to ensure a controlled slow leak of aqueous humor at the margins of the scleral flap.

Because of the critical nature of attaining sufficient and appropriate aqueous flow, different techniques have been used to enable scleral flap suture removal in the early postoperative period (1–2 weeks after surgery).

One approach is to cut the scleral flap sutures with an argon laser. Disadvantages to this method are conjunctival hemorrhage or scar tissue obscuring the suture and patient discomfort or muscle palsy limiting the ability to safely use the laser. Another technique is to place sutures that can be easily released: Instead of suturing the flap solely to the scleral bed, a nylon suture is first passed into the sclera, next through the base of the scleral flap, beneath the conjunctival insertion, and finally through the peripheral cornea. The suture is then tied with a modified slip knot so it can be easily removed at the slit lamp with a needlenose forceps or the forceps of choice. To prevent overfiltration and a flat anterior chamber, suture removal is performed postoperatively, when the chamber is deep, the eye is not hypotonous, and no sign of ciliary body shutdown is present. No good algorithms are available that define exactly when to remove releasable sutures. However, removal is typically performed within the first 2 postoperative weeks.

Once the scleral flap is sutured (with or without a releasable suture), Tenon's capsule and the conjunctiva are closed, typically with running sutures to the limbal or fornix region, depending on the style of flap. If a fornix-based flap has been used, the limbal edge of the cornea may be débrided to provide better adhesion of the conjunctiva during healing. When using antifibrotic agents, it is important to ensure that that the conjunctival closure is watertight to avoid postoperative wound leaks.

After conjunctival closure, additional balanced salt solution may be injected through the paracentesis to deepen the anterior chamber, elevate the bleb, and allow inspection for leakage around the conjunctival edges. Inspecting for a watertight closure may be assisted with the use of 2% fluorescein dye. If a leak is observed, additional conjunctival sutures are placed until leakage is no longer evident.

At the end of surgery, the pupillary sphincter and ciliary muscle should be paralyzed to minimize posterior synechiae and deepen the anterior chamber. This assists in decreasing the possibility of a flat anterior chamber and misdirection of aqueous flow behind the vitreous (malignant glaucoma). Adequate dilation can be accomplished with atropine 1% solution or ointment. In addition, a steroid-antibiotic combination ointment is often instilled at the time of surgery.

Full-Thickness (Unguarded) Trabeculectomy

In the early twentieth century, full-thickness trabeculectomy became the technique of choice for surgically lowering IOP. The procedure involved making a full-thickness hole in the sclera after creating a limbus-based conjunctival flap. The full-thickness hole was made through thermal cautery or scleral excision,[19,20] and was followed by creation of an iridectomy. This created an unrestricted channel from the anterior chamber to the subconjunctival space (see Figure 10-1A).

The full-thickness filtration procedure was and continues to be extremely successful in lowering IOP. However, it was initially abandoned for the guarded (partial-thickness) procedure because of the high rate of postoperative complications, which include hypotony, flat anterior chamber, and choroidal detachment.[21] In addition, with the advent of antimetabolites, partial-thickness procedures can now provide better long-term success rates with fewer postoperative complications.

WOUND HEALING IN GLAUCOMA FILTERING PROCEDURES

Prevention of wound healing at the fistula between the anterior chamber and the subconjunctival space is the key to achieving successful filtering surgery. In essence, this is an attempt to prevent the natural biological healing response.

Excessive scarring at the sclerostomy site or along the scleral flap can cause failure of filtration. This may occur any time from the immediate postoperative period to months and years after surgery. Surgical trauma causes the proliferation and migration of fibroblasts to the conjunctival-tenon-scleral interface. The deposition of fibroblasts leads to fibrosis, scarring, and the ultimate failure of aqueous filtration.

Adjunct Antifibrotic Agents

The limiting factor in glaucoma surgical success is often the fibroblastic activity that causes scarring and, in turn, filter failure. As a result, much attention has been focused on the use of agents that are effective in interrupting steps in the wound-healing process. The most frequently used adjuncts include pre- and postoperative corticosteroids, as well as intraoperative and postoperative antimetabolites.

Role of Corticosteroids

The frequent administration of high-dose postoperative topical steroids in glaucoma filtration surgery cannot be emphasized enough. Corticosteroids have been shown to decrease fibroblast proliferation,[22] promote bleb formation,[23] and increase aqueous flow,[24] translating to decreased IOP. The use of topical steroids is discussed in further detail in the section Postoperative Care. However, it is important to reiterate that postoperative corticosteroid use is critical to enhancing surgical success.

Preoperative injection of sub–Tenon's capsule or subconjunctival steroids remains controversial and has not definitively been shown to increase the success rate of filtration surgery.[25] Systemic steroids also have not demonstrated a significant difference in pressure-lowering effects over topical steroids.[23] Considering this lack of significant benefit and the risk of systemic side effects, the use of oral steroids is not routinely recommended.

Role of Antimetabolites

A significant advancement in filtering surgery has been the adjunct use of antimetabolite agents, also know as *antineoplastic agents*. The use of antimetabolites in conjunction with filtration surgery has been shown to increase surgical success in high-risk eyes (see Table 10-2).[26,27] Antimetabolites act to inhibit fibroblast proliferation.[28] This is critical in preventing filter failure in high-risk eyes that have an unusually vigorous healing response. Originally, antimetabolites were reserved only for use in high-risks cases. However, many glaucoma surgeons use these agents in routine cases as well. Antimetabolites can be used through postoperative subconjunctival injection and intraoperative application. The agents most commonly in use include 5-fluorouracil (5-FU) and mitomycin C (MMC).

5-Fluorouracil. Since the mid-1980s, 5-FU has been applied postoperatively through subconjunctival injections. The successful application of 5-FU in a pilot study[29] prompted numerous studies[30–32] that demonstrated a statistically significant enhancement in control of postoperative IOP (less than 21 mm Hg), a reduction in the need for postoperative antiglaucoma medication, and avoidance of reoperation for pressure control.[31]

Most commonly, 5-FU is applied postoperatively through subconjunctival injections 90–180 degrees away from the trabeculectomy site. The usual dosage of 5-FU is a 5-mg dose every day or every other day for the first 1–2 weeks after surgery.[33] The advantage of 5-FU is that doses can be titrated based on bleb appearance, development of subconjunctival fibrosis, ocular inflammation, and increasing IOP. 5-FU has also been applied intraoperatively in a manner similar to that used for MMC. The advantages over postoperative injection are a one-time intraoperative application and a significant decrease in corneal side effects. No studies clearly indicate superior efficacy and safety of 5-FU intraoperatively as compared with MMC.

Among disadvantages of postoperative 5-FU is the necessity of multiple postoperative injections, which, in turn, require good patient cooperation and compliance. Each injection carries the risk of subconjunctival hemorrhage, which may accelerate subconjunctival fibrosis. Almost all of the same potential complications exist with 5-FU and MMC. The most common complications of 5-FU injections are corneal punctate epitheliopathy, corneal epithelial defects, and primary conjunctival wound leaks secondary to 5-FU corneal and conjunctival toxicity.[30,31] Therefore, 5-FU is contraindicated in patients with underlying corneal disease. 5-FU is typically discontinued in patients if large areas of epithelial defects develop, but 5-FU may be continued in patients with superficial punctate keratitis alone.

Mitomycin C. MMC is a potent inhibitor of fibroblast proliferation[28] and has been used systemically for many years for its antitumor activity. MMC is applied intraoperatively to the filtering site via a soaked cellulose sponge. The sponge is soaked in a 0.1- to 0.5-mg/ml concentration of MMC and applied to the scleral surface after creation of the conjunctival flap. The conjunctiva is then carefully draped over the sponge for 2–5 minutes. The sponge is usually applied to the scleral surface before the scleral flap incision. It is thought that applying the sponge after the scleral incision may increase the concentrated dose to deep sclera and risk drug penetration into the anterior chamber, where it can result in prolonged ocular hypotony.[34,35] After the sponge is removed, the surgical site is copiously irrigated. The trabeculectomy is then completed in the usual fashion with

sclerostomy, iridectomy, and appropriately tightened scleral-flap closure to maintain a formed anterior chamber and a watertight conjunctival closure. Releasable sutures may be used to assist in creating tight wound closure to avoid early postoperative hypotony.

Postoperatively, MMC blebs can have a very distinct, avascular, chalky-white appearance (Color Plate 29). Often, these blebs appear thin-walled, and the area of whitening tends to be focal. The size of the bleb may be determined by the size of the MMC sponge application area.[36] The thin nature of the MMC blebs makes them susceptible to conjunctival dehiscence, which, in turn, increases the risk for wound leak and endophthalmitis.

The advantage of MMC over 5-FU postoperative injections is the single intraoperative application and the lack of corneal epithelial toxicity.[37] Although intraocular penetration of MMC through the scleral flap can result in irreversible corneal endothelial damage, careful surgical technique has rendered this complication essentially nonexistent.[38] Aside from the potential postoperative complications listed in the previous section, MMC may result in an increased incidence of bleb encapsulation formation[39] and prolonged ocular hypotony with maculopathy[40] compared with 5-FU.

The use of MMC or 5-FU has demonstrated effectiveness in increasing the success rate of high-risk filtering surgery. In some studies, MMC and 5-FU produced similar degrees of IOP control.[41,42] In one study, comparison between MMC and 5-FU at 5-year follow-up exhibited a similar late complication rate, although the pressure-lowering effect of MMC appeared to be greater than those of 5-FU.[39] Therefore, MMC may be a better choice in eyes that require a significant lowering of IOP, such as normal-tension glaucoma or endstage glaucoma. Ultimately, the decision regarding choice of antimetabolite should be based on the evaluation of each individual patient and the inherent risk of filter failure, including a previous history of filter failure.

VARIATIONS ON STANDARD GLAUCOMA FILTRATION SURGERY

Combined Surgery

The surgical management of coexistent cataract and glaucoma basically consists of three options: cataract extraction alone, glaucoma filtering surgery alone followed by cataract extraction as a second procedure (two-stage approach), or glaucoma filtering procedure combined with cataract extraction (combined procedure). The indications for performing a combined procedure include an eye with moderate to advanced glaucomatous vision loss and a visually significant cataract. These procedures are also performed to hamper an acute IOP rise after surgery or to achieve a chronic reduction of IOP below preoperative levels.[43] Control of IOP on glaucoma medications, along with consideration of medication tolerance and compliance with therapy, should also be incorporated into the decision-making process.

Cataract extraction in combined procedures is most commonly performed with phacoemulsification. This enables the posterior capsule to remain intact so vitreous incarceration into the sclerostomy site can be prevented. As opposed to intracapsular cataract extraction, these techniques also allow placement of a posterior chamber intraocular lens. The combination of glaucoma filtering surgery, cataract extraction, and insertion of a posterior chamber intraocular lens is commonly referred to as a *triple procedure.*

A combined operation is clearly a more risky procedure than filtering surgery alone because it carries the complications of both cataract and glaucoma surgery. A common complication in patients with elevated IOP preoperatively and advanced glaucomatous damage[44] is a postoperative IOP spike. The mechanism is similar to that following standard trabeculectomy and involves inadequate aqueous drainage into the filtration bleb in the early postoperative period.[45] In addition, combined procedures are at increased risk of transient bleb leaks, hyphemas, hypotony, intraocular lens capture, and astigmatism secondary to suture tightening at the trabeculectomy site or the cataract wound site.

Despite the increased risk of complications, combined procedures are a sound alternative in patients with progressive glaucomatous damage and a visually significant cataract. Although controversial, the adjunct use of antimetabolites may have an added benefit in improving long-term success in these cases.

Drainage Implants

Use of glaucoma drainage implants is generally reserved for complicated glaucomas that have not responded to conventional filtering surgery and the adjunct use of antimetabolites, or in eyes with marked conjunctival scarring where filtration surgery is thought not to be possible. Thus, they provide a useful alternative in the treatment of various refractory glaucomas, including those associated with aphakia, pseudophakia, neovascularization of the iris or angle, uveitis, prior unsuccessful filtering surgery, iridocorneal endothelial syndrome, trauma, and youth.

The basic design of most implant devices is the same. A silicone tube inserted into the anterior chamber through a scleral fistula, shunts aqueous to a reservoir positioned at the equatorial region of the globe. The bleb is a fibrous capsule surrounding a synthetic plate or band. The band is sutured to the episcleral surface posterior to the rectus muscle insertions. Once fibrous tissue encapsulates the plate, the resultant bleb cavity serves as a subconjunctival reservoir to which aqueous humor is shunted via the silicone tube.[46]

Glaucoma implants have been successful in achieving filtration in eyes at high risk for filter failure. However, significant complications occur in 50–70% of cases.[47] Complications can occur early or late in the postoperative period and are due to the type of procedure and the advanced nature of the disease. Despite the high incidence of complications, glaucoma implants have had reported success rates between 70% and 90% using multiple types of devices,[48] and, therefore, offer a valuable alternative to the treatment of refractory glaucoma.

Cyclodestructive Procedures of the Ciliary Body

The indications for any type of cyclodestructive procedure are similar to those for glaucoma implant surgery, namely refractory glaucomas. The procedures typically incorporate the application of cryotherapy or laser energy slightly posterior to the limbal region. The mechanism is believed to be the destruction of the ciliary epithelium, which thereby decreases aqueous production.

A high rate of complications exists with cyclodestructive procedures.[49,50] Common ocular complications include iritis, which is usually responsive to medical therapy, postoperative pain that may require temporary narcotic analgesia, and conjunctival burns, which heal quickly without sequelae. With these procedures, a 52% risk of developing vision loss and a 12% risk of phthisis exist.[51] A variety of mechanisms may cause vision loss, including a postoperative rise in IOP and cystoid macular edema. Therefore, the procedure is generally limited to individuals with poor visual potential or those cases in which the goal is to relieve pressure-induced pain.

POSTOPERATIVE CARE

Medical Therapy

In glaucoma filtering surgery, adequate postoperative medical management directly and dramatically affects the surgical outcome. Two key aspects in assisting success of filtering procedures are compliance with therapy by the patient and avoidance of the tendency to discontinue anti-inflammatory medication prematurely. Postoperative medical management incorporates the use of cycloplegic agents, topical corticosteroids, and topical antibiotics. Variations between clinicians exist regarding brands of agents used, frequency of instillation, and duration of use (Table 10-3).

Cycloplegic agents act to deepen the anterior chamber and decrease ciliary spasm, thereby providing symptomatic relief to the patient. These agents also maintain the blood-aqueous barrier, which decreases the influx of white blood cells into the anterior chamber. Limiting the anterior chamber inflammation assists in

TABLE 10-3. Sample Postoperative Therapy Regimen

Treatment	Daily frequency	Duration (weeks)
Topical corticosteroids		
Prednisolone acetate	q2h	0–2
	q4h	2–4
	q.i.d.	4–6
	t.i.d.	6–8
	b.i.d.	8–10
	qd	10–12
Cycloplegics		
Atropine 1%	b.i.d.	0–1
Homatropine 5%	b.i.d.	1–3*
Topical antibiotic		
Broad-spectrum antibiotic	q.i.d.	0–2

*Cycloplegic should be continued until the anterior chamber is without cell and flare.
Note: This table is a sample postoperative therapeutic regimen that assumes an uncomplicated course after filtration surgery. Alteration of frequency and duration of medication is required in cases with such complications as excessive inflammation, shallow anterior chamber, and choroidal effusions.

preventing posterior synechia, which could lead to pupillary block, high IOP, and failed filtration surgery if not prevented.

Cycloplegics are used between 1 and 4 weeks postoperatively. Either atropine 1%, scopolamine 0.25%, or homatropine 5% is used because of their longer-acting ability. Typically, patients are started on a q.i.d. schedule, tapered to b.i.d., and finally to once at bedtime (qhs). Cycloplegics may be discontinued when the anterior chamber is free of inflammation.

The administration of frequent and high-dose postoperative topical steroids in glaucoma filtration surgery is essential for surgical success. Corticosteroids are shown to decrease fibroblast proliferation,[22] promote bleb formation,[23] and increase aqueous flow,[24] translating to decreased IOP. Prednisolone acetate 1% is initially prescribed every 1 or 2 hours on the first postoperative day. It is then typically tapered to every 2 hours for the next 2 weeks, and then gradually tapered over the next 2–3 months. The frequency and schedule of tapering depend on the anterior chamber inflammation and the conjunctival inflammation around the filtering bleb.

Considering that subconjunctival fibrosis is the primary cause of filter failure and that little else can be done to influence it, discontinuing steroids prematurely should only be considered in cases of wound leaks or if other steroid complications develop. If, at any time, ocu-

lar inflammation increases, frequency of administration of topical corticosteroids should also be increased. Table 10-3 is a sample therapy regimen that assumes a non-complicated postoperative course.

Topical corticosteroid therapy carries the usual risk of steroid-induced ocular hypertension in susceptible eyes. In these cases, the risk-benefit ratio of using the steroids to create long-term IOP control versus intolerance of high IOP must be considered. Theoretically, a decrease in trabecular outflow from a steroid response should be compensated by an increase in outflow through the filtering site.

Like corticosteroids, no mutual consensus exists regarding the duration of antibiotic treatment. Antibiotic therapy acts as prophylaxis against postoperative infection and endophthalmitis. It is best to use a broad-spectrum antibiotic that is nonirritating to the conjunctiva. Therefore, aminoglycosides should be avoided. Postoperatively, an antibiotic can be used anywhere from 1 week to 1 month to once a day indefinitely. Most clinicians prescribe antibiotics for a 1- to 4-week period and reinstitute therapy if signs of a wound leak or infection appear.

Evaluation Frequency

Examination of the patient should occur more frequently in the early postoperative period because of the greater incidence of sight-threatening complications. Frequency of follow-up, duration, and type of postoperative medical therapy varies based on the clinician, individual risk factors of the patient (e.g., first surgery of an older patient with simple glaucoma versus repeat surgery on a young patient with advanced uveitic glaucoma), and whether complications occurred intraoperatively or postoperatively (e.g., hyphema, wound leak, or conjunctival hemorrhage). Typically, patients are evaluated on the first and third postoperative day, and an additional visit during the next postoperative week to ensure adequacy of filtration and absence of any serious complications.

Assuming no complications develop within the first postoperative week, follow-up can be extended to weekly visits, then bimonthly, monthly, and eventually 3–6 month intervals once the eye is stable without inflammation. Patients should be instructed to call their doctor immediately should they experience a red, painful, or traumatized eye (possible indicators of endophthalmitis or a choroidal hemorrhage).

During follow-up, patients should also be informed when it is safe and appropriate for the patient to perform strenuous tasks or lift heavy items, and when they may discontinue wearing the eye shield at bedtime. A good rule of thumb is to allow patients to resume normal activities and discontinue wearing an eye shield at 1 month after surgery in noncomplicated cases.

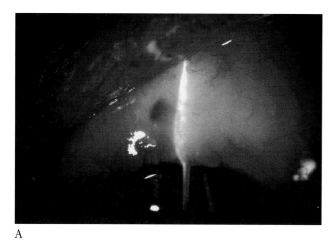

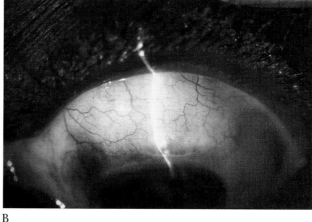

A   B

FIGURE 10-3. Functioning filtering blebs can have a variety of clinical appearances. In general, they tend to be elevated, lack significant vascularity, and contain microcysts in the overlying conjunctiva. (A) Example of a thin-walled bleb. (B) Example of a thicker-walled bleb.

Ocular Evaluation

A methodical postoperative evaluation helps ensure that important details are not overlooked. Like any evaluation, it should begin with the recording of a chief complaint, list of current ocular and systemic medications, and measuring the visual acuity. It is common within the first postoperative weeks to find acuity significantly reduced from the preoperative acuity. This usually occurs from the corneal edema, which typically resolves during the first postoperative month. However, it is important to rule out more serious complications, such as infection, wound leak, or macular edema, that can also cause reduced vision.

Biomicroscopic examination should include evaluation of the conjunctival integrity and inflammation, bleb appearance, corneal clarity, and anterior chamber depth and inflammation. Ideal bleb appearance (Figure 10-3) is a bleb that is elevated and extends a few clock hours, providing the greatest surface area over which aqueous can drain into the conjunctiva. The bleb should be nonvascularized (ischemic) and thin-walled, indicating the absence of a healing mechanism and associated fibrous tissue proliferation. Microcystic changes on the surface of the bleb or the limbal margin are excellent indicators pointing to percolation of aqueous into the conjunctiva. These negative-staining microcysts are most easily viewed when fluorescein dye is applied.

The anterior chamber should be carefully evaluated and the depth graded, as discussed in the section Early Postoperative Complications. IOP should be measured and gonioscopy only performed in the early postoperative period if suspicion of a blocked sclerostomy site exists. If performing gonioscopy is necessary, the clinician should minimize the pressure placed with the lens on the eye. Finally, the eye should be dilated and examined for the presence of a choroidal detachment, suprachoroidal hemorrhage, optic disc swelling, and macular edema.

COMPLICATIONS OF FILTERING SURGERY

Complications of glaucoma filtering surgery can be divided into three phases: intraoperative, early postoperative, and late postoperative. As with any potential surgical complication, the earlier these complications are detected and therapy is begun, the greater the likelihood of successful intervention.

Intraoperative Complications

Intraoperative complications include conjunctival perforation, hemorrhage, scleral flap perforation, corneal damage, lens damage, vitreous loss, choroidal effusion, and cyclodialysis cleft. Because of the emphasis on early and late postoperative management, detailed examination of the intraoperative complications is left for another discussion.

Early Postoperative Complications (First 2 Weeks Postoperative)

In evaluating early complications (first 2 weeks postoperative), it is important to keep in mind the big picture. Each ocular sign and its interrelationship become critical in how each complication affects another. Therefore, evaluating the eye postoperatively in a meticulous manner enables the clinician to determine and treat the root problem, rather than the associated symptoms.

Shallow Anterior Chamber

Success of filtering surgery can be seriously and permanently compromised by a postoperative flat anterior chamber. To determine the cause of a shallow chamber, the bleb appearance and IOP must be carefully evaluated (Table 10-4).

TABLE 10-4. Differential Diagnosis of Postoperative Shallow Anterior Chamber

With low intraocular pressure	With high intraocular pressure
Conjunctival wound leak	Malignant glaucoma (ciliary block)
Overfiltration of the bleb	
Ciliochoroidal detachment	Pupillary block
Hypotony	Choroidal hemorrhage
Cyclodialysis	Choroidal detachment causing angle closure

TABLE 10-5. Shallow Anterior Chamber Classification

Grade 1	Peripheral iris-cornea touch
Grade 2	Iris sphincter-cornea touch
Grade 3	Lens-cornea or vitreous-cornea touch

The classification system commonly used to grade anterior chamber depth is listed in Table 10-5. Grade 1 (peripheral iris-corneal touch) shallow chambers typically reform spontaneously without peripheral anterior synechiae formation. Management of grade 2 (iris sphincter–corneal touch) chambers tends to be more variable and depends on the etiology. Grade 2 chambers can be monitored conservatively with the continued use of cycloplegic agents and corticosteroids. With proper medical management, the chamber usually deepens in 1–2 weeks.[52] The other option with a grade 2 shallow chamber is reformation of the chamber with an injection of a viscoelastic agent, saline, air, or expandable gases.

Grade 3 (lens-cornea or vitreous-cornea touch) chambers usually require immediate surgical treatment. Lens-cornea touch carries the risk of filter failure, persistent corneal edema secondary to endothelial cell loss, anterior and posterior synechiae, and cataract formation in phakic eyes. Because choroidal detachments are frequently associated with grade 3 chambers, both are typically addressed in the treatment. Drainage of suprachoroidal fluid, along with the reformation of the anterior chamber with air, saline, expandable gases, or a viscoelastic agent, should usually be promptly performed in these cases.[53]

Shallow Anterior Chamber with Low IOP. If the IOP is low, the anterior chamber may be shallow because of a wound leak, overfiltration, ciliochoroidal detachment, or a cyclodialysis cleft. The clinician should first examine for the presence of a wound leak, which can be easily determined through a Seidel test. Treating the wound leak (see the next section) should obviate the need for re-forming the chamber surgically.

Wound Leak. A leaking bleb is a potential complication of glaucoma filtering surgery both in the early and late postoperative periods.[54,55] Bleb leaks can be caused by an undetected buttonhole in the conjunctival flap created during the time of surgery, postoperative wound conjunctival dehiscence, a perforation in the conjunctival flap of a thin-walled bleb, or even by trauma to the bleb months to years after surgery. If not

adequately treated, wound leaks place an eye at increased risk for a shallow anterior chamber, hypotony, macular edema, choroidal detachment, and endophthalmitis.

Should a conjunctival tear or buttonhole occur intraoperatively, addressing it during the surgery becomes essential. If detected early enough in the procedure, a new surgical site may be chosen. However, if the scleral flap has already been incised, the break must be tightly sutured. If a perforation is not repaired during the time of surgery, a wound leak is observed in the early postoperative period.

Clinical signs of a bleb leak include a low IOP, a shallow anterior chamber, and a flat bleb. To confirm the presence of a wound leak, a Seidel test should be carefully performed. This is typically done by placing a small amount of 2% fluorescein dye on the superior conjunctiva over the presumed area of leakage. The clinician should then elevate the lid and have the patient look down so that the entire bleb and the adjacent limbus is visible biomicroscopically. If a wound leak is present, a darker-colored stream of diluted aqueous is seen flowing down from the leakage site within the lighter-green dye (Figure 10-4).

If the bleb does not appear to be leaking, the clinician should very gently press on the eye to see if leakage occurs with pressure. In some cases, the eye is so hypotonous that much of the aqueous has already escaped out of the eye. Once a positive Seidel test is determined,

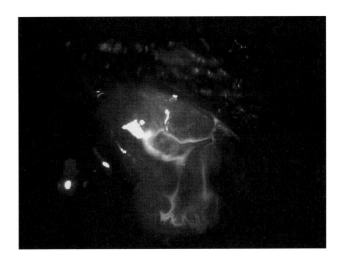

FIGURE 10-4. Positive Seidel test in a patient with a bleb wound leak. Note expanding dark flow of aqueous from the leaking site.

treatment must be instituted based on the location and extent of the leak.

In the early postoperative period, leaks are often a result of poor wound healing or opening of the sutures. If wound dehiscence occurs along the edge of the conjunctival flap or if the leak is extensive, the eye is at risk of severe complications from a grade 3 shallow anterior chamber and infection. In these situations, immediate surgical revision is often warranted.

Bleb leaks seen as a late complication are usually a result of excessive thinning of the conjunctival flap.[56] Often these leaks are small. Whether the wound leak is in the early or late postoperative period, conservative medical management may be considered first if the leak is small and no imminent threat exists of hypotony and a flat anterior chamber.

Initial medical therapy may include the use of aqueous suppressants, temporary reduction in frequency of corticosteroid instillation, antibiotics, and pressure patching or a large-diameter soft contact lens. The intent of medical intervention is to stop transconjunctival filtration through the bleb leak, which, in turn, allows sealing of the wound. Often, beta blockers or carbonic anhydrase inhibitors are used to reduce flow of aqueous across the wound, thereby allowing epithelial proliferation across the defect. Antibiotics in these cases should be used frequently to prevent infection. Aminoglycosides, such as gentamycin or tobramycin, have been thought to be an added benefit in that they can induce an allergic or irritant-type conjunctival inflammation, which would also stimulate wound healing. The last component is the application of a patch or oversized contact lens to avoid constant lid movement over the wound site. Patching can be effective, although it makes the application of aqueous suppressants and antibiotics more difficult. Most important, patching may raise the risk of infection and therefore create the need to monitor these patients on a daily basis.

The use of a large-diameter soft contact lens (e.g., 15–25 mm) is an alternative to patching. To be effective, the lens must be large enough to cover the leakage site and comfortable enough to be tolerated by the patient.[57] Typically a large-diameter soft contact lens should remain in the eye for at least 1 week. These patients should always receive concurrent antibiotic therapy and frequent follow-up because of the increased risk of infection. After 1 week, the lens should be removed and a Seidel test performed again. If a wound leak is still evident, the lens can be replaced for 2–3 weeks without removal to allow for epithelial migration. Again, antibiotic therapy and close follow-up is critical.

A slightly more involved and controversial treatment is the use of a Simmons shell, which is made out of hard polymethyl methacrylate approximately 20 mm in diameter. The shell has an internal platform that is intended to lie over the bleb to tamponade aqueous outflow from the sclerostomy site. This tends to be significantly more uncomfortable than a soft contact lens and usually requires a torpedo pressure patch over the shell. These patients need to be monitored daily for signs of infection and ocular surface abnormalities. At the first sign of corneal toxicity (abrasion or epithelial loss), the Simmons shell should be removed.[58]

Before surgical intervention, cyanoacrylate tissue adhesive or injection of autologous blood can be used to seal leaking filtration blebs. Both have shown some success and are alternatives in that they can prevent an additional surgical procedure.[59–61]

Overfiltration of the Bleb. Overfiltration of the bleb can be evidenced by a low postoperative IOP and a large, well-formed bleb. Overfiltration more commonly occurs in full-thickness procedures, where a scleral flap is not present to create resistance to aqueous flow. It may, however, occur in partial-thickness procedures, where scleral flap suture tension is inadequate. Left untreated, overfiltration can lead to anterior chamber shallowing, choroidal detachments, and hypotony.

When detected early, overfiltration is best treated conservatively. External tamponade through the use of patching can assist in slowing the flow of aqueous across the filtration site. Typically, the best option is a symblepharon ring because it can successfully tamponade the flow of aqueous while creating minimal patient discomfort.[62] Unlike a Simmons shell, a symblepharon ring allows for retention and testing of vision because the cornea remains uncovered and evaluation of IOP and intraocular examination can be carried out without removal of the ring. An added benefit of the ring is that it does not require suturing to the conjunctiva. Symblepharon rings come in multiple internal and external diameters, enabling trial fitting to ensure that the area of excessive flow is adequately covered by the ring.

With the advent of postoperative laser suture lysis and releasable sutures, the risk of overfiltration is decreased. The surgeon will tie the scleral flap sutures more tightly intraoperatively and titrate the flow postoperatively through controlled suture removal during the first 2 weeks.

Choroidal Detachment. Choroidal (ciliochoroidal) detachments frequently occur at the subclinical level after filtering surgery. A choroidal detachment occurs when hypotony yields transudation of fluid across the capillary walls of the choroid and collects in the potential space between the uvea and sclera.[63,64] This may cause a shallowing of the anterior chamber and, on rare occasions, may be responsible for a flat anterior chamber. Choroidal detachments can occur as a late complication to filter surgery and have even been reported to be recurrent in certain cases.[65]

Clinically, choroidal detachments appear as smooth, dome-shaped, orange to gray-brown elevations in the reti-

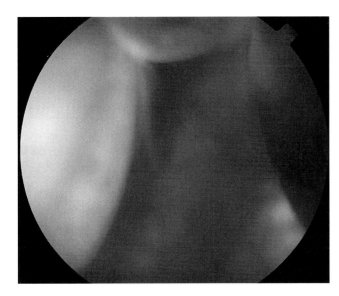

FIGURE 10-5. Ciliochoroidal detachments appear as orange, smooth, dome-shaped elevations in the retinal periphery. They are a common feature in the early postoperative period when the IOP is very low. They tend to resolve over the first 2 weeks as the ciliary body starts to produce aqueous and the IOP increases above 10 mm Hg.

nal periphery (Figure 10-5). They are frequently associated with a low IOP. Choroidal detachments can be classified from *low*, in which the elevations are shallow and in the far periphery, to *large*, in which the detachments touch from opposite retinal quadrants. The latter are often referred to as *kissing choroidals*.

Choroidal detachments are most commonly transient in nature. Most resolve spontaneously within a 2-week period without additional treatment. Because intraocular inflammation has been implicated as a causative agent, either topical or systemic steroids and cycloplegic agents have been suggested as treatment.[66] In most instances, surgical drainage of the choroidal detachment is usually unnecessary. In certain cases, however, such as those with chronic flat anterior chambers and associated choroidal hemorrhage or kissing choroidals, surgical intervention is indicated.

Shallow Anterior Chambers with High Intraocular Pressure. Table 10-4 identifies the causes of shallow anterior chambers with high IOP. One caveat in the differential diagnosis is that in eyes with grade 3 chambers, tonometry may be unreliable because of the force of the lens against the cornea.[67] In these cases, tactile IOP evaluation may assist in accurate diagnosis.

Suprachoroidal Hemorrhage. Suprachoroidal hemorrhage is one of the most difficult complications to manage in the postoperative period. A suprachoroidal hemorrhage can occur intraoperatively, in which case the eye is immediately sutured closed, the anterior cham-

ber is reformed, and attempts are made to lower the IOP using intravenous mannitol or acetazolamide if necessary. More commonly is the occurrence of postoperative or *delayed* choroidal hemorrhage. Suprachoroidal hemorrhage as a complication of filtering surgery occurs in as many as 2% of eyes. Risk factors for suprachoroidal hemorrhage include prolonged postoperative hypotony,[68,69] ciliochoroidal effusion,[70] high preoperative IOP,[71] prior vitrectomy,[70,71] history of systemic vascular disease, aphakia,[70-72] and myopia.[73]

Signs of delayed suprachoroidal hemorrhage commonly include an acute onset of severe ocular and cranial pain associated with a profound loss of vision and shallowing of the anterior chamber. On examination, corneal edema may or may not be present. The diagnosis is confirmed by indirect ophthalmoscopy, in which a large, dark choroidal elevation is evident. Treatment becomes dependent on the depth of the anterior chamber, the IOP, and the extent of the choroidal hemorrhage. If the IOP is only mildly elevated, the anterior chamber is formed, and the hemorrhage is limited, the condition typically resolves and conservative management is appropriate. If, however, a grade 3 flat chamber, retinal detachment,[73] severe hypotony, or vitreous hemorrhage is present, surgical intervention with drainage of the hemorrhage and reformation of the anterior chamber may be warranted.

Malignant Glaucoma (Aqueous Misdirection Syndrome). If the IOP is elevated, the bleb flat, and the peripheral iridectomy patent, malignant glaucoma, also known as *aqueous misdirection syndrome* or *ciliary block glaucoma*, must be considered, although it is relatively rare. In these cases, aqueous fluid becomes entrapped behind the vitreous, causing forward displacement of the vitreous body. This, in turn, applies pressure to the lens, iris, and ciliary body, causing severe shallowing of both the central and peripheral anterior chamber and high IOP.

The important differential diagnosis in these cases is pupillary block. Although pupillary block is rare when a patent iridectomy is present, pupillary block and malignant glaucoma can often show similar findings. Conservative medical treatment of malignant glaucoma includes the use of cycloplegic and aqueous suppressant therapy. Often, medical therapy is inadequate, and argon laser treatment of visible ciliary processes, neodymium:yttrium-aluminum-garnet (Nd:YAG) anterior hyaloidotomy, or posterior capsulotomy may be performed. A vitrectomy becomes necessary if all medical and laser surgery fails.

Hyphema

Small amounts of blood in the anterior chamber in the very early postoperative period are relatively common and do not present a significant threat to the success of the filtering surgery. Typically, hyphemas resorb within days after the surgery and do not require surgical intervention. In rare instances, surgical intervention may be required, such as in eyes with elevated IOP and large, nonclearing hyphemas.

Retinal Complications

Decompression retinopathy consists of postoperative retinal and occasional suprachoroidal hemorrhage and is a relatively uncommon complication of filtering surgery.[74] It is believed to be caused by a sudden decrease in IOP, causing a transient increase in retinal and choroidal blood flow. The inability of the capillary bed and the venous system to support the increase in capacity forces the blood into the extravascular space through endothelial leaks. Clinically, this appears as dot-and-blot hemorrhages in the midperipheral retina, a picture similar to a vein occlusion. In these cases, conservative therapy is recommended and the prognosis for vision recovery is relatively good.

As mentioned earlier, choroidal detachment and choroidal hemorrhage are both potential postoperative complications. Serous retinal detachment may be associated with these conditions and usually resolves concurrently.

Macular folds, also known as *hypotony maculopathy*, occur in eyes with low postoperative IOP. *Low* is patient-dependent and, therefore, difficult to define numerically. Some patients can tolerate an IOP of 4 mm Hg without damaging signs of hypotony, whereas others exhibit choroidal detachments, flat anterior chambers, and maculopathy. Hypotony maculopathy typically resolves once the IOP is normalized for the individual eye. The risk of hypotony maculopathy increased with the adjunctive use of MMC.

Late Postoperative Complications (Later Than 2 Weeks Postoperative)

Filtration Failure

A significant complication of glaucoma surgery is filter failure. Regardless of the surgical technique used, between 10% to 40% of all filtration operations fail to achieve adequate lowering of IOP. Failure rates hinge on risk factors specific to the individual case and the success of managing postoperative complications. Because risk factors are an uncontrollable variable, excellent surgical technique and conscientious management become critical in evading filter failure both in the early and late postoperative periods.

In the first 2 postoperative weeks, the eye is healing with the greatest activity. Therefore, close follow-up and meticulous examination are critical in identifying a potentially failing filter. As mentioned earlier, biomicroscopic examination should include evaluation of the bleb appearance, surrounding conjunctiva, depth and inflammation of the anterior chamber, and gonioscopic appearance of the internal sclerostomy site as indicated.

Filter failure can occur at any time postoperatively and is typically classified into two anatomic categories: internal (sclerostomy site) and external (conjunctival-Tenon-scleral interface). Internal blockage leads to a gradual or sudden increase in IOP and eventual filter failure if not treated timely. In the early postoperative period, iris, ciliary body, ciliary processes, lens, or vitreous may occlude the sclerostomy site, thereby preventing the flow of aqueous into the bleb. In the late postoperative period, blockage is more likely to occur from membrane proliferation or fibrovascular tissue growth over the sclerostomy site. Careful gonioscopic examination should be performed to ascertain whether blockage at the sclerostomy site is present. Digital pressure to the globe may then be applied to determine the extent of blockage. Digital pressure can be applied by pushing up from the lower lid with the thumb while the patient is looking up. Firm, constant pressure should be applied for 10 seconds and then stopped for 10 seconds. This cycle can be repeated up to three times (totaling 60 seconds); at each application the bleb size and IOP should be re-evaluated. If the bleb elevates or enlarges on pressure and the IOP is lowered, digital pressure may be instituted to encourage flow and maintain patency of the opening. If, however, the blockage is extensive and digital pressure is ineffective, a combination of argon or Nd:YAG lasers can sometimes be used to reopen the sclerostomy site.[75,76]

If the IOP is not controlled in the first few postoperative days and no obstruction is evident on gonioscopic examination, failure is likely resulting from resistance at the conjunctival-Tenon-scleral interface. This may be caused by the scleral flap being sutured too tightly, the presence of adhesions underneath the flap, or aqueous hyposecretion. All impede the flow of aqueous into the bleb and allow contact between the conjunctiva and the episclera. If the conjunctiva and episclera remain in contact, vascularization, cell infiltration, and fibroblast proliferation cause eventual scarring at the interface and permanent impedance to aqueous outflow resulting in eventual filter failure (Figure 10-6). Clinical signs become evident before total failure; they include an increase in IOP, conjunctival injection, bleb vascularization, and thickening and flattening of the bleb (Color Plate 30). If detected early, these eyes should be treated aggressively with topical steroids to prevent inflammation and with digital pressure to maintain flow and bleb height.

With the advent of laser suture lysis and releasable sutures, titration of aqueous flow postoperatively has become much easier. In the first few days to 2 weeks after surgery, scleral flap sutures can be released. This allows an increase in aqueous flow into the bleb and a reduction in IOP. If adhesions are suspected, digital pressure can be very effective in breaking adhesions and promoting aqueous outflow through the sclerostomy site. If

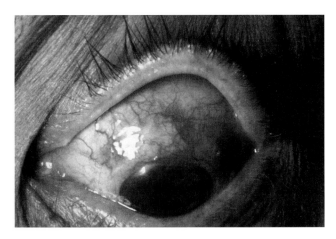

FIGURE 10-6. Subconjunctival fibrosis. Patient with a flat nonfunctioning bleb secondary to subconjunctival fibrosis.

external blockage goes untreated early or late in the postoperative period, scarring will likely occur beneath the conjunctiva or scleral flap.

Bleb Encapsulation

Encapsulated filtering bleb, also known as Tenon's cyst, typically forms in week 2 through 12 after filtering surgery, with a reported incidence between 8% and 28%.[77,78] Characteristically, an encapsulated bleb is a localized, highly elevated (domelike), opalescent, thick-walled bleb with moderate to marked vascular engorgement (Color Plate 31). IOP is usually elevated in these cases, and the patient may be symptomatic from corneal drying adjacent to the elevated bleb.

Although the etiology and mechanism are not completely understood, it is theorized that encapsulated blebs develop after trabeculectomy from the proliferation of noncontractile collagen-producing fibroblasts. This is thought to be different from the mechanism that produces bleb scarring. Therefore, the use of an antimetabolite does not decrease the incidence of this complication.[79]

Management of these patients should occur in a stepwise fashion, first with medical therapy, and second with surgery if the encapsulated bleb is not responsive to conservative therapy. The goal of therapy is to encourage the aqueous humor that is trapped in the cystic cavity to enter the subconjunctival space and to prevent adhesions, which ultimately lead to scarring and failed filtration surgery.[80] The use of digital pressure and topical corticosteroid therapy have a beneficial effect in many cases and lead to resolution of the encapsulated bleb. Digital pressure should first be performed by the doctor at the slit lamp. A positive sign of effectiveness is the spreading of fluid from the cyst into the surrounding subconjunctival space and a decrease in IOP. If either of these signs are apparent, digital pressure should be applied several times weekly in the office. Digital pressure performed at home by the patient is somewhat con-

troversial because patients may apply pressure in inappropriate amounts and in the wrong locations despite education. Digital pressure performed in the office, in conjunction with continued or increased application of topical corticosteroids to reduce the inflammatory response, often leads to spontaneous resolution. Use of aqueous-suppressing agents for a limited period has also been advocated. The decrease in aqueous production and IOP is thought to allow for remodeling of the cyst and eventually improving aqueous flow across the cyst.[81] The disadvantage in using aqueous suppressants is that they may limit the extent of bleb formation because less aqueous is available to percolate into the bleb.

If medical therapy fails, a bleb-needling procedure or surgical revision may be necessary. Both procedures create an opening in the fibrous wall beneath the conjunctiva and have been shown to be successful.[82] The risk in these procedures is perforation of the conjunctiva overlying the cystic space and bleb infection.

Vision Loss

Filtering surgery can result in sudden or gradual vision loss occurring over a period of months to years after surgery. Sudden vision loss immediately after surgery is not very common and is often related to complications occurring during the time of surgery (e.g., retrobulbar injection causing damage to the optic nerve or sudden opening of the eye intraoperatively causing hypotony, leading to choroidal hemorrhage).[83]

The etiology of progressive gradual vision loss is often more difficult to discern. One potential cause is progressive loss of visual field, leading to "snuffing out" of the central vision. This can occur if IOP is not low enough to prevent further damage, and it even occurs in cases in which control over the IOP is good. In the latter cases, progressive visual field loss may be secondary to a perfusion problem of the optic nerve or a mechanical stress on the optic nerve. Another cause of gradual reduction in visual acuity is cataract formation.

Cataract

Cataract formation is believed to be a common occurrence after filtering surgery. It may develop in as many as one-half of filtered patients in the first 5 years after surgery. The risk of cataract development varies based on individual patient risk factors, the surgical technique used, postoperative use of topical and systemic corticosteroid therapy, and the presence of postoperative hypotony with a flat anterior chamber. The time and amount of cataract progression are difficult to ascertain before surgery. However, it has been shown that when a cataract is present before surgery, a much greater likelihood exists that significant progression of that cataract will occur, compared with eyes in which no cataract was found preoperatively.[84]

Bleb Leaks

As discussed more extensively in the section Early Postoperative Complications, bleb leaks can occur at any time after filtration surgery. When leaks do occur months to years after surgery, they are most commonly caused by trauma or excessive thinning of the bleb. When bleb leaks occur late, conservative medical management with such treatments as aqueous suppressants, antibiotics, patching, large-diameter contact lens, autologous blood injection, and fibrin glue can be instituted. In many of these cases, however, the bleb becomes so fragile and brittle that surgical revision with a conjunctival graft is necessary.

Endophthalmitis

Endophthalmitis is a catastrophe that can occur early, but usually appears late in the postoperative period. When it occurs early, the organism is likely to have entered the eye during the time of surgery, as opposed to late infection, in which the organism is believed to enter the eye via the bleb.[85] Risk factors for infection include contact lens wear, thin-walled blebs, bleb leaks, and blebs positioned inferiorly.[86,87]

Signs of infection include conjunctival injection around the filtering site, a milky or purulent bleb (blebitis; Color Plate 32), intraocular inflammation, and hypopyon. Patients typically report pain at onset and worsening of vision. If the infection is detected early, the infecting organism may be confined to the bleb alone. However, because the bleb has a direct channel to the anterior chamber and, in turn, the vitreous, infection can spread quickly, causing a fulminant endophthalmitis. If the infection is limited to the bleb, patients are treated initially with topical, periocular, and systemic antibiotics, and later with topical corticosteroids to prevent scarring at the filtration site. If this is ineffective or the patient presents with vitreous involvement, more aggressive treatment, such as a vitrectomy and injection of intravitreal antibiotics, is warranted. As with any high-risk ocular infection, treatment should be initiated on detection, and, if necessary, altered on receipt of culture results.

Because of the devastating effects of endophthalmitis, all patients who have the procedure performed must be counseled extensively on the associated signs and symptoms. Should any patient experience a red or painful eye, they should be seen immediately for evaluation.

Dellen

Large or overhanging blebs can cause drying and dellen formation on the adjacent corneal surface. Patients may report a foreign-body or drying sensation. These cases are best managed with lubricating agents, such as artificial tears.

CONCLUSION

Filtration surgery has afforded tremendous advancements in the management of glaucoma. With excellent surgical technique and meticulous postoperative management, trabeculectomy surgery can effectively provide long-term control of IOP. In many cases, it can result in stability of visual field and optic nerve damage without the adjunct use of medical therapy.

However, much research still needs to be done to better define surgical outcomes and the impact on a patient's quality of life after undergoing glaucoma surgery. As we learn more about the etiology of glaucoma, we also learn how to modify surgical technique and timing of intervention so as to better manage the individual patient and the overall disease process.

REFERENCES

1. Shin DH. Trabeculectomy. Int Ophthalmol Clin 1981;21:47–68.
2. Smith RJH. Medical vs surgical therapy in glaucoma simplex. Br J Ophthalmol 1972;56:277–283.
3. Johnson DH, Yoshikawa K, Brubaker RF, Hodge DO. The effect of long-term medical therapy on the outcome of filtration surgery. Am J Ophthalmol 1994;117:139–148.
4. Sherwood M, Grierson I, Miller L, Hitchings R. Long-term effects of antiglaucoma drugs on the conjunctiva and Tenon's capsule in glaucomatous patients. Ophthalmology 1989;96:327–335.
5. Broadway D, Grierson I, Hitchings R. Adverse effects of topical antiglaucomatous medications on the conjunctiva. Br J Ophthalmol 1993;77:590–596.
6. Broadway DC, Grierson I, O'Brien C, Hitchings RA. Adverse effects of topical antiglaucoma medication. II. The outcome of filtration surgery. Arch Ophthalmol 1994;112:1446–1454.
7. Lavin MJ, Wormald RP, Migdal CS, Hitchings RA. The influence of prior therapy on the success of trabeculectomy. Arch Ophthalmol 1990;108: 1543–1548.
8. Boyd TAS. A comparison of surgical and conservative treatment in glaucoma simplex. Trans Ophthalmol Soc U K 1955;75:541.
9. Jay JL. Earlier trabeculectomy. Trans Ophthalmol Soc U K 1983;103:35–38.
10. Migdal C, Hitchings R. The role of early surgery for open angle glaucoma. Ophthalmol Clin North Am 1991;4:853.
11. Sherwood MB, Migdal CS, Hitchings RA. Filtration surgery as the initial therapy for open-angle glaucoma. J Glaucoma 1993;2:64.
12. Sherwood MB, Migdal CS, Hitchings RA, et al. Initial treatment of glaucoma: surgery or medications. Surv Ophthalmol 1993;37:293–305.

13. Jay JL, Allan D. The benefit of early trabeculectomy versus conventional management in primary open angle glaucoma relative to severity of disease. Eye 1989;3:528–535.

14. Quigley HA. A reevaluation of glaucoma management. Int Ophthalmol Clin 1984;24:1–11.

15. Schwartz AL, Anderson DR. Trabecular surgery. Arch Ophthalmol 1974;92:134–138.

16. Wolner B, Liebmann JM, Sassani JW, et al. Late bleb-related endophthalmitis after trabeculectomy with adjunctive 5-fluorouracil. Ophthalmology 1991;98:1053.

17. Reichert R, Stewart W, Shields MB. Limbus-based versus fornix-based conjunctival flaps in trabeculectomy. Ophthalmic Surg 1987;18:672–676.

18. Shuster JN, Krupin T, Kolker AE, Becker B. Limbus v. fornix-based conjunctival flap in trabeculectomy. A long-term randomized study. Arch Ophthalmol 1984;102:361–362.

19. Scheie HG. Retraction of scleral wound edges: a fistulizing procedure for glaucoma. Am J Ophthalmol 1958;45:220.

20. Iliff CE, Haas JS. Posterior lip sclerectomy. Am J Ophthalmol 1962;54:668.

21. Blondeau P, Phelps CD. Trabeculectomy vs thermosclerostomy. A randomized prospective clinical trial. Arch Ophthalmol 1981;99:810–816.

22. Sugar HS. Surgical anatomy of glaucoma. Surv Ophthalmol 1968;13:143–151.

23. Starita RJ, et al. Short and long-term effects of postoperative corticosteroids on trabeculectomy. Ophthalmology 1985;92:938–946.

24. Kronfeld P. The effect of topical steroid administration on intraocular pressure and aqueous flow after fistulizing operations. Trans Am Ophthalmol Soc 1964;62:375.

25. Ball SF. Effects of triamcinolone injection. Arch Ophthalmol 1986;104:1749–1750.

26. Costa VP, Spaeth GL, Eiferman RA, Orengo Nania S. Wound healing modulation in glaucoma filtration surgery. Ophthalmic Surg 1993;24:152–170.

27. Dietze PJ, Feldman RM, Gross RL. Intraoperative application of 5-fluorouracil during trabeculectomy. Ophthalmic Surg 1992;23:662–665.

28. Yamamoto T, Varani J, Soong HK, Lichter PR. Effects of 5-fluorouracil and mitomycin C on cultured rabbit subconjunctival fibroblasts. Ophthalmology 1990;97:1204–1210.

29. Heuer DK, Parrish RK II, Gresssel MG, et al. 5-Fluorouracil and glaucoma filtering surgery. II: A pilot study. Ophthalmology 1984;91:384–394.

30. Fluorouracil Filtering Surgery Study Group. Fluorouracil Filtering Surgery Study one year follow-up. Am J Ophthalmol 1989;108:625–635.

31. Fluorouracil Filtering Surgery Study Group. Three year follow-up of the Fluorouracil Filtering Surgery Study. Am J Ophthalmol 1993;115:82–92.

32. Goldenfeld M, Krupin T, Ruderman JM, Wong PC. 5-Fluorouracil in initial trabeculectomy, a prospective, randomized, multicenter study. Ophthalmology 1994;101:1024–1029.

33. Liebmann JM, Ritch R, Marmor M, et al. Initial 5-fluorouracil trabeculectomy in uncomplicated glaucoma. Ophthalmology 1991;98:1036–1041.

34. Mattox C. Glaucoma filtration surgery and antimetabolites. Ophthalmic Surg Lasers 1995;26(5):473–480.

35. Letchinger SL, Becker B, Wax MB. The effects of subconjunctival administration of mitomycin C on intraocular pressure in rabbits. Invest Ophthalmol Vis Sci 1992;33(suppl):736.

36. Bank A, Allingham RR. Application of mitomycin C during filtering surgery. Am J Ophthalmol 1993;116(3):377–379.

37. Skuta GL, Beeson CC, Higginbotham EJ, et al. Intraoperative mitomycin versus postoperative 5-fluorouracil in high-risk glaucoma filtering surgery. Ophthalmology 1992;99:438–444.

38. Derick RJ, Pasquale L, Quigley HA, Jampel H. Potential toxicity of mitomycin C. Arch Ophthalmol 1991;109:1635.

39. Katz GJ, Higginbotham EJ, Lichter PR, et al. Mitomycin C versus 5-fluorouracil in high-risk glaucoma filtering surgery. Ophthalmology 1995;102(9):1263–1268.

40. Zacharia PT, Deppermann SR, Schuman JS. Ocular hypotony after trabeculectomy with mitomycin-C. Am J Ophthalmol 1993;116:314–326.

41. Lewis RA, Phelps CD. Trabeculectomy v. thermosclerostomy—a five year follow-up. Arch Ophthalmol 1984;102:533–536.

42. Spaeth GL. A prospective, controlled study to compare the Scheie procedure with Watson's trabeculectomy. Ophthalmic Surg 1980;11:688–694.

43. Stewart WC. Clinical Practice of Glaucoma. Thorofare, N.J.: Slack Inc., 1990;229–239, 340–341.

44. Savage JA, Thomas JV, Belcher CD, et al. Extracapsular cataract extraction and posterior chamber intraocular lens implantation in glaucomatous eyes. Ophthalmology 1985;92:1506–1516.

45. Johnson D. Extracapsular cataract extraction, intraocular lens implantation, and trabeculectomy: the combined procedure. Int Ophthalmol Clin 1990;30:209–214.

46. Sidoti PA, Baerveldt G. Glaucoma drainage implants. Curr Opin Ophthalmol 1994;5:85–98.

47. Melamed S, Cahane N, Gutman I, et al. Postoperative complications after Molteno implant surgery. Am J Ophthalmol 1991;111:319–322.

48. Molteno ACB, Anker E, Van Biljon G. Surgical technique for advanced juvenile glaucoma. Arch Ophthalmol 1984;102:51–57.

49. Badeeb O, Trope GE, Mortimer C. Short-term effects of neodymium-YAG transscleral cyclocoagulation in patients with uncontrolled glaucoma. Br J Ophthalmol 1988;72:615–617.

50. Maus M, Katz LJ. Choroidal detachment, flat anterior chamber, and hypotony as complications of neodymium:YAG laser cyclophotocoagulation. Ophthalmology 1990;97:69–72.

51. Brindley G, Shields MB. Value and limitations of cyclocryotherapy. Graefe's Arch Clin Exp Ophthalmol 1986;224:545.

52. Stewart WC, Shields MB. Management of anterior chamber depth after trabeculectomy. Am J Ophthalmol 1988;106:41–44.

53. Fourman S. Management of cornea-lens touch after filtering surgery for glaucoma. Ophthalmology 1990;97:424–428.

54. Sugar S. Treatment of hypotony following filtration surgery for glaucoma. Am J Ophthalmol 1971;71:1023–1033.

55. Tomlinson CP, Belcher CD, Smith PD, et al. Management of leaking filtering blebs. Ann Ophthalmol 1987;19:405–408.

56. Melamed S, Hersh P, Kersten D, et al. The use of glaucoma shell tamponade in leaking filtration blebs. Ophthalmology 1986;93:839–842.

57. Blok MDW, Kok JHC, van Mil C, et al. Use of the Megasoft Bandage Lens for treatment of complications after trabeculectomy. Am J Ophthalmol 1990;110:264–268.

58. Rajeev B, Thomas R. Corneal hazards in use of Simmons shell. Aust N Z J Ophthalmol 1991;19(2):145–148.

59. Zalta AH, Wieder RH. Closure of leaking filtering blebs with cyanoacrylate tissue adhesive. Br J Ophthalmol 1991;75:170–173.

60. Leen MM, Moster MR, Katz LJ, et al. Management of overfiltering and leaking blebs with autologous blood injection. Arch Ophthalmol 1995;113:1050–1055.

61. Smith MF, Magauran R, Doyle JW. Treatment of postfiltration bleb leak by bleb injection of autologous blood. Ophthalmic Surg 1994;25:636–637.

62. Hill RA, Aminlari A, Sassani JW, Michalski M. Use of a symblepharon ring for treatment of over-filtration and leaking blebs after glaucoma filtering surgery. Ophthalmic Surg 1990;21:707–710.

63. Berke SJ, Bellows R, Shingleton BJ, et al. Chronic and recurrent choroidal detachment after glaucoma filtering surgery. Ophthalmology 1987;94:154–162.

64. Capper SA, Leopold IH. Mechanism of serous choroidal detachment: a review and experimental study. Arch Ophthalmol 1956;55:101–113.

65. Burney EN, Quigley HA, Robin AL. Hypotony and choroidal detachment as late complications of trabeculectomy. Am J Ophthalmol 1987;103:685–688.

66. Stewart WC, Crinkley CMC. Influence of serous suprachoroidal detachments on the results of trabeculectomy surgery. Acta Ophthalmol 1994;72:309–314.

67. Wright MM, Grajewski AL. Measurement of intraocular pressure with a flat anterior chamber. Ophthalmology 1991;98:1854–1857.

68. Canning CR, Lavin M, McCartney AC, Hitchings RA. Delayed suprachoroidal haemorrhage after glaucoma operations. Eye 1989;3;327–331.

69. Givens K, Shields MB. Suprachoroidal hemorrhage after glaucoma filtering surgery. Am J Ophthalmol 1987;103:689–694.

70. Gressel MG, Parrish RK II, Heuer DK. Delayed nonexpulsive suprachoroidal hemorrhage. Arch Ophthalmol 1984;102:1757–1760.

71. Fluorouracil Filtering Surgery Study Group. Risk factors for suprachoroidal hemorrhage after filtering surgery. Am J Ophthalmol 1992;113:501–507.

72. Ruderman JM, Harbin TS Jr, Campbell DG. Postoperative suprachoroidal hemorrhage following filtration procedures. Arch Ophthalmol 1986;104:201–205.

73. Reynolds MG, Haimovici R, Flynn HW Jr, et al. Suprachoroidal hemorrhage. Clinical features and results of secondary surgical management. Ophthalmology 1993;100:460–465.

74. Fechtner RD, Minckler D, Weinreb RN, et al. Complications of glaucoma surgery ocular decompression retinopathy. Arch Ophthalmol 1992;110:965–968.

75. Ticho U, Ivry M. Reopening of occluded filtering blebs by argon laser photocoagulation. Am J Ophthalmol 1977;84:413–418.

76. Drake M. Complications of glaucoma filtration surgery. Int Ophthalmol Clin 1992;32:115–130.

77. Ophir A. Encapsulated filtering bleb. A selective review—new deductions. Eye 1992;6:348–352.

78. Richter CU, Shingleton BJ, Bellows AR, et al. The development of encapsulated filtering blebs. Ophthalmology 1988;95:1163–1168.

79. Ophir A, Ticho U. Encapsulated filtering bleb and subconjunctival 5-fluorouracil. Ophthalmic Surg 1992;23:339–341.

80. Van Buskirk EM. Cysts of Tenon's capsule following filtration surgery. Am J Ophthalmol 1982;94:522–527.

81. Scott DR, Quigley HA. Medical management of a high bleb phase after trabeculectomies. Ophthalmology 1988;95:1169–1173.

82. Pederson JE, Smith SG. Surgical management of encapsulated filtering blebs. Ophthalmology 1985;92:955–958.

83. Martinez JA, Brown RH, Lynch MG, et al. Risk of postoperative vision loss in advance glaucoma. Am J Ophthalmol 1993;115:332–337.

84. Watson PG, Jakeman C, Ozturk M, et al. The complications of trabeculectomy (a 20-year follow-up). Eye 1990;4:425–438.

85. Katz LJ, Cantor LB, Spaeth GL. Complications of surgery in glaucoma. Ophthalmology 1985;92:959–963.

86. Brown RH, Yang LH, Walker SD, et al. Treatment of bleb infection after glaucoma surgery. Arch Ophthalmol 1994;112:57–61.

87. Bellows AR, McCulley JP. Endophthalmitis in aphakic patients with unplanned filtering blebs wearing contact lenses. Ophthalmology 1981;88:839–843.

Glaucoma Management

CHAPTER 11

Glaucoma Management and Treatment

Anthony B. Litwak

The management of patients with glaucoma or glaucoma suspects is case specific. General guidelines can be incorporated into the management decisions, but each patient should be evaluated individually. My general philosophy on deciding which patients to treat with intraocular pressure (IOP)-lowering agents is based on objective evidence of glaucomatous damage to the optic nerve or retinal nerve fiber layer (NFL), or an abnormal visual field test consistent with glaucoma damage. The visual field test should corroborate the optic nerve damage, but the visual field may appear normal on white-on-white perimetry if the optic nerve damage is mild. Likewise, if the visual field is abnormal, a corresponding change should be seen at the optic disc and retinal NFL. Many patients exhibit an initial visual field defect that disappears on subsequent testing due to a learning curve phenomenon. Repeating the initial visual field test within a month to uncover learning curves and to establish an accurate baseline is recommended.

The first objective of glaucoma management is to differentiate patients with glaucomatous optic nerve damage from patients who may exhibit risk factors for the disease but do not show evidence of physical damage to the optic nerve (glaucoma suspect). Identifying early glaucoma damage can be arduous. However, by careful inspection of the optic nerve (see Chapter 5), evaluation of the retinal NFL (see Chapter 6), and incorporation of new diagnostic techniques, such as short-wavelength automated (blue-on-yellow) perimetry (see Chapter 7), it is possible to establish an earlier diagnosis of glaucoma than with conventional white-on-white perimetry. Patients with evidence of glaucoma damage are generally treated with IOP-lowering therapy, whereas the majority of glaucoma suspects are periodically observed without treatment after baseline documentation (stereoscopic optic nerve and NFL photographs, threshold visual field tests) has been gathered.

SETTING A TARGET INTRAOCULAR PRESSURE

The goal of glaucoma treatment is to maintain functional vision so that patients can perform desired visual tasks throughout the rest of their lives and to limit the side effects and costs of glaucoma treatment. Most patients with mild to moderate glaucoma damage are generally asymptomatic and can function visually without compromise. Therefore, the goal of treatment in these patients is not necessarily to halt glaucoma progression (although that would be ideal), but to keep the patient visually functional in daily occupational and personal needs. The doctor needs to know the patient's occupation and understand his or her visual needs. The age of the patient at diagnosis is also very important in determining the aggressiveness of therapy. Younger patients diagnosed with glaucoma have more years to become visually impaired from their disease and warrant more aggressive treatment than an elderly patient presenting with the same degree of damage. Diagnosis of glaucoma at an earlier age may also infer that the rate of progression is more rapid because the damage is appearing at a younger age.

Glaucoma patients exhibit different rates of progression, and the patient's target pressure must be continually adjusted based on the rate of progression once it can be established. The doctor must also be vigilant for potential systemic or ocular side effects from treatment that

TABLE 11-1. Setting Target Pressures Based on Optic Nerve, Nerve Fiber Layer (NFL), and Visual Field Loss

Degree of damage[a]: desired target IOP reduction (%)	Optic nerve	Retinal NFL	Visual field[b]
Mild: 20–30	Relative thinning of the superior or inferior rim compared with temporal rim. No notches present.	Slit defects. No wedges. OR mild diffuse loss (D1) in superior and/or inferior arcade.	MD <–6 dB. AND <18 points below 5% level and <10 points below 1% level on pattern deviation plot. AND no central points[c] <20 dB.
Moderate: 30–40	Early notch in one pole of the optic nerve (rim tissue thinner in the superior or inferior pole compared with temporal pole). OR relative thinning in both the superior and inferior rims.	Early wedge defect (W1). OR moderate diffuse (D2) loss in superior or inferior arcade.	MD –6 to –12 dB. OR 18–36 points below 5% level or 10–20 points below 1% level on pattern deviation plot. OR central points between 10–20 dB in one hemifield.
Severe: 40–50	Early notching of both superior and inferior pole. OR complete notch in either the superior or inferior pole.	Complete wedge NFL defect (W2). OR severe diffuse loss (D3) in superior or inferior arcade OR moderate diffuse loss (D2) in both arcuate bundles.	MD >–12 dB. OR >36 points below 5% level or >20 points below 1% level on pattern deviation plot. OR <20 dB in both hemifields in central 5 degrees OR any point in central 5 degrees has a value of <10 dB.

IOP = intraocular pressure; MD = mean deviation.

Note: The degree of visual field damage is based on Zeiss Humphrey's 30-2 Full Threshold perimetry.

[a]Damage based on highest level of damage in any of the three categories.

[b]Modified from E Hodapp, RK Parrish, DR Anderson. Clinical Decisions in Glaucoma. St. Louis: Mosby, 1993;53–59.

[c]Central points represent the four tested points within 5 degrees of fixation.

may affect the patient's quality of life. It is counterproductive to overtreat a patient with mild glaucoma damage showing a slow rate of progression with medications that adversely affect the patient's quality of life. The benefits of treatment for preventing or slowing down the rate of significant vision loss must balance against the side effects, lifestyle compromises, and costs of glaucoma therapy.

At target pressure, the benefits of preserving vision are balanced against the safety of treatment. Once the diagnosis of glaucoma is established, quantification of the amount of glaucomatous damage helps to determine an initial target pressure (a theoretical IOP at which optic nerve damage is not likely to continue or will progress so slowly that it does not affect the patient's quality of life). In general, the greater the amount of damage present, the greater the percentage of IOP lowering required. A simplified approach for setting a target pressure based on Full Threshold (before the development of Swedish Interactive Thresholding Algorithm [SITA]) visual field analysis on the Humphrey Field Analyzer (Zeiss Humphrey

Systems, Dublin, CA) was established by Hodapp, Parrish, and Anderson.[1] They classify the amount of visual field loss as *mild*, *moderate*, or *severe loss* based on set visual field criteria (Table 11-1). The classification criteria for visual field loss should also be dependent on the visual field program because certain testing programs are less fatiguing than others. Running a 24-2 pattern instead of a 30-2 or using SITA instead of Full Threshold testing results in a less taxing test and usually in a less abnormal visual field (see Figures 7-3 and 7-7). Table 11-2 classifies visual field loss by the testing program used.

As an initial target pressure guideline, patients with mild visual field loss require 20–30% IOP reduction; with moderate loss, 30–40% IOP reduction; and with severe loss, 40–50% IOP reduction. The target pressures should also be based on the clinical assessment of the optic nerve and retinal NFL (see Table 11-1). A minority of patients, despite extensive optic nerve damage, may test surprisingly well on white-on-white perimetry. This most likely occurs because of an overlap

TABLE 11-2. Grading Glaucoma Damage and Setting Target Pressures Based on Different Visual Field Strategies

Visual field loss: set TP (%) lower than baseline IOP	30-2 Full Threshold	24-2 Full Threshold	30-2 SITA Standard	24-2 SITA Standard
Mild: 20–30	MD <–6 dB. AND <18 points below 5% level and <10 points below 1% level on pattern deviation plot. AND no central points* <20 dB.	MD <–6 dB. AND <14 points below 5% level and <8 points below 1% level on pattern deviation plot. AND no central points* <20 dB.	MD <–5 dB. AND <18 points below 5% level and <10 points below 1% level on pattern deviation plot. AND no central points* <20 dB.	MD <–5 dB. AND <14 points below 5% level and <8 points below 1% level on pattern deviation plot. AND no central points* <20 dB.
Moderate: 30–40	MD –6 to –12 dB. OR 18–36 points below 5% level or 10–20 points below 1% level on pattern deviation plot. OR central points between 10–20 dB in one hemifield.	MD –6 to –12 dB. OR 14–28 points below 5% level or 8–16 points below 1% level on pattern deviation plot. OR central points between 10–20 dB in one hemifield.	MD –5 to –10 dB. OR 18–36 points below 5% level or 10–20 points below 1% level on pattern deviation plot. OR central points between 10–20 dB in one hemifield.	MD –5 to –10 dB. OR 14–28 points below 5% level or 8–16 points below 1% level on pattern deviation plot. OR central points between 10–20 dB in one hemifield.
Severe: 40–50	MD >–12 dB. OR >36 points below 5% level or >20 points below 1% level on pattern deviation plot. OR <20 dB in both hemifields in central 5 degrees OR any point in central 5 degrees has a value <10 dB.	MD >–12 dB. OR >28 points below 5% level or >16 points below 1% level on pattern deviation plot. OR < 20 dB in both hemifields in central 5 degrees OR any point in central 5 degrees has a value <10 dB.	MD >–10 dB. OR >36 points below 5% level or >20 points below 1% level on pattern deviation plot. OR <20 dB in both hemifields in central 5 degrees OR any point in central 5 degrees has a value <10 dB.	MD >–10 dB. OR >28 points below 5% level or >16 points below 1% level on pattern deviation plot. OR <20 dB in both hemifields in central 5 degrees OR any point in central 5 degrees has a value <10 dB.

IOP = intraocular pressure; MD = mean deviation; SITA = Swedish Interactive Thresholding Algorithm; TP = target pressure.

*Central points represent the four tested points within five degrees of fixation.

of receptor fields in the retina and explains why 20–50% of the optic nerve can be damaged before a reproducible visual field defect occurs.[2,3] I observe this phenomenon in younger patients, who tend to be more alert testers during the visual field examination.

Frequently, the degree of optic nerve or NFL damage may exceed the degree of vision loss. In these cases, it is imperative to set the target pressures based on the amount of optic nerve damage (see Table 11-1 and Chapter 18, Case 1) and to follow the patient closely for progressive loss. Notching of the neuroretinal rim tissue, complete wedge NFL defects, or severe diffuse NFL thinning is indicative of advanced glaucomatous damage. Therefore, evaluation of the optic nerve and retinal NFL along with visual field interpretation is used to quantify the degree of damage and set a target pressure. Judging the degree of optic nerve damage based on the cup-to-disc ratio can be misleading in some cases because of the variation in physiologic disc size. For example, a cup-to-disc

ratio of 0.8 can be a normal physiologic cup in a patient with a large disc (see Color Plate 18), or a 0.8 cup can represent extensive glaucoma damage if the patient started with a small cup in a small physiologic disc. When assessing the cup-to-disc ratio, it is important to also assess the physiologic size of the optic disc (see Figure 5-10).

Other determinants of target pressures include the level of IOP, the race and age of the patient, and family ocular history of blindness from glaucoma. African-American patients are more likely to show progression of their disease than age-matched white patients.[4,5] Patients with a definitive family history of blindness from glaucoma or a sibling with glaucoma also warrant more aggressive therapy.[6] A young patient has a longer life span (and more time in which to go blind from the disease) and also requires more aggressive treatment. A patient who is monocular, unable to perform reliable visual field testing, or has other optic nerve or retinal diseases likely to affect the ability to

TABLE 11-3. Checklist for Setting Target Pressures Once Diagnosis of Glaucoma Is Made

1. Establish baseline intraocular pressure (at least three readings).

2. Classify amount of glaucoma damage as *mild, moderate,* or *severe* (see Tables 11-1 and 11-2).

3. Use the highest intraocular pressure reading and set target pressure 20–30% lower for mild damage, 30–40% lower for moderate damage, and 40–50% lower for severe damage.

4. Consider lowering target pressure an additional 10% if patient is younger than 50 years, African American, monocular, or has a sibling with advanced glaucoma.

follow the patient for progression may require more aggressive treatment.

A patient with poor compliance in taking medications or returning for follow-up appointments requires a different approach in therapy. Laser trabeculoplasty (LTP) should be discussed as a viable option for a patient who is noncompliant with medications and is showing mild to moderate damage. Surgical trabeculectomy should be considered in a case of poor compliance in a patient with moderate to severe glaucoma damage

or showing documented progression. Each patient is unique, so glaucoma management cannot be cook-booked. Patients exhibit different risk factors, degrees of damage, rates of progression, contraindications to therapies, and other variables associated with this condition. It is the doctor's responsibility to assess risk factors, clinical findings, degree of damage, systemic health, reliability, visual needs, compliance, level of patient anxiety, and quality of life issues when customizing management plans for each patient. (Table 11-3 offers a checklist for setting target pressures.)

MANAGING GLAUCOMA SUSPECTS

Patients with risk factors for glaucoma damage without evidence of optic nerve, retinal NFL, or visual field abnormalities are diagnosed as glaucoma suspects (Table 11-4). The management of glaucoma suspects is also case-specific. Most patients with mildly elevated IOP (mid or low 20s) without objective optic nerve damage can be observed without treatment based on the observation that only 1–2% of these patients per year develop visual field loss from glaucoma.[7,8] Treating all patients who have ocular hypertension may needlessly expose them to the side effects of medications, inconvenience of instilling eye drops, and expense of the medicine. However, it is impor-

TABLE 11-4. Factors Affecting the Clinical Decision Regarding When to Treat Glaucoma Suspects[a]

Average level of IOP (mm Hg)	Risk factors present[b]	Status of optic nerve, NFL, and visual field	Treatment decision[c]
<20	No	Equivocal[d]	Follow
<20	Yes	Normal	Follow
<20	Yes	Equivocal	Follow
20–24	No	Normal	Follow
20–24	Yes	Normal	Follow
20–24	No	Equivocal	Patient option[e]
20–24	Yes	Equivocal	Patient option
25–29	No	Normal	Follow
25–29	No	Equivocal	Treat
25–29	Yes	Normal	Patient option
25–29	Yes	Equivocal	Treat
>30			Treat all patients unless significant complications are likely

IOP = intraocular pressure; NFL = nerve fiber layer.

[a]*Glaucoma suspect* is defined as a patient with risk factors for glaucoma or suspicion of glaucoma damage to the optic nerve, NFL, or visual field, but without definitive glaucoma damage.

[b]Risk factors include a strong family history of blindness or visual field loss from glaucoma, or African American racial status. Diabetes, hypertension, and myopia are considered less significant risk factors.

[c]Target IOP should be set to reduce the IOP 20–30% or below 30 mm Hg, whichever is lower.

[d]*Equivocal* is defined as an optic nerve, NFL, or visual field that is suspicious but not definitive for glaucoma damage.

[e]*Patient option* refers to allowing the patient to decide whether he or she prefers treatment or observation when the clinical findings do not definitively show glaucoma damage.

tant to remember that visual field testing with white-on-white perimetry is not the most sensitive technique to pick up early glaucoma damage. A normal visual field on white-on-white perimetry excludes advanced glaucoma, but does not necessarily exclude the diagnosis of early glaucoma (see Chapter 18, Case 6). Testing more likely to identify early damage includes stereoscopic optic nerve evaluation (see Chapter 5), NFL evaluation (see Chapter 6), and short-wavelength automated perimetry (see Chapter 7). Establishing damage with these more sensitive tests changes the diagnosis from glaucoma suspect to glaucoma. More definitive information on the benefits of treating patients with ocular hypertension will be available from the Ocular Hypertensive Treatment Study. This study is a multicenter clinical trial of patients with elevated IOP and normal visual fields who are randomized to IOP-lowering agents versus placebo and followed with serial optic disc photographs and visual fields.

Because patients with glaucoma and glaucoma suspects are patients for life, documenting the optic nerve appearance with a set of stereoscopic disc photographs is beneficial. Photographs compared over a period of time can establish a diagnosis of glaucoma in the presence of a normal visual field test (see Color Plate 28). Early glaucoma diagnosis allows for early treatment intervention. Scanning laser ophthalmoscopes (HRT [Heidelberg Engineering, Heidelberg, Germany] and TOPSS [Laser Diagnostic Technologies, San Diego, CA]) are commercially available instruments used to measure optic nerve topography and quantify neuroretinal rim tissue. The GDx (Laser Diagnostic Technologies, San Diego, CA) along with Optical Coherence Tomography (Zeiss Humphrey System, Dublin, CA) are instruments that quantify NFL thickness. Some of these companies have developed or are developing software programs to compare results with a database of age- and race-matched controls to help interpret the vast array of data obtained with these devices. These instruments may prove to be clinically validated for earlier diagnosis and determining progression of glaucoma. However, they are expensive and do not have long-term published data to prove effectiveness in clinical practice.

Some glaucoma suspects may warrant treatment even though they do not exhibit objective signs of glaucoma damage. Patients with IOP consistently over 35 mm Hg are at a greater than 50% risk of developing glaucoma damage.[9,10] Both young and elderly patients with elevated IOP may also be at a higher risk for developing a central retinal vein occlusion, an irreversible event with high ocular morbidity.[11,12] Therefore, patients with IOP consistently higher than 30 mm Hg, even without physical evidence of glaucoma optic nerve damage, are usually treated with IOP-lowering agents. It is probably not necessary to achieve a target pressure below 20 mm Hg in a patient without optic nerve compromise. Target IOP for patients with elevated pressure without optic nerve dam-

age is usually set at 20% reduction from baseline or below 30 mm Hg, whichever is lower. Other factors—a monocular or noncompliant patient, presence of an anomalous optic disc, concurrent optic neuropathy or retinopathy besides glaucoma, or an unreliable visual field tester—can also influence whether the benefits of treatment to prevent glaucoma damage outweigh the risks of potential side effects from medications.

As mentioned earlier, patients with IOP higher than 30 mm Hg, regardless of optic nerve status or age, are generally started on IOP-lowering therapy to reduce the risk of future glaucoma damage and venous occlusive disease. Target pressures are set lower than 30 mm Hg or 20% reduction from baseline. Patients who present with a central retinal vein occlusion in one eye and elevated IOP in the fellow eye are also generally treated to achieve a target IOP lower than 20 mm Hg in both eyes. No proven prospective clinical trials are available to prove that lowering IOP reduces the risk of vein occlusions, but given the high morbidity of vein occlusions and their irreversibility, the potential benefits of glaucoma treatment appear to outweigh most drawbacks. Once the target pressure is achieved, it is also important to monitor the IOP in the fellow eye of a patient with a central retinal vein occlusion because of diurnal fluctuations of 10 mm Hg or higher.[12]

Patients without optic nerve damage and IOP in the upper 20s mm Hg may be considered for treatment after risk factors have been assessed and the risks and benefits of treatment have been discussed. The patient should play a part in the treatment decision process, especially in these borderline cases. Some patients prefer to be started on medication if any significant risk of developing glaucoma damage exists, whereas some patients prefer not to be put on any medication unless there is an absolute certainty that glaucoma damage is present or likely to develop. I encourage patients to be involved in management decisions and find that an informed patient is much more likely to be a compliant patient.

INITIATING THERAPY

Before starting a patient on medication, establishing a baseline set of IOP measurements is imperative. The IOP in glaucoma patients varies more than 20% from the highest to the lowest IOP reading.[13] At least three IOP readings should be obtained, preferably two in the morning and one in the afternoon. This can be accomplished on the initial visit, at the visual field appointment, and at the next follow-up visit. Without knowledge of how the IOP fluctuates when the patient is not taking medications, establishing an accurate target pressure and judging the effectiveness of medications are laborious. After establishing a target pressure determined by the baseline IOP (at least three IOP readings while the patient is off of medications) and the degree of glaucoma damage (based on optic nerve, NFL, and visual field; see Table 11-1), institution of therapy is begun. I believe that glaucoma damage is more likely to occur from the spikes in IOP rather than the average IOP. Therefore, I use the highest IOP reading, rather than the average of the three baseline measurements, to set the target pressure. Initial treatment is typically topical medications followed by LTP followed by filtering surgery. Some debate exists as to whether medications, LTP, or filtering surgery should be the initial treatment for glaucoma. The advantages of filtering surgery are the ability to achieve lower IOP and better control of IOP fluctuations, and some studies show less visual field progression after filtering surgery.[14,15] The success rate is approximately 65% and as high as 85% in phakic primary open-angle glaucoma.[16] Filtering surgery may also provide a better quality of life by eliminating the potential side effects and inconvenience of instilling eyedrops on a daily basis.

Some studies indicate that the success rate for filtering surgery decreases with previous use of glaucoma topical medications.[17] It is believed that chronic use of topical beta blocker or adrenergic agonists may alter the conjunctival tissue and promote conjunctival scarring. However, surgery is not without drawbacks. Complications, such as endophthalmitis, hypotony maculopathy, wound leaks, choroidal detachment, and suprachoroidal hemorrhage, although rare, can result in significant ocular morbidity. Acceleration of cataract formation is the most common complication, and it is estimated that cataract surgery is required in more than 40% of filtering patients within 5 years of glaucoma surgery.[18] The Collaborative Initial Glaucoma Treatment Study is evaluating the initial treatment regimen (topical medicines followed by LTP and filtering surgery versus filtering surgery first) for newly diagnosed glaucoma patients. The study is also looking at quality-of-life issues by using a detailed questionnaire to interview the patients in the study to determine how glaucoma therapy affects their well-being.

LTP has also been evaluated as an initial treatment for newly established glaucoma patients. The results of the Glaucoma Laser Trial (GLT) indicate that LTP is as effective as medications, although the success rate with LTP declines with time, and most patients require adjunctive medical therapy after 2 years.[19,20] LTP should be considered as an initial treatment in patients with poor compliance, inability to administer eye drops, or contraindication to the topical antiglaucoma medications. Certain types of glaucoma are more likely to have a favorable response to LTP. These include pseudoexfoliative and pigmentary glaucoma, and primary open-angle glaucoma in patients older than 50 years. LTP is less effective and probably should not be attempted in uveitic glaucoma, traumatic glaucoma (with angle scarring), and steroid-induced glaucoma.

My clinical approach to newly diagnosed glaucoma patients is to discuss treatment options with the patient. I usually start topical medical therapy first and use LTP as adjunctive treatment after the patient is on two or three topical medications. I consider more aggressive treatment, including filtering surgery, at the first sign of confirmed progression of damage in a patient with moderate or severe disease. Determining progression can be a difficult task and in some cases requires multiple visual field tests (see Chapter 7). Patients should always have confirmed documentation of progression before surgical intervention is initiated. Patients who are initially diagnosed with confirmed severe glaucomatous damage should also be candidates for filtering surgery if an estimated target pressure cannot or is unlikely to be obtained with medicines and LTP.

MEDICAL THERAPY

For a full description of glaucoma medications, including contraindications and side effects, see Chapter 8. The clinician has many choices for topical therapeutic treatment of glaucoma. Therapy is directed at lowering IOP, which is one of the few risk factors for glaucoma that can be changed or altered. New therapies designed to directly treat (blood-flow enhancers) or prevent (neuroprotective agents) damage to the optic nerve are being investigated. These agents may change the way we treat glaucoma in the future, but they are still in early clinical trials.

Topical Medications

Beta Blockers

Beta blockers are my initial treatment in the majority of new glaucoma patients without systemic contraindications. These medications have been thoroughly studied since Timoptic (timolol maleate) was introduced in the late 1970s. In fact, all new glaucoma IOP-lowering agents are clinically evaluated against Timoptic for effectiveness. Topical beta blockers are effective in lowering IOP, generally well tolerated by the patient, and cost-effective. The latter is an important consideration in a cost-controlled managed care environment. The cost of nonselective beta blockers has decreased substantially because of increased competition and the availability of generics.

When prescribing topical beta blockers, the doctor must scrutinize the patient's medical history to avoid prescribing a beta blocker to a patient with pulmonary or cardiac problems. Documentation in the patient's chart for negative contraindications (i.e., denies shortness of breath, asthma, bronchitis, emphysema) and recording a resting pulse and blood pressure is mandatory. The patient should be questioned about symptoms of shortness of breath, history of asthma, emphysema, bronchitis, heart block, or overt cardiac failure. The patient's current medications should be evaluated for any that may indicate a potential pulmonary or cardiac contraindication to topical beta blockers. These medicines include β-agonist oral inhalers (e.g., albuterol, isoproterenol); breathing medications, such as theophylline or oral prednisone in

TABLE 11-5. Advantages and Disadvantages of Different Topical Beta Blockers for the Treatment of Glaucoma

Topical beta blocker	Concentration (%)	Advantages	Disadvantages
Timolol maleate (Timoptic)	0.25 and 0.50	Most studied beta blocker 27% IOP reduction Generic available	Expensive
Timolol maleate (Timoptic XE)	0.25 and 0.50	Gel formation allows qd dosage Generic available	Expensive Gel temporarily blurs vision
Timolol hemihydrate (Betimol)	0.25 and 0.50	Pseudogeneric of timolol maleate Less cost, same effectiveness Good drop size	
Levobunolol hydrochloride (Betagan)	0.25 and 0.50	Same effectiveness as timolol maleate Longer duration of action than other beta blockers Generic available	Large drop size compared with other bottles increases cost per drop
Betaxolol hydrochloride (Betoptic)	0.25 (suspension)	β_1 selective—may be used with caution in patients with mild breathing problems, but should not be used in patients with moderate or severe breathing problems	Expensive Stinging Suspension must be shaken Poor drop size Less IOP reduction compared with timolol maleate
Metipranolol hydrochloride (Optipranolol)	0.3	Inexpensive	Reported 0.5% incidence of granulomatous iritis
Carteolol hydrochloride (Ocupress)	1.0	ISA prevents less cardiac and pulmonary side effects May have less effect on HDL Efficient drop size	Expensive Slightly less IOP reduction compared with timolol maleate

IOP = intraocular pressure; ISA = intrinsic sympathomimetic activity; HDL = high-density lipoproteins.

patients with chronic obstructive pulmonary disease; and heart medications, such as digitalis drugs for patients with congestive heart failure. If the resting pulse is lower than 60 or reveals an irregular heart rate, then beta blockers should be avoided unless clearance is given from the patient's primary care or cardiac doctor. Patients who routinely participate in athletic activities should be warned that their exercise tachycardia may be reduced and affect performance. Male patients treated for impotency should also avoid topical beta blockers. Patients with diabetes who experience frequent bouts of hypoglycemia may have symptoms of tachycardia masked by topical beta blockers. Beta blockers may also conceal symptoms of thyrotoxicosis.

The lowest concentration of beta blocker should be prescribed because the dose-response curve shows slight difference between 0.25% and 0.5% timolol.[21] The usual starting dosage is twice daily, although once-a-day therapy may provide 24-hour coverage.[22] If once-a-day therapy is initiated, the practitioner should arrange for IOP checks at the 24-hour time frame to ensure 24-hour IOP

control. The choice of which beta blocker to use is practitioner-dependent. Each may have a specific advantage or disadvantage (Table 11-5). Timoptic XE is a gelrite formulation of timolol and is prescribed once daily.[23] Betaxolol (Betoptic), a selective β_1 blocker, can sometimes be used with caution in patients with mild breathing problems. However, evidence exists of a crossover effect to β_2 receptors with betaxolol.[24] With the advent of other effective glaucoma medications available, such as latanoprost (Xalatan) and brimonidine (Alphagan), I am less inclined to prescribe even a selective beta blocker, such as betaxolol, for a patient with any type of breathing problem. With beta blockers and other topical medications, it is beneficial to instruct the patient on punctal occlusion with eyelid closure to reduce systemic absorption and to improve ocular penetration and effectiveness.

Latanoprost (Xalatan). New medications introduced in 1996 have challenged the beta blockers as the initial drug used to treat glaucoma. Latanoprost 0.005% by Pharmacia in Peapack, New Jersey, is a topical prostaglandin agonist that decreases IOP by increasing uveoscleral outflow.[25] The drug should be refrigerated if the period of use is expected to be longer than 6 weeks. It is prescribed once a day in the evening with peak IOP lowering achieved 8–12 hours after instillation. Once-a-day therapy has been shown to be more effective than twice-a-day therapy.[26] Latanoprost shows long-term efficacy and safety.[27] In comparative studies with timolol 0.5%, it reduced IOP 35% versus 27% for timolol.[26] Adding latanoprost to a topical beta blocker resulted in an additional 20% IOP reduction. The primary IOP-lowering mechanism of beta blockers is a decrease in aqueous production. Medications that increase outflow, such as latanoprost (uveoscleral outflow) or pilocarpine (trabecular outflow), may be more additive to beta-blocker (aqueous-suppressant) therapy than medications that also decrease aqueous production (α agonists, carbonic anhydrase inhibitors [CAIs]). Therefore I generally use latanoprost as my first second-line drug if a patient has not reached target IOP on a beta blocker alone. Latanoprost is also an ideal drug for primary therapy if the patient has a contraindication to beta blockers because of its high effectiveness and the convenience of once-a-day treatment.

The reported systemic side effects of latanoprost have been minor. The drug does not appear to exacerbate breathing problems in patients with treated asthma.[28] An increase in iris pigmentation occurred in approximately 10% of patients.[29] The patients most likely to exhibit this iris color change had hazel, mixed-color (blue-green color in the iris periphery with a light brown pupillary collarette) irises. The change in iris color results from an increase in the size of the iris melanocyte, and not from an increase in number of melanocytes. The change is often irreversible. Another unusual side effect of latanoprost is an increase in growth and thickness of eyelashes.[30] The U.S. Food and Drug Administration approved the use of latanoprost as adjunctive therapy or primary therapy when the patient has failed to achieve a target pressure on other glaucoma medications or has contraindications to these medications. Latanoprost may be approved as initial glaucoma therapy after more clinical experience is gained and the long-term effects on iris color change are better understood.

In patients with normal-tension glaucoma (NTG), latanoprost lowered IOP by 21%.[31] Because latanoprost lowers pressure by increasing uveoscleral outflow and is not limited by episcleral venous pressure, it may be an ideal drug for patients with NTG. Latanoprost also appears to have a more favorable effect on ocular perfusion pressure than timolol in patients with NTG.[32]

Many questions about the clinical use of latanoprost remain:

Can latanoprost be used in patients with uveitic glaucoma? Latanoprost is a prostaglandin agonist that may exacerbate the inflammatory component of the uveitis. In most cases with a uveitic component, I do not prescribe latanoprost.

Should latanoprost be used in patients with glaucoma and pseudophakia? There may be an increased risk of developing cystoid macular edema because of latanoprost's prostaglandin activity. Approximately 5% of eyes developed anterior uveitis and 1% of eyes developed cystoid macular edema while on latanoprost in one study.[33] In pseudophakic patients with glaucoma, I try to avoid latanoprost.

Should latanoprost be used in patients with pigmentary glaucoma? If latanoprost changes the size of the melanocyte in certain patients, does this eventually lead to a worsening of pigment blockage in the trabecular meshwork? No good data are available on this question, but I would be cautious in using latanoprost in pigmentary glaucoma.

Should latanoprost be used in patients with angle closure or significant peripheral anterior synechiae in the angle? Latanoprost appears to lower IOP by a mechanism other than increasing trabecular outflow. However, the onset of action with latanoprost is generally longer than with beta blockers, and latanoprost may exacerbate the inflammation usually associated with acute angle closure, so I generally do not use it.

Answers to many of these situations will be uncovered with further clinical trials and experience with latanoprost.

Another theoretical issue concerns the use of latanoprost with pilocarpine. Miotics, such as pilocarpine, inhibit uveoscleral outflow, which may reduce the effectiveness of latanoprost. In a small clinical trial of patients on maximal medical therapy with pilocarpine, approximately 63% showed an additional 20% reduction in IOP, compared with a response of 83% of patients on maximal medical therapy who were not taking pilocarpine.[34] If latanoprost is added to the regimen of a patient already on pilocarpine, I examine a series of IOP readings with and without latanoprost. If the IOP is reduced 20%, I continue both medicines. If it is not significantly reduced, I discontinue the pilocarpine and observe the IOP. This situation of using pilocarpine and latanoprost occurs with less frequency because pilocarpine is not as often prescribed with the advent of newer glaucoma medications (brimonidine [Alphagan], dorzolamide [Trusopt], brinzolamide [Azopt]).

Latanoprost and Timolol Combination (Xalcom). The Food and Drug Administration has issued an approvable letter for the investigational fixed combination of latanoprost and timolol (Xalcom) to treat glaucoma. The medication will be administered once a day and should be used for patients who have failed to achieve a target pressure on latanoprost or timolol alone.

α_2 Agonists

Brimonidine (Alphagan). Brimonidine is a selective α_2 agonist by Allergan Pharmaceutical in Irvine, California that was approved as an initial glaucoma medication in 1996. It may possess neuroprotective properties in rat models,[35] but no clinical proof exists of neuroprotection in glaucoma patients. It is approved as a t.i.d. medication but has b.i.d. effectiveness.[36] The peak IOP reduction (2 hours after instillation) is similar to timolol 0.5%, although the trough IOP reading (12 hours after instillation) is less effective compared with timolol 0.5% through the first year of use.[37] Brimonidine lowers IOP by 27% by decreasing aqueous production and increasing uveoscleral outflow.[36] Brimonidine is similar to apraclonidine (Iopidine) but is 30 times more selective to the α_2 receptor.[38] Brimonidine has less reported incidence of allergy, tachyphylaxis, mydriasis, and lid retraction than apraclonidine. Patients who develop allergy with apraclonidine can successfully be switched to brimonidine without allergy in 90% of cases.[39] Because the medication passes the blood-brain barrier, patients should be monitored for systolic blood pressure lowering.[40] Reports have been made of central nervous system depression (hypotension, bradycardia, apnea) in infants receiving topical brimonidine.[41] Other reported side effects include allergy (10%), conjunctival blanching and follicles, dry mouth, fatigue, and depression.[42] Brimonidine further lowers IOP by 20% when added to topical beta blockers.[43] When added to a topical beta blocker, it should be prescribed on a b.i.d. dosage. However, when brimonidine is used as initial therapy, t.i.d. dosing may be required.[37,44–46] If b.i.d. dosing is used as primary therapy, then 12-hour trough IOP readings should be scheduled. Brimonidine has also been shown to be effective in preventing postoperative IOP spikes after laser procedures.[47–50]

Apraclonidine (Iopidine). Apraclonidine (Alcon Pharmaceutical, Fort Worth, TX) is another α_2-adrenergic agonist; it was first introduced as a 1% concentration used to prevent IOP spikes in patients undergoing laser procedures (LTP, laser peripheral iridotomy, yttrium-aluminum-garnet [YAG] capsulotomy).[51] In 1995, 0.5% apraclonidine was approved for short-term use (less than 3 weeks) in chronic open-angle glaucoma for patients on maximal medical therapy. It is approved for t.i.d. dosage but has b.i.d. effectiveness. Long-term studies with 0.5% apraclonidine show that the clinical response is variable. Approximately one-fourth of patients on the drug develop tachyphylaxis, and one-fourth of the patients

develop ocular allergy. Brimonidine is a better α_2 agonist for chronic glaucoma therapy because it does not appear to lead to the development of tachyphylaxis or as high an incidence of ocular allergy. Apraclonidine is better suited for short-term IOP reduction and the prevention of postoperative IOP spikes associated with laser procedures.

Patients receiving chronic α_2 agonist therapy for glaucoma may experience a higher incidence of IOP spikes after laser procedures (LPI, LTP, YAG capsulotomy) despite the use of apraclonidine immediately before and after the laser procedure.[52] The proposed mechanism is saturation of the α_2 receptor from chronic α-agonist therapy. The clinician must take this into account before contemplating laser treatment in patients receiving chronic α_2-agonist treatment and be prepared to manage post-laser IOP spikes if they occur. Switching medications a few weeks before laser treatment and treating only 180 degrees of trabecular meshwork for LTP at a time may be prudent if the patient is on an α_2-agonist drug.

Topical Carbonic Anhydrase Inhibitors

Dorzolamide (Trusopt). Dorzolamide 2% is a topical CAI introduced by Merck (West Point, PA) in 1995. It is a sulfa derivative and was approved by the U.S. Food and Drug Administration as a t.i.d. medication, but it has b.i.d. effectiveness. It is less effective than oral CAIs but has fewer systemic side effects.[53] Ocular allergy, bitter taste, and stinging are the most frequent reported side effects. No reports have been made of aplastic anemia associated with dorzolamide. Dorzolamide may affect corneal endothelial permeability[54] and should probably not be used in patients with corneal compromise. It does not appear to affect corneal thickness or function in normal corneas.[55] Dorzolamide is additive to beta blockers (10–20% additional IOP lowering) and better tolerated than pilocarpine.[56–58] When dorzolamide is added to a topical beta blocker, it should be prescribed on a b.i.d. dosage. Studies show similar IOP reduction on b.i.d. and t.i.d. dosing, and the cost can be reduced by one-third if the drug is prescribed b.i.d. However, the cost is still significantly greater than with dipivefrin, pilocarpine, or acetazolamide tablets. Dorzolamide is not additive to oral CAIs, so topical and oral CAIs should not be used concurrently.[59]

Timolol and Dorzolamide Combination (Cosopt). A combination drug of 0.5% timolol and 2% dorzolamide called Cosopt (Merck) is available as a b.i.d. drug and has been shown to have IOP-lowering action similar to the administrations of its separate components.[60] I would not recommend Cosopt as initial therapy but would consider it if a patient did not achieve target pressure with a topical beta blocker alone.

Brinzolamide (Azopt). Brinzolamide 1% (Alcon, Fort Worth, TX) is another topical CAI that is approved for t.i.d. dosing but used b.i.d. for adjunctive therapy. It is a suspension that must be shaken before instillation. Clinical studies show similar effectiveness as dorzolamide for IOP reduction (approximately 20%).[61] Less occurrence is reported of stinging and bitter taste compared with dorzolamide, but a greater incidence of temporary blurred vision after instillation because of the suspension formulation.

Less Frequently Prescribed Glaucoma Medications

Older adjunctive glaucoma medications, such as epinephrine (Glaucon/Epifrin) or dipivefrin (Propine), pilocarpine (and other cholinergics), and oral CAIs (Diamox/Neptazane) are prescribed with less frequency in the treatment of glaucoma with the introduction of the newer glaucoma medications. This occurred because the newer medications have greater effectiveness, fewer side effects, and less frequent dosing schedules. The cost of the newer medications is much greater than the older medicines. When cost or affordability of medications is a patient issue, then the older glaucoma medications may be considered along with LTP as alternative therapies.

Dipivefrin (Propine) and Other Epinephrine Drugs

Dipivefrin 0.1% (Allergan Pharmaceuticals, Irvine, CA) is a prodrug of epinephrine that has fewer ocular and systemic side effects than epinephrine drugs (Glaucon [Alcon, Fort Worth, TX] and Epifrin [Allergan, Irvine, CA]). Dipivefrin is not very additive to nonselective beta blockers and has a high incidence of ocular allergy and rebound conjunctival hyperemia. Dipivefrin is more additive to betaxolol than other nonselective beta blockers.[62] It can be used as initial therapy in a patient who has a contraindication to a beta blocker and for whom cost of medication is an issue. Dipivefrin is available as a generic.

Pilocarpine and Other Cholinergics

Pilocarpine is additive to the beta blockers, but its dosage is q.i.d., and the ocular side effects of dim vision, accommodative spasm, and brow ache limit patient compliance. Patients older than 60 years have fewer problems with accommodative spasm and brow ache and are more likely to tolerate pilocarpine therapy than a younger patient. Initiation of pilocarpine therapy should always begin with a break-in schedule regardless of the patient's age. This technique involves using low-dose pilocarpine, either 0.5% or 1%, at bedtime only. The patient can take acetaminophen

(Tylenol) approximately 45 minutes before instillation if he or she is experiencing significant brow ache. After a few days, the patients can use the drop b.i.d., and then t.i.d and q.i.d. The build-up schedule to q.i.d. should take 2–3 weeks. If the patient is re-examined and the target pressure has not been reached, then the next-higher dose is substituted for the current concentration. The 0.5% concentration of the drug can be switched to 1%, 1% can be changed to 2%, and 2% can be changed to 4%. I rarely prescribe higher than 2% pilocarpine in patients with light-colored irises, or 4% in patients with dark-colored-irises.

Patient education about pilocarpine's side effects and break-in schedule can improve pilocarpine tolerance. With other glaucoma medications available, I rarely use pilocarpine in a patient younger than age 60 years, unless cost is an issue. However, many patients may be able to tolerate the side effects of pilocarpine by using a sustained-released form of the drug. Pilopine gel 4% is a ointment form of pilocarpine that is prescribed before bedtime. The patient inserts a 0.25-in. strip of the gel into the lower cul-de-sac before retiring. The accommodative spasm occurs during sleep, but the IOP lowering can last up to 24 hours. Checking the IOP in the late afternoon to ensure 24-hour effectiveness is prudent. A supplemental drop of pilocarpine may be prescribed in the early evening to provide 24-hour coverage. Another sustained-release form of pilocarpine is the Ocusert. This depot formulation of pilocarpine comes in 20- and 40-μg concentrations. It is inserted into the lower cul-de-sac and can last for as long as a 1 week. Patient satisfaction varies with these sustained-release forms of pilocarpine. Stronger cholinergics, such as carbachol and phospholine iodine, traditionally were substituted for pilocarpine therapy if the desired target pressure was not obtained. However, these drugs have greater systemic and ocular side effects and are rarely prescribed in newly diagnosed glaucoma patients. With the advent of newer glaucoma medications that have fewer ocular side effects, pilocarpine and other cholinergic drugs are not used as often in the therapy of glaucoma.

Oral Carbonic Anhydrase Inhibitors

Methazolamide (Neptazane) (Lederle, Wayne, NJ), acetazolamide (Diamox) (Lederle, Wayne, NJ), and dichlorphenamide (Daranide) (Merck, West Point, PA) are oral CAIs that are additive to the beta blockers but have multiple systemic side effects, such as paresthesias, fatigue, stomach upset, loss of appetite and libido, and depression. CAIs are sulfa derivatives, and patients may experience sulfa allergy. Kidney stones, potassium and sodium loss, and blood dyscrasias are potential systemic complications of oral CAIs. Methazolamide is generally better tolerated than acetazola-

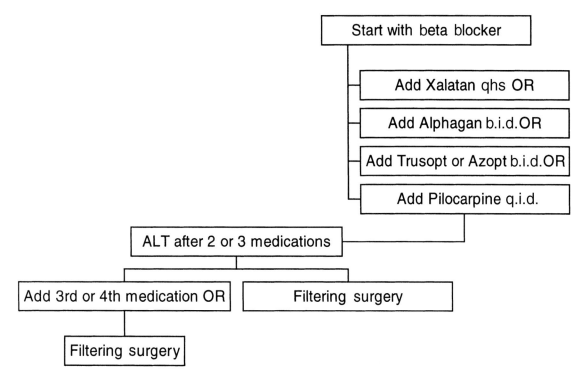

FIGURE 11-1. Flow chart of glaucoma management in a patient without contraindications to any glaucoma therapy. (ALT = argon laser trabeculoplasty.)

mide or dichlorphenamide and is less likely to cause kidney stones. Methazolamide is more expensive than acetazolamide. Methazolamide is prescribed 25- or 50-mg b.i.d. or t.i.d. Acetazolamide is prescribed in 125- to 250-mg tablets q.i.d., and a 500-mg sustained-release Sequel (Lederle, Wayne, NJ) for b.i.d. dosing is available, but at a higher cost than acetazolamide tablets. With the advent of topical CAIs, dorzolamide and brinzolamide, I generally use oral CAIs for short-term emergency IOP reduction or in patients who have difficulty instilling eyedrops until laser or filtering surgery can be performed.

Glaucoma Therapy

Glaucoma therapy is case-specific (cases differing in such factors as type of glaucoma, systemic contraindications, age, compliance) and influenced by the doctor's prior experience with medicines and modes of therapy. This section presents my general approach to a newly diagnosed glaucoma patient who does not have any contraindications to the use of any glaucoma medications (Figure 11-1). I will also give the patient a medication dosing schedule (Figure 11-2) to improve compliance.

Beta blockers remain the mainstay of initial glaucoma treatment in the majority of glaucoma patients who do not have pulmonary or cardiac contraindications. They are generally well tolerated, can be prescribed qd or b.i.d., and are the most cost-effec-

tive drug for treating glaucoma. Second-line therapy has taken a new direction with the addition of latanoprost, brimonidine, dorzolamide, and brinzolamide. If a patient has failed to achieve the desired target pressure on a beta blocker alone, I generally add latanoprost qhs or brimonidine b.i.d. I use brinzolamide or dorzolamide if the patient has not responded to latanoprost or brimonidine or develops an intolerable side effect. Once a patient is on two or three glaucoma medications, I consider LTP as my next line of therapy if the patient is still not at the desired IOP. Pilocarpine remains an effective, inexpensive, additive glaucoma agent, although the ocular side effects can limit its effectiveness, especially in patients younger than 60 years. Dipivefrin (because of its poor additivity to beta blockers) and oral CAIs (because of their systemic side effects) play a less significant role in the medical management of glaucoma. The advantages and disadvantages of these medications are summarized in Table 11-6.

Determining the Effectiveness of Medications

When prescribing glaucoma medications, it is important to judge the effectiveness of each drug. Medicines that do not significantly lower IOP should be discontinued and another medication or procedure substituted. Judging the effectiveness of glaucoma medications is not a simple task and requires an understanding of the factors that can affect the IOP. First,

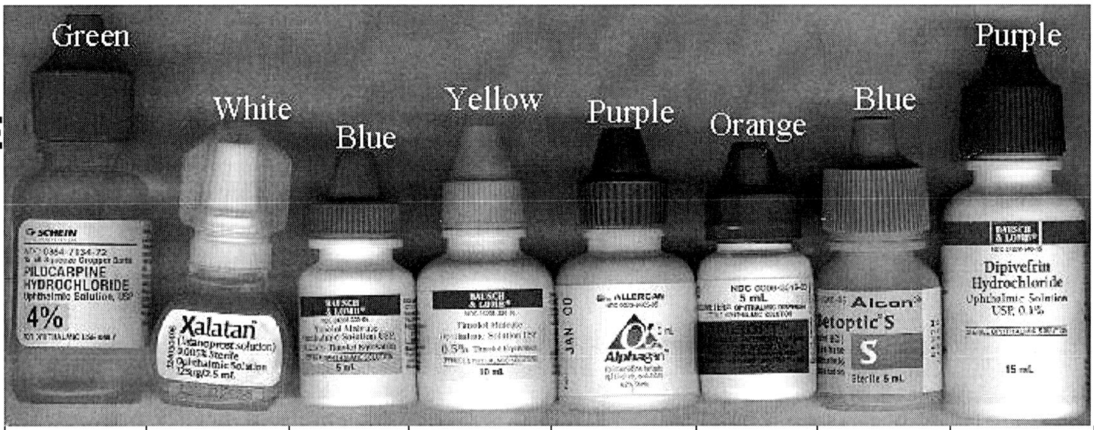

	Pilocarpine	Xalatan	Timolol 0.25 %	Timolol 0.5%	Alphagan	Trusopt	Betoptic	Propine
Breakfast								
Lunch								
Dinner								
Bedtime								

Always wait FIVE minutes between drops.

FIGURE 11-2. Patient medication dosing schedule. (Designed by Peter A. Lalle, OD., Department of Veterans Affairs, Maryland Health Care System, Baltimore, MD.)

patients exhibit different responses to medications; some patients may respond better to beta blockers than latanoprost or α agonists, and vice versa. This outcome cannot be predicted other than by trial and error. Second, glaucoma patients are more likely to exhibit wide diurnal fluctuations in IOP. IOP spikes can occur at a similar time in the day or they can be sporadic. The clinician must consider whether a given IOP reading is at the patient's peak or trough diurnal curve. The best way to determine the amount of IOP variation is through diurnal curves or by sampling a number of IOP readings taken at different times of the day. It is important that these readings are taken before the patient is started on glaucoma medications. Third, adrenergic agents, such as beta blockers and α agonists, have crossover effects to the fellow eye if used in one-eye trials.

The effectiveness of glaucoma medications can be judged in several ways, each with certain limitations. Monocular trials evaluate the effectiveness of a medication by comparing the IOP between the two eyes when only one eye has been treated. This is a popular technique and one that I frequently use when judging the effectiveness of latanoprost, because latanoprost does not produce a contralateral IOP lowering. However, erroneous interpretations can occur from monocular trials because of the crossover effect exhibited by topical beta blockers and other adrenergic agonists (brimonidine). Also, uniocular trials do not account for diurnal IOP spikes that may be more pronounced in one eye.[13] For this reason, I prefer to establish a baseline set of at least three IOP readings (to establish the diurnal fluctuation) before the patient is started on treatment, and then compare this group of IOP readings with a set of readings taken while the patient is

TABLE 11-6. Advantages and Disadvantages of Adjunctive Medications for the Treatment of Glaucoma

Medication	Concentration (%)	Advantages	Disadvantages
Latanoprost (Xalatan)	0.005	Dosage is qd	Expensive
		Additive to beta blockers Few systemic side effects	Iris color change in hazel irises (3–12%)
			May induce iritis, may cause cystoid macular edema in pseudophakes
Brimonidine tartrate (Alphagan)	0.2	Additive to beta blockers	As primary therapy, administered t.i.d.
		Can be prescribed b.i.d. as adjunctive therapy	Expensive Large drop size increases cost per drop
		Generally well tolerated	
		May have neuroprotective properties	Ocular allergy (10–20%) Depression of the central nervous system in infants
Dorzolamide hydrochloride (Trusopt)	2.0	Fewer systemic side effects than oral carbonic anhydrase inhibitors	Expensive, allergy (10%)
		Has b.i.d. effectiveness as adjunctive therapy	Only 10–20% additive to beta blockers
			Stinging
			Bitter taste
Brinzolamide (Azopt)	1.0	Fewer systemic side effects than oral carbonic anhydrase inhibitors	Expensive, allergy (10%) Temporary blurred vision from suspension
		Dosage for adjunctive therapy is b.i.d.	
		Same effectiveness as dorzolamide hydrochloride with less stinging	
Pilocarpine (Pilocar)	0.5, 1.0, 2.0, 3.0, 4.0, 6.0	Inexpensive Additive to beta blockers	Dosage is q.i.d. Miosis
			Accommodative spasm
			Brow ache
Dipivefrin hydrochloride (Propine)	0.1	Inexpensive More additive to betaxolol hydrochloride (Betoptic) than nonselective beta blockers	Not additive to nonselective beta blockers
			Ocular allergy (>20%) Rebound hyperemia
Apraclonidine (Iopidine)	0.5	Good for short-term IOP lowering	Expensive Tachyphylaxis
			Ocular allergy (>20%)

IOP = intraocular pressure.

on medications (see Chapter 18, Case 1). I treat both eyes when using adrenergic agents (assuming both eyes have glaucoma) rather than just one because of the crossover effect. In general, the clinician is looking for a 20–30% reduction with a beta blocker or first-line therapy. If this reduction is not achieved, the patient can be treated with a higher concentration of the beta blocker (e.g., a shift from 0.25% to 0.50% concentration). A second alternative would be to switch to another beta blocker or different class of medication (e.g., change from a beta blocker to latanoprost or brimonidine). For additive therapy, an additional 15–20% IOP reduction is desired. Again, this can be assessed by comparing a series of IOP readings before and after the new medication is added. However, because of the potential wide diurnal IOP fluctuations in glaucoma patients, assessment of effectiveness should be based on at least two and preferably three readings before a medication is judged ineffective.

Laser Trabeculoplasty

Chapter 9 offers a full description of the argon laser trabeculoplasty (ALT) procedure, patients most likely to benefit, pre- and postoperative management, complications, and long-term effectiveness. LTP was demonstrated in the GLT to be as effective as medications for the initial treatment of glaucoma.[19,63] However, the effectiveness of LTP decreases with time. Therefore, in most cases, LTP does not obviate the need for topical medications. LTP lowers the mean IOP approximately 22% and may also reduce the incidence of diurnal IOP spikes in glaucoma patients.[64] I consider LTP similar to an effective topical glaucoma medication. I recommend LTP as initial treatment for patients who cannot tolerate medical therapy because of side effects, contraindications, or an inability to physically administer the eyedrops. LTP is an ideal therapy for patients who are noncompliant in taking their medications. In patients tolerant and compliant with medical therapy, I recommend LTP after the patient is on two or three medications and still has not reached the desired target pressure. Patients on more than three medications are less likely to be compliant, and the inconvenience of multiple instillations may have an impact on their quality of life.

LTP is more effective when used in patients with certain characteristics and types of glaucoma. Elderly patients respond to LTP better than younger patients. LTP is more effective in chronic open-angle, pigmentary, and pseudoexfoliative glaucomas and is less effective in uveitic, traumatic, or steroid-induced glaucomas. The response in patients after cataract surgery is variable. LTP should not be attempted in patients with extensive peripheral anterior synechiae or angle neovascularization.

The decision to treat the entire 360 degrees in one session or 180 degrees in divided sessions is debatable. In one study, a higher incidence of IOP spikes was seen after treatment of a full 360 degrees compared to 180 degrees, but the IOP-lowering effect was greater when 360 degrees were treated.[65] With pre- or post-treatment using apraclonidine or brimonidine, the occurrence of IOP spikes has been dramatically reduced, whether treatment was of 180 or 360 degrees.[50,66,67] Treating 360 degrees prevents any delay in further intervention, if LTP is not successful in meeting a target pressure. (Generally, waiting 4–6 weeks is necessary to assess the effectiveness of LTP.) Proponents of treating 180 degrees advocate that the other 180 degrees can be treated at a later date to lower the IOP when needed. Patients on chronic α_2-agonist therapy probably should have only 180 degrees treated in one session because of the higher incidence of post-laser IOP spikes despite the pre- and postoperative use of apraclonidine.[52]

Eventual loss of IOP control is the rule with LTP; approximately 19% fail after 1 year, and an additional 10% fail each year, reaching a 65% failure rate at 5 years.[68] After 360 degrees of treatment has been performed, retreatments are less likely to control progression of glaucoma[69] and are generally not performed.

Glaucoma Filtering Surgery

See Chapter 10 for a full description of filtering surgery, including surgical techniques, patient selection, pre- and postoperative management, complications, and long-term effectiveness. Glaucoma filtering surgery has been traditionally considered a last resort for endstage glaucoma patients. With improvement in surgical technique, adjunctive antifibrotic medications, and vigilant postoperative care, the success rate of glaucoma filtering surgery in phakic primary open-angle glaucoma has improved to 80–90%. Complications, although rare, do occur and are more frequent with the use of antimetabolite agents, such as mitomycin C and 5-fluorouracil. Acceleration of cataract formation occurred in nearly one-half of glaucoma surgery patients after 5 years in one study.[18]

Filtering surgery should not be delayed to the point at which the patient develops severely constricted visual fields (see Chapter 18, Case 7). The indications for filtering surgery should be documented progression or likely progression despite maximal tolerated medical and laser therapy (MMT). This definition has many interpretations. First, what is the definition of *progression*? The NTG study indicates that it may take five visual field tests before glaucoma progression can be determined because differentiating actual visual field loss progression from long-term visual field fluctuation is difficult (see Chapter 7). Comparison of serial stereoscopic optic nerve photographs and NFL photographs can also be used to diagnose glaucoma progression, although serial visual field testing is more likely to identify glaucoma progression.[18] The definition of MMT is also variable, but usually includes at least two or more topical medications and 360 degrees of LTP. Filtering surgery should not be delayed once documented progression is established and the patient is on MMT. Filtering surgery should also be considered early in the treatment regimen in a patient who presents with severe glaucomatous damage or in a patient who is unlikely to achieve a target pressure through medical or laser therapy. The age of the patient is also an important consideration. A young patient diagnosed with glaucoma has more years to go blind from the disease and may warrant more aggressive treatment, such as filtering surgery. A patient with poor compliance or inability to instill eye drops should also be considered for laser or surgical intervention.

CLINICAL TRIALS AND GLAUCOMA MANAGEMENT

Several clinical trials in glaucoma have been completed or are pending completion. Information from these trials should be incorporated into the management of glaucoma patients as it becomes available.

Collaborative Normal-Tension Glaucoma Study

The Collaborative Normal-Tension Glaucoma Study is a completed clinical trial that showed lowering of IOP reduces the rate of glaucoma progression in patients with NTG.[18] One hundred and forty NTG patients (with demonstrated visual field progression or visual field defects threatening fixation, or with new disc hemorrhages) were randomly assigned to an untreated group (n = 79) or to a group being treated with medical or surgical intervention to achieve a 30% reduction in IOP (n = 61). Neither eye of patients in this latter group was treated with beta blockers or adrenergic agonists because of the potential cardiovascular, vasoconstrictive, and crossover effects that could confound the data. Glaucoma progression was seen in 35% of the control eyes versus 12% of the treated eyes. Of the treated group, almost one-half maintained a 30% IOP reduction with topical medication, LTP, or both, without the need for filtering surgery. These results demonstrate that a 30% reduction in IOP slows the rate of progression of NTG. However, 65% of untreated NTG patients showed no progression during a follow-up period of 5 years or more. Additionally, 12% of the NTG patients continued to progress despite a 30% IOP reduction.

Ocular Hypertension Treatment Study

The Ocular Hypertension Treatment Study is an ongoing trial that will determine whether medical reduction of IOP in ocular hypertensive patients reduces the risk of developing glaucomatous nerve or visual field damage. This study will also produce natural history data on developing glaucoma and which patients are most likely to benefit from early treatment.

Early Manifest Glaucoma Trial

The Early Manifest Glaucoma Trial, an ongoing clinical trial, is similar to the Ocular Hypertension Treatment Study, but patients in this trial already have documented early glaucoma damage. Patients are randomized to medical reduction of IOP versus observation. They will be followed with serial visual fields and optic nerve photographs to compare the rate of glaucoma progression.

Glaucoma Laser Trial and Glaucoma Laser Trial Follow-Up Study

The GLT study compared medicines versus ALT as first-line treatment for newly diagnosed glaucoma patients.[19,63] The study has been completed and showed that initial use of ALT was at least as effective as initial use of medicines in lowering IOP and producing stability of optic nerve and visual fields. The Glaucoma Laser Trial Follow-Up Study reported that eyes initially treated by laser had a 1.2-mm HG greater reduction in IOP and a 0.6-dB greater improvement in the visual field compared to the group initially treated with medicines.

Collaborative Initial Glaucoma Treatment Study

The Collaborative Initial Glaucoma Treatment Study is an ongoing clinical trial that compares filtering surgery as an initial treatment of glaucoma to medicines as initial treatment followed by LTP followed by filtering surgery. Quality-of-life issues, such as convenience of treatments and ability to perform daily visual tasks, in addition to visual acuity and field progression, will be monitored throughout the study.

Advanced Glaucoma Intervention Study

A completed clinical trial, the Advanced Glaucoma Intervention Study (AGIS), investigated the next line of therapy when a patient has failed MMT. Patients were randomized to LTP followed by filtering surgery or filtering surgery followed by LTP.[70] If the patient still was not at target IOP or was progressing, the patient underwent a second trabeculectomy procedure. In AGIS, none of the trabeculectomy procedures was performed with antimetabolites, such as 5-fluorouracil or mitomycin C. The results of this trial showed a difference in outcome based on the race of the patient.[71] African-American patients retained better visual acuity and visual fields throughout the study with initial use of LTP followed by filtering surgery. However, white patients had better long-term visual outcome with filtering surgery before LTP after failing MMT. The study was not intended to measure a difference in treatment modalities based on the patient's race, and therefore the treatment groups were not initially matched based on race.[72] Differences in age, degree of glaucoma damage, education, systemic hypertension and diabetes, and cataract status were seen. Also, a significantly greater incidence of cataract development was seen in the group receiving filtering surgery. The impact of cataract formation and the slight differences in the treatment groups based on race may have affected the final outcome of AGIS.

The conclusion of the authors of the study were that African-American patients benefited more from having LTP before filtering surgery after they have exhausted MMT, and white patients did better with filtering surgery before LTP. However, another way to interpret the data from this study is that African-American patients and white patients responded equally well to LTP, but the success rate for filtering surgery is much better in white than in African-American patients. This finding might imply that LTP should be the next line of therapy in both groups (because of fewer potential complications). However, when trabeculectomy is recommended, African Americans are at a greater risk of filter failure that may warrant the adjunctive use of antimetabolites. Antimetabolites are not without additional risks (see Chapter 10), and each case must be individually evaluated.

FUTURE OF GLAUCOMA THERAPY

The future of glaucoma therapy probably will be much different from the traditional approach to lowering IOP. It would be logical to direct our treatment approach to the optic nerve, where glaucoma damage is occurring, and adjunctively lower the IOP if it is elevated. In cases in which IOP does not appear to be a primary contributing factor in the disease process, optic nerve treatment would be the primary therapy. The exact physiologic event causing optic nerve damage is still unknown. The damage may be the result of an insufficient blood supply, a compression of ganglion cell axons, poor structural support of axons, or a release of toxic biochemical substances. Some evidence suggests that once ganglion cell axons are damaged, they release a chemical substance (glutamate or nitric oxide) that may be toxic to remaining healthy axons. This may explain why some glaucoma patients continue to show progressive visual field loss despite achieving low target pressures. Agents are under study that are directed at inhibiting the release of glutamate or other free radical ions via the blockade of the N-methyl-D-aspartate receptors.

Evidence also exists to suggest that glutamate or lack of neurotrophins may trigger a cell process called *apoptosis*. Apoptosis is a process in which the ganglion cell turns on a genetic program that causes the cell to commit suicide. The cell quickly dies without inducing inflammation or leaving any cellular debris. This process seems to fit the glaucoma model of losing axons without inflammation or exudation. Neurotrophins are agents that can inhibit apoptosis, and they are being investigated for use in glaucoma treatment. In the future, we will look to enhance the "survival signals" of the ganglion cells and try to suppress the "death signals."

Our approach to glaucoma in the future may be to combat the disease on different fronts. Genetics has already isolated one gene on chromosome 1 that accounts for up to 3% of glaucoma. Gene therapy may be able to prevent the disease from ever occurring. Agents also exist that alter the sito-skeleton of the trabecular meshwork matrix. These agents can increase aqueous outflow out of the eye.

New technologies may allow us to measure blood flow to the optic nerve. Investigational studies are already in place to examine blood flow enhancers. Agents such as calcium channel blockers dilate blood vessels and may increase blood flow, although systemic side effects of hypotension may limit their effectiveness. Certainly, new agents will be investigated that can increase profusion pressure to the optic nerve.

I am optimistic about the future of glaucoma therapy. It is exciting to be able to combat glaucoma from different fronts (gene therapy, blood-flow enhancers, neuroprotectors) and not just by lowering the IOP. Hopefully, we will be able to identify which glaucoma patients are most likely to benefit from these future therapies. Glaucoma therapy in the future may be specific for the inciting factors causing the disease. Until this new wave of treatments is developed, the clinician still needs to improve diagnostic skills and incorporate new technologies to better diagnose patients with glaucoma. Current treatment for glaucoma will continue to be directed at lowering the IOP. Better therapeutic and surgical modalities will allow us to achieve our target pressures with fewer side effects and complications. Evaluating the effectiveness of our therapies will be directed at serial optic nerve, NFL, and visual field analysis. The vast majority of glaucoma patients will be able to maintain functional vision to accomplish their daily visual tasks. Future technologies and therapies will hopefully eradicate blindness as a sequela of glaucoma.

REFERENCES

1. Hodapp E, Parrish RK, Anderson DR. Clinical Decisions in Glaucoma. St. Louis: Mosby, 1993.

2. Quigley HA, Addicks EM, Green WR. Optic nerve damage in human glaucoma. III. Quantitative correlation of nerve fiber loss and visual field defect in glaucoma, ischemic neuropathy, papilledema, and toxic neuropathy. Arch Ophthalmol 1982;100:135–146.

3. Quigley HA, Dunkelberger BS, Green WR. Retinal ganglion cell atrophy correlated with automated perimetry in human eyes with glaucoma. Am J Ophthalmol 1989;107:453–464.

4. Tielsch JM, Sommer A, Katz J, et al. Racial variations in the prevalence of primary open-angle glaucoma. The Baltimore Eye Survey. JAMA 1991;266:369–374.

5. Sommer A, Tielsch JM, Katz J, et al. Racial differences in the cause-specific prevalence of blindness in East Baltimore. N Engl J Med 1991;325:1412–1417.

6. Tielsch JM, Katz J, Sommer A, et al. Family history and risk of primary open angle glaucoma. The Baltimore Eye Survey. Arch Ophthalmol 1994;112:69–73.

7. Quigley HA, Enger C, Katz J, et al. Risk factors for the development of glaucomatous visual field loss in ocular hypertension. Arch Ophthalmol 1994; 112:644–649.

8. Kitazawa Y, Horie T, Aoki S, et al. Untreated ocular hypertension. A long-term prospective study. Arch Ophthalmol 1977;95:1180–1184.

9. Pohjanpelto PEJ, Palva J. Ocular hypertension and glaucomatous optic nerve damage. Acta Ophthalmol 1974;52:194.

10. Kass MA, Hart WM Jr., Gordon M, et al. Risk factors favoring the development of glaucomatous visual field loss in ocular hypertension. Surv Ophthalmol 1980;25:155–162.

11. Luntz MH, Schenker HI. Retinal vascular accidents in glaucoma and ocular hypertension. Surv Ophthalmol 1980;25:163–167.

12. Chew EY, Trope GE, Mitchell BJ. Diurnal intraocular pressure in young adults with central retinal vein occlusion. Ophthalmology 1987;94:1545–1549.

13. Geerts L, Litwak AB. IOP fluctuation in glaucoma patients. Submitted for publication. 1999.

14. Migdal CS, Hitchings RA. Control of chronic simple glaucoma with primary medical, surgical and laser treatment. Trans Ophthalmol Soc U K 1986;105:653–656.

15. Jay JL, Allan D. The benefit of early trabeculectomy versus conventional management in primary open angle glaucoma relative to severity of disease. Eye 1989;3:528–535.

16. Veldman E, Greve EL. Glaucoma filtering surgery, a retrospective study of 300 operations. Doc Ophthalmol 1987;67:151–170.

17. Johnson DH, Yoshikawa K, Brubaker RF, et al. The effect of long-term medical therapy on the outcome of filtration surgery. Am J Ophthalmol 1994;117:139–148.

18. Collaborative Normal-Tension Glaucoma Study Group. Comparison of glaucomatous progression between untreated patients with normal-tension glaucoma and patients with therapeutically reduced intraocular pressures. Am J Ophthalmol 1998; 126:487–497.

19. Glaucoma Laser Trial Research Group. The Glaucoma Laser Trial (GLT) and Glaucoma Laser Trial Follow-up Study: 7. Results. Am J Ophthalmol 1995;120:718–731.

20. Shingleton B, Richter C, Dharma SK. Long-term efficacy of argon laser trabeculoplasty. A 10-year follow-up study. Ophthalmology 1993;103:1482–1484.

21. Zimmerman TJ, Kaufman HE. Timolol: dose response and duration of action. Arch Ophthalmol 1977;95:605–607.

22. Soll DB. Evaluation of timolol in chronic open-angle glaucoma: once-a-day vs twice-a-day. Arch Ophthalmol 1980;98:2178–2181.

23. Levy NS, Alsbury C. Evaluation of timolol in gellan gum: a new vehicle to extend its duration of action. Ann Ophthalmol Glaucoma 1994;26:166–169.

24. Harris LS, Greenstein MD, Bloom AF. Respiratory difficulties with betaxolol. Am J Ophthalmol 1986;102:274–275.

25. Patel SS, Spencer CM. Latanoprost. A review of its pharmacological properties, clinical efficacy and tolerability in the management of primary open-angle glaucoma and ocular hypertension. Drugs Aging 1996;9:363–378.

26. Alm A, Stjernschantz J. Effects of intraocular pressure and side effects of 0.005% latanoprost applied once daily, evening or morning. A comparison with timolol. Scandinavian Latanoprost Study Group. Ophthalmology 1995;102:1743–1452.

27. Watson PG. Latanoprost. Two years' experience of its use in the United Kingdom. Latanoprost Study Group. Ophthalmology 1998;105:82–87.

28. Hedner J, Svedmyr N, Lunde H, Mandahl A. The lack of respiratory effects of the ocular hypotensive drug latanoprost in patients with moderate steroid-treated asthma. Surv Ophthalmol 1997;41(suppl 2):S111–S115.

29. Watson P, Stjernschantz J. A six-month, randomized, double-masked study comparing latanoprost with timolol in open-angle glaucoma and ocular hypertension. The Latanoprost Study Group. Opthalmology 1996;103:127–137.

30. Johnstone MA. Hypertrichosis and increased pigmentation of eyelashes and adjacent hair in the region of the ipsilateral eyelids of patients treated with unilateral topical latanoprost. Am J Ophthalmol 1997;124:544–547.

31. Rulo AH, Greve EL, Geijssen HC, Hoyng PF. Reduction of intraocular pressure with treatment of latanoprost once daily in patients with normal-pressure glaucoma. Ophthalmology 1996;103:1276–1282.

32. Drance SM, Crichton A, Mills RP. Comparison of the effect of latanoprost 0.005% and timolol 0.5% on the calculated ocular perfusion pressure in patients with normal tension glaucoma. Am J Ophthalmol 1998;125:585–592.

33. Warwar RE, Bullock JD, Ballal D. Cystoid macular edema and anterior uveitis associated with latanoprost use. Experience and incidence in a retrospective review of 94 patients. Ophthalmology 1998;105:262–268.

34. Strier SE. The additive effect of latanoprost 0.005% in patients on maximally tolerated medical therapy. Clin Eye Vis Care 1997;9:189–196.

35. Yoles E, Wheeler LA, Schwartz M. Alpha 2-adrenoreceptor agonists are neuroprotective in a rat model of optic nerve degeneration. Invest Ophthalmol Vis Sci 1999;40:65–73.

36. Walters TR. Development and use of brimonidine in treating acute and chronic elevations of intraocular pressure: a review of safety, efficacy, dose response, and dosing studies. Surv Ophthalmol 1996;41(suppl):S19–S26.

37. Schuman JS. Clinical experience with brimonidine 0.2% and timolol 0.5% in glaucoma and ocular hypertension. Surv Ophthalmol 1996;41(suppl):S27–S37.

38. Burke J, Schwartz M. Preclinical evaluation of brimonidine. Surv Ophthalmol 1996;41(suppl):S9–S18.

39. Shin DH, Glover BK, Cha SC, et al. Long-term brimonidine therapy in glaucoma patients with apraclonidine allergy. Am J Ophthalmol 1999;127:511–515.

40. Nordlund JR, Pasquale LR, Robin AL, et al. The cardiovascular, pulmonary, and ocular hypotensive effects of 0.2% brimonidine. Arch Ophthalmol 1995;113:77–83.

41. Carlesen JO, Zabriskie NA, Kwon YH, et al. Apparent central nervous system depression in infants after the use of topical brimonidine. Am J Ophthalmol 1999;128:255–256.

42. Adkins JC, Balfour JA. Brimonidine. A review of its pharmacological properties and clinical potential in the management of open-angle glaucoma and ocular hypertension. Drugs Aging 1998;12:225–241.

43. Schwartzenberg GW, Buy YM. Efficacy of brimonidine 0.2% as adjunctive therapy for patients with glaucoma inadequately controlled with otherwise maximal medical therapy. Ophthalmology 1999;106:1616–1620.

44. Schuman JS, Horwitz B, Choplin NT, et al. A 1-year study of brimonidine twice daily in glaucoma and ocular hypertension. Arch Ophthalmol 1997;115:847–852.

45. LeBlanc RP. Twelve-month results of an ongoing randomized trial comparing brimonidine tartrate 0.2% and timolol 0.5% given twice daily in patients with glaucoma or ocular hypertension. Brimonidine Study Group 2. Ophthalmology 1998;105:1060–1067.

46. Katz LJ. Brimonidine tartrate 0.2% twice daily vs timolol 0.5% twice daily: 1-year results in glaucoma patients. Brimonidine Study Group. Am J Ophthalmol 1999;127:20–26.

47. Brimonidine-ALT Study Group. Effect of brimonidine 0.5% on intraocular pressure spikes following 360 degree argon laser trabeculoplasty. Ophthalmic Surg Lasers 1995.

48. David R, Spaeth GL, Clevenger CE, et al. Brimonidine in the prevention of intraocular pressure elevation following argon laser trabeculoplasty. Arch Ophthalmol 1993;111:1387–1390.

49. Barnebey HS, Robin AL, Zimmerman TJ, et al. The efficacy of brimonidine in decreasing elevations in intraocular pressure after laser trabeculoplasty. Ophthalmology 1993;100:1083–1088.

50. Barnes SD, Campagna JA, Dirks MS, Doe EA. Control of intraocular pressure elevations after argon laser trabeculoplasty: comparison of brimonidine 0.2% to apraclonidine 1.0%. Ophthalmology 1999;106:2033–2037.

51. Robin AL. Effects of ALO 2145 on intraocular pressure following argon laser trabeculoplasty. Arch Ophthalmol 1987;105:646–650.

52. Chung HS, Shin DH, Birt CM, et al. Chronic use of apraclonidine decreases its moderation of post-laser intraocular pressure spikes. Ophthalmology 1997;104:1921–1925.

53. Maus TL, Larsson LI, McLaren JW, Brubaker RF. Comparison of dorzolamide and acetazolamide as suppressors of aqueous humor flow in humans. Arch Ophthalmol 1997;115:45–49.

54. Egan CA, Hodge DO, McLaren JW, Bourne WM. Effect of dorzolamide on corneal endothelial function in normal human eyes. Invest Ophthalmol Vis Sci 1998;39:23–29.

55. Kaminski S, Hommer A, Koyuncu D, et al. Influence of dorzolamide on corneal thickness, endothelial cell count and corneal sensitivity. Acta Ophthalmol Scand 1998;76:78–79.

56. Laibovita R, Boyle J, Snyder E, et al. Dorzolamide versus pilocarpine as adjunctive therapies to timolol: a comparison of patient preference and impact on daily life. Clin Ther 1996;18:821–832.

57. Strahlman ER, Vogel R, Tipping R, Clineschmidt CM. The use of dorzolamide and pilocarpine as adjunctive therapy to timolol in patients with elevated intraocular pressure. Dorzolamide Additivity Study Group. Ophthalmology 1996;103:1283–1293.

58. Wayman L, Larsson LI, Maus T, et al. Comparison of dorzolamide and timolol as suppressors of aqueous humor flow in humans. Arch Ophthalmol 1997;115:1368–1371.

59. Rosenberg LF, Krupin T, Tang LQ, et al. Combination of systemic acetazolamide and topical sorzolamide in reducing intraocular pressure and aqueous humor formation. Ophthalmology 1998;105:88–92.

60. Hutzelmann J, Owens S, Shedden A, et al. Comparison of the safety and efficacy of the fixed combination of dorzolamide/timolol and the concomitant administration of dorzolamide and timolol: a clinical equivalence study. International Clinical Equivalence Study Group. Br J Ophthalmol 1998;82:1249–1253.

61. Silver LH. Clinical efficacy and safety of brinzolamide (Azopt), a new topical carbonic anhydrase inhibitor for primary open-angle glaucoma and ocular hypertension. Brinzolamide Primary Therapy Study Group. Am J Ophthalmol 1998;126:400–408.

62. Allen RC, Epstein DL. Additive effect of betaxolol and epinephrine in primary open angle glaucoma. Arch Ophthalmol 1986;104:1178–1184.

63. Glaucoma Laser Trial Research Group. The Glaucoma Laser Trial (GLT). Results of argon laser trabeculoplasty versus topical medicines. Ophthalmology 1990;97(11):1403–1413.

64. Greenidge KC, Spaeth GL, Fiol-Silva Z. Effect of argon laser trabeculoplasty on the glaucomatous diurnal curve. Ophthalmology 1983;90(7): 800–804.

65. Honrubia FM, Ferrer EJ, Leciñena J, Torron C, Gomez ML. Long term follow-up of the argon laser trabeculoplasty in eyes treated 180 degrees and 360 degrees of the trabeculum. Int Ophthalmol 1992;16(4–5):375–379.

66. Threlkeld AB, Assalian AA, Allingham RR, et al. Apraclonidine 0.5% versus 1% for controlling intraocular pressure elevation after argon laser trabeculoplasty. Ophthalmic Surg Lasers 1996;27:657–660.

67. David R, Spaeth GL, Clevenger CE, et al. Brimonidine in the prevention of intraocular pressure elevation following argon laser trabeculoplasty. Arch Ophthalmol 1993;111(10):1387–1390.

68. Spaeth GL, Baez KA. Argon laser trabeculoplasty controls one third of cases of progressive, uncontrolled, open angle glaucoma for 5 years. Arch Ophthalmol 1992;110:491–494.

69. Richter CU, Shingleton BJ, Bellows AR, et al. Retreatment with argon laser trabeculoplasty. Ophthalmology 1987;94(9):1085–1089.

70. Advanced Glaucoma Intervention Study (AGIS). 1. Study design and methods and baseline characteristics of study patients. Control Clin Trials 1994; 15:299–325.

71. Advanced Glaucoma Intervention Study (AGIS). 4. Comparison of treatment outcomes with race. Seven year results. Ophthalmology 1998;105:1146–1164.

72. Advanced Glaucoma Intervention Study (AGIS). 3. Baseline characteristics of black and white patients. Ophthalmology 1998;105:1137–1145.

Follow-Up Schedule

Anthony B. Litwak

The follow-up schedule for glaucoma patients (Tables 12-1 to 12-5) is based on the severity of damage to the optic nerve (interpreted through optic nerve, nerve fiber layer [NFL], and visual field assessment), the achievement of a target intraocular pressure (IOP), and the stability of the optic nerve and visual field status. Tables 12-1 to 12-5 are meant only to give the clinician guidelines for monitoring glaucoma patients. Glaucoma management and follow-up should be individualized for each patient.

Determining the stability of glaucoma requires establishing accurate baseline data. This should include baseline IOP off medications (at least three readings), stereoscopic optic disc photographs, NFL photographs, and baseline visual fields. The majority of patients exhibit a visual field learning curve (see Figure 7-6). It is important to identify visual field learning curves and to discard these tests when establishing a visual field baseline. Some patients may require two or more visual field tests to establish a reliable, accurate baseline, and some patients may not be able to provide accurate visual field results. The easiest visual field testing program should be used for patients who are poor visual field testers. Swedish Interactive Thresholding Algorithm (SITA), SITA Fast, or FASTPAC testing strategies or frequency-doubling perimetry should be chosen instead of Full Threshold strategy, and a 24-2 pattern should be used instead of a 30-2 testing pattern (see Figures 7-3 and 7-7).

Patients who cannot perform reliable visual field tests require comparison of stereoscopic optic nerve and NFL photographs to follow progression. This technique may not be as sensitive in determining glaucoma progression and therefore may necessitate a 10% further reduction of the calculated target pressure. The clinician should correlate the visual field loss with the optic nerve status to determine accuracy of the visual field result. A visual field result that does not correlate to the amount of optic nerve and NFL damage should be suspected as an unreliable visual field test. SITA threshold testing greatly improves the efficiency of obtaining reliable baseline visual fields because of the shorter testing times compared with Full Threshold testing. Newly diagnosed glaucoma or glaucoma suspect patients are started on SITA threshold testing if available. If the patient is unreliable on SITA testing or is a poor visual field candidate, then the SITA Fast threshold strategy should be used.

It is important not to compare visual field tests using different testing strategies. Full Threshold, FAST-PAC, SITA, and SITA Fast should not be intermixed when making interpretations. The 30-2 and 24-2 test patterns should also not be intermixed when making interpretations (see Chapter 7).

MANAGEMENT OF A NEWLY DIAGNOSED GLAUCOMA PATIENT

After a patient is diagnosed with glaucoma and the baseline IOP and the degree of glaucoma damage are established, a target pressure is set (see Chapter 11). In most cases, medical therapy is chosen as first-line treatment. Medications should be instituted one at a time, starting with the lowest concentration. An exception to this practice would be a patient with endstage disease and extremely elevated IOP, who would require multiple medications to achieve a desirable target pressure. In this case, the patient may be started on two or three

TABLE 12-1. Follow-Up Schedule for a Newly Diagnosed Glaucoma Patient Once a Target Pressure Is Set

Degree of damage	Follow-up visit for intra-ocular pressure check
Mild	Within 1 mo
Moderate	Within 2–3 wks
Severe	Within 1 wk

TABLE 12-4. Follow-Up Schedule for a Progressing Glaucoma Patient Once a New Target Pressure Is Set

Degree of damage	Follow-up visit for intra-ocular pressure check
Mild	Within 1 mo
Moderate*	Within 2–3 wks
Severe*	Within 1 wk

*Progressing patients with moderate to severe damage should be considered candidates for glaucoma filtering surgery.

medicines and followed on a daily basis. Most non-end-stage patients are asked to return in 1–4 weeks depending on the degree of damage and the amount of IOP lowering required (see Table 12-1). If there is a 20% decrease from the highest baseline pressure reading but the patient is not at the desired target pressure, then a higher concentration of the initial medication (e.g., timolol 0.25% to timolol 0.5%) can be used or a second medication can be added. The same follow-up schedule (see Table 12-1) is used. If there is not a 20% decrease from the highest baseline IOP reading and the patient has been correctly taking medications, then either a second IOP reading should be obtained (especially if a wide diurnal fluctuation of the baseline IOP was seen), or the medication should be switched because of limited effectiveness. This is one of the most important reasons to take at least three IOP readings before the initiation of medicines to help establish how much diurnal fluctuation is present. If multiple baseline IOP measurements are not performed, then many medications may be deemed nonresponsive, when, in fact, the medication was effective but masked by a diurnal spike in the patient's pressure.

If little change is noted after several comparisons of IOP while the patient is on and off medication, then beta blockers can be changed to other beta blockers. In general, timolol, levobutanol and timolol hemihydrate (Betimol) are slightly more effective than carteolol, metipranolol, or betaxolol. Beta blockers can also be switched to other classes of medications, such as the prostaglandins or α agonists. The same follow-up process is instituted. In general, I look for a 20–30% reduction in IOP from the highest baseline pressure reading from primary therapy and at least a 15–20% reduction for adjunctive therapy.

At each follow-up visit, it is important to establish when the patient last took the medication, whether the patient has been compliant with the dosing schedule, and whether the patient is experiencing any side effects or has any concerns. The patient is probably most likely to be compliant with medications on the day of the doctor's visit. This may explain why some patients show documented progression of disease despite seemingly good IOP control. The clinician must investigate for possible poor compliance. Patients with early or moderate optic nerve damage are typically more symptomatic from the side effects of medications than from the disease. Thus, patients may discontinue their medications without their doctor's knowledge. Determining compliance is discussed in Chapter 13.

TABLE 12-2. Follow-Up Schedule for a Newly Diagnosed Glaucoma Patient Once a Target Pressure Is Achieved

Degree of damage	Intraocular pressure check	Dilated fundus examination	Visual fields*
Mild	q4mo	q1yr	q1yr
Moderate	q3mo	q6–12mo	q6–12mo
Severe	q2mo	q6mo	q6mo

*After baseline visual fields are established.

TABLE 12-3. Follow-Up Schedule for a Stable Glaucoma Patient*

Degree of damage	Intraocular pressure check	Dilated fundus examination	Visual fields
Mild	q4–6mo	q1yr	q1yr
Moderate	q3–4mo	q9–12mo	q9–12mo
Severe	q3mo	q6–12 mo	q6–12mo

*Stable is defined as no documented optic nerve or visual field progression over last year of follow-up and intraocular pressure at desired target pressure. Gonioscopy and stereoscopic disc photographs should be performed every 1–2 years.

TABLE 12-5. Follow-Up Schedule for a Progressing Glaucoma Patient after a New Target Intraocular Pressure Is Achieved

Degree of damage	Intraocular pressure check	Dilated fundus examination	Visual fields
Mild	q3mo	q6mo	q6mo
Moderate	q2–3mo	q4–6mo	q4–6mo
Severe	q1–2mo	q3–6mo	q3–6mo

After baseline visual field data are obtained and the desired target IOP is achieved, the newly diagnosed glaucoma patient should be seen at 2–4 month intervals for IOP checks (see Table 12-2). If the desired target IOP is not obtained, then changing or adding medications and laser trabeculoplasty should be contemplated. The patient should have repeat tonometry readings within 1 month if the desired target pressure is not satisfied. More advanced glaucoma damage should be followed within 1 week if the desired target pressure is not achieved.

Dilation of the pupils in a newly diagnosed glaucoma patient is performed every 6–12 months after the initial diagnosis. Dilation should be scheduled to occur after a recent visual field test has been performed, so that the doctor can correlate the visual field results with the optic nerve and NFL appearance. If the glaucoma damage is classified as *moderate* or *severe*, then the repeat visual field test is scheduled for 6 months. If the damage is mild to moderate, then the repeat visual field should be performed yearly (see Table 12-3).

Gonioscopy should be performed initially and on a yearly basis for all glaucoma patients or suspects. If the patient has narrow angles or has recently started pilocarpine, then gonioscopy should be performed at each visit. Patients with cataracts may exhibit swelling of the lenses resulting in a forward displacement, shallowing of the anterior chamber, and narrowing of the angle. These patients may become candidates for laser peripheral iridotomy (see Chapter 16). Patients at risk for angle neovascularization (e.g., status post central retinal vein occlusion, proliferation diabetic retinopathy) or peripheral anterior synechia (e.g., history of chronic or recurrent iritis) should have gonioscopy performed at each visit (see Chapters 15 and 17).

Stereoscopic optic disc photographs should be performed every 2 years or sooner if a change to the optic nerve is suspected. If the visual field test has shown progression, I also take photographs to establish a new baseline for subsequent comparisons. Clinically, visual field testing is more sensitive in uncovering glaucoma progression than serial optic nerve comparisons. However, approximately 10% of patients show progression on serial comparison of optic nerve photographs without a confirmable visual field change.[1] There are two other caveats: Some patients cannot perform reliable visual fields and some patients will just have a "bad" visual field day. It is therefore prudent to always repeat the visual field to confirm progression.

FOLLOW-UP SCHEDULE FOR AN ESTABLISHED, STABLE GLAUCOMA PATIENT

When a patient has had 1 year of follow-up from the initial diagnosis, the target pressures have been achieved, and the optic nerve and visual field status is stable, then the patient can be followed at slightly longer intervals. IOP checks are usually scheduled every 3–6 months, whereas dilated examination of the optic nerves and NFL and visual field testing are repeated once or twice a year, depending on the severity of damage (see Table 12-3).

FOLLOW-UP SCHEDULE FOR AN ESTABLISHED PROGRESSING GLAUCOMA PATIENT

If progression of glaucoma has been documented by visual field or optic nerve comparisons, then compliance with medications must be explored (see Chapter 13). If compliance has been poor, then re-education with medications or laser or surgical intervention should be considered. If compliance is good, then more aggressive therapy should be instituted. The new target pressure should be lowered an additional 20–30%. At a minimum, I try to achieve target pressures lower than 15 mm Hg in a patient with moderate to severe damage and lower than 18 mm Hg in a patient with mild to moderate damage. These target pressures may need to be lower depending on what level of IOP has caused the patient's disease to progress. IOP lowering may be achieved by additional medications, laser trabeculoplasty, or surgical trabeculectomy. Patients with moderate or severe glaucoma damage should be considered for trabeculectomy if progression of the disease has been documented. Trabeculectomy should not be delayed until the patient has only tunnel visual fields remaining. The potential complications of filtering surgery must be considered and discussed with the patient (see Chapter 10), but a patient progressing into moderate or severe glaucoma damage despite medical therapy is a strong candidate for surgical intervention.

The follow-up schedule for a patient who is progressing should be based on the severity of glaucoma damage and the difference between current IOP and the new, desired target IOP (see Tables 12-4 and 12-5). Treatment modifications should be initiated after the confirming visual field test to establish a new baseline for future comparisons. Tonometry checks should be scheduled within 1 month after a new target IOP is set and within 1 week if the patient has moderate to severe damage. Patients with mild to moderate loss should have visual field testing repeated in 6 months, and patients with moderate to severe loss should have visual field testing repeated in 3–6 months.

Flow charts are an excellent device for summarizing patient data over a period of time (Figure 12-1). The charts used in our clinic have spaces to record the date and time of the appointment, the patient's IOP, the calculated target pressure, current medications, and the last time the medications were used. These serial recordings allow the doctor to judge the effectiveness of medications and the level of IOP correlated with the stability or progression of the optic nerve and visual field. This information is invaluable in determining the effectiveness of therapy and establishing a new target IOP.

There are also spaces on the flow chart to record the stereoscopic assessment of the optic nerve (cup-to-disc ratio, size of the optic disc), the grading of the retinal NFL, and gonioscopy. The dates of the visual fields, disc photographs, and dilated fundus examination are also recorded. This allows the doctor at a glance to decide which tests need to be scheduled or performed. An area is also marked on the flow chart to record systemic or ocular conditions, contraindications to medications, and allergic reactions. Under a "comments" section, information concerning compliance or side effects from medications can be recorded.

DETERMINING PROGRESSION

Determining progression of glaucoma damage is one of the most arduous tasks of glaucoma management. The most important aspect of determining progression is to obtain accurate baseline data. This includes baseline visual field testing (learning-curve adjusted) and stereoscopic optic disc photography. The optic disc photographs are routinely repeated every 2 years. If the suspicion for progression is high or if the patient is an unreliable visual field tester, then the photographs should be repeated yearly. The photographs should be a stereoscopic pair and viewed with a stereo viewer on a light box. The clinician should note the contour of the neuroretinal rim tissue and estimate the amount of remaining tissue, especially in the superior and inferior temporal poles of the optic nerve. The photographs should be viewed at the time of the dilated fundus examination to judge for changes. However, viewing a series of photographs side by side makes it easier to determine change than judging prior photographs with the clinical examination of the optic nerve.

Judging progression by comparing recorded cup-to-disc ratios in the patient's chart suffers from poor interobserver variability. A skilled observer using the same stereoscopic technique may be able to detect change by comparing a recorded disc drawing, but the accuracy is always better if photographs are compared (see Color Plate 28). Therefore, stereoscopic optic disc photographs are an essential part of following glaucoma patients for progression. Changes in the NFL can also be documented by comparing the color optic disc photographs, but black-and-white photographs are usually much easier to evaluate (see Figure 6-14). Appearance of a disc hemorrhage (Drance hemorrhage) is also an objective sign of glaucoma progression (see Color Plate 26).

Serial visual field testing remains the primary method to determine glaucoma progression. However, unlike comparing optic disc or NFL photographs for change, which is objective, the interpretation of serial visual fields for progression is much more difficult. For a full description of determining visual field progression, see Chapter 7.

Several variables must be understood in visual field analysis. First, patients exhibit learning curves, which may mean that two or more visual field tests are necessary to establish a baseline (see Figure 7-6). Second, patients can have a bad visual field day (fatigue artifacts) that is not related to the disease (see Figure 7-13). This usually shows improvement with repeat testing. Third, glaucoma patients, especially those with advanced loss, have higher short- and long-term fluctuations in visual field tests and tend to demonstrate wide variability that is not necessarily a sign of progression (see Figure 7-27). The Glaucoma Change Probability (GCP) program in the Humphrey STATPAC analysis attempts to compensate for long-term fluctuation (LTF) in glaucoma patients. This program uses the first two visual fields to create a baseline and then compares all subsequent field with this baseline. The program contains a database of age-matched controlled glaucoma patients. Comparing the amount of change in the patient's visual field with the amount of LTF in an age-matched stable glaucoma patient can help determine whether the patient's field is progressing or just exhibiting LTF (see Figure 7-28). The GCP is limited to a rather small database of controlled glaucoma patients. Glaucoma patients with very mild or very severe visual field loss are not included in the database. Thus, a small "x" can appear in the GCP printout, which indicates that there are not enough patients in the database to determine a statistical probability of whether a point is progressing (see Figure 7-29).

When comparing serial visual fields, it is important to incorporate the same testing strategy in each test. Switching from a Full Threshold strategy to SITA testing may show an apparent improvement in the visual field due to lower patient fatigue (see Figure 7-7). Likewise, a 24-2 test tends to show an improved visual field

GLAUCOMA FLOW SHEETS

Name _____ DOB _____ ID number _____

Diagnosis: _____ Risk Factors: _____

Date/Time	Medications/Time	IOP		Target		C/D		
		OD	OS	OD	OS	OD	OS	
								Vertical Disc Diameter with 60D:
								Gonioscopy:
								NFL:
								Laser/Surgery:
								Dates of DFE:
								Dates of Visual Fields:
								Dates of Photographs:

CONTRAINDICATIONS:	COMMENTS:
INTOLERANCE:	

FIGURE 12-1. Glaucoma flow charts. Flow charts are a convenient way to document the vital characteristics of the glaucoma or glaucoma suspect patient. Included are serial tonometry readings; recording target pressures; current glaucoma medications; gonioscopy results; cup-to-disc (C/D) ratios; optic disc size; nerve fiber layer (NFL) grading; and dates of dilated fundus examinations (DFE), visual fields, stereoscopic photos, and laser or surgical procedures. Also included is a "comments" section to document contraindications or side effects from medicines, allergies, and poor compliance. (DOB = date of birth; IOP = intraocular pressure; OD = right eye; OS = left eye.)

TABLE 12-6. Reviewing the Visual Field to Determine
  Progression

1. Print out overview of all fields.

   - Inspect for reliability.

   - Determine when target pressure is reached and
     exclude prior fields.

   - Select two or three fields to form a baseline.

   - Inspect grayscales and probability plots for worsening.

   - Correlate suspected areas with threshold values.

2. Print out glaucoma change probability analysis after
   selecting appropriate baseline tests.

   - Review grayscale and total deviation plots again.

   - Review difference in dB from baseline and identify
     nonedge points (include four most nasal points)
     that have decreased by 10 dB.

   - Correlate suspected points with change probability plot;
     two or three contiguous points are a significant cluster.

3. Suspected defect should be present on a minimum of two
   successive fields.

compared with a 30-2 test (see Figure 7-3). This phenomenon is believed to be due to less stressing (fatiguing) of
the damaged ganglion cell axon when a shorter and easier
testing strategy is used. It is important to always use the
same testing pattern and strategy when making visual
field comparisons. If a new test strategy is used, then a
new baseline must be established for future comparisons.

To account for these discrepancies in visual field
interpretation, the clinician should scrutinize the first
several visual fields to uncover a learning curve
improvement and discard these early visual fields. If this
is not done, then subsequent visual fields may be interpreted as being much better than they actually are. If a
visual field looks as if it is getting worse, it should
always be repeated. Patients can have a bad testing day
for a variety of reasons, including not feeling well, not
being well rested, and feeling anxious about the test.
Accounting for changes in pupil size (start of miotic
therapy) or changes in media opacities (cataracts) is
also important. Glaucoma patients, especially those
with advanced disease, exhibit high short- and long-
term fluctuation between points, and differentiating this
from actual progression can be difficult.

The criteria for determining visual field progression
(Table 12-6; see Chapter 7) should incorporate interpretation of both the overview and GCP printouts. First, all of
the visual fields should be printed in the overview mode
and inspected for reliability. Unreliable visual fields (determined by reliability indexes) and learning curves should
be removed from the analysis. Avoid mixing 24-2 and 30-
2 patterns or using different threshold strategies (e.g., Full
Threshold with SITA or FASTPAC). The clinical history
should be reviewed to determine when the most recent

target pressure was achieved, and baseline fields should be
selected that correspond to that time. Next, changes in the
grayscale and the total and pattern probability plots
should be reviewed. Remember that once points in the
probability plots have declined to a P value of <.5%, the
probability plots will not show any further progression.
However, the grayscales and the numeric values can be
followed until the numeric values decline to 0 dB.

The GCP should also be printed out using the
appropriate baseline visual fields determined from the
overview inspection. The grayscale and the total deviation
plots should be reviewed. The "change in decibels from
baseline" plot for follow-up fields should be examined,
and nonedge, contiguous points that have decreased by at
least 10 decibels should be identified. Correlate these
points to the change probability plots. Consider two or
three contiguous P values <5% (dark triangles) points as
necessary to form a significant cluster. Beware of the small
letter "x" in the GCP plot indicating that there are not
enough points in the database to make a statistical comparison. In these cases, look at the "change in decibels
from baseline plot" and locate the corresponding value. A
change of 10 dB or more that is not an edge point should
be viewed as a significant change. Any suggestion of
visual field loss progression should be confirmed with at
least two and preferably three visual field tests. Despite all
this effort, whether the field is stable or has progressed
may not be clearly evident. In addition to reviewing the
visual fields, the clinician should also evaluate the corresponding IOPs during the corresponding time interval, as
well as optic nerve and NFL appearance, and compliance
with medications and follow-up. In the final analysis, the
clinician's judgment must determine whether the patient's
disease is stable or progressing.

SUMMARY

Glaucoma management and follow-up should be individualized for each patient. It should be designed based on
the severity of the disease, the stability of progression,
and the response to treatment. Glaucoma management
also includes patient education, maintaining compliance,
and monitoring for side effects and other related issues
(cost, dosing schedule, visual demands) that may affect
the patient's quality of life. When indicated, referral for
surgical or second opinion, social services counseling,
blind rehabilitation, or low-vision consultation should be
provided.

REFERENCE

1. Collaborative Normal Tension Glaucoma
Study Group. Comparison of glaucomatous progression between untreated patients with normal tension
glaucoma and patients with therapeutically reduced
intraocular pressures. Am J Opthalmol 1999;127:120.

Maintaining Compliance and Patient Education

Paul C. Ajamian and Steven J. Boeyink

Compliance with medical therapy is an issue that should be of constant concern for health professionals in many fields. The problem is especially critical for eye doctors who manage patients with glaucoma, because the nature of this particular disease fosters noncompliance. Patients are usually asymptomatic in the early, moderate, and sometimes even advanced stages of their disease. Patients with glaucoma do not get better, and they may get worse despite the best efforts of the clinician. Patients expect some benefit from medication, either in the form of improved vision or comfort, but rarely achieve it. When patients feel they do not benefit from a medication, they may ignore our instructions and can potentially lose visual function because of it. Too often it is incorrectly assumed that writing a prescription is a guarantee that eye drops will get into a patient's eyes. Despite the impressive array of antiglaucoma medications available, they are of little value if the patient does not follow the recommended regimen.

On the positive side, glaucoma is a disease that can be treated effectively, with most patients retaining adequate sight throughout their lives. With proper diagnosis, treatment, and patient education, eye doctors can play a major role in the positive outcomes of many glaucoma patients. Because medical intervention is still the main form of therapy, practitioners must use their influence to be sure that eye drops are instilled in a proper and timely manner. However, all patients are potential defaulters.[1] We can never assume that compliance will simply happen. To this end, patient education and a solid doctor-patient relationship are the most critical but most often overlooked components of glaucoma management. This chapter reviews the epidemiology of noncompliance, along with the reasons for noncompliance and the clinical detection of the problem. Methods for improving compliance are examined, including patient tips and office protocols.

DEFINING THE PROBLEM

Compliance is defined as the degree to which patients adhere to their doctor's advice. *Noncompliance* lies along a spectrum of increasing deviation from the intended treatment plan. Just how much a patient must deviate from the prescribed plan to be considered noncompliant is debatable. Some think that one missed dose per month is technically noncompliance, and others give patients the freedom to make a few mistakes and reserve the term for regular offenders. These differences in definition yield different estimates of the magnitude of the noncompliance problem.

ESTIMATES OF INCIDENCE

The exact magnitude of noncompliance in glaucoma will never be known, but clinical experience and a review of the literature indicates that it probably lies somewhere between 25% and 50%. Kass has done a number of compliance studies.[2–7] His group found that 24% of patients on pilocarpine were noncompliant, whereas those on timolol were noncompliant in 18% of cases.[3,4] An interesting finding in this study was that the average patient on q.i.d. therapy instilled an average of only 2.6 drops per day.[3] Vincent found that 58% of his patients were noncompliant.[8] A similar finding of 59% noncompliance was reported by Chang and associates in a study of compliance caps and their effect on drop usage.[9] A comprehensive study of aging and its effect on compliance showed that a large study population did not take prescribed therapy for 30% of the 12-month follow-up period.[10] An interesting finding within this study was that patients with more complex ocular medication schedules actually showed *greater* compliance, perhaps because the severity of their condition had been impressed on them more than it is on the average patient. No matter how compliance is measured or what the incidence really is, we know that noncompliance is a significant problem for doctors who manage or comanage glaucoma.

FORMS OF NONCOMPLIANCE

A noncompliant patient is one who fails to follow his or her physician's advice. Specifically, this treatment failure can be broken down into at least five different forms:

1. **Failure to take medication as often as prescribed.** Failure to take medication is what most people think of as noncompliance, which includes missing doses, cessation of treatment, and the inability to get the drop into the eye.

2. **Improper dose timing.** Improper timing often occurs because patients are not aware of the duration of action of their medication and instill drops when it is most convenient for them based on their lifestyle. This is especially prevalent with those medications requiring more frequent instillation. A study using an electronic medication monitor showed that patients tended to skip their noon dose and to space the other doses closer together, apparently to make it easier to remember those doses.[11] The problem of dosage timing underscores the need for the practitioner to be flexible when recommending times that drops be instilled, and creative in tying those instillations to daily activities, such as meals, brushing teeth, waking up, and going to bed.

3. **Excessive use of medication.** Excessive medicating often occurs because patients aren't explicitly told to take a single drop, and they adopt the "more is better" strategy. This can also include patients with poor instillation technique who waste drops in an effort to get at least one dose into the eye.

4. **Taking the medication for the wrong reason.** This form of noncompliance could include patients using glaucoma medications to treat their red, itchy eyes or using a previously purchased bottle of tetrahydrozoline hydrochloride (Visine) or antibiotic to treat their glaucoma before obtaining their next glaucoma prescription refill.

5. **Filling prescriptions.** A certain percentage of patients never get the initial prescription filled because of the cost of the medication or the lack of perceived need to take it. Others do not make the effort to refill a prescription when the bottle is empty because the patient experienced no benefit from the first bottle of drops. These patients are also less likely to keep their follow-up appointments. These patients often return several years later with symptoms of vision loss from severe progression of their disease.

DETECTING NONCOMPLIANCE

An interesting finding that has emerged from various studies is that doctors are very poor at determining which of their patients are noncompliant. Aside from asking the patient outright, most methods of detection are not ideal in their accuracy, practicality, or objectivity. Patients may also try to avoid detection by taking drops just before an office visit.

The most common techniques for detecting noncompliance are[12]:

- Patient interview
- Clinical outcome
- Calculation of drops used and prescriptions filled

Patient Interview

Although not always reliable, the patient interview is probably the most practical method for assessing compliance in the clinical setting. Kass and colleagues interviewed 141 patients and reported that they admitted to missing only 3% of drop administrations.[5] In other studies, 31–50% of patients admitted incorrect or inadequate use of medications.[8,13] From this, it can be assumed that many patients do not acknowledge their missed treatments. Appropriate interviewing techniques can still be very valuable, however, in assessing noncompliance and bringing the truth to light. Open-ended questions rather than statements are helpful: "How are you using your drops, Mrs. Jones?" may be a more useful question than "Are you still taking your yellow-top drop twice a day?" More specific questions can help in eliciting other forms of noncompliance, such as improper spacing, excessive treatment, and improper instillation technique. The Kass study found major differences between patient accounts of how medication was used and direct observation of actual instillation. This finding emphasizes the value of watching patients instill the drops on occasion and reviewing instillation techniques on follow-up visits.

Clinical Outcome

Monitoring clinical results, both objectively and subjectively, is probably the best way to detect noncompliance. This involves careful evaluation of the optic nerve, visual field changes, and intraocular pressure (IOP) from visit to visit. Determining glaucoma control with IOP readings alone can be misleading, because some patients may only take the medications on the day of the doctor's visit. If the IOP is at or below the desired target pressure, yet progression of cupping or field defects is noted, poor compliance may be the cause. When the desired target pressure has been achieved and the IOP is uncharacteristically elevated on follow-up visits, then noncompliance is also possible. However, this can be difficult to distinguish from loss of effect of medication or from diurnal fluctuations that are known to commonly occur in patients with glaucoma.

Another way to determine compliance is the observation of secondary effects of a certain medication. For example, cholinergic agents, such as pilocarpine, cause fixed, miotic pupils. Epinephrine drugs, such as dipivefrin, can result in adrenochrome deposits in the lower palpebral conjunctiva with chronic use.

Calculation of Drops Used and Prescriptions Filled

In a study by Gurwitz et al., prescription fills were monitored within the New Jersey Medicaid system. It was revealed that the average patient was without therapy for 112 days of the year.[10] Another study used an electronic medication monitor to record the installation of drops by patients on pilocarpine.[6] Although this concept is interesting, affording total objectivity, such studies are very impractical in all but research settings. Another method of assessing compliance is the diligent recording of refill requests in the patient's record. This can be valuable information, but it requires the assistance of office staff and often is not practical. The simplest method for determining whether refills have been dispensed is to stay in close touch with the patient's pharmacist. Ask the pharmacist when the last refill was dispensed, and whether the patient picks up refills on a monthly basis. Recent federal legislation encourages more active involvement by pharmacists in patient counseling and compliance, so many pharmacists may be willing to provide you with this information.

REASONS FOR NONCOMPLIANCE

A reason almost always exists, legitimate or otherwise, for noncompliance, and it is the doctor's duty to make an earnest effort to ascertain and address those issues.

Some of the most common causes of noncompliance are:

1. Side effects (ocular and systemic)
2. Cost
3. Frequency of instillation
4. Lack of understanding of disease and medication instructions
5. Use of multiple medical conditions (polypharmacy)
6. Miscellaneous factors

Side Effects

Many patients complain of bothersome ocular side effects of topical glaucoma medications, the most common being stinging and redness. Dry-eye patients who experience symptoms *before* glaucoma therapy may notice an exacerbation of symptoms once glaucoma drops are added. In a study involving patients with pigmentary glaucoma,[14] 80% of those on timolol, 82% on dipivefrin, and 100% on pilocarpine reported adverse effects. These effects, when combined with the absence of any observable benefit, may discourage patients from complying.

Systemic absorption of topical glaucoma medications can result in a variety of side effects (see Chapter 8). It is important to continually reinforce the reasons for taking glaucoma medications. The patient should be taught that vision loss from glaucoma is never regained, and the purpose of the medications is to preserve the remaining vision. The doctor should also warn the patient of potential ocular and systemic symptoms from the medications. Patients should be encouraged to report side effects immediately so that medications can be adjusted in a timely manner. On each visit, review the progressive nature of glaucoma and emphasize that the disease is being controlled with ongoing use of the drops.

Cost

Cost can be a major factor in patient noncompliance and can be addressed to some extent by the substitution of "interchangeable" medications. Examples include prescribing a lower-cost beta blocker as the first-line drug. Generics are more commonly being substituted for brand names, even if "dispense as written" or "brand necessary" is indicated. Be aware that there is a great deal of price variation between pharmacies, making it worthwhile to do an occasional telephone-shopping comparison so that patients can be steered in the right direction. Drop size and number of drops per bottle, which determine how long a bottle lasts, also vary significantly (Table 13-1). For those not able to afford medication, patient assistance programs are available through the large pharmaceutical companies, assuming the patient meets certain financial criteria. An open discussion with patients about the cost of medications is important so that they can be made aware of these resources. General questions, such as "Are you able to get your medicine, Mrs. Jones? I know the drops are fairly expensive," or "If I prescribed a less expensive medication, would that help?" can lead to the discovery that the patient is having problems affording the drug(s). Managed care has altered the way we prescribe medication as well. We may hesitate to prescribe a prostaglandin analog because of its cost, but if the patient is on a drug plan as part of a health

TABLE 13-1. Cost Comparison of Glaucoma Medications

Product	Labeled volume (ml)	Actual volume (ml)	Drops/ ml	Drops/ bottle	Drops/ day	Days/ bottle	Cost ($) (Average wholesale price)	Cost ($)/ day	Estimated intraocular pressure decrease (mm Hg)	Cost/mm Hg of decrease/ 30 days
Newer agents										
Latanoprost (Xalatan)	2.5	3.0	34.5	103.5	1	51.75	42.48	0.82	8.4	2.93
Brimonidine (Alphagan)	10.0	10.2	25.4	259.08	2	64.77	48.00	0.74	6.48	3.43
Dorzolamide hydrochloride (Trusopt)	5.0	5.5	26.3	144.65	2	36.16	22.64	0.63	4.8	3.94
Beta blockers										
Levobunolol hydrochloride (Betagan 0.5%)	5.0	5.2	20.4	106.08	2	26.52	19.99	0.75	6.72	3.35
Timolol maleate (Timoptic 0.5%)	5.0	5.4	37.9	204.66	2	51.17	19.79	0.39	6.72	1.74
Timolol hemihydrate (Betimol 0.5%)	5.0	5.4	26.3	142.02	2	35.51	13.94	0.39	6.72	1.74
Timolol maleate (Timoptic XE 0.5%)	5.0	5.9	22.6	133.34	1	66.67	28.88	0.43	6.72	1.92
Betaxolol hydrochloride (Betoptic S)	5.0	4.9	25.4	124.46	2	31.12	22.94	0.74	5.28	4.20

Source: Modified from R Fiscella. Costs of glaucoma medications. Am J Health Syst Pharm 1998;55;272–275.

maintenance organization, it only costs them a small copay. Another consideration is that most health maintenance organizations have a drug formulary, and a medication chosen because of its convenient dosage or lack of side effects may not be covered by the plan. All of these issues may eventually affect compliance and should be contemplated by the doctor when therapeutic regimens are prescribed.

Frequency of Instillation

Frequency of instillation may also have an impact on compliance. Although it might make intuitive sense that compliance decreases when the dosage is increased, Kass and coworkers found only marginally improved compliance in patients on b.i.d. timolol versus q.i.d. pilocarpine.[4] In patients in whom drop instillation is difficult for whatever reason, a qd beta blocker or prostaglandin might be preferable to the b.i.d. medication.

However, patients are less likely to miss both instillations of a b.i.d. medication than the single instillation of a qd drug. Thus, patients on a qd drug miss a full day of medication if they miss a single dose.

Lack of Understanding

Poor patient understanding has a negative impact on compliance and is, to some extent, under the control of the doctor. Patients may not comprehend the severity of the disease. They need to be told that the medication they are taking reduces eye pressure to avoid loss of peripheral vision, and that just because they see well does not mean that their disease is under control. Education regarding drop dosage and instillation technique is also of critical importance, and this is the responsibility of doctor and staff alike. Kass and colleagues found that only 20% of patients in their study reported being instructed on how to instill their drops.[7]

Polypharmacy

Patients with multiple medical conditions tend to be less compliant.[15] *Polypharmacy*, as it is sometimes called, can lead to deletion of medications that patients think are less important. For example, if given a choice between affording or remembering to take a heart medication or an eye drop, the patient may logically choose the heart medication. The practitioner can talk with the patient about where glaucoma should be on their priority list of conditions, and why.

Miscellaneous

Other factors that have been implicated as reasons for noncompliance are increasing age,[10] gender (male patients have been shown to be less compliant),[15] race, increased time in the waiting room,[16] and having administration schedules that do not correlate well with patients' personal schedules.[11] Patients who dislike their physicians also tend to be less compliant.

Practitioners should operate on the premise that a significant percentage of the patient population will be noncompliant to some extent at one time or another. No doctor should assume that he or she always knows when a patient is noncompliant. It is essential to keep the lines of communication open, gain each patient's trust, and be willing to bring up the subject of compliance in an open and compassionate manner.

INCREASING COMPLIANCE: THE PHYSICIAN'S DUTY

The most important factor affecting compliance is the time that doctor and staff spend in educating patients. This may seem obvious, but many doctors merely tell patients that they "see signs of glaucoma" and that the patient "will need to use drops twice a day." From that point on, any deviation from the intended treatment plan is viewed as an annoyance or as the "patient's problem." With a little time, effort, and a caring manner, the doctor can proactively improve compliance in many patients.

Ways to increase compliance include:

1. Proper handling of the initial office visit
2. Initial and ongoing patient education
3. Assessment of compliance
4. Providing written instructions (large print when needed) and reminders
5. Establishing a relationship with patients that inspires trust, responsibility, and the willingness to compromise

The initial office visit is a crucial time for setting the stage for compliance. The manner in which the patient is handled by the doctor on the first visit may have signifi-

cant ramifications for future success of treatment. The doctor must impress on the patient the severity of glaucoma and the mechanism of the disease in a firm but caring way. In our office, we use visual aids to show a sequence of increasingly cupped optic nerves with corresponding visual field loss. A discussion of how treatment prevents such loss by lowering the pressure should also be undertaken, with emphasis that lowered eye pressure will not be felt by the patient, but must be measured by the doctor. It may also be useful to involve family members in this discussion whenever possible. We encourage family members to sit in during the examination, as well as during the final consultation, so that they understand the patient's condition. They become involved in the patient's care from the outset, which can be helpful later in the treatment phase as they observe changes in patient behavior, energy level, and compliance with the medication regimen.

Once a drug is selected, possible adverse ocular and systemic side effects should be discussed. Instructions should be given to call their doctor immediately if the patient experiences any side effects from taking the eye drops. In this way, patients are less likely to discontinue treatment for extended periods between visits. Discuss with them what to do if they accidentally forget a dosage, telling them to put a drop in as soon as they remember, and then simply get back on the original schedule. Offer to provide two prescriptions for the same medication, one for home and one for work, to increase convenience.

DROP INSTILLATION

Proper drop instillation technique should be taught on the first visit as well, and followed up with additional training at future visits. This can be delegated and should be periodically assessed by responsible staff. Some patients do better instilling drops in a seated position with head tilted back, whereas others can be encouraged to lie down. Keeping drops refrigerated allows a positive feedback mechanism as the cold drop enters the eye. Teaching nasolacrimal occlusion using digital pressure at the time of installation is also advocated. This technique enhances drug delivery to the eye and minimizes systemic absorption. With fewer symptoms, compliance is hopefully enhanced. Patients using multiple drops should also be instructed to wait 5 minutes between instilling each one. Remember the importance of occasionally asking patients to demonstrate their instillation techniques. Patients may not perceive that they have a problem getting drops into the eye, so they may not mention it. However, many patients, if asked, do report problems, such as:

- Handling the container. This can be a significant problem in arthritic patients.

How to use your eye drops

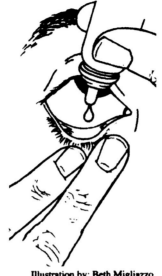

Illustration by: Beth Migliazzo
Overland Park, KS

1. Wash your hands well with soap and water.

2. Stand in front of a mirror.

3. Using your forefinger and thumb, gently pull down your lower lid to form a pocket, or pull your lower lashes forward to create a pocket.

4. Tilt your head back and look up.

5. Place one drop in the pocket. Do not let the tip of the bottle touch your finger, eye, or other surface.

6. Continue to hold your lower lid down a few seconds to let the drop settle.

7. Close your eye and move your eyeball from side to side.

8. With closed eyes, gently apply pressure with your index finger to the inside corner of your eye. This puts pressure on the tear duct and helps keep the medication in contact with your eye.

9. Repeat the steps for your other eye.

10. If you have trouble, ask your eye care professional's staff for help.

FIGURE 13-1. Diagram and description of proper eyedrop instillation. (Reprinted with permission from CibaVision Novartis Co. Glaucoma Questions and Answers Pamphlet. Atlanta, GA 1996.)

- Blinking just as the drop contacts the eye.
- Missing the eye altogether.
- Worrying about whether the correct amount got into the eye.

Ongoing patient education is essential. Patients rarely comprehend everything about their disease and medication schedule on the initial visit. Even if they understand at the time, they may be apt to forget. Repeated reinforcement over time and written instructions are the keys to success. In selected patients, showing them their visual fields and comparing them to normal visual fields or to previous fields from that patient can be a useful educa-

tional tool. Discussing IOP readings can be very illustrative of treatment success, but this must be done with caution. Patients need to be educated that a higher or lower pressure reading from one visit to the next is less important than the overall stability of the optic nerve and visual field.

Written information on the proper instillation of eye drops is beneficial to improve compliance for all glaucoma patients (Figure 13-1). Instruction that emphasizes tying doses to events of the day, can improve compliance. Some patients may benefit by setting a digital watch or alarm clock. Written instructions and drop schedules can be very valuable, especially as the com-

Medication Dosing Schedule

Name_____

	Left Eye	Right Eye
Breakfast	1 drop timolol .5% (yellow cap)	1 drop timolol .5% (yellow cap)
Lunch		
Dinner	1 drop timolol .5% (yellow cap)	1 drop timolol .5% (yellow cap)
Bedtime	1 drop latanoprost .005% (clear cap)	1 drop latanoprost .005% (clear cap)

Comments: Close eyelids immediately after instilling eyedrops and keep eyelids closed for 2–3 minutes. This allows the medication to work in the eye and decreases the risk of systemic side effects.

When taking more than one eyedrop at the same time, wait at least 5 minutes before instilling the next drop.

DO NOT run out of your eye medications. Refill your prescription approximately 1 week before you expect to run out of your eyedrops. If you need a refill before your next scheduled appointment, please call the eye clinic.

Call the clinic with any questions or concerns with your eye medications or glaucoma.

FIGURE 13-2. These medication dosing forms instruct the patient to take timolol in the morning and at dinnertime in both eyes and latanoprost in both eyes before bedtime.

plexity of therapeutic regimens increases. These instructions can be designed individually or a preprinted form can be used (Figure 13-2; see Figure 11-2). Space at the bottom of a form can be used for individualized instruction and reminders. Any written schedules should also refer to medications by cap color if possible. Additionally, the doctor can help patients tailor the scheduling of drops to their daily routines. This should include mealtimes, bedtime, breaks at the jobs, and any other activities that are done on a daily basis at a desirable time for drop administration.[17] Lastly, the patient should be asked to bring the drops with them on each follow-up visit, and occasionally asked to describe and demonstrate how the drops are used. This gives the practitioner a better sense of compliance than simply assuming that instructions are being followed (see Case 8 in Chapter 18).

Assessing compliance at each visit is critical. We ask patients directly whether they are using their drops. Indirect investigation can help confirm the answer. For example, patients should be asked to bring the drops with them at each visit, and the bottles examined to see whether they look used or brand new. They can be asked about when they used their drops

Rx Refill Request

Patient Name_____

Date Last Seen_____

Medication(s) Needed_____

_____

_____

_____

• •

☐ **Refill OK**   **Number of refills 1 2 3 4 5**

☐ **Refill Denied**

☐ **Schedule Return Visit   Appt Date/Time**_____

FIGURE 13-3. Medication refill request form.

last and the time recorded; if they say they have not used the drops for 1 day, gently ask them whether they miss the drops at other times during the month, and if so, how often. One way to keep track of medication use and to ensure compliance with follow-up visits is to have a system to carefully track prescription refill requests. The doctor should write out a number of refills for each medication that will last just until the next scheduled follow-up examination. The doctor should be certain that the patient has adequate refills so that the medication does not run out prematurely. Some medications may last longer than others because of drop size and packaging of the bottle. A patient who requests refills for their prescription at a follow-up appointment is probably compliant. A patient who replies that a new prescription is not necessary should be further questioned about why the refills from the previous prescription have not been exhausted.

The office or clinic should have a protocol for telephone refills. A refill should never be approved without the knowledge of the practitioner. We use a form that the staff fills out, attaches to the chart, and brings to us for review (Figure 13-3). This is an opportunity to see when the patient was last seen, whether any visits have been missed, and whether they are using the appropriate quantity of drops. Tracking glaucoma patients to be sure they keep appointments is critical. We mark all glaucoma charts with a fluorescent green

sticker, so that at the end of the day, if a scheduled glaucoma patient missed the appointment, that patient is handled with priority. Calls are made and the patient's status is reported to the doctor, so that further action can be taken. A personal call from the practitioner or a registered letter may be necessary to get a patient back in for a follow-up visit. We use a special form (Figure 13-4) for no-show patients and keep it in the chart to document the steps taken to reschedule the missed visit.

NONCOMPLIANT PATIENTS

Some patients, despite our best efforts, do not comply with the medical regimen prescribed. These patients should be considered for laser or surgical therapy. More studies are pointing to these techniques as first-line treatment when it appears that medications are not or cannot be used. Most insurance companies cover laser trabeculoplasty or surgical trabeculectomy, but they may not cover the cost of medications. If a patient is being referred for surgical consultation, be sure to make the appointment for the patient, rather than leaving that responsibility to the patient. Write down the appointment time and date in the patient chart, as well as on a card given to the patient. If the patient refuses to let your staff make the appointment, document this as well. Send a letter to the specialist summarizing the case and outlining the reason for the referral, along with your observations of noncompliance.

Patient No Show Status Report

Date/Time of Appt Missed_____

Diagnosis:_____

Action Taken:

☐ **Spoke to Patient on**_____. **Comments**_____

☐ **Rescheduled appt** <u>for</u>_____ **@**_____ **am/pm**

☐ **Left message on answering machine on** _____

☐ **Called pt on** _____**but no answer. Try again on** _____

☐ **Sent certified letter on** _____

FIGURE 13-4. Missed appointment record sheet.

CONCLUSION

One of the greatest variables affecting compliance with glaucoma therapy is the doctor's interaction and communication with the patient. Glaucoma is a chronic disease that requires lifelong therapy and surveillance. We must educate our glaucoma patients with compassion and understanding and be willing to spend the extra time necessary to help our patients fully understand their disease. The more active a role we play in our patients' management, the greater the success in treating this chronic and potentially sight-threatening disease.

REFERENCES

1. Porter AWM. Drug defaulting in general practice. BMJ 1969;1:218.

2. Kass MA, Becker B. Compliance to Ocular Therapy. In IH Leopol, RP Burns (eds). Symposium on Ocular Therapy (vol 9). New York: John Wiley and Sons, Inc., 1976;119.

3. Kass MA, Meltzer DW, Gordon M, et al. Compliance with topical pilocarpine treatment. Am J Ophthalmol 1986;101:515.

4. Kass MA, Gordon M, Morley RE Jr, et al. Compliance with topical timolol treatment. Am J Ophthalmol 1987;103:188.

5. Kass MA, Hodapp E, Gordon M, et al. Part I. Patient administration of eyedrops: interview. Ann Ophthalmol 1982;14:775.

6. Kass MA, Meltzer DW, Gordon MO. A miniature compliance monitor for eyedrop medication. Arch Ophthalmol 1984;102:1550.

7. Kass MA, Hodapp E, Gordon M, et al. Part II. Patient administration of eyedrops: observation. Ann Ophthalmol 1982;14:889.

8. Vincent D. Patient's viewpoint of glaucoma therapy. Sight Sav Rev 1972;42:213–221.

9. Chang JS Jr, Lee DA, Petursson G, et al. The effect of a glaucoma medication reminder cap on patient compliance and intraocular pressure. J Ocular Pharmacol 1991;7:117.

10. Gurwitz JH, Glynn RJ, Monane M, et al. Treatment for glaucoma: adherance by the elderly. Am J Pub Health 1993;83(5):711–716.

11. Granstrom PA. Glaucoma patients not compliant with their drug therapy: clinical and behavioral aspects. Br J Ophthalmol 1982;66:464.

12. Goldberg I. Compliance. In Ritch R. The Glaucomas. St Louis: Mosby 1996;1375–1382.

13. Spaeth GL. Visual loss in a glaucoma clinic. I. Sociologic considerations. Invest Ophthalmol 1970;9:73.

14. Lehto I. Side effects of topical treatment in pigmentary glaucoma. Acta Ophthalmol Copenh 1992;70(2):225–227.

15. Bloch S, Rosenthal AR, Friedman L, et al. Patient compliance in glaucoma. Br J Ophthalmol 1977;61:531.

16. Kass MA. Non-compliance to ocular therapy. Glaucoma reports. Ann Ophthalmol 1978;10:1244.

17. Fingeret M, Schuettenberg SP. Patient drug schedules and compliance. J Am Optom Assoc 1991;62(6):478–480.

Normal Tension Glaucoma

14

Normal Tension Glaucoma

Mitchell W. Dul

A growing fraction of glaucoma specialists believe that normal tension glaucoma (NTG) is simply a continuum of high-tension glaucoma, and not a separate disease entity. This chapter discusses the management of patients with glaucoma damage and statistically normal intraocular pressure (IOP) separately because there may be alternative approaches to treatment compared to those used for high-tension glaucoma. Some evidence suggests that nonselective beta blockers may be contraindicated in NTG because of their effect on the blood supply to the optic nerve.[1-4] Data are available from the Collaborative Normal Tension Glaucoma Study that showed IOP lowering decreases the risk of visual field loss progression, but specifically excluded the use of all beta blockers.[5] Because there may be alternative treatment protocols developing for NTG, it is beneficial to discuss the epidemiology, clinical features, and treatment trial results for patients with glaucoma damage and normal IOP. At the same time, we should consider NTG to be a common entity and similar in the majority of clinical features to primary open-angle glaucoma (POAG),[6,7] with the exception of the level of IOP.

Since its first description by von Graefe in 1857,[8] various definitions of *normal tension glaucoma* have been suggested. The literature remains cluttered with a variety of definitions of this disease. A 1998 survey of 63 articles pertaining to NTG published between 1973 and 1997 revealed that the range of maximum IOP levels acceptable for categorization of NTG was broad, from 17 mm Hg to 26 mm Hg.[9] In more than 40% of these studies, including the Collaborative Normal Tension Glaucoma Study Group, patients with IOP higher than 21 mm Hg were acceptable for study inclusion. For the purposes of this discussion, *normal tension glaucoma* is defined as a disease in which the anterior chamber angle is normal, the IOP on diurnal testing never exceeds 21 mm Hg (2 SD from the statistical norm), and changes in the optic nerve head (ONH) and visual field occur that are consistent with glaucoma.

EPIDEMIOLOGY

There is a wide discrepancy in the literature regarding the prevalence of NTG because any assessment relies on a consistent definition of the disease and reliable observations of the optic nerve and visual field. Previously thought to be rare, NTG is now known to be a common form of glaucoma that is not commonly detected.[10] As such, it is surely an under-reported condition. NTG probably accounts for approximately 25–30%[11,12] of all open-angle glaucoma cases, although greater variability is seen when race is factored in. In the Baltimore Eye Survey, consisting primarily of African Americans and white Americans,[13] 16.7% of glaucomatous eyes never had a recorded IOP exceeding 21 mm Hg. However, 55% had an initial IOP reading 21 mm Hg or lower, highlighting the need for multiple IOP measurements in the differential diagnosis of NTG. In a population of 21,000 Japanese workers, 151 cases of open-angle glaucoma were diagnosed, of which 99 (55%) were NTG.[14]

Shiose and colleagues[15] also estimated that, in seven regions throughout Japan, the prevalence of NTG in patients older than 40 years is approximately 2.04%, and only 0.5% for patients with POAG. The high prevalence of NTG and low prevalence of POAG in this population might reflect a racial peculiarity in the age-specific trend of the IOP. It is noteworthy that although the prevalence of NTG in Japan increases with age, a concurrent decrease in IOP is seen.

Refractive Error

In the United States and Europe, myopia is believed to be a possible risk factor for the development of NTG,[16] although evidence to the contrary also exists.[17] In Japan, high myopia is thought to be a risk factor for NTG.[18]

Gender

Whether NTG affects one gender more than another is not clear. Many reports suggest that women are more at risk.[19] Others report an equal likelihood of either gender manifesting NTG.[12] There is some evidence[20] suggesting that men are more severely affected in the early stages of the disease, while women have an overall worse prognosis.[19]

Age

NTG is unusual in people younger than 50 years, although it does occur.[21]

PATHOPHYSIOLOGY OF NORMAL TENSION GLAUCOMA

Role of Blood Flow in Normal Tension Glaucoma

The principal arterial blood supply to the anterior optic nerve is via the short posterior ciliary arteries. The prelaminar and laminar region of the anterior optic nerve is supplied by direct branches of these vessels and by vessels originating from the arterial circle of Zinn-Haller. The retrolaminar region is primarily supplied by branches of the pial arteries and the short posterior ciliary arterial system. Although longitudinal anastomoses of capillaries throughout the anterior optic nerve could be viewed as a protective mechanism against regional ischemic insult, flow resistance may be high enough in these fine capillaries to limit collateral flow.[22] Hayreh reminds us that there is no one standard pattern of blood supply to the optic nerve.[23] The blood supply to the nerve is very complex, and marked interindividual variation is seen. These complexities may be responsible for some of the problems in the understanding of NTG and other vascular optic nerve diseases.

Many variables influence blood flow to the ONH in the general population. These include, but are not limited to: local autoregulation and vasospasm; IOP; blood viscosity; intraluminal pressure; venous outflow; and physiologic individual variation in the blood supply to the ONH. Although certainly a great deal of overlap exists between these variables in the general population, some evidence suggests that the vasculature and blood flow of the ONH in patients with NTG differs from that of patients with POAG and nonglaucomatous patients. With the use of color Doppler ultrasound imaging to measure systolic and diastolic blood flow velocities of the ret-

robulbar vessels in NTG, POAG, and controls, a significant increase in vascular resistance and a decrease in blood flow velocity (especially end-diastolic velocity) are seen in the ophthalmic artery, central retinal artery, and posterior ciliary arteries of patients with NTG or POAG.[24-27] Because artificially increasing IOP only affects the hemodynamics of the central retinal artery,[28] factors other than IOP likely play a role in the pathogenesis of glaucomatous optic neuropathy.[27,29] Although it is true that low-grade ischemia can lead to optic atrophy, the relationship of that atrophy to glaucoma remains unproven. No substantiated clinical evidence exists that ischemia directly causes glaucomatous optic atrophy in POAG or NTG. Additionally, Doppler imaging is limited to measurements of blood velocity, and calculations of vascular resistance are theoretical. Therefore, interpretation of these measurements is difficult, as blood flow velocity may not be analogous to optic nerve perfusion.[22]

Optic Nerve Head Profusion: Role of Nocturnal Blood Pressure

Nocturnal hypotension, particularly when superimposed on other vascular risk factors (e.g., patients taking antihypertensive agents at bedtime), may reduce the flow of blood to the ONH below a critical point. This may be a factor in the pathogenesis of glaucomatous optic neuropathy.[30] The level of the nocturnal blood pressure dip appears to be significantly greater in NTG than in POAG and controls.[31-33] Nocturnal blood pressure parameters tend to be even lower in patients with progressive visual field defects compared with NTG and POAG patients who were stable.[34]

Role of Other Parameters in the Pathogenesis of Normal Tension Glaucoma

Miller and Quigley in human studies[6] and Iwata in monkey studies[35] suggest that a primary weakness of the lamina cribrosa, to a point at which even statistically "normal" IOP could deform it and cause secondary mechanical damage to the ganglion cell axons of the optic nerve, may play an etiologic role in the pathogenesis of NTG.

CLINICAL FEATURES

Intraocular Pressure

Population studies show that the IOP in the general population more or less respects a Gaussian (bell) curve that is skewed toward higher IOP (possibly due to the presence of glaucoma patients in the general population). The statistical average IOP is 15.5 ± 2.6 mm Hg. It is important to understand that the phrase *normal intraocular pressure* is used for IOP that is "normal" in the statistical sense, within

2 SD of this statistical average, and is not meant to imply "normal" in the sense of being "free of disease." To have statistically abnormal pressure and be free of glaucoma (ocular hypertensive) and to have statistically normal pressure and manifest glaucoma damage are both quite possible.[36] As a reference point, 21 mm Hg (2 SD from the mean) will be considered the upper limit of statistically "normal" IOP. In a significant percentage of cases of NTG, the untreated IOP is in the high teens (19 mm Hg),[37] which is statistically higher than the average "normal" IOP.

Age seems to play a role in the distribution of IOP in a population. In general, the older the population, the greater the average IOP and the greater the standard deviation. The exception to this appears to occur in the Japanese population, where IOP statistically decreases with age overall, and more so in men than women. This is noteworthy in light of the increased prevalence of NTG in Japan, especially among the elderly, compared with other nations.

Diurnal Fluctuation in Intraocular Pressure

The average diurnal range of IOP in the nonglaucomatous population is 5 mm Hg and usually only peaks once in a 24-hour period. It is generally highest in the early morning and lowest at night, but this is only a statistical trend. IOP has a significant probability of peaking at any time of day,[38] although that time of day is usually consistent in a given patient. In POAG, the diurnal IOP fluctuation is generally higher than in the nonglaucoma population, and it is not unusual to observe IOP spikes of more than 10 mm Hg.

The 24-hour IOP range in populations with NTG is similar to the nonglaucomatous population[39-41] and peak IOPs in NTG patients often occur during office hours.[42] It is noteworthy that most studies of diurnal IOP in NTG are conducted with the patient in the sitting position. When IOP is measured with the patient in a supine position, some NTG patients' IOP exceed 21 mm Hg.[43] In the Baltimore Eye Study, more than one-half of the patients diagnosed with glaucoma optic nerve damage and an initial IOP below 21 mm Hg had a subsequent IOP reading higher than 21 mm Hg. This finding highlights the need for multiple IOP readings to establish an accurate baseline before initiating medical therapy.

Role of Corneal Thickness in Intraocular Pressure

Evidence exists that patients with NTG have significantly thinner central corneas (521 ± 31 µ) when compared with controls (555 ± 34) and patients with POAG (556 ± 35).[44,45] No significant difference was seen in corneal curvature, and gender did not influence the data. By accounting for corneal thickness,[46] we may be underestimating the IOP in NTG patients by an average of 2.3

mm Hg and possibly more.[47] In one study,[44] when corneal thickness was taken into account, 31% of the NTG patients met the diagnostic criteria for POAG. Central corneal thickness may play a significant role in the division between normal and increased IOP at a cutoff point of 21 mm Hg.[48] The mean corneal thickness in a Japanese population was 503 ± 27,[49] which is significantly less than that reported in Hong Kong, Chinese,[50] and elderly white Americans.[48] This racial difference may account, in part, for the increased prevalence of NTG in the Japanese population. If the 21 mm Hg cut off definition of NTG is strictly adhered to, then central corneal pachymetry should be included in the workup of NTG.

Effects of Myopic Photorefractive Surgery on Central Corneal Thickness and Intraocular Pressure

Patients who have had excimer myopic photorefractive surgery with the corresponding thinning of the central cornea associated with the procedure have statistically lower IOP when compared with preoperative findings.[51-55] This decrease is in the magnitude of 2–3 mm Hg. Consequently, peripheral (temporal cornea) applanation tonometry readings[51] or pneumotonometry readings[52] may be a more accurate measure of true IOP in these cases. These measurements were consistent with preoperative central applanation readings.[51,52]

Role of Intraocular Pressure in the Pathogenesis of Normal Tension Glaucoma

The role of IOP in the pathogenesis of NTG is incompletely understood. Cartwright and Anderson demonstrated that in 12 of 14 cases of NTG with asymmetric IOP, the glaucomatous damage to the optic nerve and the visual field was greater in the eye with the higher IOP.[56] In contrast, Chen studied a group of 24 patients with monocular early glaucomatous damage secondary to NTG and found no significant difference in IOP between the two eyes.[57] Orgul and Flanner studied 23 bilateral but asymmetric cases of NTG and showed that 12 patients had more severe visual field loss in the eye with the higher IOP, whereas 11 had more severe loss in the eye with the lower IOP.[58] Haefliger and Hitchings studied the relationship between asymmetry of visual fields and IOP differences in an untreated NTG population and concluded that patients with NTG may be divided into those in whom IOP could be important in the pathogenesis of the visual field defect, and a majority in whom this relationship is less likely.[59] In a population of 59 NTG patients, Crichton and colleagues found that 47 patients had asymmetric visual field defects, but only 13 of these also had asymmetric IOP.[60] In most cases, the eye with the higher IOP had the more pronounced vision loss, but the

TABLE 14-1. Summary of the Results of the Collaborative Normal Tension Glaucoma Study, 1998

Question: Does a 30% or greater lowering of intraocular pressure, achieved by medical or surgical means, change the rate of progression of normal tension glaucoma?

Group	Rate of progression of normal tension glaucoma (%)	Rate of cataract development (%)
Untreated group (n = 79)	35	14
Treated group (n = 61)	12	38*

Answer: Lowering intraocular pressure by 30% significantly reduces the risk of progression in normal tension glaucoma. However, 65% of untreated patients did not progress, and 12% of patients progressed despite intraocular pressure lowering.

*Seventy percent of the cataracts that occurred in the treated group were in patients that received filtering surgery. Filtering surgery significantly increases the development of cataracts (P = .0001). No statistically significant difference in cataract development was seen in the untreated and medically treated groups (P = .18).

majority (n = 34) of the 47 cases of asymmetric visual field loss had equal IOP in each eye. These data suggest that IOP is not the predominant factor in developing glaucomatous damage in patients with NTG. Collectively, these studies suggest that factors other than IOP play a role in the pathogenesis of NTG.

Effects of Intraocular Pressure Reduction on Normal Tension Glaucoma Progression

In the late 1990s, evidence showed that lowering IOP, both surgically[61] and medically,[5] probably slows the rate of progression of NTG. Bhandari and associates studied 17 patients with progressive bilateral NTG.[61] Each received a unilateral trabeculectomy. The untreated eye served as a control. The rate of visual field loss progression was significantly less in the treated eye.[61]

The Collaborative Normal Tension Glaucoma Study Group is the first multicenter, prospective, randomized, untreated control clinical trial to provide evidence that IOP reduction is effective in any type of chronic glaucoma (Table 14-1).[10] One hundred forty NTG patients (with demonstrated visual field loss progression or visual field defects threatening fixation, or with new disc hemorrhages) were randomly assigned to an untreated group (n = 79) or to a group receiving a 30% reduction in IOP by medical or surgical intervention (n = 61). Neither eye in the latter group was treated with beta blockers or adrenergic agonists because of the potential cardiovascular, vasoconstrictive, and crossover effects that could confound the data. Glaucoma progression was seen in 35% of the control eyes versus 12% of the treated eyes. Of the treated group, almost one-half maintained a 30% IOP reduction with topical medication, laser trabeculoplasty, or both, without the need for filtering surgery.[62] These results demonstrate that a 30% reduction in IOP slows the rate of progression of NTG. However, 65% of untreated NTG patients showed no progression during a follow-up

period of 5 years or more. Additionally, in 12% of the NTG patients, despite a 30% IOP reduction, visual field loss continued to progress.

Optic Nerve Head in Normal Tension Glaucoma

Whether using traditional ophthalmoscopic analysis or digitized imaging systems, it is safe to say that glaucomatous optic nerves still are not differentiated from nonglaucomatous optic nerves with certainty. Our clinical capabilities leave us with an enormous overlap between what is physiologic and what is glaucomatous. Although we have learned to focus greater attention on the optic nerve and nerve fiber layer, particularly in the presence of statistically "normal" IOP, the optic nerve evaluation is a skill acquired through accumulated experience. The optic nerve anatomy consists of vascular, neural, and connective tissue, all of which, to varying degrees, play a role in the pathogenesis of NTG, but none of which is understood in sufficient detail. As a result, all that can be stated with certainty is that patients with NTG represent a heterogeneous group.

Taken as a group, some characteristics of the optic nerve of patients with NTG appear to present with greater frequency when compared with nonglaucomatous eyes or the optic nerve of patients with POAG (Table 14-2). The clinical value of these findings in a given patient is much less compelling because of the tremendous overlap in appearance between nonglaucomatous and glaucomatous optic nerves.

Size of the Optic Nerve Head

Some evidence suggests that the average optic disc area is larger in patients with NTG than in patients with POAG.[63–65] The clinical relevance of these observations is weak because of high individual physiologic variation in disc size. Compared with patients with POAG, patients with NTG tend to have thinner neuroretinal rim tissue

TABLE 14-2. Optic Nerve and Retinal Nerve Fiber Layer
Characteristics Suggestive of Normal Tension Glaucoma
versus Primary Open Angle Glaucoma

Optic nerve head
- Larger disc
- Thinner temporal neuroretinal rim tissue
- Acquired pit of the optic nerve
- Disc hemorrhage
- Peripapillary atrophy

Retinal nerve fiber layer
- Focal nerve fiber layer loss (intraocular pressure ≤18 mm Hg)
- Diffuse nerve fiber layer loss (intraocular pressure >18 mm Hg)

located in the inferior and inferior temporal quadrant[66] and in the temporal quadrant.[67]

Acquired Pits of the Optic Nerve

Acquired pits of the optic nerve (APONs) are discrete, focal areas of excavation within the lamina cribrosa at the base of the optic cup (see Color Plate 24). There is greater visibility of laminar dots within the optic pit.[68] APONs may represent a structural weakness of the lamina cribrosa,[69] a focal or localized area of nonperfusion, or both.[66] APONs were reported by Javitt and colleagues to occur in 74% of a population with NTG and in 15% of a population with POAG.[70] They are usually located in the inferior quadrant (70%) or the superior quadrant (30%) of the optic cup.[71] Dense visual field defects with steep borders correlate with the location of APONs in the majority of patients. Cashwell and Ford retrospectively studied the visual fields of 97 patients who had APONs and found that in 82% of the cases, one of the most central test points (within 3 degrees of fixation) was severely depressed (P <.5).[72] This suggests that the presence of an APON may represent a greater threat to fixation in glaucoma patients.

Optic Disc Hemorrhages (Drance Hemorrhage)

In several retrospective studies, the prevalence of optic disc hemorrhage in NTG varied from 10% (n = 77 eyes)[73] to 64% (n = 50 eyes).[74] The average is approximately 25%. One prospective study reported a prevalence of 43% (n = 58 patients) in NTG patients.[75] Disc hemorrhages are more likely to occur in cases of NTG than in POAG.[76–78] In advanced glaucoma, the location of the disc hemorrhage correlates with neuroretinal rim notching and peripapillary atrophy (see Color Plate 26).[78] Disc hemorrhages can also represent an early sign of glaucoma damage and may precede visible glau-

comatous change in the nerve fiber layer, the visual field, and the topography of the disc (see Figure 5-14).[79] They may forecast greater progression of ONH damage and visual field loss.[80] Therefore, the presence of a disc hemorrhage in a glaucoma suspect patient or glaucoma patient generally indicates a need for the start of or increase in medical therapy.

Retinal Nerve Fiber Layer Defects

Localized (slit or wedge) NFL defects, as opposed to diffuse NFL loss, have been reported to occur more commonly in NTG than in POAG.[81,82] When IOP was higher than 18 mm Hg, NTG patients were more likely to have diffuse nerve fiber layer loss compared with NTG patients whose IOP never exceeded 18 mm Hg. The latter group was more likely to exhibit focal NFL loss (see Figures 6-6 and 6-7).[83]

Peripapillary Atrophy

PPA appears to be associated with functional and structural optic nerve damage in glaucoma,[84] and its progression is associated with progressive optic disc damage and visual field loss. PPA tends to develop in an area of thinning of the neuroretinal rim tissue of the optic nerve (see Figure 5-13). It occurs more commonly in NTG than POAG, but the finding is not specific for glaucoma damage.[85] It may occur as a normal senile aging change. The pathophysiology of PPA in glaucoma is unknown; vascular ischemia to the choroidal circulation has been proposed. The posterior ciliary arteries are the main blood supply to the optic nerve and peripapillary choroid. This suggests that an anomaly of the optic nerve head circulation may play some role in the pathogenesis of PPA associated with glaucoma (with or without elevated IOP).[22]

Visual Field Loss in Normal Tension Glaucoma

As is the case with the ONH, the patterns of visual field defects in NTG represent a wide spectrum of presentations. The overlap in appearance between visual fields in patients with NTG and POAG is high, and drawing precise conclusions based on visual field characteristics is difficult. That being said, statistical trends suggest that the visual fields in patients with NTG may have some distinguishing characteristics. Compared with their POAG counterparts, the visual fields of patients with NTG tend to manifest more localized defects,[86–89] a steeper slope of the defect,[90,91] and a defect closer to central fixation.[92,93] Whether a propensity exists for the visual field defects associated with NTG to be more prevalent in the inferior or superior hemifield remains controversial.

Progression of Visual Field Loss in Normal Tension Glaucoma

Some evidence suggests that the progression of disease in NTG may also be distinct from that in POAG. Of 57 NTG eyes studied by Gliklich and associates,[94] 53% showed progression of visual field loss after 3 years of follow-up, and 62% had progressed by 5 years. A dense scotoma extending from the nasal periphery toward fixation was the most common visual field defect. Noureddin and colleagues reported that one-half of 84 NTG patients showed visual field progression with a mean follow-up period of 28 months.[95] No statistically significant difference was seen between patients with progression and nonprogression with respect to age or IOP. In contrast, higher IOP, larger cup-to-disc ratios, and increased ratio of area of PPA to disc area were found to have significant influence on the progression of visual field changes in NTG.[96] The Collaborative Normal Tension Glaucoma Study Group demonstrated that in NTG patients with visual field progression or a visual field defect that threatened fixation, a 30% reduction in IOP had a statistically significant effect of slowing the progression of optic nerve damage and visual field loss.[5] A minority of patients (12%) continued to progress despite IOP lowering. However, 65% of the patients in the observation group did not progress over a 5-year follow-up period. There is no reliable way to predict which patients with NTG will progress and which will remain stable.

TREATMENT

The Collaborative Normal Tension Glaucoma Study (NTGS) showed that lowering IOP by 30% significantly reduced the rate of progression in patients with NTG in whom fixation was threatened or with visual field progression. In this study, beta blockers and epinephrine drugs were not used because of theoretical concerns of affecting blood flow to the optic nerve. The triage of therapy was pilocarpine, laser trabeculoplasty, and filtering surgery to achieve a 30% reduction from the baseline IOP. Medications such as topical prostaglandins, α_2 agonists, and carbonic anhydrase inhibitors were not available at the start of the trial and were not studied. The NTGS also did not include NTG patients with less damaged optic nerves.

Many unanswered questions remain regarding the treatment of NTG. Despite the plethora of claims regarding the potential benefits of specific ocular topical drugs to enhance anterior optic nerve blood flow, no consistent clinical studies have demonstrated that eye drops adversely affect optic nerve blood flow (Table 14-3) or that blood flow is even important. Clinical studies using primarily laser and ultrasound Doppler techniques suggest anomalies of the blood flow in some populations of glaucoma patients, but it has been difficult to corre-

late those clinical findings with possible ischemia within the optic nerve itself.[22] Additionally, the accuracy of laser Doppler technology has come into question.[97] Other factors may also contribute to glaucomatous optic neuropathy, including excitotoxicity, neurotrophic deprivation, and autoimmunity. Like ischemia, these may occur with or without elevated IOP. In the future, preventing retinal ganglion cell death, independent of the cause of NTG, may be an additional means of therapeutic intervention.

NTG patients with fixation threatened or with progressive visual field loss should have their IOP lowered by at least 30% (Table 14-4). Patients with lesser degrees of damage should be treated on an individual basis. If the benefits of treatment outweigh the risks, then most NTG patients should have their IOP lowered. Nonselective beta blockers and epinephrine drugs should be avoided because of the potential concern of reducing the blood flow to the optic nerve.[1-4] Because the majority of the β-adrenergic receptors in the anterior optic nerve and nerve head appear to be of the β_2 subtype,[98] β_1-selective glaucoma medications should, in theory, have less of an effect on ONH profusion. Betaxolol has been reported to have no influence on ONH blood flow,[2,99] although Graf-Grauwiller and coworkers[100] and Arend and associates[101] reported that it increased peripheral blood flow. In patients with NTG, Harris and colleagues found that betaxolol may have an ocular vasorelaxant effect independent of any influence on IOP.[102]

Latanoprost may be an ideal medication for patients with NTG because it can lower the IOP below the episcleral venous pressure and only has to be given once a day. It also does not appear to change the blood velocity in retrobulbar vessels.[4] Brimonidine is a selective α_2 agonist that does not appear to affect blood flow to the optic nerve. However, apraclonidine, another α_2 agonist, does appear to decrease blood velocity and increase resistance in retrobulbar vessels.[103] Topical carbonic anhydrase inhibitors, although less effective in lowering IOP than latanoprost and brimonidine, may increase ocular blood flow.[28] Topical pilocarpine appears to have no effect on ONH profusion pressure in nonglaucoma patients[1,99] or in POAG patients.[104] Pilocarpine was the primary topical medication used in the NTGS.

Argon laser trabeculoplasty is effective in lowering IOP in NTG and has few side effects. It was one of the primary modes of treatment in the NTGS. Filtering surgery is another mode of therapy that was used in the NTGS. However, filtering surgery has a greater complication rate than topical or laser treatments. As many as one-half of the patients in the NTGS who had filtering surgery required cataract extraction. The risk-benefit ratio should be contemplated for each mode of treatment in patients with NTG.

TABLE 14-3. Summary of Effects of Antiglaucoma Medications on Blood Flow to the Optic Nerve

Drug	Route	Subjects	Vascular site	Method	Results	Author (date)
Beta blockers						
Timolol 0.5% (20 days)	Topical	Rabbit	Optic nerve head	Laser speckle tissue circulation analyzer	Increased peripheral blood velocity in optic nerves	Tamaki et al.,[109] (1997)
Timolol 0.5% (1 wk)	Topical	Human	Retrobulbar	Color Doppler	No change	Nicolela et al.,[4] (1996)
Timolol 0.5%	Topical	Human	Retinal/retro-bulbar	Pulsation amps, Doppler ultrasound	Decreased choroidal and optic nerve head blood flow	Schmetterer et al.,[1] (1997)
Timolol 0.5%	Topical	Human	Choroidal	Laser Doppler velocimetry	Decreased choroidal blood flow	Yoshida et al.,[3] (1991)
Timolol 0.5%	Topical	Human	Ophthalmic and central retinal artery	Oculo-oscillo dynamography	No change	Pillunat et al.,[99] (1988)
Timolol 0.5% (12 mos)	Topical	Open-angle glaucoma	Choroidal/retinal	Langham ocular blood flow system	Decreased pulsatile blood flow	Carenini et al.,[2] (1994)
Timolol 0.5%	Topical	NTG	Retinal	Two-part fluorometry	Slight increase in arterial and venous velocity	Truckenbrodt et al.,[110] (1992)
Timolol 0.5%	Topical	NTG	Retrobulbar	Color doppler	No change	Harris et al.,[102] (1995)
Betaxolol 0.5%	Topical	Human	Retinal/retro-bulbar	Pulsation amps, Doppler ultrasound	No change in optic nerve head or choroidal blood flow	Schmetterer et al.,[1] (1997)
Betaxolol 0.5%	Topical	Human	Ophthalmic central retinal artery	Oculo-oscillo dynamography	No change	Pillunat et al.,[99] (1988)
Betaxolol 0.5%	Topical	NTG	Retrobulbar	Color Doppler	Less resistance	Harris et al.,[102] (1995)
Betaxolol 0.5% (12 mos)	Topical	Open-angle glaucoma	Choroidal/retinal	Langham ocular blood flow system	Stable	Carenini et al.,[2] (1994)
Levobunolol 0.5% (1 wk, b.i.d).	Topical	Human	Retinal	Laser Doppler velocimetry	Slight increase in flow	Bloom et al.,[111] (1997)
Levobunolol 0.5%	Topical	Human	Retinal/retrobulbar	Pulsation amps, Doppler ultrasound	No change	Schmetterer et al.,[1] (1997)
Carteolol 2% (20 days)	Topical	Human	Optic nerve head	Laser speckle tissue circulation analyzer	Increased blood velocity	Tamaki et al.,[112] (1998)
Carteolol 2%	Topical	Human	Ophthalmic and central retinal artery	Oculo-oscillo dynamography	Decrease in perfusion	Pillunat et al.,[99] (1988)
Prostaglandins						
Latanoprost 0.005% (1 wk)	Topical	Human	Retrobulbar	Color Doppler	No change	Nicolela et al.,[4] (1996)

continued

TABLE 14-3. *(continued)*

Drug	Route	Subjects	Vascular site	Method	Results	Author (date)
Carbonic anhydrase inhibitors						
Dorzolamide 2% (2 gtt)	Topical	Human	Retinal	Scanning laser	Accelerates blood velocity	Harris et al.,[28] (1996)
			Retrobulbar	Color Doppler	No effect	
Dorzolamide 2% (1 gtt)	Topical	Human	Retinal	Laser Doppler	No effect	Grunwald et al.,[113] (1997)
Acetazolamide (750 mg)	Oral	Human	Ophthalmic and central retinal artery	Oculo-oscillo dynamography	No effect	Pillunat et al.,[99] (1988)
Adrenergics						
Dipivefrin	Topical	Human	Retinal/retro-bulbar	Pulsation amps, Doppler ultrasound	Decreased choroidal and optic nerve head blood flow	Schmetterer et al.,[1] (1997)
Apraclonidine 1%	Topical	Human	Retrobulbar	Color Doppler ultrasound	Decreased velocity, increased resistance	Celiker et al.,[103] (1996)
Brimonidine 0.2%	Topical	Ocular hyperten-sion	Retrobulbar	Color Doppler ultrasound	No change	Lachkar et al.,[114] (1998)
Miotics						
Pilocarpine (1 wk)	Topical	Human	Choroidal/retinal	Langham ocular blood flow system	No change in pulsa-tile blood flow	Claridge et al.,[104] (1993)
Pilocarpine	Topical	Human	Retinal/retro-bulbar	Pulsation amps, Doppler ultrasound	No change	Schmetterer et al.,[1] (1997)
Calcium channel blockers						
Verapamil	Topical	Human	Anterior optic nerve	Laser Doppler	Increased capillary blood speed	Netland et al.,[115] (1996)
Nifedipine	Oral	Human	Retrobulbar	Langham ocular blood flow system	If cold exposure test is negative, no change	Schmidt et al.,[116] (1997)
					If cold exposure test is positive (vasospas-tic), increased pulse amplitude	

NTG = normal tension glaucoma.

EFFECTS OF CALCIUM CHANNEL BLOCKERS ON THE PROGRESSION OF NORMAL TENSION GLAUCOMA

Calcium channel blockers may decrease vasospasm and increase capillary dilation. The benefits of oral nifedipine (and other calcium channel blockers) on the clinical course of glaucoma are unclear. Liu and associates reported no apparent difference in the stability of the visual fields or optic discs for patients with NTG who were taking cal-cium channel blockers for nonophthalmic diseases com-pared with NTG patients who were not taking these drugs.[105] In contrast, Netland and coworkers reported that fewer NTG patients on calcium channel blocker ther-apy showed any significant progression of visual field defects or optic nerve damage compared with NTG patients who were not taking calcium channel blockers.[106] As more and more research on the effects of calcium chan-nel blockers on ONH circulation and the clinical course of the disease emerges, the role of this classification of drug in the management of NTG may become more clear. No clear evidence yet exists of an advantageous role of oral calcium channel blockers in NTG, and these medications have significant systemic side effects (hypotension).

TABLE 14-4. Treatment Protocol for Normal Tension Glaucoma

1. Set target pressure 30% from the highest intraocular pressure reading after a series of pretreatment intraocular pressure readings.

2. Use latanoprost, brimonidine, dorzolamide, brinzolamide, betaxolol, or pilocarpine as primary agents.

3. Determine effectiveness of medicines by a 20% or greater intraocular pressure reduction from baseline. If a 20% reduction not achieved, discontinue medication and try a different medication.

4. Avoid nonselective beta blockers and epinephrine drugs because of potential vasoconstrictive properties.

5. If target pressure (of 30% or more decrease) is not achieved on two medications, consider argon laser trabeculoplasty.

6. If target intraocular pressure is not achieved with argon laser trabeculoplasty and medications and the patient has fixation threatened, then consider filtering surgery. Consider filtering surgery with confirmed progressive visual field loss despite medical and laser therapy.

DIFFERENTIAL DIAGNOSIS OF NORMAL TENSION GLAUCOMA

The most common differential diagnosis of NTG is POAG, in which the circadian range of IOP exceeds normal limits at times other than when the patient is tested. This can be differentiated from NTG by using serial pretreatment IOP readings or diurnal curves. Patients with large physiologic cupping and alleged early visual field loss that is no longer apparent in subsequent visual field testing due to a learning curve can also be misdiagnosed with NTG. All visual field defects, especially when they do not correlate to the optic nerve, should be confirmed with subsequent tests. Close scrutiny of the parameters suggestive of NTG in the patient history, the ONH, and visual fields assist in the differential diagnosis.

Undetected high levels of IOP may also be present in cases of intermittent angle-closure glaucoma, uveitic glaucoma, steroid-induced glaucoma, or "burned-out" pigmentary glaucoma. In general, these conditions can be effectively ruled out by a careful history, slit-lamp examination, serial tonometry, and gonioscopy (Table 14-5).

TABLE 14-5. Differential Diagnosis of Normal Tension Glaucoma Versus Other Types of Glaucoma

History	Slit lamp	Diurnal pressures	Gonioscopy
Intermittent angle closure (see Chapter 16)			
Intermittent pain, blurred vision, halos surrounding lights, conjunctival injection, more frequent in dim illumination (when pupil is dilated), more common in hyperopia versus myopia	Narrow angle, evidence of posterior synechiae, previous peripheral iridotomy, glaucomflecken	Intermittent spikes; post-mydriatic intraocular pressure may reveal spike	Narrow angle; peripheral anterior synechiae, especially in superior angle
Uveitic glaucoma (see Chapter 15)			
Previous episodes or history of treatment for uveitis and/or glaucoma	Low grade iritis, posterior synechiae, old keratic precipitates	Intermittent spikes with active iritis	Peripheral anterior synechiae, especially in the inferior angle; angle scarring, pigment clumping in angle
Steroid-induced glaucoma (see Chapter 15)			
History of corticosteroid use	Normal	High when patient is on steroids	Normal
Systemic conditions associated with steroid use:			
Allergic disorders			
Dermatologic disorders			
Atopic dermatitis			
Pruritus			
Lung disease			
Asthma			
Chronic obstructive pulmonary disease			

continued

TABLE 14-5. (*continued*)

History	Slit lamp	Diurnal pressures	Gonioscopy
Arthritis and musculoskeletal disorders			
Gout			
Rheumatoid arthritis			
Systemic lupus erythematosus			
Polyarteritis nodosa			
Sarcoidosis			
Polymyositis-dermatomyositises			
Giant cell arteritis			
Liver disease			
Alcoholic hepatitis			
Following organ transplant			
Pigmentary glaucoma (see Chapter 15)			
Younger (<40 years)	Krukenberg's spindle	Intermittent spikes	Open angle
Myopia	Concave iris contour		
Male	Iris transillumination Pigment in anterior chamber especially with dilation or exercise		Heavily pigmented trabecular meshwork

Nonglaucomatous Conditions That Mimic Normal Tension Glaucoma

Any condition that yields glaucomatous optic nerves or visual field abnormalities without raised IOP can be confused with NTG (Table 14-6). Optic disc anomalies, such as large physiologic cups or myopic discs with PPA, present diagnostic challenges. Physiologic cups are diagnosed only after careful assessment of the optic nerve (including measuring the optic disc size; see Figure 5-10), nerve fiber layer, visual field, and IOP over time. Myopic discs can be particularly difficult to assess because they are often inserted obliquely and contrast cues afforded by the adjacent retinal grounds are confounded by the presence of PPA. This makes the assessment of the neuroretinal rim more arduous. Additionally, a significant percentage of these patients manifest some level of visual field loss, which makes the differential diagnosis even less straightforward. Other congenital anomalies, such as ONH colobomas, optic pits (see Color Plate 25), tilted discs, and optic nerve head drusen might also produce visual field defects and be confused with NTG. Diagnosis is made by careful, correlating examination of the optic nerve and the visual field.

Vascular Lesions That Mimic Normal Tension Glaucoma

The most common vascular lesion that resembles NTG is anterior ischemic optic neuropathy (AION). There are two types of AION: an arteritic form usually caused by giant cell arteritis, and a nonarteritic form associated with systemic vasculopathies, such as hypertension, diabetes, and arteriosclerosis. Like NTG, AION is generally a condition involving patients older than 50 years. It typically presents as a sudden, painless loss of vision or visual field in one eye in conjunction with swelling of the optic nerve. Visual field loss is often localized to one hemifield but may also include diffuse loss. The optic nerve, after the initial disc edema, usually becomes pale in 4–6 weeks after the initial event, representing optic atrophy. However, some cases of resolved arteritic AION (giant cell arteritis) can resemble glaucomatous cupping, and the IOP is generally within "normal" limits. The clinical profile of giant cell arteritis is an elderly patient with symptoms of headache, scalp tenderness, and jaw claudication with an elevated sedimentation rate and positive C-reactive protein.

Retinal embolic disease (e.g., cardiac, carotid) could also be mistaken for NTG. Symptoms generally are acute loss of vision or visual field and evidence of retinal arterial plaques or sclerosed retinal vessels. The ONH, although possibly excavated in a manner akin to glaucoma, may appear pale from retrograde atrophy of the ganglion cell axons. The blood supply to the ONH may also be compromised in the presence of blood loss (e.g., during surgery), blood dyscrasias (e.g., sickle cell disease), or carotid artery disease. Midperipheral dot-and-blot hemorrhages suggest ocular ischemic syndrome secondary to carotid artery disease.

TABLE 14-6. Differential Diagnosis of Normal Tension Glaucoma

Clinical finding	Diagnosis
Glaucoma damage to the optic nerve/visual field loss with normal IOP	
IOP spikes on serial IOP readings or diurnal curve	POAG
Concurrent systemic use of:	Masked POAG
Beta blockers	
Calcium channel blockers	
Clonidine	
Previous PRK/LASIK:	Masked POAG
Thin cornea (pachometry)	
Previous increase in IOP:	
History of corticosteroid use	Steroid-induced glaucoma
Evidence of anterior chamber inflammation	Uveitic glaucoma
Evidence of pigment dispersion	Pigmentary glaucoma
Diurnal normal IOP and ONH/nerve fiber layer suggestive of glaucomatous optic neuropathy	
With ONH pallor of rim tissue (disproportionate with cupping)	Nonglaucomatous optic atrophy
	Anterior ischemic optic neuropathy
	Optic neuritis
	Leber's optic neuropathy
	Toxic optic neuropathy
	Congenital disc anomaly
	Optic pit
	Optic nerve coloboma
	Optic nerve head drusen
	Tilted disc
	Hypoplastic disc
Without rim pallor	Measure disc size (vertical diameter >2 mm: consider large physiologic cup)
Visual field loss and diurnal normal IOP	
Repeat visual field test	No visual field loss on repeat visual field test: learning curve
Repeated visual field defects respect vertical midline	Rule out chiasmal/posterior chiasmal lesion
	Pituitary tumor
	Meningioma
	Craniopharyngioma
	Cerebral vascular accident
Repeated visual field defects do not respect vertical midline	Rule out anterior chiasm disease
	Branch retinal artery occlusion/branch retinal vein occlusion
	Retinal scar
	Other optic neuropathy (anterior ischemic optic neuropathy, optic neuritis, compressive, disc drusen), look for disc pallor

IOP = intraocular pressure; POAG = primary open-angle glaucoma; ONH = optic nerve head; PRK = photorefractive keratectomy.

TABLE 14-7. Findings Suggestive of Neurologic Disease in the Workup of Normal Tension Glaucoma

1. Younger age (<50 years)
2. Visual acuity disproportionately worse than the appearance of optic nerve head.
3. Optic nerve head pallor (see Color Plate 23) or swelling.
4. Visual field respecting vertical midline (see Figure 7-17).

Neurologic Conditions That Mimic Normal Tension Glaucoma

Neurologic conditions that could be confused with NTG include meningioma of the optic nerve, pituitary adenoma, craniopharyngioma, opticochiasmic arachnoiditis, empty-cell syndrome, and Leber's optic neuropathy.[37] Kupersmith and Krohn demonstrated lesions compressing the anterior visual pathway in 16 patients with "normal" IOP.[107] The visual fields in most patients revealed a bitemporal visual field defect and Snellen acuity loss out of proportion to the extent of the optic cupping. Greenfield and associates studied 52 eyes of 29 patients with NTG and 44 eyes of 28 control patients with compressive lesions.[108] They found that none of the patients diagnosed with glaucoma had neuroradiologic evidence of a mass lesion involving the anterior visual pathway. Patients with compressive disease tended to be younger, have lower levels of visual acuity, have visual fields that respected the vertical midline, and display neuroretinal rim pallor. Detailed assessments of the optic disc, visual acuity, visual fields, and the age of the patient should provide ample information to rule out compressive lesion of the optic nerves or chiasm and NTG. Neuroimaging studies are not required for typical cases of NTG (in which no evidence of disc pallor is found, no vertical midline respect is seen on visual field, and optic cupping is proportional to visual field loss) (Table 14-7).

SUMMARY

There is much to be learned about the characteristics and treatment of NTG. It is a diagnosis of exclusion after a careful history and diagnostic assessment. Several clinical findings may be more prevalent in NTG than in other forms of open-angle glaucoma (e.g., disc hemorrhage, APONs, visual fields with steeper slopes that are closer to fixation), but these are not unique to NTG. The role of the optic nerve vasculature in the pathogenesis and treatment of NTG is incompletely understood. Treatment should be aimed at arresting progression and may, in the future, be targeted at enhancing blood flow or preventing ganglion cell death.

In the past, there was no evidence of the benefit of lowering IOP in patients who present with glaucomatous optic nerve damage and IOP in the statistically nor-

mal range. However, the NTGS showed that patients with NTG and progressing visual field loss or visual field loss close to fixation attained a threefold reduction in the risk of progression when IOP was decreased by 30%. The study did not address which methods of therapy are most effective in preventing visual field loss progression. Newer topical medications, such as topical prostaglandins, α agonists, and topical carbonic anhydrase inhibitors, were not available at the time of the study design. The NTGS did show that cataract acceleration was a significant complication of filtering surgery.

Patients with obvious damage from glaucoma and normal IOP should have their IOP reduced. A 30% reduction would be a logical initial target pressure based on the NTGS, but each mode of therapy required to achieve a target pressure should be weighed against the potential side effects of the treatment. NTG patients with less definitive damage should be given a choice between treatment and close observation. In the NTGS, 65% of nontreated patients did not progress over a 5-year follow-up period. Nonselective beta blockers and epinephrine drugs should be avoided in NTG patients because of the potential adverse effect on blood supply to the optic nerve. Latanoprost, topical carbonic anhydrase inhibitors, and brimonidine are effective in lowering IOP and do not appear to alter the blood supply to the optic nerve. These drugs can be used as the initial treatment for NTG, although they were not studied in the NTGS. Pilocarpine was the primary medication used in the NTGS. It can be used as a primary or secondary agent in NTG. Argon laser trabeculoplasty is also an attractive treatment option when the desired target pressure is not met with the use of one or two topical medications. Filtering surgery is advocated when a patient shows documented, confirmed progression of the visual field loss or optic nerve defect despite medical and laser therapy, or if central fixation is threatened and the IOP cannot be lowered 30% with medications and argon laser trabeculoplasty.

REFERENCES

1. Schmetterer L, Strenn K, Findl O, et al. Effects of antiglaucoma drugs on ocular hemodynamics in healthy volunteers. Clin Pharmacol Ther 1997; 61(5): 583–595.

2. Carenini AD, Sibour G, Boles Carenini B. Differences in the longterm effect of timolol and betaxolol on the pulsatile ocular blood flow. Surv Ophthalmol 1994;38(suppl):S118–S124.

3. Yoshida A, Feke GT, Ogasaware H, et al. Effect of timolol on human retinal, choroidal and optic nerve head circulation. Ophthalmic Res 1991;23(3):162–170.

4. Nicolela MT, Buckley AR, Walman BE, Drance SM. A comparative study of the effects of timolol and

latanoprost on blood flow velocity of the retrobulbar vessels. Am J Ophthalmol 1996;122(6):784–789.

5. Collaborative Normal-Tension Glaucoma Study Group. Comparison of glaucomatous progression between untreated patients with normal-tension glaucoma and patients with therapeutically reduced intraocular pressures. Am J Ophthalmol 1998;126:487–497.

6. Miller KM, Quigley HA. Comparison of optic disc features in low-tension and typical open-angle glaucoma. Ophthalmic Surg 1987;18(12):882–889.

7. Wang XH, Stewart WC, Jackson GJ. Differences in optic discs in low-tension glaucoma patients with relatively low or high pressures. Acta Ophthalmol Scand 1996;74(4):364–367.

8. Von Graefe A. Amaursos mit Sehnervenexcavation. Archiv Ophthalmol 1857;68:389.

9. Lee BL, Renuka B, Weinreb RN. The definition of normal-tension glaucoma. J Glaucoma 1998;7:366–371.

10. Caprioli J. Editorial: the treatment of normal-tension glaucoma. Am J Ophthalmol 1998;126(4):578–581.

11. Sommer A. Glaucoma: facts and fancies. Eye 1996;10:295–301.

12. Klein BEK, Klein R, Sponsel WE, et al. Prevalence of glaucoma: the Beaver Dam Eye Study. Ophthalmology 1992;99:1499–504.

13. Sommer A, Tielsch JM, Katz J, et al. Relationship between intraocular pressure and primary open angle glaucoma among white and black Americans. The Baltimore Eye Survey. Arch Ophthalmol 1991;109:1090–1095.

14. Shiose Y. Prevalence and clinical aspects of low-tension glaucoma. In Henkind P (ed). Acta XXIV International Congress of Ophthalmology. Philadelphia: JB Lippincott, 1983;587–591.

15. Shiose Y, Kitazawa Y, Tsukahara S, et al. Epidemiology of glaucoma in Japan: a nationwide glaucoma survey. Jpn J Ophthalmol 1991;35(2):133–155.

16. Leighton DA, Tomlinson A. Ocular tension and axial length of the eyeball in open-angle glaucoma and low-tension glaucoma. Br J Ophthalmol 1973;57(499):499–502.

17. Bengtsson B. Findings associated with glaucomatous visual field defects. Acta Ophthalmol 1980;58(20):20–32.

18. Huang L, Zhou W. The relationship of structure in vivo of low tension glaucoma and myopia. Yen Ko Hsueh Pao 1990;6(3–4):58–59.

19. Levene R. Low tension glaucoma: a critical review and new material. Surv Ophthalmol 1980;61:621–664.

20. Orgul S, Gaspar AZ, Hendrickson P, Flammer J. Comparison of the severity of normal-tension glaucoma in men and women. Ophthalmologica 1994;208(3):142–144.

21. Werner EB. Low Tension Glaucoma. In R Ritch, MB Shields, T Krupin (eds). The Glaucomas. St. Louis: Mosby, 1989;804.

22. Wang L, Cioffi GA, Van Buskirk EM. The vascular pattern of the optic nerve and its potential relevance in glaucoma. Curr Opin Ophthalmol 1998; 9(11):24–29.

23. Hayreh SS. Inter-individual variation in blood supply of the optic nerve head. Its importance in various ischemic disorders of the optic nerve head, and glaucoma, low-tension glaucoma and allied disorders. Doc Ophthalmol 1985;59(3):217–246.

24. Kaiser HJ, Schoetzau A, Stumpfig D, Flammer J. Blood-flow velocities of the extraocular vessels in patients with high-tension and normal-tension primary open-angle glaucoma. Am J Ophthalmol 1997;123:320–327.

25. Nicolela MT, Hnik P, Drance SM. Scanning laser Doppler flowmeter study of retinal and optic disk blood flow in glaucomatous patients. Am J Ophthalmol 1996;122:775–783.

26. Yamazaki Y, Drance SM. The relationship between progression of visual field defects and retrobulbar circulation in patients with glaucoma. Am J Ophthalmol 1997;123:287–295.

27. Cellini M, Possati GL, Sbrocca M, Caramazza N. Correlation between visual field and color Doppler parameters in chronic open angle glaucoma. Int Ophthalmol 1996;20:215–219.

28. Harris A, Joos K, Kay M, et al. Acute IOP elevation with scleral suction: effects on retrobulbar hemodyamics. Br J Ophthalmol 1996;80:1055–1059.

29. Harris A, Spaeth G, Wilson R, et al. Nocturnal ophthalmic arterial hemodyamics in primary open-angle glaucoma. J Glaucoma 1997;6:170–174.

30. Hayreh SS, Zimmerman MB, Podhajsky P, Alward WL. Nocturnal arterial hypotension and its role in optic nerve head and ocular ischemic disorders. Am J Ophthalmol 1994;15;117(5):603–624.

31. Muzyka M, Nizankowska MH, Koziorowska M, Zajac-Pytrus H. Occurrence of nocturnal arterial hypotension in patients with primary open-angle glaucoma and normal tension glaucoma. Klin Oczna 1997;99(2):109–113.

32. Kaiser HJ, Flammer J, Graf T, Stumpfig D. Systemic blood pressure in glaucoma patients. Graefes Arch Clin Exp Ophthalmol 1993;231(12):677–680.

33. Meyer JH, Brandi-Dohrn J, Funk J. Twenty-four hour blood pressure monitoring in normal tension glaucoma. Br J Ophthalmol 1996;80(10):864–867.

34. Graham SL, Drance SM, Wijsman K, et al. Ambulatory blood pressure monitoring in glaucoma. The nocturnal dip. Ophthalmology 1995;102(1):61–69.

35. Iwata K. Primary open angle glaucoma and low tension glaucoma—pathogenesis and mechanism of optic nerve damage. Nippon Ganka Gakkai Zasshi 1992;96(12):1501–1531.

36. Van Buskirk EM. Editorial: the tale of normal-tension glaucoma. J Glaucoma 1998;7:363–365.

37. Geijssen HC. Studies on Normal-Pressure Glaucoma, Amstelveen, New York: Kugler Publications, 1991.

38. Zeimer RC, Wilensky JT, Gieser DK, et al. Application of a self-tonometer to home tonometry, Arch Ophthalmol 1986;104(48):49–53.

39. De Viver C, O'Brien C, Lanigan L, Hitchings R. Diurnal intraocular pressure variations in low-tension glaucoma. Eye 1994;8:521–523.

40. Yamagami J, Araie M, Shirato S, Ishii R. Diurnal variation of intraocular pressure in low tension glaucoma. Nippon Ganka Gakkai Zasshi 1991;95(5):495–499.

41. Ido T, Tomita G, Kitazawa Y. Diurnal variation of intraocular pressure of normal-tension glaucoma. Influence of sleep and arousal. Ophthalmology 1991;98(3):296–300.

42. Yamagami J, Araie M, Aihara M, Yamamoto S. Diurnal variation in intraocular pressure of normal tension glaucoma eyes. Ophthalmology 1993;100(5):643–650.

43. Mardin CY, Jonas J, Michelson G, Junemann A. Are there genuine and pseudo-normal pressure glaucomas? Body position–dependent intraocular pressure values in normal pressure glaucoma. Klin Monastsbl Augenheilkd 1997;211(4):235–240.

44. Morad Y, Sharon E, Hefetz L, Nemet P. Corneal thickness and curvature in normal tension glaucoma. Am J Ophthalmol 1998;125:164–168.

45. Copt RP, Thomas R, Mermoud A. Corneal thickness in ocular hypertension, primary open-angle glaucoma, and normal tension glaucoma. Arch Ophthalmol 1999;117:14–16.

46. Ehlers N, Bramsen T, Sperling S. Applanation tonometry and central corneal thickness. Acta Ophthalmol (Copenh) 1975;53:34–43.

47. Whitacre MM, Stein RA, Hassanein K. The effect of corneal thickness on applanation tonometry. Am J Ophthalmol 1993;115:592–596.

48. Wolfs RC, Klaver CC, Vingerling JR, et al. Distribution of central corneal thickness and its association with intraocular pressure: The Rotterdam Study. Am J Ophthalmol 1997;123:767–772.

49. Wada I. Ultrasound biomicroscopic corneal thickness measurement for corneal thickness mapping. Jpn J Ophthalmol 1997;41(1):12–18.

50. Lam AK, Douthwaite WA. The corneal-thickness profile in Hong Kong Chinese. Cornea 1998;17(4):384–388.

51. Schipper I, Senn P, Niesen U. Are we measuring the right intraocular pressure after excimer laser photorefractive laser keratoplasty in myopia? Klin Monatsbl Augenheilkd 1995;206(5):322–324.

52. Abbasoglu OE, Bowman RW, Cavanagh HD, McCulley JP. Reliability of intraocular pressure measurements after myopic excimer photorefractive keratectomy. Ophthalmology 1998;105(12):2193–2196.

53. Mardelli PG, Piebenga LW, Whitacre MM, Siegmund KD. The effect of excimer laser photorefractive keratectomy on intraocular pressure measurements using the Goldmann applanation tonometer. Ophthalmology 1997;104(6):945–948.

54. Chatterjee A, Shah S, Bessant DA, et al. Reduction in intraocular pressure after excimer laser photorefractive keratectomy. Correlation with pretreatment myopia. Ophthalmology 1997;104(3):355–359.

55. Rosa N, Cennamo G, Breve MA, La Rana A. Goldmann applanation tonometry after myopic photorefractive keratectomy. Acta Ophthalmol Scand 1998;76(5):550–554.

56. Cartwright MJ, Anderson DR. Correlation of asymmetric damage with asymmetric intraocular pressure in normal-tension glaucoma (low-tension glaucoma). Arch Ophthalmol 1988;106(7):898–900.

57. Chen RY. Intraocular pressure and optic nerve damages in monocular early glaucoma: a comparative study of primary open angle glaucoma and low tension glaucoma. Chung Hua Yen Ko Tsa Chih 1992; 28(4):217–220.

58. Orgul S, Flammer J. Interocular visual field and intraocular pressure asymmetries in normal tension glaucoma. Eur J Ophthalmol 1994;4(4):199–201.

59. Haefliger IO, Hitchings RA. Relationship between asymmetry of visual field defects and intraocular pressure difference in an untreated normal (low) tension glaucoma population. Acta Ophthalmol (Copenh) 1990;68(5):564–567.

60. Crichton A, Drance SM, Douglas GR, Schulzer M. Unequal intraocular pressure and its relation to asymmetric visual field defects in low tension glaucoma. Ophthalmology 1989;96(9):1312–1314.

61. Bhandari A, Crabb DP, Poinoosawmy D, et al. Effect of surgery on visual field progression in normal tension glaucoma. Ophthalmology 1997;104:1131–1137.

62. Schulzer M, and the Normal Tension Glaucoma Study Group. Intraocular pressure reduction in normal tension glaucoma patients. Ophthalmology 1992;99:1469–1470.

63. Tuulonen A, Airaksinen PJ. Optic disc size in exfoliative, primary open angle, and low-tension glaucoma. Arch Ophthalmol 1992;110(2):211–213.

64. Burk RO, Rohrschneider K, Noack H, Volcker HE. Are large optic nerve heads susceptible to glaucomatous damage at normal intraocular pressure? A three-dimensional study by laser scanning tomography. Graefes Arch Clin Exp Ophthalmol 1992;230(6):552–560.

65. Jonas JB. Size of glaucomatous discs. Ger J Ophthalmol 1992;1(1):41–44.

66. Caprioli J, Spaeth GL. Comparison of the optic nerve head in high- and low-tension glaucoma. Arch Ophthalmol 1985;103(8):1145–1149.

67. My Li. Comparison between the optic nerve heads in low tension glaucoma and primary open angle glaucoma. Chung Hua Yen Ko Tsa Chih 1989; 25(6):322–325.

68. Stutman RS. Acquired pits of the optic nerve in glaucoma. Clin Eye Vis Care 1996;8:215–223.

69. Radius RL, Maumenee AE, Green WR. Pit-like changes of the optic nerve head in open-angle glaucoma. Br J Ophthalmol 1978;62:389–393.

70. Javitt JC, Spaeth GL, Katz LJ, et al. Acquired pits of the optic nerve. Increased prevalence in patients with low-tension glaucoma. Ophthalmology 1990;97(8):1038–1043.

71. Aduaguba C, Ugurlu S, Caprioli J. Acquired pits of the optic nerve in glaucoma: prevalence and associated visual field loss. Acta Ophthalmol Scand 1998;76(3):272–277.

72. Cashwell LF, Ford JG. Central visual field changes associated with acquired pits of the optic nerve. Ophthalmology 1995;102(9):1270–1278.

73. Chumbley LC, Brubaker RF. Low-tension glaucoma. Am J Ophthalmol 1976;81:76.

74. Tuulonen A, Airaksinene PF, Alanko HI. Optic disc size in eyes with and without an optic disc hemorrhage. Invest Ophthalmol Vis Sci 1992;33(suppl):883.

75. Kitazawa Y, Shirato S, Yamamoto T. Optic disc hemorrhage in low-tension glaucoma. Ophthalmology 1986;93:853–857.

76. Gloster J. Incidence of optic disc haemorrhages in chronic simple glaucoma and ocular hypertension. Br J Ophthalmol 1981;65(7):452–456.

77. Airaksinen PJ, Mustonen E, Alanko HI. Optic disc hemorrhages. Analysis of stereophotographs and clinical data of 112 patients. Arch Ophthalmol 1981;99(10):1795–1801.

78. Sugiyama K, Tomita G, Kitazawa Y, et al. The association of optic disc hemorrhage with retinal nerve fiber layer defect and peripapillary atrophy in normal-tension glaucoma. Ophthalmology 1997;104(11):1926–1933.

79. Drance SM. Disc hemorrhages in the glaucomas. Surv Ophthalmol 1989;33(5):331–337.

80. Siegner SW, Netland PA. Optic disc hemorrhages and progression of glaucoma. Ophthalmology 1996;103(7):1014–1024.

81. Jonas JB, Bennis S. Localised wedge shaped defects of the retinal nerve fibre layer in glaucoma. Br J Ophthalmol 1994;78:285–290.

82. Yamazaki Y, Koide C, Miyazawa T, et al. Comparison of retinal nerve-fiber layer in high- and normal-tension glaucoma. Graefes Arch Clin Exp Ophthalmol 1991;229:517–520.

83. Yamazaki Y, Koide C, Takahashi F, Yamada H. Diffuse nerve fiber layer loss in normal-tension glaucoma. Int Ophthalmol 1992;16:247–250.

84. Park KH, Tomita G, Liou SY, Kitazawa Y. Correlation between peripapillary atrophy and optic nerve damage in normal-tension glaucoma. Ophthalmology 1996;103(11):1899–1906.

85. Uchida H, Ugurlu S, Caprioli J. Increasing peripapillary atrophy is associated with progressive glaucoma. Ophthalmology 1998;105(8):1541–1545.

86. Drance SM, Douglas GR, Airaksinen PJ, et al. Diffuse visual field loss in chronic open-angle and low-tension glaucoma. Am J Ophthalmol 1987;104(6):577–580.

87. Zeiter JH, Shin DH, Juzych MS, et al. Visual field defects in patients with normal-tension glaucoma and patients with high-tension glaucoma. Am J Ophthalmol 1992;114(6):758–763.

88. Araie M, Yamagami J, Suzuki Y. Visual field defects in normal-tension and high-tension glaucoma. Ophthalmology 1993;100(12):1808–1814.

89. Samuelson TW, Spaeth GL. Focal and diffuse visual field defects: their relationship to intraocular pressure. Ophthalmic Surg 1993;24(8):519–525.

90. Hitchings RA, Anderton SA. A comparative study of visual field defects seen in patients with low-tension glaucoma and chronic simple glaucoma. Br J Ophthalmol 1983;67(12):818–821.

91. Caprioli J, Spaeth GL. Comparison of visual field defects in the low-tension glaucomas with those in the high-tension glaucomas. Am J Ophthalmol 1984;97(6):730–737.

92. Takada M, Araie M, Suzuki Y, et al. The central field defects in low-tension glaucoma. A comparison of the central visual field defects in low-tension glaucoma with those in primary open angle glaucoma. Nippon Ganka Gakkai Zasshi 1993;97(11):1320–1324.

93. Koseki N, Araie M, Suzuki Y, Yamagami J. Visual field damage proximal to fixation in normal- and high-tension glaucoma eyes. Jpn J Ophthalmol 1995;39(3):274–283.

94. Gliklich RE, Steinmann WC, Spaeth GL. Visual field change in low-tension glaucoma over a five-year follow-up. Ophthalmology 1989;96(3):316–320.

95. Noureddin BN, Poinoosawmy D, Fietzke FW, Hitchings RA. Regression analysis of visual field progression in low tension glaucoma. Br J Ophthalmol 1991;75(8):493–495.

96. Araie M, Sekine M, Susuki Y, Koseki N. Factors contributing to the progression of visual field damage in eyes with normal-tension glaucoma. Ophthalmology 1994;101:1440–1444.

97. Tsang AC, Harris A, Kagemann L, et al. Brightness alters Heidelberg retinal flowmeter measurements in an in vitro model. Invest Ophthalmol Vis Sci 1999;40(3):795–799.

98. Dawidek GM, Robinson MI. Beta-adrenergic receptors in human anterior optic nerve: an autoradiographic study. Eye 1993;7:122–126.

99. Pillunat L, Stodtmeister R. Effect of different antiglaucomatous drugs on ocular perfusion pressures. J Ocul Pharmacol 1988;4(3):231–242.

100. Graf-Grauwiller T, Stumpfig D, Flammer J. Do beta-blockers cause vasospasm? Ophthalmologica 1993;206(1):45–50.

101. Arend O, Harris A, Arend S, et al. The acute effect of topical beta-adrenoreceptor blocking agents on retinal and optic nerve head circulation. Acta Ophthalmol Scand 1998;76(1):43–49.

102. Harris A, Spaeth GL, Sergott RC, et al. Retrobulbar arterial hemodynamic effects of betaxolol and timolol in normal-tension glaucoma. Am J Ophthalmol 1995;120(2):168–175.

103. Celiker UO, Celebi S, Celiker H, Celebi H. Effect of topical aproclonidine on flow properties of central retinal and ophthalmic arteries. Acta Ophthalmol Scand 1996;74(2):151–154.

104. Claridge KG. The effect of topical pilocarpine on pulsatile ocular blood flow. Eye 1993;7:507–510.

105. Liu S, Araujo SV, Spaeth GL, et al. Lack of effect of calcium channel blockers on open-angle glaucoma. J Glaucoma 1996;5(3):187–190.

106. Netland PA, Chaturvedi N, Dryer EB. Calcium channel blockers in the management of low-tension and open-angle glaucoma. Am J Ophthalmol 1993;115(5):608–613.

107. Kupersmith MJ, Krohn D. Cupping of the optic disc with compressive lesions of the anterior visual pathway. Ann Ophthalmol 1984;16(10):948–953.

108. Greenfield DS, Siatkowski RM, Glaser JS, et al. The cupped disc. Who needs neuroimaging? Ophthalmology 1998;105:1866–1874.

109. Tamaki Y, Araie M, Tomita K, Tomidokoro A. Effect of topical timolol on tissue circulation in optic nerve head. Jpn J Ophthalmol 1997;41(5):297–304.

110. Truckenbrodt C, Klein S, Vilser W. Does timolol modify retinal hemodynamics in patients with normal pressure glaucoma? Ophthalmology 1992;89(6):452–454.

111. Bloom AH, Grunwald JE, DuPont JC. Effect of one week of levobunolol Hcl 0.5% on the human retinal circulation. Curr Eye Res 1997;16(3):191–196.

112. Tamaki Y, Araie M, Tomita K, Tomidokoro A. Effect of topical carteolol on tissue circulation in optic nerve head. Jpn J Ophthalmol 1998; 42(1):27–32.

113. Grunwald JE, Mathur S, DuPont J. Effect of dorzolamide hydrochloride 2% on the retinal circulation. Acta Ophthalmol Scand 1997;75(3):236–238.

114. Lachkar Y, Migdal C, Dhanjil S. Effect of brimonidine tartrate on ocular hemodynamic measurements. Arch Ophthalmol 1998;116(12):1591–1594.

115. Netland PA, Feke GT, Konno S, et al. Optic nerve head circulation after topical channel blocker. J Glaucoma 1996;5(3):200–206.

116. Schmidt KG, von Ruckmann A, Geyer O, Mittag TW. Effect of nifedipine on ocular pulse amplitude in normal pressure glaucoma. Klin Monatsbl Augenheilkd 1997;210(6):355–359.

Secondary Open-Angle Glaucoma

15

Secondary Open-Angle Glaucoma

Anthony A. Cavallerano

The secondary glaucomas are a group of disorders that result from an elevation in intraocular pressure (IOP) arising from an abnormal ocular or systemic condition. The resultant rise in IOP has the potential to adversely affect the nerve fibers, the optic nerve, and the visual field in much the same way as primary glaucoma. A variety of ocular, systemic, and congenital disorders can result in an elevated IOP, and the clinician must first identify the cause for the elevated IOP as part of the treatment and management strategy. Many factors influence the status of the IOP, and often the diagnosis of a secondary glaucoma relates to features other than the appearance of the optic nerve or the visual field examination.

In some cases, the distinction between primary and secondary glaucoma remains unclear. The criteria for defining secondary glaucoma rest with the cause for the resultant IOP elevation, and the guidelines for initiating treatment in primary glaucoma must be expanded so that therapy is instituted in a timely and often more aggressive manner. Sometimes the management plan varies significantly from the standard treatment regimens of primary open-angle glaucoma. Eliminating the underlying cause of the elevated IOP often is the first step in appropriate treatment of a secondary glaucoma.

The diagnosis of secondary glaucoma frequently depends on tonometric findings, slit-lamp biomicroscopic examination of the anterior segment, and gonioscopic evaluation of the anterior chamber angle. However, other ocular and systemic factors play an important role in the final diagnosis. To understand their complexity, it is necessary to define and classify the secondary glaucomas, recognize risk factors for this class of disorders, and devise a rationale for therapeutic intervention.

CLASSIFICATION OF THE SECONDARY GLAUCOMAS

The secondary glaucomas are separated into two categories: secondary open-angle and secondary narrow- or closed-angle glaucoma (Table 15-1). Further classification of each type is based on the clinicopathology or the mechanism of IOP elevation. This chapter covers the more common secondary open-angle glaucomas; chapter 17 discusses the secondary angle-closure glaucomas.

PSEUDOEXFOLIATION SYNDROME

Overview

Pseudoexfoliation (PXF) *syndrome* and *pseudoexfoliation glaucoma* are terms that have been applied to an asymptomatic secondary glaucoma that results from the diffuse deposition of white dandruff-like flecks on the anterior segment structures of the eye. The PXF material represents an abnormal protein synthesis and has been recovered from the corneal endothelium, the lens capsule, the ciliary zonules, and the trabecular meshwork. Elevated IOP may result from the obstruction to aqueous outflow in susceptible individuals. The term *pseudoexfoliation syndrome* was adopted to distinguish it from delamination of the anterior lens capsule (exfoliation), a condition that usually results from thermal injury to the crystalline lens.[1-4]

PXF is thought to be indigenous to Scandinavian populations,[5-7] but the disorder varies widely in incidence and reportedly has widespread distribution throughout the world. Although the syndrome is more prevalent in women, glaucoma with PXF tends to occur in both sexes equally.[8]

TABLE 15-1. Overview of the Secondary Glaucomas

Secondary open-angle glaucoma

Exfoliative/pseudoexfoliative glaucoma

Pigmentary glaucoma

Uveitic/inflammatory glaucoma

Corticosteroid-induced glaucoma

Glaucomatocyclitic crisis (Posner-Schlossman syndrome)

Fuchs' heterochromic iridocyclitis

Phacolytic glaucoma

Lens particle glaucoma

Phacoanaphylactic glaucoma

Aphakic/pseudophakic glaucoma

Traumatic glaucoma

Glaucoma associated with hyphema

Glaucoma associated with intraocular hemorrhage

Secondary Angle-Closure Glaucoma (see Chapter 17)

Phacomorphic glaucoma

Ectopia lentis

Aphakic/pseudophakic pupillary block glaucoma

Uveitic/inflammatory glaucoma (pupillary block from 360
  degrees of posterior synechiae)

Neovascular glaucoma

Iridocorneal endothelial syndrome

Ciliary block (malignant) glaucoma

Iris cysts and ciliary body cysts

Intraocular tumors

Ciliochoroidal effusion

**Glaucoma associated with developmental/systemic
  disorders**

Aniridia

Axenfeld-Rieger syndrome

Peter's anomaly

Sturge-Weber syndrome

von Hippel-Lindau syndrome

Oculodermal melanocytosis

Bourneville syndrome

Louis-Bar's syndrome

Racemose angioma of the retina

Diffuse congenital hemangiomatosis

Thyroid disease

Amyloidosis

The prevalence of PXF syndrome increases significantly with age, first appearing after the fifth decade and reaching a maximum incidence in the seventh decade.[9,10] Approximately one-half of the cases of PXF syndrome are unilateral or asymmetric between the two eyes.[9-11] Most cases become bilateral eventually, usually within 10 years of detection.[9-11] Heredity does not seem to be a factor in the development of PXF syndrome, and no underlying systemic predilection to the disorder has been seen. Cataract, when present, has no causal relationship and is merely an accompanying age-related disorder.

The incidence of glaucoma with PXF syndrome varies widely because of the variability of uncontrolled studies and the lack of proper patient selection. The incidence of PXF syndrome in the open-angle glaucoma population varies from 3% in most populations to 75% in Sweden.[12] Patients with PXF syndrome have a greater risk of developing glaucomatous damage.[11] Among patients with PXF, 5% develop elevated IOP within 5 years of diagnosis, increasing to 15% of patients within 10 years.[8,13] In most cases, IOP elevation develops in the fellow eye within 6 years.[14] Glaucoma occurs in approximately 7–20% of patients with PXF syndrome, and the IOP in PXF patients tends to be higher and more difficult to control than in patients with primary open-angle glaucoma.[8,11,15]

Clinicopathogenesis

PXF syndrome occurs when ocular tissue in the anterior segment synthesizes an abnormal protein. The detritus, which is amyloid-like in nature, may result from disturbances in the biosynthesis of basement membrane structures, and the relationship between the deposited material and glycosaminoglycans has been recognized.[16,17] Other sources of the PXF material include the nonpigmented ciliary epithelium and the iris pigment epithelium.[18,19] Amyloid protein deposits have also been recovered from the lining of the lungs, gastrointestinal tract, and other systemic organs in patients with PXF syndrome.

The mechanism for the development of glaucoma with PXF syndrome is not well understood.[20,21] Elevated IOP probably results from a combination of obstructed outflow through the trabecular meshwork by PXF material and pigment liberated from the iris, and by dysfunction of the trabecular cells or endothelial cells of the canal of Schlemm. Hypoperfusion of the iris vessels is apparent on iris fluorescein angiography, and neovascular-like clumps of iris vessels are sometimes observed.[22,23] The role that these vascular abnormalities play in PXF syndrome remains unclear.

Clinical Findings

PXF material may be found on most structures of the anterior segment of the eye, including the corneal endothelium, the pupillary border, and the anterior surface of

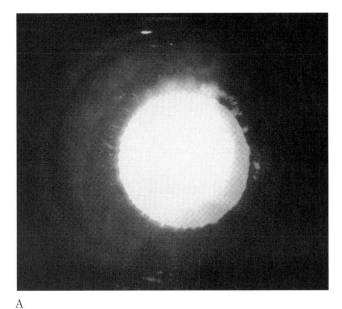

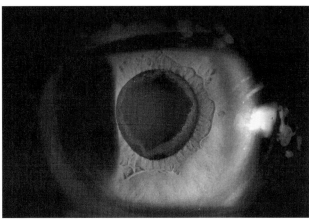

A   B

FIGURE 15-1. (A) In pseudoexfoliation syndrome, pupillary iris transillumination defects are often present. (B) The anterior lens capsule in pseudoexfoliation syndrome with the concentric zones of varying translucency and gray-white granular material.

the iris, where it is more easily seen in blue irides (see Color Plate 4). Transillumination defects of the iris are present, beginning at the pupillary border and extending to the midperipheral iris (Figure 15-1A). In contrast, the iris transillumination defects seen in pigmentary dispersion syndrome (PDS) commence at the midperiphery and progress to the periphery (see Color Plate 3). The pupillary border of the iris takes on a typical moth-eaten appearance best observed by retroillumination with the slit-lamp biomicroscope (see Figure 15-1A).

The distinctive appearance of gray-white granular material on the anterior lens capsule is the hallmark of this disorder. A central translucent zone is often surrounded by a clear zone that corresponds to an area of rubbing on the anterior lens capsule by the posterior surface of the iris at the pupillary border (Figure 15-1B and Color Plate 5). The peripheral and central zones may be connected by a bridge of material or may be totally separate. Rarely, posterior synechiae may be present, resulting in a secondary angle-closure glaucoma from pupillary block.

Pigment liberation and dispersion into the anterior chamber may occur after dilation, and a postdilation pressure spike is common.[23,24] Pigment may be deposited on the corneal endothelium, and although pigmentation of the trabecular meshwork is a consistent feature of PXF syndrome, it can be differentiated from that seen in PDS by the patchy nature and lack of homogeneous appearance of the pigment in the trabecular meshwork.[12,25] Pigment in the trabecular meshwork may represent the earliest sign of PXF syndrome, and its appearance may predate the capsular lens changes.[26] Sampaolesi's line, a pigmented line anterior to Schwalbe's line, can often be seen in PXF syndrome.

The deposition of PXF material on the ciliary processes and zonules may weaken their attachment, thus increasing the technical difficulty of the surgical technique during extracapsular cataract extraction. Intraoperative and postoperative surgical complications are more likely to occur in patients with PXF syndrome, including rupture of the posterior capsule, dislocation of the lens, and displacement of the intraocular lens implant.[27,28] Weakening of the ciliary zonules and the customary iris changes associated with PXF can also result in iridodonesis and phacodonesis.

The diagnosis of PXF syndrome is made by observation of its characteristic features by slit lamp biomicroscopic examination of the anterior segment of the eye and by gonioscopy. Distinct pigmentation of the corneal endothelium, gray-white deposits at the iris pupillary border or on the anterior lens surface after dilation, or dense pigmentation of the trabecular meshwork should alert the clinician to the possibility of PXF syndrome. Due to the likelihood of a postdilation pressure rise, repeat tonometry before the patient is dismissed is recommended. Careful examination and photodocumentation of the optic nerve using stereoscopic techniques and threshold visual field tests should be obtained. If the tests are normal, the patient should be monitored with 4–6 month IOP checks and yearly dilated fundus evaluation.

Differential Diagnosis

The differential diagnosis of glaucoma with PXF syndrome includes PDS and true exfoliation of the anterior lens capsule. True exfoliation, or capsular delamination,

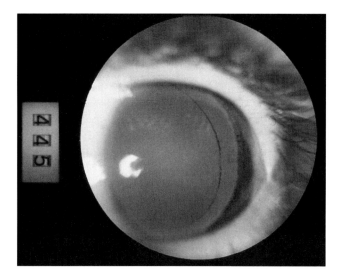

Figure 15-2. Pigmentation on anterior surface of crystalline lens sometimes referred to as *Zentmayer's ring*.

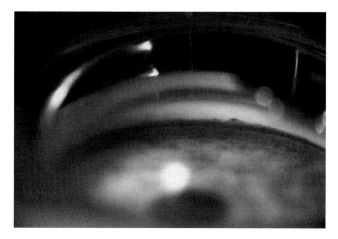

Figure 15-3. Gonioscopic view of a densely pigmented trabecular meshwork in pigmentary dispersion glaucoma. Note Sampaolesi's line anterior to Schwalbe's line.

which results from exposure to extremely high temperatures, is almost always associated with cataract but rarely with glaucoma. Pigmentary dispersion syndrome can be differentiated from PXF syndrome by the appearance of Krukenberg's spindle, a denser, more homogeneous deposition of pigment in the trabecular meshwork and peripheral iris transillumination defects. PXF syndrome is seen more commonly in elderly patients, and PDS is found in younger patients.

Treatment and Management

Nonselective topical beta blockers are generally the first-line treatment for PXF glaucoma, if no systemic contraindications are present. Topical α agonists, carbonic anhydrase inhibitors, and pilocarpine are alternative or adjunctive medications. Latanoprost (Xalatan) should be used with caution because of the pigmentary dispersion component of PXF syndrome. Latanoprost may increase the size of melanocyte, which may affect aqueous outflow through the pigmented trabecular meshwork. IOP is often higher in PXF glaucoma and more refractory to treatment compared to patients with primary open-angle glaucoma.[2]

Argon laser trabeculoplasty (ALT) has been shown to be very effective in lowering IOP in PXF glaucoma; however, the effect may be ephemeral, and patients require constant observation.[29,30] Apraclonidine (Iopidine) can be administered prophylactically to prevent postlaser IOP spikes.[31] Medical therapy usually must also be maintained after ALT to ensure adequate control of the IOP. Filtration surgery can also be performed in the treatment of PXF glaucoma and demonstrates results similar to or better than those reported for patients with primary open-angle glau-

coma.[2] Periodicity of follow-up is dependent on the control of IOP, stability of the optic nerve and visual field, and compliance with medications and follow-up appointments.

PIGMENTARY GLAUCOMA

Overview

PDS is characterized by the liberation of pigment particles from the posterior iris pigment epithelium (see Figure 3-9).[32] The pigment particles are carried by aqueous convection currents and deposited on the corneal endothelium, anterior surface of the iris, anterior surface of the crystalline lens (Figure 15-2), ciliary zonules, and the trabecular meshwork (Figure 15-3). Elevated IOP can result from the obstruction of aqueous outflow by pigment granules that deposit in the trabecular spaces.[33,34] Elevated IOP can lead to glaucomatous damage to the optic nerve (pigmentary glaucoma).

An autosomal dominant mode of transmission may exist, but inheritance is independent of sex or iris color.[33,35] Most patients with pigmentary dispersion are white, and the disorder is rare in blacks or Asians.[33]

PDS typically affects young myopic individuals who are anatomically disposed by having a posterior concave iris contour. Men and women have similar rates of PDS, however, pigmentary glaucoma is more prevalent in men. The age of onset is slightly younger in men, 35–45 years compared to a decade later for women, especially in higher degrees of myopia.[32,36,37] Pigmentary glaucoma accounts for 1.0–1.5% of all glaucomas.[32] The liberation of pigment appears to diminish with age, and the incidence of pigmentary glaucoma also decreases with advancing age.[34]

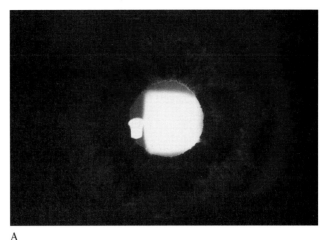

A

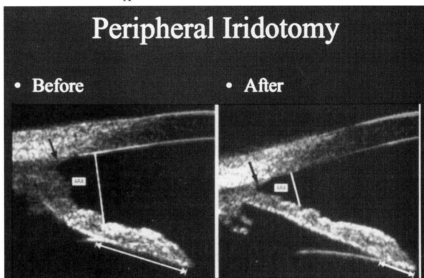

B

FIGURE 15-4. (**A**) Example of advanced peripheral iris transillumination defects in a patient with pigmentary dispersion syndrome. (**B**) Ultrasound biomicroscopy shows a concave iris contour before peripheral iridotomy and a straighter contour after peripheral iridotomy because the pressure is more equalized between the anterior and posterior chambers. (Photo courtesy of Samuel F. Boles, MD, Omni Eye Specialists, Baltimore, MD.)

Clinicopathology

PDS is characterized by a loss of pigment from the pigment epithelium of the iris. This loss of pigment may be the result of degeneration or atrophy of the tissue, aided by the back-and-forth rubbing of the posterior iris surface by the ciliary zonules.[38] The corresponding loss of pigment has been corroborated by iris transillumination, where the loss occurs in the midperipheral to peripheral zone of the iris (see Color Plate 3 and Figure 15-4A). This is in contradistinction to PXF, in which transillumination defects occur more often in the pupillary or middle zone of the iris (see Figure 15-1A). The anterior chamber angle in pigment dispersion is deeper and appears to bow posteriorly in a concave configuration toward the periphery (Figure 15-4B), thus promoting the mechanical contact of the posterior iris surface with the ciliary zonules.[39,40]

The mechanism for the development of elevated IOP in PDS remains unclear. The most popular theory of pigmentary glaucoma is that the pigment granules accumulate in the trabecular meshwork and eventually cause a dysfunction of trabecular endothelial cells.[41,42] These cells are responsible for the phagocytosis of pigment granules and cellular debris. With the build-up of pigment and cellular debris, the outflow of aqueous through the trabecular meshwork becomes obstructed.[41,42] Patients with pigmentary glaucoma are also prone to a bolus release of iris pigment via changes in pupil dilation or exercise. The acute release of pigment can cause dramatic elevations in the IOP. However, a significant number of PDS patients do not demonstrate an acute elevation of IOP with pigment release into the anterior chamber.[43,44] Studies have also shown that dense pigmentation of the trabecular meshwork can occur in the absence of elevated IOP.[45]

Iris fluorescein angiography studies in pigmentary dispersion have demonstrated vascular hypoperfusion of the iris, decreased iris vessels, and leakage of fluorescein, especially at the pupillary border.[33] Pigmentary dispersion has also been reported after retinal detachment, but whether the association rests with the higher frequency of retinal detachment found in myopia is not clear.[33,46]

Clinical Findings

Pigmentary dispersion is characterized by a liberation and accumulation of pigment on the corneal endothelium (i.e., Krukenberg's spindle; see Figure 3-9). Pigment granules, whether liberated spontaneously or after pupillary mydriasis, can be seen floating in the anterior chamber due to the convection currents of the aqueous. The pigment granules eventually deposit on the corneal endothelium, iris surface, and trabecular meshwork, which can be observed more prominently in the inferior angle due to the effects of gravity (see Figure 15-3 and Color Plate 1). Pigment can also be seen on the ciliary zonules and on the surface of the crystalline lens (referred to as *Zentmayer's ring* or *Scheie's line*)[47] (see Figure 15-2). Radial transillumination defects of the iris arranged in a spoke-like configuration are present; these may be isolated slit-like defects, or they may coalesce to involve the entire iris (see Color Plate 3 and Figure 15-4A). The anterior chamber angle is wide open, and the iris has a concave appearance approaching the periphery (see Figure 15-4B). Dense homogeneous pigmentation of the trabecular meshwork is observed by gonioscopy, and a pigmented Schwalbe's line can sometimes be observed (Sampaoelesi's line).

The diagnosis of PDS and glaucoma is made by careful slit-lamp biomicroscopic and gonioscopic examination of the anterior structures of the eye, tonometry, optic nerve head evaluation, and visual field tests. Understanding the risk factors and paying careful attention to anatomic details of the iris aid in the detection and diagnosis of pigmentary dispersion. Stereoscopic examination of the optic nerve head and visual fields are also required to detect glaucomatous changes in the optic nerve.

Typically, the patient is asymptomatic, but if the IOP is significantly elevated, patients with pigment dispersion or pigmentary glaucoma occasionally complain of blurred vision and haloes around lights. Postdilation pressure elevation can occur with PDS, especially if a shower of pigment into the anterior chamber has occurred as a result of the pupillary mydriasis. As with PXF, it is advisable to repeat tonometry after dilation before dismissing the patient with PDS. Vigorous exercise can also cause a liberation of pigment and IOP spikes, so patients at risk should be educated of this phenomenon. Patients with PDS without glaucoma should be followed according to the level of IOP and status of the optic nerve and visual fields. The relatively young age of the typical pigmentary glaucoma patient is a concern because they theoretically have more years to become visually impaired from their disease.

Differential Diagnosis

In the differential diagnosis of PDS, any abnormality of the anterior segment that results in the liberation of cellular material, such as pigment and inflammatory debris (e.g., PXF, uveitis, ciliary body or iris cysts) and the liberation of pigment subsequent to intraocular surgery or trauma should be considered. Iris chafing syndrome after intraocular lens implantation, especially when an intraocular lens implant is placed in the scleral sulcus, can result in PDS and glaucoma as a late complication of the surgery.[48,49]

PDS is most easily confused with PXF. Patients with PDS are typically younger than patients with PXF. The trabecular meshwork pigmentation is more dense and homogeneous in PDS, and the iris transillumination defects characteristically begin at the midperiphery of the iris rather than at the pupillary border as is seen in PXF syndrome.

Treatment and Management

Medical therapy of pigmentary glaucoma requires adherence to the same principles established for primary open-angle glaucoma. In the early stages of treatment, patients with pigmentary glaucoma may be subject to wide fluctuations in the IOP, especially in those younger age groups.[33] Beta blockers, α agonists, and topical carbonic anhydrase inhibitors have been proven effective in the treatment of pigmentary glaucoma, either alone or in combination. Prostaglandin analogs may be contraindicated based on their tendency to increase the size of melanocytes.

Cholinergic drugs, such as pilocarpine, are very effective in lowering the IOP in patients with pigmentary glaucoma. Cholinergic agents increase aqueous outflow and also minimize the iris to ciliary zonule brushing effect by constricting the pupil and increasing the separation between these structures. This may decrease the liberation of pigment; however, miotics are not well tolerated by young individuals because of brow ache, ciliary spasm, and blurring of vision. Low-dose (0.5% and 1.0%) or sustained-release forms of pilocarpine (Ocusert, Pilopine Gel) can be used with some success to minimize these unwanted side effects. Patients with PDS have a higher incidence of retinal detachment, and a thorough stereoscopic peripheral retinal examination to look for lesions, such as lattice retinal degeneration and retinal breaks, is warranted before instituting cholinergic therapy.[33,46] Oral carbonic anhydrase inhibitors are generally not well tolerated and therefore should only be used to control acute IOP spikes.

ALT is also an option for patients with pigmentary glaucoma. ALT produces a satisfactory IOP lowering in most patients, but it is generally less effective in young patients. Filtering surgery is an option for patients with pigmentary glaucoma that cannot be controlled with medications and ALT. However, young patients are more likely to develop scarring of the filtering bleb resulting in a higher rate of failure. Antimetabolites, such as mitomycin C, can be considered in patients with a higher risk for filter failure.

Laser peripheral iridotomy (LPI) is a controversial treatment for patients with PDS or pigmentary glaucoma. The rationale for its use is to relieve the reverse pupillary block component caused by the presence of a higher IOP in the anterior chamber than in the posterior chamber. This IOP asymmetry results in further posterior bowing of the iris and greater iris-zonule contact and pigment release. Peripheral iridotomy is thought to equalize the pressure in the anterior and posterior chambers, resulting in a less concave iris contour and less pigment release. The effectiveness of the procedure may not be known for several months, until the trabecular cells have a chance to phagocytize the pigment already released into the meshwork. LPI is generally recommended for patients with marked iris concavity on slit-lamp, gonioscopy or ultrasound biomicroscopic examination (see Figure 15-4B). The timing of the procedure and the identification of patients for whom it is suitable is still debatable. Some advocate the use of LPI on any PDS patient with a concave iris contour, regardless of the optic nerve or IOP status. Others only use the procedure on pigmentary glaucoma patients whose IOP elevation is not controlled with topical medications and ALT. Finally, some do not recommend the procedure in any PDS or pigmentary glaucoma patient. Further clinical studies may indicate when and in which patients LPI is most beneficial.

UVEITIC GLAUCOMA

Overview

Uveitis can produce a secondary open- or closed-angle glaucoma. Chronic, recurrent, or severe acute inflammation has the potential to produce an elevation in IOP and glaucomatous damage to the optic nerve. Elevated IOP is seen more frequently in chronic than in acute inflammatory processes. In most ocular inflammatory disease states, especially acute stages, the IOP is typically reduced because of a decrease in aqueous production.[47]

The etiology of uveitis is frequently unknown, but the condition can be associated with certain systemic diseases, such as sarcoidosis, lupus erythematosus, ankylosing spondylitis, syphilis, tuberculosis, Reiter's syndrome, and rheumatoid arthritis.[50,51] Common viral causes for uveitis and secondary glaucoma include herpes simplex, herpes zoster ophthalmicus, and rubella. Uveitis may occur after trauma or intraocular surgery, or may be the result of a primary ocular disorder such as Fuchs' heterochromic iridocyclitis or glaucomatocyclitic crisis (Posner-Schlossman syndrome).

TABLE 15-2. Mechanisms of Elevated Intraocular Pressure in Uveitis

Obstruction of trabecular meshwork by inflammatory cells and debris

Swelling and dysfunction of trabecular meshwork (trabeculitis)

Scarring of outflow channels

Elevated episcleral venous pressure

Peripheral anterior synechiae formation

Iris bombé from posterior synechiae

Angle neovascularization from iris ischemia

Clinicopathology

The mechanism for uveitic glaucoma is generally understood (Table 15-2). Inflammation causes a change in the blood-aqueous barrier that results in the liberation of protein and cellular matter into the anterior chamber and the vitreous. This is followed by a reduction of aqueous outflow because of obstruction at the trabecular meshwork or the intertrabecular cellular level. A trabeculitis (inflammation of the trabecular meshwork) can also result in less aqueous outflow. Pressure spikes are common in patients with chronic uveitis. Chronic inflammation can result in permanent ocular structural changes, such as iris atrophy, peripheral anterior synechiae, posterior synechiae, and cataract. Once peripheral anterior synechiae have formed in the angle, less trabecular meshwork is available to drain aqueous. Pupillary block and a secondary angle-closure glaucoma can result from extensive (360 degrees) posterior synechiae. This can be differentiated from primary angle closure glaucoma by examination of the fellow eye, which will also have a narrow anterior chamber angle (see Chapter 16).

Clinical Findings

The clinical symptoms of anterior uveitis include complaints of pain, photophobia, and blurred vision. However, some patients with mild or chronic uveitis may not present with any subjective symptoms. Clinical findings of uveitis may include circumlimbal hyperemia (see Color Plate 6), cells and flare in the anterior chamber or vitreous, keratitic and trabecular precipitates (see Color Plate 7), peripheral anterior synechiae (see Color Plate 8), and posterior synechiae (see Figure 3-13). Signs of chronic or recurrent uveitis include iris atrophy, peripheral anterior synechiae, posterior synechiae, cataract, and pigment accumulation on the corneal endothelium or pigment clumping in the angle.

Treatment and Management

The first step in the management of glaucoma resulting from anterior uveitis is medical control of the inflamma-

TABLE 15-3. Laboratory Tests Used in the Etiologic Diagnosis of Uveitis

Suspected etiology	Laboratory test
Ankylosing spondylitis	Sacroiliac joint x-ray film
	HLA testing
Histoplasmosis	Chest x-ray film
Tuberculosis	Purified protein derivative skin test
	Chest x-ray film
Sarcoidosis	Serum angiotensin–converting enzyme
	Serum lysozyme
	Limited gallium scan
	Biopsy of suspected lesion (skin, conjunctiva, lacrimal gland)
	Chest x-ray film
Syphilis	Fluorescent treponemal antibody absorption test
	VDRL test
Lupus erythematosus	Antinuclear antibody
Rheumatoid conditions	Rheumatoid factor
	Erythrocyte sedimentation rate
	HLA testing
Toxocara	Enzyme-linked immunosorbent assay (ELISA)
Toxoplasmosis	Fluorescent antibody test
	ELISA
Juvenile rheumatoid arthritis	Antinuclear antibody
	Erythrocyte sedimentation rate
Reiter's syndrome	HLA testing
	Sacroiliac joint x-ray film
Behçet's disease	HLA testing

tion and prevention of complications arising from the inflammation. A mydriatic and cycloplegic agent, such as homatropine 5% b.i.d.–q.i.d., should be used to prevent or break posterior synechiae and reduce the discomfort caused by photophobia and ciliary spasm. Cycloplegic agents have also been shown to lower IOP by increasing uveoscleral outflow and to help stabilize the permeability of the iris vasculature. Topical corticosteroids inhibit the inflammatory response and decrease capillary permeability, thus restoring the blood-aqueous homeostasis and reducing the release of cellular exudates and protein. Topical prednisolone acetate 1% can be administered every 1–4 hours during the acute stages of the inflammation, depending on the severity of the anterior chamber reaction. The steroids are gradually tapered based on the decrease in intraocular inflammation. It is important not to taper the steroids too quickly, to reduce the likelihood of a rebound inflammation.

Penetration of topical corticosteroids is increased because of the inflammatory response, but if topical agents prove to be ineffective, sub–Tenon's capsule steroid injection or systemic steroids may be administered. Topical and systemic corticosteroids can result in ocular complications including posterior subcapsular cataract, steroid-induced IOP elevation, and opportunistic infections. Steroid injections can be associated with acute IOP spikes. Immunosuppressive therapy has been used in the treatment of chronic refractory uveitis in an attempt to avoid the complications of long-term corticosteroid therapy. Cyclosporine A, methotrexate, and chlorambucil have been used with moderate success in the treatment of anterior uveitis.[51] A medical workup and treatment for underlying systemic conditions are required in the patient with chronic, recurrent, or bilateral uveitis (Table 15-3).

Control of the anterior uveitis with topical steroids is the first step in treating a patient with uveitic glaucoma. Aqueous-suppressing agents, such as beta blockers, α agonists, and topical carbonic anhydrase inhibitors, can be used in conjunction to lower the IOP.[52] Topical prostaglandins and miotic agents should be avoided because of their propensity to exacerbate the inflammation or increase the likelihood of posterior synechiae. ALT is not effective in uveitic glaucoma and may exacerbate the inflammation.[53] Peripheral iridotomy is indicated if a risk of pupillary block from 360 degrees of posterior synechiae exists. Filtration surgery usually requires adjunctive use of antimetabolites or setons because of the higher risk of filter scarring in patients with uveitic glaucoma.

CORTICOSTEROID-INDUCED GLAUCOMA

Both topical and systemic corticosteroids can result in permanent ocular tissue changes, such as posterior subcapsular cataracts. Corticosteroid-induced glaucoma must be considered in patients on long-term steroid therapy. IOP elevation has been detected as early as 1 week and as late as several months after treatment is initiated.[29,46,54] The amplitude of IOP increase is dose-related and is allied closely to the potency, frequency, and route of administration and the susceptibility to steroid response on the part of the patient. When corticosteroids are used to treat ocular inflammation, steroid-induced glaucoma may be misdiagnosed as uveitic glaucoma and vice versa. Therefore, distinguishing steroid-induced elevated IOP from elevated IOP as a result from anterior chamber inflammation is important.

In general, if a patient with uveitis is treated with steroids and the anterior chamber reaction improves but the IOP increases, then a steroid-induced mechanism should be suspected. The steroids should be gradually tapered and the IOP controlled with aqueous-suppressing agents until the steroids can be discontinued. The steroids should not be tapered too quickly, causing a rebound inflammation, especially in a patient with a history of recurrent uveitis. Rimexelone (Vexol) is a "soft" topical steroid that is less likely to cause a steroid response than prednisolone acetate.

If a uveitic patient presents with an acute severe or increased anterior chamber reaction and IOP is also elevated, then the uveitic component is probably the primary cause of the elevated IOP. In this situation, the steroids should be increased in addition to aqueous-suppressing agents. The management of uveitic glaucoma is often complex and challenging. Patients need to be followed closely, sometimes on a daily basis, depending on the severity of the inflammation and the level of the IOP. Uveitis patients should be routinely followed at 3- to 6-month intervals, even during times of quiescence. The patients should have gonioscopy performed to rule out peripheral anterior synechiae and should be periodically dilated to rule out posterior synechiae, which are often not apparent when the patient is in a nondilated state.

GLAUCOMATOCYCLITIC CRISIS

Glaucomatocyclitic crisis, referred to as the *Posner-Schlossman syndrome*, produces significant elevation in IOP in association with recurrent episodes of mild anterior uveitis.[55] Patients have relatively few symptoms in spite of the episodic and marked elevation of IOP. The clinical features of this rare disorder include ciliary flush, IOP as high as 60 mm Hg, faint flare, fine keratitic precipitates, and open angles without peripheral anterior synechiae. The elevated IOP is probably caused by a trabeculitis, possibly involving prostaglandins, and can last from hours to weeks. The disorder is recurrent in nature, and the patient should be monitored for visual field defects and optic nerve changes. Glaucomatocyclitic crisis is treated with topical corticosteroids, beta-blockers, α agonists, and topical carbonic anhydrase inhibitors.[56] Topical prostaglandin, miotic agents, and laser trabeculoplasty should be avoided. Occasionally, filtration surgery is required to control the IOP, but it does not control the recurrence of the inflammation.

FUCHS' HETEROCHROMIC IRIDOCYCLITIS

Fuchs' heterochromic iridocyclitis is a form of anterior uveitis associated with secondary cataract and glaucoma.[57] Most cases are unilateral, affect men and women equally, and typically have onset in the fourth decade of life.[58] Increased IOP is seen in 13–59% of patients.[59] The disorder is characterized by a mild anterior uveitis with minimal cell and flare, round or stellate keratitic precipitates, hypochromia, gray-white nodules on the anterior surface of the iris, and opacities in the vitreous.[59] Toldeo de Abreu and associates[60] reported chorioretinal scars that are suggestive of toxoplasmosis. The etiology for the elevated IOP is poorly understood, but the anterior chamber angle is open in the absence of peripheral anterior synechiae. Neovascular-like vessels may appear on the iris surface and in the anterior chamber angle. It has been suggested that the chronic inflammation causes permanent scarring of the outflow channels.[59] Treatment options include topical beta-blocking agents, α agonists, carbonic anhydrase inhibitors, corticosteroids, and cycloplegic agents to treat the uveitis component. The IOP elevation often does not respond well to antiglaucoma or corticosteroid therapy. Filtration surgery yields disappointing results and often is associated with postoperative hyphema.[60] Cataract surgery is often combined with a filtering procedure because of the development of cataract from the chronic inflammation.

LENS-INDUCED SECONDARY OPEN-ANGLE GLAUCOMA

A variety of disorders of the crystalline lens can result in a secondary open- or closed-angle glaucoma (Table 15-4). The secondary angle-closure glaucomas are covered in Chapter 17.

The diagnosis of lens-induced glaucoma can be made by a careful history and meticulous examination

TABLE 15-4. Conditions Associated with Ectopia Lentis

Hereditary disorders
Isolated ectopia lentis
Spontaneous late subluxation of lens
Ectopia lentis et pupillae
Microspherophakia
Marfan syndrome
Weill-Marchesani syndrome
Homocystinuria
Secondary ocular causes
Exfoliation syndrome
High myopia
Intraocular tumors
Uveitis
Extraocular causes
Surgery
Trauma

Source: Modified from R Ritch, MB Shields, T Kruppin (eds). The Glaucomas. St. Louis: Mosby, 1989.

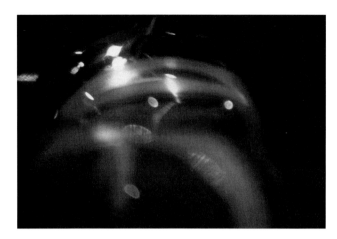

FIGURE 15-5. Increased ciliary body band width in a patient with angle recession after blunt trauma to the globe.

of the crystalline lens and the anterior chamber at the pupillary plane. Phacolytic glaucoma can occur when protein leaks from the lens of a hypermature or mature cataract, causing an inflammatory response replete with macrophages, and obstructs aqueous outflow. This type of lens-induced glaucoma should not be confused with retained cortical lens particles or debris after cataract surgery that can also lead to an inflammatory response and increased IOP. Another situation causing lens-induced glaucoma follows neodymium:yttrium-aluminum-garnet (Nd:YAG) laser capsulotomy, when free-floating lens particles obstruct aqueous outflow. If lens material is isolated within the eye, true anaphylaxis may develop from the leaking lens protein; this can occur when a cataractous lens spontaneously leaks protein or if protein leaks after trauma. Traumatic leakage of protein is rare, and the clinical differentiation from phacolytic glaucoma is difficult.

The management of these patients is aimed at controlling the ocular inflammation with topical steroids and treating the elevated IOP with aqueous-suppressing agents. Once the eye is quiet and the IOP is lowered, the cataract or lens material should be surgically removed.

TRAUMATIC GLAUCOMA

Blunt trauma to the eye, orbit, or craniofacial region can result in a number of ocular complications that lead to an increase in IOP and glaucomatous damage to the optic nerve. The rise in IOP after trauma is unpredictable and can occur immediately or be delayed for years after the injury. Acute rises in IOP after trauma are usually associated with uveitis, hyphema, or lens dislocation. The rise in IOP can also have an insidious onset due to chronic degeneration and dysfunction of the trabecular meshwork from previous trauma. The clinician should be vigilant for clinical signs of prior trauma, which include asymmetric or rosette cataract (see Color Plate 12), iris sphincter tears (see Figure 3-3), iridodialysis (splitting of the iris root away from the angle; see Figure 3-14), angle recession (Figure 15-5; see Color Plate 14), pigment clumping in the angle (see Color Plate 15), and cyclodialysis (see Figure 4-17). Although none of these signs represents a stage of secondary glaucoma development, all are associated with trauma significant enough to cause angle recession or trabecular meshwork damage. Patients with a history or physical evidence of ocular trauma should be carefully evaluated and periodically monitored for the development of glaucoma.

ANGLE-RECESSION GLAUCOMA

Angle recession (see Figure 15-5) occurs when a blunt object impacts the eye and causes a posterior dislocation of the ocular contents. On recovery, the cornea and sclera reform rapidly, but the greater density of the crystalline lens prevents it from returning as quickly, resulting in opposing forces that can cause a tear between the longitudinal and circular muscles of the ciliary body. The same process can cause tearing of the ciliary zonules, resulting in lens dislocation, iridodialysis, anterior and basal vitreous detachment, retinal tears, and retinal detachment.[61]

The visibility of an angle recession suggests concurrent damage to the trabecular meshwork. In addition to altered anatomic structure, there is also the elimination of the tractional effect of the ciliary muscle pulling of the scleral spur to increase aqueous outflow through the trabecular meshwork. Over time, the trabecular meshwork function may further deteriorate, creating more obstruction to outflow that results in late-onset secondary glaucoma.

Gonioscopic evaluation of the anterior chamber angle structures reveals a difference in angle depth when comparing eyes (see Figure 4-16). The key feature is the widening of the ciliary body band in one or more quadrants of the angle in the affected eye. A variable ciliary body width on gonioscopic slit-lamp examination may indicate the possibility of angle recession. The greater the circumference and depth of the angle recess, the greater the likelihood that a secondary glaucoma will develop.[62] However, visualizing an angle recession with gonioscopy is not necessary to diagnose traumatic glaucoma.

Management

Medical management of traumatic or angle-recession glaucoma consists of aqueous-suppressing agents, such as topical beta blockers, α agonists, and carbonic anhydrase inhibitors. Miotics may be of limited value because the tractional effects of the ciliary body on the trabecular meshwork are minimized by the tear between the two structures. Topical prostaglandins should be initially avoided if a traumatic iritis is present, but they can be tried in the treatment of late-onset glaucoma. ALT is less successful in traumatic glaucoma and may increase the risk of postlaser IOP spikes. Filtering surgery may be required in intractable cases. Aggressiveness of therapy depends on the level and control of IOP, the degree of optic nerve damage, and the amount of visual field loss.

GLAUCOMA ASSOCIATED WITH HYPHEMA

Hyphema secondary to blunt trauma to the globe may create an acute rise in IOP because of the blood and blood products that obstruct the trabecular meshwork. Elevated IOP is more common if the hyphema is greater than 50% of the anterior chamber. A hyphema this significant is usually secondary to a rebleed, which most often occurs 3–5 days after the injury. At this point, clotting may occur in the form of an 8-ball or dumbbell.

Management

Management of elevated IOP secondary to hyphema is best achieved by use of topical beta blockers, α agonists, oral or intravenous carbonic anhydrase inhibitors, and oral or intravenous hyperosmotic agents. Miotics and prostaglandin agents should be avoided. If the eye is severely inflamed, topical corticosteroids may be of value. Strong cycloplegics, such as 1% atropine, may be used to prevent posterior synechiae and limit iris movement. It appears that the standard management of hospitalization and bed rest does little to prevent the likelihood of a rebleed.[61,63,64] Some studies have demonstrated that the use of oral aminocaproic acid administered 100 mg/kg every 4 hours for a maximum dosage of 30 g, along with limiting physical activity, decreased the possibility of a rebleed.[65] Patients should be followed on a daily basis and IOP monitored until the hyphema resolves.

Surgical evacuation of the hyphema is sometimes necessary, but evidence suggests that a delay is advisable to minimize complications. Surgery is indicated in cases of intractable pain, severely elevated IOP (50–60 mm Hg for 4–5 days), blood staining of the cornea,[63] and hyphemas that remain longer than 9 days.[53] Should evacuation be indicated, the ideal time seems to be on the fourth day after the appearance of the hyphema to maximize total removal, minimize adherence, and avoid rebleed.[66] Another important consideration in the management of hyphema is that trauma producing hyphema is often sufficient enough to damage the trabecular meshwork causing a late-onset traumatic glaucoma.

GLAUCOMA ASSOCIATED WITH INTRAOCULAR HEMORRHAGE

Vitreous hemorrhage may also result in a secondary glaucoma, referred to as *ghost cell glaucoma*. During resorp-

tion of a vitreous hemorrhage, erythrocytes degenerate over a 3-week period from red cells to rigid ghost cells. These ghost cells stay within the vitreous cavity unless the anterior hyaloid face is ruptured, in which case the ghost cells travel forward into the anterior chamber and cause obstruction of the trabecular meshwork, a process that usually occurs weeks to months after the injury. The ghost cells in the anterior chamber are tan in color and may be confused with the cells of anterior uveitis.[67]

Management

Ghost cell glaucoma is treated in a manner similar to hyphema, with aqueous-suppressing agents; however, if the IOP cannot be adequately controlled, surgical evacuation of the cells in the anterior chamber may be necessary.

SUMMARY

Management of the secondary glaucomas represents a diagnostic and therapeutic challenge for the primary care doctor. Identification of the underlying cause of the elevated IOP is sometimes confounded by a variety of interrelated factors that may complicate the final diagnosis and delay appropriate treatment. The clinician should be familiar with the wide array of distinct clinical entities that can produce an elevation in IOP and result in a secondary glaucoma. Surveillance of the optic nerve and visual field for signs of glaucoma damage should be influenced by an understanding of the mechanisms of the secondary glaucoma.

Management entails the elimination or treatment of the underlying cause of the elevated IOP. Although the treatment consisting of lowering IOP may be similar to that for primary open-angle glaucoma, exceptions occur when a particular therapeutic agent is ineffective or contraindicated (e.g., miotics or prostaglandins in uveitic glaucoma) in a secondary glaucoma. Management and treatment should therefore be tailored to each patient. The frequency of examination is predicated by the success of IOP control, the amount of glaucoma damage to the optic nerve, and the stability of the visual field.

REFERENCES

1. Sugar HS, Harding C, Barsky D. The exfoliation syndrome. Ann Ophthalmol 1976;10:1165–1181.

2. Layden WE. Exfoliation Syndrome. In R Ritch, MB Shields (eds). The Glaucomas. St. Louis: Mosby, 1996;993–1022.

3. Jones WJ. True exfoliation. Clin Eye Vis Care 1989;3:166–167.

4. Brodrick D, Tate GW. Capsular delamination (true exfoliation) of the lens. Arch Ophthalmol 1979; 97:1693–1698.

5. Dell WM. The epidemiology of the pseudoexfoliation syndrome. J Am Optom Assoc 1985;56:113–119.

6. Ohrt V, Nehen JH. The incidence of glaucoma capsulare based on a Danish hospital material. Acta Ophthalmol 1981;59:888–893.

7. Forsius H. Prevalence of pseudoexfoliation of the lens in Finns, Lapps, Icelanders, Eskimos and Russians. Trans Ophthalmol Soc U K 1979;99:296–298.

8. Henry JC, Krupin T, Schmitt M, et al. Long-term follow-up of pseudoexfoliation and the development of elevated intraocular pressure. Ophthalmology 1987;94:545–552.

9. Hiller R, Sperduto RO, Krueger DE. Pseudoexfoliation, intraocular pressure, and senile lens changes in a population-based survey. Arch Ophthalmol 1982;100:1080–1082.

10. Hansen E, Sellevold OJ. Pseudoexfoliation of the lens capsule. Development of the exfoliation syndrome. Acta Ophthalmol 1969;47:161–173.

11. Kozart DM, Yanoff M. Intraocular pressure status in 100 consecutive patients with exfoliation syndrome. Ophthalmology 1982;89:214–218.

12. Layden WE, Shaffer RN. Exfoliation syndrome. Am J Ophthalmol 1974;78:835–841.

13. Slagsvold JE. The follow-up in patients with pseudoexfoliation of the lens capsule with and without glaucoma. 2. The development of glaucoma in persons with pseudoexfoliation. Acta Ophthalmol 1986; 64:241–245.

14. Brooks AM, Gillies WE. The presentation and prognosis of glaucoma in pseudoexfoliation of the lens capsule. Ophthalmology 1988;95:271–276.

15. Sugar S. Pigmentary glaucoma associated with the exfoliation-pseudoexfoliation syndrome: update. The Robert N. Shaffer lecture. Ophthalmology 1984;91:307–310.

16. Ringvold A, Husby G. Pseudoexfoliation material—an amyloid like substance. Exp Eye Res 1973;17:289.

17. Harnisch JP, Barrach HJ, Hassell HR, Sinha PK. Identification of basement membrane proteoglycan in exfoliation material. Graefes Arch Klin Exp Ophthalmol 1981;215:273–278.

18. Streeten BW, Gibson SA, Dark AJ. Pseudoexfoliative material contains an elastic microfibrillar-associated glycoprotein. Trans Am Ophthalmol Soc 1986; 84:304–320.

19. Dark AJ, Streeten BW, Conward CC. Pseudoexfoliative diseases of the lens: a study in electron microscopy and histochemistry. Br J Ophthalmol 1977;61:462–472.

20. Toriyama K, Maezawa N. Electron microscopic study on the trabecular tissues in glaucoma capsulare. Acta Soc Ophthalmol Jpn 1976;80:780–789.

21. Richardson TM, Epstein DL. Exfoliation glaucoma: a quantitative perfusion and ultrastructural study. Ophthalmology 1981;88:968–980.

22. Brooks AM, Gillies WE. The development of microneovascular changes in the iris in pseudoexfoliation of the lens capsule. Ophthalmology 1987;94:1090–1097.

23. Krause U, Hine J, Frisius H. Pseudoexfoliation of the lens capsule and liberation of iris pigment. Acta Ophthalmol 1978;56:329–334.

24. Roth M, Epstein D. Exfoliation syndrome. Am J Ophthalmol 1980;89:477–481.

25. Wishart PK, Spaeth GL, Poryzees EM. Anterior chamber angle in the exfoliation syndrome. Br J Ophthalmol 1985;69:103–107.

26. Prince AM, Streeten BW, Ritch R, et al. Preclinical diagnosis of pseudoexfoliation. Arch Ophthalmol 1987;105:1076–1082.

27. Gillies WE. Effect of lens extraction in pseudoexfoliation of the lens capsule. Br J Ophthalmol 1973;57:46–51.

28. Radian AB, Radian AL. Senile pseudoexfoliation in aphakic eyes. Br J Ophthalmol 1975;59:577–579.

29. Lieberman MF, Hoskins HD, Hetherington J. Laser trabeculoplasty and the glaucomas. Ophthalmology 1983;90:790–795.

30. Higginbotham EJ, Richardson TM. Response of exfoliation glaucoma to laser trabeculoplasty. Br J Ophthalmol 1986;70:837–839.

31. Tuulonen A, Airaksinen PJ. Laser trabeculoplasty in simple and capsular glaucoma. Acta Ophthalmol 1983;61:1009–1015.

32. Sugar HS, Babour FA. Pigmentary glaucoma: a rare clinical entity. Am J Ophthalmol 1949;32:90–92.

33. Richardson TM. Pigmentary Glaucoma. In R Ritch, MB Shields, T Kruppin (eds). The Glaucomas. St. Louis: Mosby, 1989;981–985.

34. Scheie HG, Cameron JD. Idiopathic atrophy of the epithelial layers of the iris and ciliary body. Arch Ophthalmol 1958;59:216–228.

35. Mandelkorn RM, Hoffman ME, Olander KW, et al. Inheritance and the pigmentary dispersion syndrome. Ann Ophthalmol 1983;15:577–582.

36. Bick MW. Pigmentary glaucoma in females. Arch Ophthalmol 1957;58:483–494.

37. Berger A, Ritch R, McDermott JA, et al. Pigmentary dispersion, refraction and glaucoma. Invest Ophthalmol Vis Sci 1987;28:114–119.

38. Rodriques MM, Spaeth GL, Weinreb S, et al. Spectrum of trabecular pigmentation in open angle glaucoma: a clinicopathologic study. Trans Am Acad Ophthalmol Otolaryngol 1976;81:258–276.

39. Davidson JA, Brubaker RF, Ilstrup DM. Dimension of the anterior chamber in pigment dispersion syndrome. Arch Ophthalmol 1983;101:81–83.

40. Campbell DG. Pigment dispersion syndrome and glaucoma: a new theory. Arch Ophthalmol 1979;97:1667–1672.

41. Lichter PR. Pigmentary glaucoma: current concepts. Trans Am Acad Ophthalmol Otolaryngol 1974;78:309–313.

42. Richter CU, Richardson TM, Grant WM. Pigmentary dispersion syndrome and pigmentary glaucoma: a prospective study of the natural history. Arch Ophthalmol 1986;104:211–215.

43. Epstein DL, Boger WP, Grant WM. Phenylephrine provocative testing in the pigmentary dispersion syndrome. Am J Ophthalmol 1978;85:43–50.

44. Kristensen P. Mydriasis-induced pigment liberation in the anterior chamber associated with acute rise in intraocular pressure in open-angle glaucoma. Acta Ophthalmol 1965;43:714–724.

45. Lichter PR, Shaffer RM. Diagnostic and prognostic signs in pigmentary glaucoma. Trans Am Acad Ophthalmol Otolaryngol 1970;74:984–998.

46. Syrdalen P. Intraocular pressure and ocular rigidity in patients with retinal detachment. Acta Ophthalmol 1970;48:1036–1044.

47. Becker B, Shaffer RN. Secondary Open Angle Glaucoma. In HD Hoskins, MA Kass (eds). Diagnosis and Therapy of the Glaucomas. St. Louis: Mosby, 1989;308–350.

48. Woodhams JT, Lester JC. Pigmentary dispersion glaucoma secondary to posterior chamber intraocular lenses. Ann Ophthalmol 1984;16:852–854.

49. Cataract Surgery Combined with Glaucoma Surgery or Keratoplasty. Jaffe NS, Jaffe MS, Jaffe GF (eds). Cataract Surgery and Its Complications. St. Louis: Mosby, 1989;317–333.

50. Smith ME, Zimmerman LE. Contusive angle recession in phacolytic glaucoma. Arch Ophthalmol 1965;7:65:799–804.

51. Jabs DA, Johns CJ. Ocular involvement in chronic sarcoidosis. Am J Ophthalmol 1986;102:297–301.

52. Zegarra H, Gutman FA, Conforto J. The natural course of central retinal vein occlusion. Ophthalmology 1979;86:1931–1939.

53. Robin AL, Pollack IP. Argon laser trabeculoplasty in secondary forms of open-angle glaucoma. Arch Ophthalmol 1983;101:382–384.

54. Simmons RJ, Depperman SR, Dueker DK. The role of goniophotocoagulation in neovascularization of the anterior chamber angle. Ophthalmology 1980;87:79–82.

55. Kass MA, Becker B, Kolker AE. Glaucomatocyclic crisis and primary open-angle glaucoma. Am J Ophthalmol 1973;75:668–673.

56. Hung PT, Chang JM. Treatment of glaucomatocyclic crisis. Am J Ophthalmol 1974;77:169–172.

57. Kimura SJ, Hogan MJ, Thygeson P. Fuchs' syndrome of heterochromic cyclitis. Arch Ophthalmol 1971;71:1289.

58. Franceschetti A. Heterochromic cyclitis (Fuchs' syndrome). Am J Ophthalmol 1955;39:50–58.

59. Liesgang TJ. Clinical features and prognosis in Fuchs' uveitis syndrome. Arch Ophthalmol 1982;100:1622–1626.

60. Toledo de Abreu MT, Belfort R Jr, Hirata PS. Fuchs' heterochromic cyclitis and ocular toxoplasmosis. Am J Ophthalmol 1982;93:739–744.

61. Kaufmann JH, Tolpin DW. Glaucoma after traumatic angle recession. Am J Ophthalmol 1974;78:648–654.

62. D'Ombrain AW. Traumatic monocular chronic glaucoma. Trans Ophthalmol Soc Aust 1945;5:116–121.

63. Eagling EM, Roper-Hall MJ. Eye Injuries. An Illustrated Guide. Philadelphia: Lippincott, 1986;5–9.

64. Rakusin W. Traumatic hyphema. Am J Ophthalmol 1972;74:284–292.

65. Read J. Traumatic hyphema: surgical vs. medical management. Ann Ophthalmol 1975;7:659–670.

66. Kitazawa Y. Management of traumatic hyphema with glaucoma. Int Ophthalmol Clin 1979; 21:167–181.

67. Campbell DG. Ghost Cell Glaucoma. In R Ritch, MD Shields (eds). The Secondary Glaucomas. St. Louis: Mosby, 1982;320–327.

CHAPTER 16

Primary Angle-Closure Glaucoma

Jimmy Jackson

CLASSIFICATION

The classification of angle-closure glaucoma (ACG) is based on the presence or absence of pupillary block and whether the angle closure mechanism is primary or secondary. With pupillary block, the normal flow of aqueous through the pupil from the posterior chamber to the anterior chamber is restricted. This leads to increased pressure in the posterior chamber that pushes the peripheral iris forward (iris bombé) until it blocks the trabecular meshwork (Figure 16-1). The trabecular meshwork is presumed to be functioning normally but may be damaged by appositional contact with the iris.

Primary angle-closure glaucoma (PACG) with pupillary block exists when a predisposing anatomic basis for the condition is present, such as a narrow angle. PACG may be further subdivided into suspect, subacute, acute, and chronic forms. ACG can also occur in the absence of pupillary block. PACG without pupillary block, or *plateau iris*, is a clinical entity in which the central anterior chamber depth is normal, the iris plane is flat, the ciliary body is anatomically displaced anterior, no ciliary sulcus is present, and the peripheral anterior chamber angle is extremely narrow or closed (Figure 16-2). Gonioscopy is required to make the diagnosis and reveals that the peripheral iris makes a sharp turn posteriorly (like a plateau) before inserting into the ciliary body. Secondary ACG is always associated with some other primary disease process (examples include 360 degrees of posterior synechiae from anterior chamber inflammation, rubeosis irides, and ciliochoroidal effusion).[1] Examination of the fellow eye is helpful in differentiating primary from secondary ACG. In PACG, both angles are anatomically narrow, whereas in secondary ACG the fellow eye typically has an open angle.

EPIDEMIOLOGY OF PRIMARY ANGLE-CLOSURE GLAUCOMA

PACG is relatively uncommon in the United States and accounts for less than 10% of all diagnosed cases of glaucoma.[2-4] In other populations, however, ACG occurs more frequently and may exceed the incidence of open-angle glaucoma (OAG). Examples of populations with high incidences of ACG include the Mongoloid peoples of East Asia,[5] Greenland and Alaskan Eskimos,[6-8] Sri Lankans,[9] Eastern Indians,[10,11] and Asians.[12] The prevalence of ACG within a particular population also depends on a number of variables. Primary among these are race, family history, age, sex, and refractive error (Table 16-1).

CLINICAL BACKGROUND

Most cases of PACG involve some form of pupillary block and occur in eyes with narrow angles.[2,13-17] A small degree of relative pupillary block is always present in phakic individuals as the iris rests against the anterior surface of the lens. This contact is usually of little significance. However, circumstances can arise that increase the contact force between the iris and lens. This iris-lens apposition increases resistance of aqueous flow from the posterior chamber through the pupil and leads to an increase in the pressure within the posterior chamber. Eventually, sufficient force may be generated from the posterior chamber to displace the peripheral iris forward. The peripheral iris may then balloon forward (iris bombé) and occlude the trabecular meshwork, inhibiting aqueous drainage. Aqueous production continues, resulting in a rapid and marked elevation in intraocular pressure (IOP).

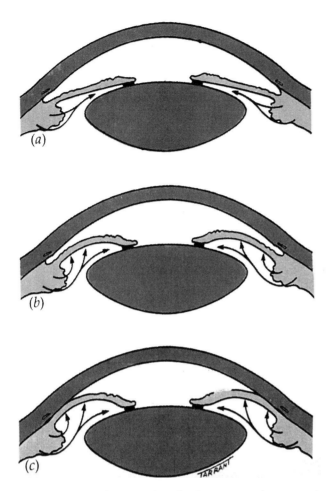

FIGURE 16-1. Mechanism of angle closure: (a) relative pupil block, (b) iris bombé, and (c) iridotrabecular contact. Iridotomy relieves the block and opens the angle. (Reprinted with permission from JJ Kanski, JA McAllister, JF Salmon. Glaucoma [2nd ed]. Oxford: Butterworth–Heinemann, 1996;59.)

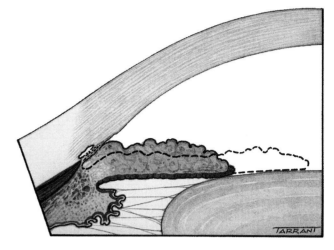

FIGURE 16-2. Mechanism of angle closure in plateau iris. Pupillary dilation causes bunching of the peripheral iris occluding the trabecular meshwork. (Reprinted with permission from JJ Kanski. Clinical Ophthalmology [3rd ed]. Oxford: Butterworth–Heinemann, 1994;257.)

Only certain eyes have anterior chamber depths small enough and angles narrow enough to undergo primary angle closure. These susceptible eyes may undergo pupillary block spontaneously or, more commonly, have it precipitated by pupillary dilation. Dilation, with resultant pupillary block in at-risk individuals, may occur naturally after emotional upset or in dim illumination (restaurant or theater), or may be induced pharmacologically by a variety of systemic and topical medications. The greatest iris-to-lens contact occurs when the pupil is in the mid-dilated (3.5–4.0 mm) state.[15,18,19] In contrast, when the pupil is widely dilated, little or no contact occurs between the lens and the iris, and therefore minimum pupillary block is present.[13] When induced pharmacologically, this high-risk mid-dilation state occurs briefly as the pupil achieves maximum dilation. However, as the pupil returns to its original state, the iris remains in the mid-dilated position for a longer period of time. With pharmacologic dilation, this typically occurs 1 to several hours after the dilating agent has been administered, depending on the agent used.

ACUTE PRIMARY ANGLE-CLOSURE GLAUCOMA

An acute angle closure attack is a true ophthalmic emergency, and immediate, appropriate therapy must be instituted to prevent vision loss. An acute angle closure attack that is not induced pharmacologically is usually unilateral, with the population most at risk consisting of elderly, hyperopic individuals.[5,20,21] Typical patient complaints are ocular redness, pain (may be ocular or referred), blurred vision, halos around lights, tearing, photophobia, and nausea and vomiting.

Development and progression of these symptoms is typically rapid. The level of pain experienced seems to be related more to the rapid rise in pressure than to the absolute level of the IOP increase. African-American patients may experience less pain when undergoing an acute ACG attack, and thus a relative lack of pain

TABLE 16-1. Factors That Increase the Incidence of Primary Angle-Closure Glaucoma

Factor	Population at increased risk
Age	Older (peak incidence in sixth decade)
Sex	Female
Refractive error	Hyperopes
Race	Asians (especially Chinese), Eskimos (Greenland and Alaska), Eastern Indians, Philippinos

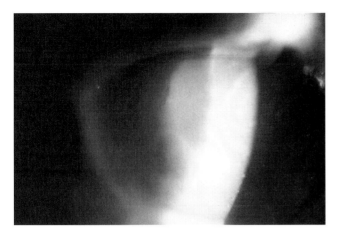

FIGURE 16-3. During an attack of acute angle-closure glaucoma, the rise in intraocular pressure is associated with infarction of the iris tissue with an associated inflammatory response. Decompensation of the corneal epithelium with the development of corneal edema occurs. Note the mid-dilated pupil.

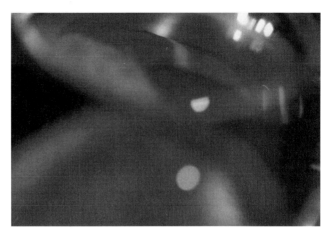

FIGURE 16-4. Gonioscopy slide shows a convex iris contour and shallow anterior chamber angle. The angle structures are not visible. This was the fellow eye of a patient who presented with an acute primary angle closure attack.

should not deter the clinician from a thorough evaluation.[22,23] Examination classically reveals circumlimbal injection, a mid-dilated nonreactive pupil, corneal edema, anterior chamber inflammation (Figure 16-3), and an IOP in the 40–90 mm Hg range. It is crucial to determine whether the patient is suffering from primary acute ACG with pupillary block rather than one of the secondary ACGs or some other cause of acute IOP rise. Conditions in the differential diagnosis include:

- POAG with unusually high IOP
- Glaucomatocyclitic crisis
- Neovascular glaucoma
- Uveal effusion with secondary angle-closure
- Malignant glaucoma
- Phacomorphic glaucoma with secondary angle-closure
- Anterior chamber angle tumor or mass
- Uveitic glaucoma with or without secondary angle closure
- Plateau iris syndrome
- Pigmentary dispersion syndrome/glaucoma
- Exfoliative glaucoma
- Iridocorneal endothelial syndrome

Appropriate management of these various conditions differs dramatically from that of acute PACG, as pupillary block plays little or no role. Gonioscopy and slit-lamp evaluations are crucial in diagnosing the etiology of an IOP rise. If the cornea is edematous (as is often the case), the use of topical glycerin may temporarily clear it enough to permit an adequate view. Alternatively, gonioscopy and slit-lamp evaluation of the fellow eye is essential, as anterior chamber anatomy is almost always similar for the right and left eyes (Figure 16-4). Possible

exceptions would be in cases of trauma, anisometropia, asymmetric cataracts, or unilateral pseudophakia.

Treatment of Acute Primary Angle-Closure Glaucoma

A review of the patient's medical history is mandatory, with particular emphasis directed toward the patient's cardiac, renal, and pulmonary status to rule out any contraindications to the medical treatment of PACG. The treatment of acute PACG with pupillary block is directed toward three main goals:

1. Decreasing the IOP and breaking the pupillary block component
2. Performing the definitive treatment of laser peripheral iridotomy (LPI) or surgical iridectomy (generally after the attack has been broken medically)
3. Evaluating the fellow eye for prophylactic treatment

Pharmaceuticals used in the management of an acute angle closure attack include topical, oral, and intravenous agents. Topical agents usually include miotics (pilocarpine), β-adrenergic blockers, α-adrenergic agonists (apraclonidine or brimonidine), topical carbonic anhydrase inhibitors (dorzolamide or brinzolamide), and steroids (to reduce inflammation). Oral agents used are CAIs and hyperosmotics. Hyperosmotics and CAIs can also be administered intravenously.

Pilocarpine

Pilocarpine serves to constrict the pupil, firm the peripheral iris, and pull the iris away from the trabecular meshwork. Concentrations stronger than 2% should be avoided because they may produce ciliary-body thickening and vascular congestion, which can shallow the anterior chamber, increase pupillary block, and aggravate rather than relieve ACG.[13,24] The recommended dosage of pilocarpine is 1 drop of 2% solution every 15–30 minutes up to a total of 3–4 doses.[13,25] Some controversy exists as to when the pilocarpine should be administered. When the IOP is higher than 40–50 mm Hg, the pupillary sphincter muscle is often ischemic and unresponsive to topical miotic agents.[26–28] Once the IOP has been reduced, normal blood flow returns to the iris sphincter, and it becomes responsive to pilocarpine therapy.[28] This has led some authorities to suggest that pilocarpine should not be administered until the pressure is reduced to approximately 40 mm Hg.[26,29,30] However, most experts still recommend that pilocarpine be given at the first diagnosis of acute PACG because this allows its immediate availability when sphincter muscle receptors regain function.[14,16,25,31,32] Care should be taken to avoid overdosing, which may produce a cholinergic crisis with nausea, vomiting, diarrhea, sweating, bradycardia, and hypotension, especially in elderly patients.[13] A predisposed fellow eye should be maintained on pilocarpine 2% q.i.d. until LPI is performed.[13]

Beta Blockers

If the patient has no pulmonary contraindications, any of the nonselective beta blockers may be used, with timolol 0.5% (Timoptic or Betimol) probably most commonly used. Betaxolol 0.25% (Betoptic S) may be used with caution in patients with mild pulmonary disease. The recommended dosage (for any beta blocker) is 1 drop every 30 minutes up to a total of 2 doses.

α-Adrenergic Agonists

Apraclonidine (Iopidine) 0.5% or 1%, which has been approved for use in anterior segment laser procedures to prevent IOP spikes, is an adjunct therapy in angle closure.[31,33,34] It is an α-adrenergic agonist that lowers IOP by decreasing aqueous production and increasing uveoscleral outflow. Usual dosage is 1–2 drops in the affected eye at the time of diagnosis, to be repeated once in 30 minutes if necessary.[1] Brimonidine 0.2% (Alphagan) is another α₂ agonist that can be substituted for apraclonidine.

Topical Carbonic Anhydrase Inhibitors

Dorzolamide (Trusopt) or brinzolamide (Azopt) are topical CAIs that decrease IOP by decreasing aqueous production. Topical CAIs can be substituted for oral CAIs if the patient is nauseous or has a systemic contraindication for oral CAIs. The recommended dosage is 1 drop every 30–60 minutes up to a total of three to four doses.[1]

Topical Steroids

Topical steroids do not directly treat the acute angle closure attack but are useful in managing secondary inflammation. Usual dosage is 1 drop of 1% prednisolone acetate four to eight times a day and tapered as the anterior chamber subsides.[1]

Oral Carbonic Anhydrase Inhibitors

An oral CAI should be given immediately on diagnosis if the patient is not nauseated. A 500-mg dose (two 250-mg tablets) of acetazolamide (Diamox) is most commonly used.[1] The 500-mg Diamox Sequel should be avoided; it is a time-release formulation and therefore has a slower onset of action. Acetazolamide should be avoided in patients with kidney problems, and methazolamide (Neptazane) becomes the CAI of choice in those patients. A dose of 100 mg of methazolamide is recommended. CAIs should be avoided in patients allergic to sulfa because they are sulfa-based drugs. Topical or intravenous CAIs may be substituted if the patient is nauseous and cannot tolerate oral CAIs.

Oral Hyperosmotic Agents

Oral hyperosmotic agents are the most effective means of lowering IOP during acute angle closure attacks. If the patient is not nauseated or vomiting and not diabetic, 50% glycerin (Osmoglyn) should be administered in a dose of 2–3 ml/kg of body weight.[1] In diabetic patients, 45% isosorbide (Ismotic, which is not broken down into free sugars) is substituted and is administered in a dose of 1.5 ml/lb of body weight.[13,26,27,31] These agents are best tolerated if given chilled (serve over crushed ice), and the entire dose should be consumed within 5 minutes.[17] When patients are nauseated, an intravenous hyperosmotic agent can be used. Intravenous hyperosmotics should be used with caution, however, because of their systemic complications (disorientation, confusion, diarrhea, seizures, dehydration, cardiovascular stress), which are the same as the oral hyperosmotics but with a more rapid onset.

Suggested Management Protocol

Immediately after the diagnosis of acute angle closure, the patient should receive the medications listed in Table 16-2, providing no contraindications exist. While attempting to break an angle closure attack, IOP readings should be checked every 30 minutes. If the IOP remains elevated after 30 minutes, all topical medications should be repeated. If the attack is not broken 1 hour after treatment is instituted, oral hyperosmotics should be administered. If the patient is still in angle closure 4–6 hours after treatment was initiated, emergency LPI or surgery iridectomy should be attempted.

TABLE 16-2. Medical Management of an Acute Primary Angle Closure Attack[a]

500 mg acetazolamide orally.[b]

One drop of 0.5% timolol.

One drop of 2% pilocarpine.

Two drops of 0.5% apraclonidine or 0.2% brimonidine.

If the angle closure attack is not broken in 30 mins, then the topical agents are repeated. If the attack is not broken in 60 mins, then oral hyperosmotic agents (50% glycerin, 2–3 ml/kg or 45% isosorbide, 1.5 ml/lb) should be given.

[a]Assuming no medical contraindications are present.
[b]One drop of 2.0% dorzolamide or 1.0% brinzolamide can be substituted if the patient cannot tolerate (nausea and vomiting) oral acetazolamide.

An acute attack of angle closure should not be considered broken until the IOP is returned to normal levels, the pupil is miotic, and the angle is open on gonioscopy. Gonioscopy also allows the assessment of peripheral anterior synechiae (PAS), which may have formed from appositional contact of the iris and trabecular meshwork (see Color Plate 8). Low pressure is not, by itself, indicative of a broken angle closure attack. If the angle is not open, the IOP can rise again to very high levels within hours to days. If the attack can be broken medically, the patient should be maintained on 2% pilocarpine q.i.d. bilaterally, and 1% prednisolone acetate four to eight times a day in the affected eye until an LPI is performed. Most clinicians also keep the patient on a topical beta blocker b.i.d. in the affected eye. Miosis (pilocarpine) helps guard against pupillary block, topical steroids treat the inflammation associated with angle closure, and a beta blocker decreases posterior chamber pressure by decreasing aqueous production. An LPI should be performed within a few days of an acute angle closure attack. This gives the eye a chance to quiet as the anterior chamber inflammation decreases and the iris congestion and corneal edema subsides.[1,13,35] An LPI should also be performed for the fellow eye.

Laser Peripheral Iridotomy

The primary indications for an LPI is ACG in which pupillary block is presumed to be the causative factor.[36,37] Prophylactic LPIs are indicated in all fellow eyes after an acute angle closure attack in the opposite eye.[36–41] Intermittent and chronic angle closure glaucoma are also considered to be indications for LPI.[37,40,41] Patients with ACG caused by iris neovascularization, inflammatory PAS, or swelling of the ciliary body (uveal effusion) are not candidates for LPI because pupillary block is not the mechanism for these conditions.

At the time of this writing, argon (thermal) and neodymium:yttrium-aluminum-garnet (Nd:YAG; photodisruptor) are the two types of lasers most commonly used for LPI (Table 16-3). Although the argon laser has the longest history of use for LPI, many practitioners feel that the Nd:YAG laser is the preferred instrument[35,42] because a lower incidence of iridotomy closure is associated with it, and its success is not dependent on the degree of pigmentation of the iris.

TABLE 16-3. Comparison of Characteristics of Nd:YAG and Argon Laser Peripheral Iridotomy

Characteristic	Nd:YAG	Argon
Iris color	Not a factor[36,37,60]	Difficulty penetrating blue iris[36,37,60]
Type of energy	Photodisruptive	Thermal
Total energy	Less energy used[37,60]	More energy used[37,60]
Iris bleed	20–60%[39,42,46,48,49]	Rare[36]
Peripheral iridotomy closure	Rare[46,50,60]	16–40%[46,47,49,50,60]
Peripheral iridotomy margins	Jagged[36,37]	Smooth[36,37]
Lens injury	More likely ±[36]	Possible
Corneal injury	Possible	Possible
Pupil distortion	Rare[60]	Common[60]
Postoperative intraocular pressure rise*	Common[39,42,46]	Common[42,55]

*Decreases with use of apraclonidine.
Source: Reprinted with permission from J Jackson. Clinical Applications of Lasers. In D Pitts, R Kleinstine (eds). Environmental Vision–Interactions of the Eye, Vision and the Environment. Stoneham, Mass.: Butterworth, 1993;239.

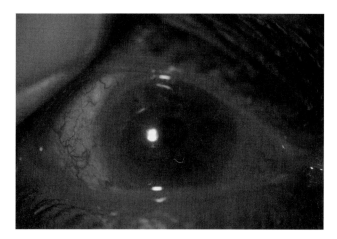

FIGURE 16-5. Peripheral iridotomy. In patients with primary angle closure glaucoma with a pupillary block component, a laser iridotomy equalizes the pressure between the anterior and posterior chamber. A patent iridotomy should transilluminate and not be obstructed with any fibrotic iris tissue.

Contraindications. Corneal edema may preclude LPI in patients with an acute angle closure attack. Managing the patient medically until the cornea clears and anterior chamber deepens before proceeding with LPI is generally preferred. In cases in which delay is judged to be unsafe, the physician can either use topical glycerin in an attempt to clear the cornea or opt for a surgical iridectomy.

General Features. The use of a contact lens with a peripheral convex button makes the creation of an LPI easier and safer with both Nd:YAG and argon lasers. The two most commonly used lenses are the Abraham Iridectomy Lens and the Wise Iridotomy Lens (Ocular Instruments, Bellevue, WA). These lenses serve to prevent lid closure, stabilize the eye, absorb heat energy away from the cornea (in conjunction with gonio solution), and minimize energy loss by reflection. Because of their high plus buttons, they also focus the laser energy at the iris while decreasing the energy delivered to the cornea and retina. Most clinicians consider the use of these lenses to be mandatory.[35–37,40,43,44]

The preparation of the patient is minimal. An explanation of the procedure with possible complications is mandatory. Written informed consent signed by the patient is recommended. Miosis serves to thin the iris and make penetration easier. Apraclonidine is used as prophylaxis against an IOP spike. Pilocarpine (generally 2–4%) and apraclonidine 0.5% or 1.0% are given 1 hour before the iridotomy. Topical anesthetic is almost always sufficient. Retrobulbar anesthesia is reserved for the rare uncooperative patient (cannot maintain fixation) or for patients with severe nystagmus.

The placement of the iridotomy should be under the superior lid to avoid secondary images and for cosmetic concerns. In most patients, this corresponds to the 11 o'clock or 1 o'clock position, because air bubbles (caused by the procedure) can accumulate at 12 o'clock and cause difficulty in completing the iridotomy. Theoretically, superiornasal is the preferred site; it has the added benefit of avoiding accidental macular exposure. Performing two iridotomies is often advantageous because it offers a measure of protection against future closure. This is particularly true for argon laser iridotomies because of the higher incidence of iridotomy closure. The iridotomy should be placed far enough peripherally to minimize exposure to the lens and far enough from the limbus to avoid a corneal burn. Generally, two-thirds of the distance from the pupillary margin to the limbus is satisfactory. Corneal arcus, as well as other corneal opacities, should be avoided because they interfere with precise focusing. If present, it is advantageous to choose an iris crypt for the iridotomy site because this represents an area of relatively thinner iris.[36,37] When using the argon laser with a lightly pigmented iris, it is helpful to find an iris freckle for the iridotomy site. The increased pigmentation absorbs laser energy and aids in penetration.[36,37] Nd:YAG lasers do not require pigmentation and therefore are preferable in patients with lightly pigmented irides.

Penetration through the iris is not always easy to confirm. The practitioner must be familiar with several techniques to evaluate a successful iridotomy. Penetration through the iris into the posterior chamber is often signaled by a "plume of pigment." This is caused by the sudden release of trapped aqueous in the posterior chamber that carries dispersed pigment with it. Transillumination (Figure 16-5) is often indicative of a patent iridotomy in medium and dark irides, but light irides can transilluminate even if complete penetration has not been obtained. Direct observation of the anterior lens capsule is clear evidence of penetration but is often difficult to ascertain. The definitive method of determining iris penetration is verification of deepening of the anterior chamber via gonioscopy.

Neodymium:Yttrium-Aluminum-Garnet Laser Peripheral Iridotomy

The Nd:YAG laser is a photodisruptor. A shock wave is created that mechanically cuts tissue. This effect is not pigment-dependent. Therefore, a decided advantage of the Nd:YAG laser is its ability to create an iridotomy regardless of iris color. The primary disadvantage of the Nd:YAG laser is the occurrence of bleeding at the iridotomy site with its use. However, this is usually self-limiting and can usually be controlled with minimal digital pressure with the iridotomy lens.

Argon Laser Peripheral Iridotomy

It is much more important when performing argon LPI (than with Nd:YAG) for a clinician to have a number of techniques in the armamentarium and retain a flexibility in approach should one technique prove to be unsuccessful. The argon laser is a photocoagulator, and the effect of laser energy varies tremendously in irides with different amounts of pigmentation. Iris color is the single most important factor in determining which argon iridotomy technique should be used. Light-colored irides are the most difficult to penetrate with the argon laser because the pigment is often insufficient to absorb the laser energy. Most clinicians recommend the use of the Nd:YAG laser in these cases. Dark-brown irides can also be quite difficult to penetrate because of their tendency to char. This charring appears as black, shiny material at the base of the iridotomy site and is a result of excessive heat generated by the absorption of laser energy by the presence of high amounts of pigment. A combination of argon and Nd:YAG lasers (the argon is used first, then the Nd:YAG) may be used to penetrate dark-brown irides. Light-brown irides are the easiest to penetrate with the argon laser.

Postprocedure Management

Immediately after the iridotomy, a second drop of apraclonidine is administered. A topical steroid, such as 1% prednisolone acetate, is prescribed four to eight times a day for 1 week to control for any anterior chamber inflammatory reaction. The patient may be placed on 2% pilocarpine four times a day for 1 week as well to prevent closure of the newly created iridotomy,[45] although miotics can exacerbate inflammation caused by the iridotomy procedure.

The IOP should be checked 1–3 hours after the iridotomy. If the pressure is under control, the patient is next seen at 1 day to 1 week after the operation, depending on any complications encountered during the procedure. If the pressure is still elevated despite a patent peripheral iridotomy, then the patient should be prescribed aqueous-suppressing agents (beta blockers, α agonists, CAIs). An attempt can be made to gradually reduce these agents as the eye quiets. After 1 week, if the iridotomy remains patent, it is recommended that the patient be dilated to prevent posterior synechiae formation and for fundus examination.

Complications

Complications after LPI, as well as all anterior segment laser procedures, are quite common but not usually sight-threatening. Postoperative IOP rise has been studied by a host of investigators.[33,39–42,48–54] A rise of 10 mm Hg or more in IOP has been reported in as many as 43% of eyes not receiving prophylactic IOP-lowering medication. Risks from the IOP rise can be minimized by use of apraclonidine and beta blockers.[33,51–54] A study by Robin[55] found that 96% of all eyes that demonstrated a post-iridotomy IOP spike did

so within 2 hours. The final 4% of IOP spikes occurred within 3 hours after the iridotomy, and no eyes without an IOP elevation during the first 3 hours developed a late (days to weeks) IOP elevation.

Iritis is a very common postoperative complication after LPI.[42,56] The iritis is usually transient and responds well to topical steroid therapy. More severe iritis may be encountered when excessive energy is used to create the iridotomy because of poor iris penetration. Higher frequency of steroid dosage (every 1–2 hours) should be prescribed for severe anterior chamber inflammation. Pigment dispersion after LPI is also common, and pigmented cells should be differentiated from inflammatory white cells when contemplating steroid dosing. Blurred vision is frequently reported after LPI secondary to released pigment or iris bleeding (with Nd:YAG laser). Rapid resolution is usually noted.

Corneal and lenticular opacities have been reported with argon and Nd:YAG lasers.[39,42,56] Use of iridotomy lenses and careful focusing prevent most corneal opacities. Corneal opacities that do occur usually resolve completely within 24–48 hours, although in eyes with marginally decompensated cornea cases of further decompensation have occurred.[57] Lenticular opacities have been found to be stable and nonprogressive[36] or to resolve altogether.[58]

Iris bleeding can occur with Nd:YAG laser iridotomies. Although the incidence is high (as much as 60% in some studies), the bleeding can usually be controlled by application of slight digital pressure to the globe with the iridotomy lens. Serious complications related to iris hemorrhaging from LPI are rare.[39,42,46,48,49,56]

Retinal or macular damage is a rare but potentially severe complication of LPI. Use of an iridotomy lens, careful focusing, and directing the iridotomy site (superior-nasal) away from the fovea minimize this risk.

Monocular diplopia or blurring can occur if the iridotomy site is not well covered by the lid.[59] Therefore, a site above the palpebral aperture should be chosen when selecting an iridotomy site. Pupil irregularities can occur with the argon laser because of contraction associated with the photocoagulative nature of the laser, but these are usually of no visual consequence.

Closure of the iridotomy site occurs in 16–40% of patients after argon LPI.[46,47,50,60] Closure is most likely to occur in the first 1–2 months and almost never after 6 months.[46,47,50] Closure with the argon laser can be minimized by performing larger peripheral iridotomies and controlling postoperative inflammation. Closure is very rare with the Nd:YAG laser,[46,50,60] and this is the main reason why many practitioners choose the Nd:YAG over the argon for LPI. Iridotomies created with a Nd:YAG laser increase in size over time, and this may be the reason for the low incidence of closure with this laser.

Surgery

Typically, if the acute ACG attack is not broken within 3–6 hours after treatment is initiated and LPI has been unsuccessful, the patient is referred for surgical iridectomy. Some eyes that develop acute PACG with pupillary block eventually require filtering surgery for IOP control.[61,62] Potential causes include extensive PAS, irreversible damage to the meshwork, and the presence of mixed-mechanism glaucoma. This has caused some authorities to recommend primary filtering surgery for eyes that have experienced severe, prolonged, or recurrent attacks of ACG.[63,64] Other studies have demonstrated that iridectomy combined with medical treatment gave results equal to those obtained by primary filtering surgery with fewer complications.[62,63,65]

Prognosis and Follow-Up

PACG patients should not be considered cured even after a successful LPI has been performed. These patients should be considered glaucoma suspects for life and receive appropriate follow-up care. Along with IOP measurement and evaluating the iridotomy for patency, gonioscopy, visual fields, and optic nerves should be monitored over the long term. Elevated pressure in the immediate post-iridotomy period can occur secondary to incomplete or closed iridotomy, inflammation, or extensive PAS, or in response to steroid therapy. Late-stage IOP rise may be a result of trabecular meshwork damage that occurred during the period of appositional closure. The development of OAG is also more common in these patients.

PLATEAU IRIS SYNDROME

Primary ACG without pupillary block is usually called *plateau iris syndrome*. Plateau iris configuration is a clinical entity in which the central anterior chamber depth is normal, the iris plane is flat, and the peripheral anterior chamber angle is extremely narrow. Gonioscopy, which is required to make the diagnosis, reveals that the peripheral iris takes a sharp turn posteriorly before inserting into the ciliary body. Pupillary dilation causes the peripheral iris to bunch and block the trabecular meshwork, preventing the drainage of aqueous (see Figure 16-2). Some clinicians diagnose plateau iris syndrome when the anterior chamber remains capable of closure with dilation in the presence of a patent iridotomy.[1,20] Patients with plateau iris configuration typically have no symptoms until they develop an acute or subacute attack of primary ACG incited by pupillary dilation. In some cases, peripheral iridotomy can cure the patient with plateau iris syndrome by preventing future attacks of primary ACG, suggesting that pupillary block plays a considerable role in the development of acute ACG in these patients.[66,67] Despite a patent iridotomy,

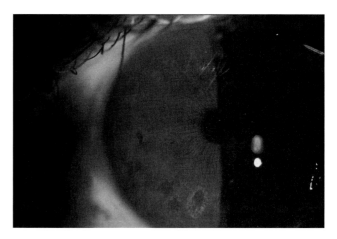

FIGURE 16-6. Laser iridoplasty. Peripheral iris burns are made with a laser to stretch the peripheral iris out of the angle.

most patients with plateau iris syndrome remain at risk for primary ACG. Treatment of this condition includes the use of chronic miotic agents (1–2% pilocarpine) or peripheral gonioplasty to prevent the peripheral iris from bunching into the angle.[67]

Argon Laser Peripheral Iridoplasty (Gonioplasty)

The argon (or diode) laser can produce significant contour changes in the iris because of its coagulative effect. Argon peripheral iridoplasty is a technique by which the peripheral iris is contracted or flattened to pull it away from the angle. This technique can be used to "open" sections of the angle and may be effective as a treatment in cases of ACG secondary to plateau iris syndrome that is not responsive to medical management.

The technique of peripheral iridoplasty consists of placing large (300–500 µm), low-power burns to the peripheral iris 1–2 mm inside the limbus (Figure 16-6). Topical anesthetic is sufficient, and most practitioners do not use a laser contact lens. Pilocarpine is used 1 hour before treatment to put the iris on stretch and make shrinking of tissue more easily visible. When iridoplasty is being used to break an attack of acute angle closure, generally only 90–180 degrees of the angle needs to be treated. Iridoplasty can induce anterior chamber inflammation (iritis) and requires postoperative topical steroid therapy. Other complications are uncommon and mirror those of laser iridotomy.

SUBACUTE ANGLE-CLOSURE GLAUCOMA

In the subacute stage of primary ACG, patients undergo incomplete angle closure that resolves spontaneously. Symptoms vary widely based on the level of IOP, the patient's pain threshold and level of awareness, and perhaps race.[1] Subacute attacks tend to increase over time, and the patient may progress to chronic primary ACG or have an acute angle closure attack. Clinical signs of prior angle closure attacks include PAS, glaucomflecken (anterior cataract formation), high tide line of pigment above Schwalbe's line in the anterior chamber angle, and posterior synechiae in conjunction with a patient who has a narrow anterior chamber angle.

CHRONIC ANGLE-CLOSURE GLAUCOMA

Chronic primary ACG is defined as permanent closure of parts of the anterior chamber by PAS from an anatomically narrow anterior chamber angle. Symptoms may be mild or absent until very late in the disease. IOP may not become elevated until one-half or three-fourths of the angle are occluded with PAS. Closure of the angle with PAS may progress slowly and therefore mimic primary OAG that becomes refractory over time to standard medical therapy (see Case 5 in Chapter 18). The differential diagnosis of primary OAG and chronic primary angle closure is made by gonioscopy.

WHEN TO RECOMMEND PROPHYLACTIC LASER PERIPHERAL IRIDOTOMY FOR NARROW ANGLES

Prophylactic LPIs are indicated in all fellow eyes after a primary acute angle glaucoma attack in the opposite eye.[36,37,39–41,43,44,51–55] Evidence of subacute angle closure attacks (i.e., PAS, high tide line in the angle, glaucomflecken) or chronic angle closure (PAS usually in the superior angle) is also considered indications for LPI.[37,40,41] Prophylactic LPIs are also indicated in eyes that on gonioscopic examination have appositional angle closure, even if IOP is normal and PAS have not yet formed.[68] LPI is not indicated if the angle is not susceptible to spontaneous closure. The difficulty lies in determining which eyes are susceptible to spontaneous closure. Provocative testing has been used in the past by some clinicians to indicate which eyes are at risk for developing angle closure. These provocative tests have included the use of various pharmacologic agents and physiologic tests, such as the mydriatic provocative test, the dark room test, the prone test, and the prone dark room test.[1,34,68] All of these provocative tests can result in false-positive and false-negative results.

Because all patients eventually need a dilated fundus evaluation, the mydriatic provocative test can be performed as part of the routine examination. In a patient who has narrow angles without signs of angle closure or PAS, a weak concentration of tropicamide (0.5%) can be instilled in one eye only (to avoid a bilateral angle closure attack). Sympathomimetics, such as phenylephrine, are not used because if a pupillary block attack does occur it may be more difficult to abort. IOP and gonioscopy should be repeated approximately 30–60 minutes after the mydriatic is instilled. If the IOP is elevated by more than 5 mm Hg and gonioscopy shows a closed or more narrow angle than before dilation, the test should be considered positive and a peripheral iridotomy scheduled. It is important to remember that a patient may exhibit an increase in IOP postdilation that is not related to a narrowing of the angle. Postdilation gonioscopy and the observation of pigment dispersion in the anterior chamber are key differentiating tests.

Any angle closure attack induced by dilation should be medically treated as described in the earlier section Acute Primary Angle-Closure Glaucoma. A pharmacologic angle closure attack is more likely to occur when the pupil is returning to its normal physiologic state from the dilated position. The time frame is generally 2–4 hours after the mydriatic drop is instilled.

Most experienced clinicians rely on the slit-lamp examination of the anterior chamber and contour of the iris along with dynamic gonioscopy to decide whether a patient is at risk for angle closure and whether a need for prophylactic LPI exists.[1,34,68,69] Clinical guidelines to determine which narrow-angle patients should have prophylactic peripheral iridotomies include:

- History of or clinical evidence of subacute angle closure attacks
- Any PAS in the angle related to appositional angle closure
- Full trabecular meshwork not viewed in at least one quadrant with goniolens tilting
- Narrow-angle patient without easy assess to medical and laser treatment if an acute angle closure attack occurs

Prognosis and Follow-Up

PACG patients should not be considered cured even after a successful LPI has been performed. A significant number of PACG patients will require IOP lowering therapy despite an open anterior chamber angle after LPI (mixed mechanism glaucoma). All PACG patients should be considered glaucoma suspects for life and receive appropriate follow-up care. Along with IOP measurement and evaluating the iridotomy for patency, gonioscopy, visual fields and optic nerves should be monitored long term. Elevated pressure in the immediate post-iridotomy period can occur secondary to incomplete or closed iridotomy, inflammation, extensive PAS, or in response to steroid therapy. Late-stage IOP rise may be a result of trabecular meshwork damage that occurred during the period of appositional closure or to non–pupillary block components of angle closure, such as plateau iris or a secondary angle-closure mechanism.

REFERENCES

1. Jackson J, Carr L, Fisch B, Malinovsky V, Talley D. Optometric clinical practice guideline. Care of the patient with primary angle-closure glaucoma. St. Louis: The American Optometric Association, 1994.

2. Van Herick W, Schaffer RN, Schwartz A. Estimation of width of angle of anterior chamber. Incidence and significance of the narrow angle. Am J Ophthalmol 1969;68:626.

3. Cockburn DM. Slit-lamp estimate of anterior chamber depth as a predictor of the gonioscopic visibility of the angle structures. Am J Optom Physiol Opt 1982;59:904.

4. Spaeth GL. The normal development of the human anterior chamber angle: a new system of descriptive grading. Trans Ophthalmol Soc U K 1971;91:709.

5. Congdon N, Wang F, Tielsch JM. Issues in the epidemiology and population-based screening of primary angle-closure glaucoma. Surv Ophthalmol 1992; 36:411.

6. Alsbirk PH. Primary angle-closure glaucoma: oculometry, epidemiology and genetics in a high-risk population. Acta Ophthalmol 1976;54(127):5.

7. Clemmesen V, Alsbirk PH. Primary angle-closure glaucoma in Greenland. Acta Ophthalmol 1971; 49:47.

8. Cox JE. Angle-closure glaucoma among the Alaskan Eskimos. Glaucoma 1984;6:135.

9. Pararajasegaram R. Glaucoma pattern in Ceylon. Trans Asia Pac Acad Ophthalmol 1968;3:274.

10. Alsbirk PH. Prevention and Control of Visual Impairment and Blindness (with Special Reference to Glaucoma) in India. World Health Organization, Consultant Report, SE Asia Region/Ophthalmology, New York: World Health Organization, 1984.

11. Linner E. Assessment of Glaucoma as a Cause of Blindness, India. World Health Organization, SE Asia Region/Ophthalmology, New York, World Health Organization, 1982.

12. Lob RCK. The problems of glaucoma in Singapore. Singapore Med J 1968;9:76.

13. Hoskins HD Jr, Kass M. Angle Closure with Pupillary Block. In HD Hoskins Jr, M Kass (eds). Becker-Shaffer's Diagnosis and Therapy of the Glaucomas (6th ed). St. Louis: Mosby, 1989;208.

14. Tomlinson A, Leithton DA. Ocular dimensions in the heredity of angle-closure glaucoma. Br J Ophthalmol 1973;57:475.

15. Chandler PA. Narrow angle glaucoma. Arch Ophthalmol 1952;47:695.

16. Wollensak J, Zeisberg B. Pathophysiology, treatment, and prophylaxis of angle-closure glaucoma. Glaucoma 1986;8:3.

17. Simmons RJ, Blecher CD, Dallow RL. Primary Angle-Closure Glaucoma. In W Tasmon, EA Jaeger (eds). Duane's Clinical Ophthalmology. Philadelphia: Lippincott, 1989;(3)53:1.

18. Lowe RF. Anatomical basis for primary angle-closure glaucoma. Br J Ophthalmol 1970;54:161.

19. Mapstone R. Mechanics of pupil block. Br J Ophthalmol 1968;52:19.

20. Fisch BM. Primary Angle-Closure Glaucoma. In BM Fisch (ed). Gonioscopy and the Glaucomas. Boston: Butterworth–Heinemann, 1993;59.

21. Bengtsson B. The prevalence of glaucoma. Br J Ophthalmol 1981;65:46.

22. Alper M, Laubach J. Primary ACG in the American Negro. Arch Ophthalmol 1968;79:663.

23. Luntz M. Primary ACG in urbanized South African caucasoid and negroid communities. Br J Ophthalmol 1973;57:445.

24. Wollensak J. Prophylaxis and treatment of narrow angle glaucoma. Glaucoma 1979;1:91.

25. Greco JJ, Kelman CD. Systemic pilocarpine toxicity in the treatment of angle-closure glaucoma. Ann Ophthalmol 1973;5:57.

26. Garnias F, Mapstone R. Miotics in closed angle glaucoma. Br J Ophthalmol 1975;59(4):205.

27. Anderson D, Davis E. Sensitivities of ocular tissues to acute pressure-induced ischemia. Arch Ophthalmol 1975;93:267.

28. Zimmerman T. Pilocarpine. Ophthalmology 1981;88:85.

29. Fingeret M, Kowal D. Acute Glaucomas: Diagnosis and Treatment. In J Classe (ed). Optometry Clinics (vol 1). Norwalk, Conn.: Appleton & Lange, 1993;165.

30. Kramer P, Ritch R. The treatment of acute angle-closure glaucoma revisited. Ann Ophthalmol 1984;16:1101.

31. Stelmack T. Angle-Closure Glaucoma. In TL Lewis, M Fingeret (eds). Primary Care of the Glaucomas. Norwalk, Conn.: Appleton & Lange, 1993;347.

32. Hillman J. Management of acute glaucoma with pilocarpine-soaked hydrophilic lens. Br J Ophthalmol 1974;58:674.

33. Robin AL, Pollack IP, deFaller JM. Effects of topical ALO 2145 (p-aminoclonidine hydrochloride) on acute intraocular pressure rise after argon iridectomy. Arch Ophthalmol 1987;105:1208.

34. American Academy of Ophthalmology. Preferred Practice Pattern. Primary Angle-Closure Glaucoma. San Francisco: American Academy of Ophthalmology 1992;1.

35. Jackson J. Clinical Applications of Lasers. In D Pitts, R Kleinstein (eds). Environmental Vision—Interactions of the Eye, Vision and the Environment. Stoneham, Mass.: Butterworth, 1993;239.

36. Ritch R, Solomol I. Laser Treatment of Glaucoma. In L'Esperance V (ed). Ophthalmic Lasers. St. Louis: Mosby, 1989;650.

37. Alward W. Laser Iridotomy. In: T Weingeist, S Sneed (eds). Laser Surgery in Ophthalmology. Norwalk, Conn.: Appleton & Lange, 1992;139.

38. Rostron C. Acute angle-closure glaucoma: surgery or laser? Glaucoma 1985;7:268.

39. Fleck B, Dhillon B, Khanna V, et al. A randomized, prospective comparison of Nd:YAG laser iridotomy and operative peripheral iridectomy in fellow eyes. Eye 1991;5:315.

40. Hoskins H, Kass M. Laser Treatment for Internal Flow Block. In H Hoskins, M Kass (eds). Becker-Shaffer's Diagnosis and Therapy of the Glaucomas. St. Louis: Mosby, 1989;499.

41. Iwata K, Abe H, Sugiyama J. Argon laser iridotomy in primary angle-closure glaucoma. Glaucoma 1985;7:103.

42. Robin A, Pollack I. A comparison of neodymium:YAG and argon laser iridotomies. Ophthalmology 1984;91:1011–1016.

43. Diekert J, Mainster M, Ho P. Contact lenses for laser applications. Ophthalmology 1984(suppl);79.

44. Quigley H. Surgery of the Glaucomas. In: T Rice, R Michels, W Stark (eds). Ophthalmic Surgery. St. Louis: Mosby, 1984;177.

45. Shields M. Textbook of Glaucoma (2nd ed). Baltimore: Williams & Wilkins, 1987;450.

46. Del Prioro L, Robin A, Pollack I. Neodymium:YAG and argon laser iridotomy. Long-term follow-up in a prospective, randomized clinical trial. Ophthalmology 1988;95:1207.

47. Assaf A. Argon laser iridectomies. Glaucoma 1985;7:75.

48. Wise J. Low-energy linear-incision neodymium:YAG laser iridotomy versus linear-incision argon laser iridotomy. A prospective, randomized clinical trial. Ophthalmology 1987;94:1531.

49. Gray R, Honre N, Ayliffe W. Efficacy of Nd:YAG laser iridotomies in acute angle-closure glaucoma. Br J Ophthalmol 1989;73:182.

50. Moster M, Schwartz L, Spaeth G, et al. Laser iridectomy: a controlled study comparing argon and neodymium:YAG. Ophthalmology 1986;93:20.

51. Krupin T, Stone R, Cohen B, et al. Acute intraocular pressure response to argon laser iridotomy. Ophthalmology 1985;92:922.

52. Schrems W, Eichelbronner O, Krieghteiin G. The immediate IOP response of Nd:YAG laser iridotomy and its prophylactic treatability. Acta Ophthalmol 1984;62:673.

53. Liv P, Hung P. Effect of Timolol on intraocular pressure elevation following argon laser iridotomy. J Ocul Pharmacol 1987;3:249.

54. King M, Richards D. Near syncope and chest tightness after administration of apraclonidine before argon laser iridotomy (letter). Am J Ophthalmol 1990;110:308.

55. Robin A. Medical management of acute postoperative intraocular pressure rise associated with anterior segment ophthalmic laser surgery. Int Ophthalmol Clin 1990;30:102.

56. Schwartz L, Moster M, Spaeth G, et al. Transient iritis following laser iridotomy. Am J Ophthalmol 1986;102:41.

57. Schwartz A, Martin N. Corneal decompensation after argon laser iridectomy. Arch Ophthalmol 1988;106:1572.

58. Higginbotham E, Ogura Y. Lens clarity after argon and Nd:YAG laser iridotomy in the rabbit. Arch Ophthalmol 1987;105:540.

59. Murphy P, Trope G. Monocular blurring: a complication of YAG laser iridotomy. Ophthalmology 1991;98:1539.

60. Prum B, Shields S, Shields M, et al. In vitro videographic comparison of argon and Nd:YAG laser iridotomy. Am J Ophthalmol 1991;111:589.

61. Bobrow J, Drews R. Long-term results of peripheral iridectomy. Glaucoma 1981;3:319.

62. Hyams S, Friedman Z, Keroub C. Mixed glaucoma. Br J Ophthalmol 1977;61(2):105–106.

63. Forbes M. Indentation gonioscopy and efficacy of iridectomy in angle-closure glaucoma. Trans Am Ophthalmol Soc 1974;72:488.

64. Gelber E, Anderson D. Surgical decisions in chronic angle-closure glaucoma. Arch Ophthalmol 1976;94:1481.

65. Murphy M, Spaaeth G. Iridectomy in primary angle-closure glaucoma. Arch Ophthalmol 1974;91:114.

66. Lowe RF, Ritch R. Angle-Closure Glaucoma. Mechanisms and epidemiology. In R Ritch, MB Shields, T Krupin (eds). The Glaucomas. St. Louis: Mosby, 1989;825.

67. Hoskins HD Jr, Kass MA (eds). Becker-Shaffer's diagnosis and therapy of the glaucomas (6th ed). St. Louis: Mosby, 1989;238.

68. Ritch R. Definitive signs and gonioscopic visualization of appositional angle closure are indications for prophylactic laser iridotomy. Surv Ophthalmol 1996;41:31.

69. Wilensky J, Kaufman P, Frohlichstein D. Follow-up of angle-closure glaucoma suspects. Am J Ophthalmol 1993;115:338–346.

Secondary Angle-Closure Glaucoma

Kelly H. Thomann

Secondary angle-closure glaucoma is a diverse group of clinical conditions associated with ocular or systemic abnormalities leading to closure of the anterior chamber angle. These conditions must be differentiated from primary angle-closure glaucoma, which results from an anatomic predisposition and may present after a precipitating event (e.g., pupil dilation or being in a darkened environment). The examination of the fellow eye is crucial in the diagnosis of secondary angle-closure glaucoma because that eye does not have an anatomic predisposition for closure as in primary angle-closure glaucoma.

Secondary angle-closure glaucoma may be divided into two groups (Table 17-1): *with pupillary block* (Figure 17-1) and *without pupillary block*. The latter may be further subdivided into conditions that cause a direct obstruction of the trabecular meshwork, such as angle neovascularization with fibrovascular membrane and peripheral anterior synechiae (PAS) (Figure 17-2), and those caused by a forward displacement of the ciliary body, most often resulting from a condition affecting the posterior segment[1] (Figure 17-3), for example ciliochoroidal effusion.

Diagnosis of secondary angle-closure glaucoma is suspected when elevated intraocular pressure (IOP) and asymmetric anterior chamber angles are found. Optic nerve damage or visual field loss is not always present when the diagnosis is made. Similar to primary angle-closure glaucoma, the eye is often painful, with visual acuity reduced. The cornea may be hazy and edematous and the conjunctiva markedly hyperemic. Gonioscopy reveals a shallow to closed peripheral anterior chamber angle, whereas the angle of the fellow eye is completely open. If

the fellow angle is very narrow or closed, then primary angle closure is a more likely diagnosis (see Figure 4-5).

Management of secondary angle-closure glaucoma varies according to the associated ocular or systemic condition, the amount of pressure elevation, and the mechanism leading to angle closure. Medical management is instituted immediately to acutely lower IOP. This includes drugs that decrease aqueous humor production, namely a topical nonselective beta blocker, topical α_2 agonist (apraclonidine or brimonidine), and an oral or topical carbonic anhydrase inhibitor (acetazolamide, 500 mg p.o.; dorzolamide; or brinzolamide). Pilocarpine may or may not be used once the IOP is lower than 40 mm Hg (when the iris becomes nonischemic), depending on the mechanism for angle closure. In some cases of secondary angle closure, pilocarpine is contraindicated, and a cycloplegic should be used to relax the ciliary muscle. If the pressure does not respond to these medications, then a hyperosmotic agent is usually added. Once the IOP is acutely managed, the mechanism of angle closure must be identified and treated. Because the management of secondary angle-closure glaucoma is case specific, it is addressed in individual sections within this chapter.

SECONDARY ANGLE CLOSURE WITH PUPILLARY BLOCK

Phacomorphic Glaucoma/Angle Closure Secondary to Ectopia Lentis

Angle-closure glaucoma can occur in an eye with a hypermature cataract or anteriorly dislocated lens. The primary mechanism for angle closure in these cases is

TABLE 17-1. Secondary Angle-Closure Glaucoma: Underlying Etiologies

With pupillary block

Phacomorphic glaucoma/lens subluxation

Ectopia lentis

Pseudophakic and aphakic pupillary block

Uveitis with 360-degree posterior synechiae

Without pupillary block

Caused by a direct obstruction of the trabecular meshwork

Neovascular glaucoma

Iridocorneal endothelial syndrome

Inflammation/uveitis/penetrating trauma with peripheral anterior synechiae

Caused by a forward displacement of the ciliary body

Ciliary block (malignant) glaucoma

Cysts of the iris or ciliary body

Intraocular tumor

Ciliochoroidal effusion

Inflammatory: scleritis, pars planitis, Harada disease

Vascular: s/p central retinal vein occlusion, nanophthalmos

Posterior intraocular tumors

Uveal effusion syndrome (idiopathic)

Postoperative: s/p panretinal photocoagulation, s/p scleral buckling surgery, suprachoroidal hemorrhage, hypotony

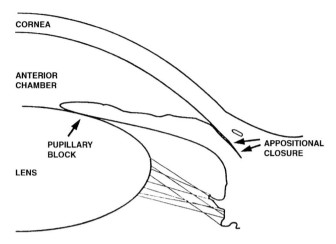

FIGURE 17-1. Pupillary block glaucoma. The iris bows forward (iris bombé) because of increased resistance between the iris and lens. Eventually, the peripheral iris occludes the angle. (Reprinted with permission from AA Cavallerano, LJ Alexander. Secondary Glaucoma. In J Classé [ed], Optometry Clin 1991;1[1]:173.)

pupillary block, in which the lens pushes the iris forward, eventually occluding the pupil and not allowing aqueous to pass into the anterior chamber (Figure 17-4). In turn, the pressure in the posterior chamber rises, causing the peripheral iris to distend forward (iris bombé), narrow the iridocorneal angle, and ultimately close it. PAS may develop from chronic peripheral iris apposition to the trabecular meshwork.

Angle closure resulting from a swollen, cataractous lens is called *phacomorphic glaucoma*. This may be a form of primary angle-closure glaucoma in which a cataractous lens enhances the narrow angle component, thus precipitating closure in an anatomically predisposed eye. However, it may also occur in an eye in which the fellow angle is open. In this case, the increased lens size is the primary mechanism.[2]

Ectopia lentis describes a lens that is completely or incompletely dislocated. The lens is displaced from its normal central position within the posterior chamber. The presence of angle closure depends on the amount and direction of displacement. Angle closure can occur if the lens moves anteriorly and blocks the surface of the iris, resulting in pupillary block and iris bombé. Vitreous may also prolapse forward and contribute to pupillary block. Prolonged, repeated, subclinical closure can ulti-

mately lead to PAS and absolute closure of the angle.[3] Ectopia lentis can be secondary to trauma, ocular disease, or hereditary conditions (Table 17-2).

Subluxation of the lens is the result of loosening or breakage of the zonules. A subluxated lens remains behind the iris and at least partially behind the pupil, but it can cause angle closure if it tilts into the pupil margin and blocks the pupil. Prolapsed vitreous can also contribute to pupillary block.

A patient with angle-closure glaucoma from a cataractous or displaced lens has clinical findings similar to a patient with primary angle-closure glaucoma. However, some clues help to differentiate these cases from primary angle closure. A history of previous trauma to the eye or systemic conditions associated with ectopia lentis may be obtained. In cases of ectopia lentis, a history of variable refractive error, irregular astigmatism, or monocular diplopia may also exist. The patient may report or previous records may indicate that visual acuity had been reduced because of a dense cataract. Iridodonesis or phacodonesis may be observed.[4] The zonules may appear stretched or thickened, or they may be visualized attached to the lens capsule, if ruptured.[3] The anterior chamber depths should be compared by gonioscopy. Because these conditions are usually asymmetric or unilateral, the anterior chamber of the fellow eye is more open. Also, a mature, hypermature, or dislocated (incomplete or complete) lens may be observed in the symptomatic eye, whereas the fellow eye may or may not have similar findings, depending on the underlying etiology.

Acute management of phacomorphic glaucoma is the same as for primary angle-closure glaucoma. The immediate goal is to quickly reduce the IOP medically

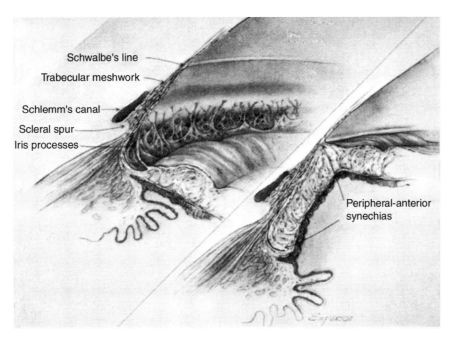

FIGURE 17-2. Schematic diagram of direct angle obstruction from peripheral anterior synechiae in angle-closure glaucoma without pupillary block. Iris neovascularization or fibrotic membrane pulls the peripheral iris into the trabecular meshwork. (Reprinted with permission from HD Hoskins, M Kass. Becker and Schaeffer's Diagnosis and Therapy of the Glaucomas [6th ed]. St. Louis: Mosby, 1989;239.)

(Table 17-3 lists specific dosages) and attempt to open the angle before cataract removal.[2] One drop every 10 minutes for 30 minutes of 1% or 2% pilocarpine should be applied if the IOP is lower than 40 mm Hg. If the IOP is higher than 40 mm Hg, miotic therapy is not effective because the sphincter muscle will be ischemic and nonresponsive. One drop of a topical nonselective beta blocker, an α_2 agonist, and an oral or topical carbonic anhydrase inhibitor may also be used initially. If no response is obtained, an oral hyperosmotic agent may be added.

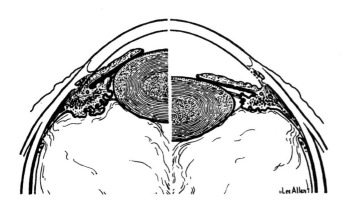

FIGURE 17-3. Schematic diagram of the forward displacement of the ciliary body, vitreous, and lens in angle-closure glaucoma without pupillary block. (Reprinted with permission from CD Phelps. Angle-closure glaucoma secondary to ciliary body swelling. Arch Ophthalmol 1974;92:287–290. © 1974, American Medical Association.)

In phacomorphic glaucoma, after the acute attack is reversed, surgical intervention is usually necessary. Laser peripheral iridotomy (PI) will reverse the pupillary block, but because the dense cataract causes a reduction of visual acuity, cataract surgery provides definitive treatment for the glaucoma and vision improvement. Both intracapsular cataract extraction (ICCE) and extracapsular cataract extraction (ECCE) have been advocated, but more surgeons prefer ECCE if the posterior capsule is intact because it allows the option of a posterior chamber implant and is also less traumatic on eyes with intumescent cataracts.[2] If cataract surgery is contraindicated, laser PI is preferred over surgical iridectomy because it carries less potential for complications. The PI should be placed as peripherally as possible on the iris. However, these patients should be monitored carefully because the angle may ultimately close again if the lens continues to swell, push the iris forward, and occlude the iridotomy. In these cases, a surgical iridectomy may be necessary.[3]

If angle closure is secondary to a noncataractous lens, which has subluxated into the anterior chamber causing pupillary block, the patient should be placed supine to help alleviate pupillary block. An oral hyperosmotic agent (e.g., 50% glycerin solution, 2–3 ml/kg p.o., or 45% isosorbide solution, 1.5 ml/lb of body weight) helps shrink the volume of the vitreous and may allow the lens to move posteriorly and decrease pupillary block.[3] One drop of a topical nonselective beta blocker, topical α_2 agonist, and oral or topical carbonic anhydrase inhibitor are also given. Weak cycloplegic/mydriatic agents (e.g., tropicamide 1% and phenylephrine

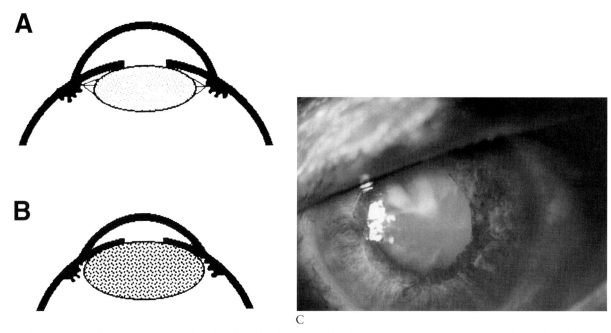

FIGURE 17-4. Schematic diagram of pupillary block with phacomorphic glaucoma. (A) In the early stage of pupillary block, the lens periphery is not in contact with the iris and an iridectomy or iridotomy can re-establish communication between the posterior and anterior chambers. (B) In the late stage of phacomorphic glaucoma, the peripheral iris is displaced forward by the swollen lens and an iridotomy or iridectomy is of no benefit. (Reprinted with permission from F Tomey Karim, AA Al-Rajhi. Neodymium:YAG laser iridotomy in the initial management of phacomorphic glaucoma. Ophthalmology 1992;99:663.) (C) Clinical slide of a patient with a hypermature cataract causing pupillary block and secondary angle closure.

2.5% topically) are used to dilate the pupil and allow the lens to return to a posterior position. Once the lens is returned to the posterior chamber, pilocarpine 1–2% ophthalmic solution, 1 drop q.i.d., should be used and continued chronically to maintain a decreased pupil aperture and prevent the lens from returning to the anterior chamber.[3] Laser PI is necessary to prevent future episodes of angle closure.[5] However, if an anteriorly displaced lens cannot be repositioned in the posterior chamber, it should be removed. A lens remaining in the anterior chamber causes corneal decompensation and becomes cataractous over a short period of time. When the lens is removed from the anterior chamber, ICCE is the required technique.

The management of a lens posteriorly subluxated into the vitreous is case specific. A lens that floats freely in the vitreous or settles inferiorly on the retina may remain indefinitely without complications.[3,5] However, complications (e.g., vitreous or retinal inflammation, retinal detachment) can also occur, necessitating its removal. Removing the lens from the posterior chamber is considered easier by some because it allows for more control of the intraocular environment and the constant infusion of fluid during the procedure.[6]

A number of opinions are available regarding whether to remove a partially subluxated lens. Some advocate a conservative approach with noncataractous subluxated lenses. In many of these cases, only a PI is necessary to release or prevent pupillary block.[5] Others advocate

removal of the lens under any condition. Surgical removal of the lens becomes necessary when vision is severely compromised or if the lens is adherent to the cornea.

TABLE 17-2. Conditions Associated with Ectopia Lentis

Heritable disorders
   Isolated ectopia lentis
   Spontaneous/late subluxation of the lens
   Ectopia lentis et pupillae
   Microspherophakia
   Marfan syndrome
   Weill-Marchesani syndrome
   Homocystinuria
Secondary ocular causes
   Exfoliation syndrome
   High myopia
   Intraocular tumors
   Uveitis
Extraocular causes
   Surgery
   Trauma

Source: Modified from R Ritch, MB Shields, T Kruppin (eds). The Glaucomas. St. Louis: Mosby, 1989.

TABLE 17-3. Acute Medical Management of Phacomorphic Secondary Angle-Closure Glaucoma

1. Pilocarpine 1–2% ophthalmic solution, 1 gtt every 10 mins × 30 mins if intraocular pressure <40 mm Hg

2. Nonselective beta blocker ophthalmic solution, 1 gtt b.i.d.

3. α_2 agonist ophthalmic solution, 1 gtt b.i.d.–t.i.d.

4. Acetazolamide, 500 mg p.o. b.i.d. or topical carbonic anhydrase inhibitor, 1 gtt b.i.d.–t.i.d.

5. Oral hyperosmotics: glycerine 50% solution, 2.0–3.0 ml/kg of body weight

   For diabetic patients: oral 45% isosorbide 1.5 ml/lb of body weight

6. Prednisolone acetate 1% ophthalmic solution, 1 gtt every 1–2 hrs (to control inflammation in preparation for cataract removal)

Pseudophakic and Aphakic Pupillary Block Glaucoma

Pupillary block glaucoma occurs rarely in patients after extracapsular or, more frequently, intracapsular cataract surgery. The pupil aperture may become blocked by the anterior vitreous face or posterior capsule after, for example, wound leak or iridocyclitis or an air bubble trapped behind the iris or the intraocular lens.[7,8] Other possible causes of pupillary block glaucoma after cataract surgery include a posterior vitreous detachment associated with pooling of retrovitreal aqueous, a dense impermeable anterior hyaloid membrane, and inadequate iris openings from a nonperforating or subsequently blocked iridectomy.[9] Pupillary block glaucoma after cataract surgery most often

occurs with an anterior chamber intraocular lens (IOL) in the absence of a functional iridectomy (Figure 17-5).[10,11] Pupillary block glaucoma is relatively rare with extracapsular surgery, but when it occurs, multiple factors most likely contribute to it. The anterior chamber angle anatomy may have been altered by the placement of the lens in the ciliary sulcus rather than the capsular bag, zonular disruption may lead to forward vitreous displacement, or there may have been a pre-existing shallow anterior chamber.[9,10] Although surgical iridectomy is always indicated after ICCE, there is controversy regarding whether surgical iridectomy should be carried out with ECCE. Some ophthalmic surgeons advocate an iridectomy in all cases, whereas others claim it carries additional surgical risk (e.g., bleeding, iridodialysis, postoperative glare).[8] Also, PI at the time of cataract extraction does not rule out the chance of pseudophakic pupillary block because the haptic of the IOL may rotate to occlude the iridectomy, or it may become occluded by other mechanisms (e.g., vitreous prolapse, inflammatory debris).[11] Also, pupillary block glaucoma can follow cataract extraction without IOL placement (in aphakes; Figure 17-6) if the vitreous face or posterior capsule causes relative or absolute block of the pupil or iridectomy.[12]

Pseudophakic pupillary block glaucoma can occur immediately after cataract surgery or several years later.[11,13] Therefore, signs and symptoms are variable. The patient may be asymptomatic or have the classic symptoms of acute angle-closure glaucoma. The eye may be injected, visual acuity reduced, and the cornea edematous and hazy.[11] The IOP is usually elevated but may be normal.[13,14] Careful slit-lamp evaluation reveals mild to prominent iris bombé configuration.[14] In cases involving an anterior chamber IOL, the peripheral iris may appear to bulge around the edges of the implant.[13]

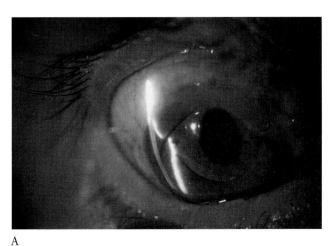

A

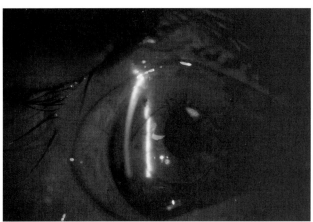

B

FIGURE 17-5. (A) Pseudophakic patient with an anterior chamber intraocular lens blocking the pupil, resulting in pupillary block. Note anterior chamber shallowing. (B) A peripheral iridotomy was performed to allow aqueous entrance into the anterior chamber, relieving pupillary block. Note deepening of the anterior chamber compared with Figure 17-5A.

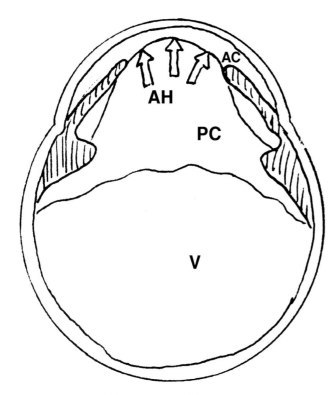

FIGURE 17-6. Aphakic pupillary block glaucoma. Aqueous humor (AH) collects behind an intact posterior lens capsule. The iris balloons forward because of the pressure from the accumulation of the aqueous humor in the posterior chamber (PC). (AC = anterior chamber; V = vitreous.)

The integrity of the cataract incision, the presence or absence of a surgical iridectomy, and notation of the haptic location in relation to the iridectomy site are also important components of the initial evaluation. Careful assessment of the anterior vitreous face in relation to the iridectomy site is critical. Gonioscopy should be done to evaluate the angle structures and also may be useful to determine the relation of the haptic to the iridectomy. Sodium fluorescein dye should be used to rule out a wound leak.[15] If a wound leak is present, indirect ophthalmoscopy and ultrasound may be useful to rule out secondary choroidal detachment.[14]

The definitive treatment of pseudophakic and aphakic pupillary block glaucoma is to re-establish the pathway between the posterior and anterior chambers through a peripheral PI.[7,14] However, medical management may be initiated if an iridotomy cannot be done immediately (Table 17-4). A hyperosmotic agent (e.g., 50% glycerin solution, 2–3 ml/kg p.o., or 45% isosorbide solution, 1.5 ml/lb of body weight p.o.) is used to help shrink the volume of the vitreous. A carbonic anhydrase inhibitor (e.g., acetazolamide 500 mg p.o. or a topical carbonic anhydrase inhibitor) is used to decrease aqueous humor production along with a topical nonselective beta blocker and α_2 agonist. Weak cycloplegic/

TABLE 17-4. Management of Pseudophakic and Aphakic Pupillary Block Glaucoma

1. Nonselective beta blocker ophthalmic solution, 1 gtt b.i.d.

2. α_2 Agonist ophthalmic solution, 1 gtt b.i.d.–t.i.d.

3. Short-acting mydriatic solution:
   - 1% tropicamide ophthalmic solution, 1 gtt and
   - 2.5% phenylephrine ophthalmic solution, 1 gtt

4. Carbonic anhydrase inhibitor:
   - Acetazolamide, 500 mg orally b.i.d., or
   - Topical carbonic anhydrase inhibitor, 1 gtt b.i.d.–t.i.d.

5. If there is no response after Steps 1–4 are carried out:
   Osmotic agents:
   - Oral 50% glycerin solution, 2–3ml/kg, or 45% isosorbide solution, 1.5 ml/lb of body weight, or
   - Intravenous mannitol

6. If Steps 1–5 fail to break pupillary block:
   - Argon or neodymium:yttrium-aluminum-garnet laser iridotomy or
   - Peripheral iridectomy

mydriatic agents (e.g., tropicamide 1% and phenylephrine 2.5% topically) may be used in an attempt to dilate the pupil so that it becomes larger than the optic of the IOL, which may allow some aqueous humor to pass into the anterior chamber. A weak agent is used because it will be necessary to constrict the pupil immediately before laser iridotomy.[14]

If laser iridotomy is not possible (e.g., the cornea is hazy), a surgical iridectomy should be performed. When iris bombé is so severe that the iris almost touches the corneal endothelium, neodymium:yttrium-aluminum-garnet (Nd:YAG) laser iridotomy is preferred to avoid corneal endothelial damage. This technique requires a minimal amount of laser energy and makes it easier to achieve iris perforation under acute conditions.[7,9]

Pupillary Block Glaucoma Secondary to Uveitis with 360-Degree Posterior Synechiae

Pupillary block glaucoma may follow severe cases of uveitis if 360 degrees of posterior synechiae form, resulting in a bound-down, secluded pupil (see Figure 3-13). This prevents the flow of aqueous from the posterior chamber to anterior chamber and ultimately leads to iris bombé and angle closure.[16] Because the pupil is blocked by the synechiae in these cases, the central anterior chamber is *not* as shallow as it is with nonpupillary block mechanisms (e.g., ciliochoroidal effusion). Pupillary block glaucoma secondary to uveitis and posterior synechiae must be treated

TABLE 17-5. Management of Secondary Angle-Closure Glaucoma Caused by Uveitis/Chronic Inflammation and Posterior Synechiae

Primary goal: reverse the pupillary block before the development of peripheral anterior synechiae

Uveitis treatment:

- Anti-inflammatory agent (e.g., prednisolone acetate 1% ophthalmic solution, 1 gtt q1h, then tapered)
- Mydriatic-cycloplegic agent (e.g., homatropine 5% ophthalmic solution, 1 gtt t.i.d.)

Glaucoma treatment:

- Aqueous suppressants: nonselective beta blocker, 1 gtt b.i.d.; acetazolamide 250 mg p.o. q.i.d., or topical carbonic anhydrase inhibitor, 1 gtt b.i.d.–t.i.d.; α_2 agonist, 1 gtt b.i.d.–t.i.d.
- Laser iridotomy
- If media are not clear: argon laser pupilloplasty to disrupt the posterior synechiae or argon laser gonioplasty to contract the peripheral iris and open the angle, followed by laser iridotomy
- If iridotomy closes: repeat to reopen existing iridotomy or surgical iridectomy

Surgical management:

- Filter with antimetabolite, with or without seton

as soon as possible to break the posterior synechiae and prevent the formation of PAS, which leads to permanent and irreversible angle closure.[17]

In these cases, the IOP may or may not be elevated, depending on the status of the ciliary body. Posterior synechiae are noted on slit-lamp examination. Gonioscopy reveals no angle structures with a forward bowing of the iris. The degree of iris bombé is variable, and its classic presentation may not be observed if only the peripheral portion of the iris bulges forward to close the angle.

The initial treatment of pupillary block glaucoma secondary to uveitis (Table 17-5) is homatropine 5% ophthalmic solution t.i.d. or atropine 1% ophthalmic solution b.i.d. topically to dilate the pupil, help reduce inflammation, and improve uveoscleral outflow. Prednisolone acetate 1% ophthalmic solution should be prescribed at one drop every 1–4 hours, depending on the amount of inflammation, and then tapered in accordance to the anterior chamber reaction. One drop of a topical nonselective beta blocker, an α_2 agonist, or both b.i.d. can be used if the IOP is elevated. A carbonic anhydrase inhibitor (e.g., acetazolamide, 500 mg b.i.d. p.o. or topical carbonic anhydrase inhibitor b.i.d.–t.i.d.) may also be added to further reduce the IOP. Miotics are avoided because they induce ciliary spasm and inflammation and enhance the formation of synechiae. Topical prostaglandins should also be avoided because they may

exacerbate the inflammatory component. Oral hyperosmotics may be less effective in achieving an osmotic gradient if the blood-aqueous barrier has been broken.[17]

A laser iridotomy should be performed in a patient with iris bombé from 360 degrees of posterior synechiae before PAS develops. Continued control of the inflammatory process is important because the iridotomy may close with continued excessive inflammation. Laser iridotomy may also be performed in the presence of extensive posterior synechiae without angle closure to prevent subsequent closure from pupillary block and iris bombé.[18] If the iridotomy fails, a large-sector surgical iridectomy should be made.[19]

Trabeculectomy with antimetabolites (mitomycin C, 5-fluorouracil), full thickness filtration procedures, or filtering surgery with setons (e.g., Molteno implant) may be useful in cases in which the IOP cannot be controlled medically.[17,18]

SECONDARY ANGLE GLAUCOMA WITHOUT PUPILLARY BLOCK CAUSED BY DIRECT OBSTRUCTION OF THE ANGLE

Neovascular Glaucoma

Neovascularization of the iris has been documented since the mid-1800s, and its association with diabetic retinopathy dates back to 1888.[20] Neovascular glaucoma is one of the most difficult types of glaucoma to manage because once secondary angle closure occurs, it is extremely difficult to reverse. Therefore, early diagnosis of iris or angle neovascularization, before neovascular glaucoma develops, is desirable to preserve vision.

Neovascularization of the iris primarily results from hypoxic retinal conditions, the most common being central retinal vein occlusion, diabetic retinopathy, and ocular ischemic syndrome from carotid artery occlusive disease (Table 17-6).[21] Although the underlying etiology of neovascularization may vary, the pathogenesis and clinical appearance of neovascular glaucoma are similar. However, onset and rate of progression vary with the underlying etiology and amount of retinal ischemia.[21] For example, anterior segment neovascularization associated with an ischemic central retinal vein occlusion may develop in a matter of weeks. The term *90-day glaucoma* is a misnomer because neovascular glaucoma can occur much sooner after an ischemic central retinal vein occlusion.

New vessel growth is stimulated by an angiogenic factor that is released by hypoxic retinal tissue. The new vessels usually begin at the pupil margin (see Color Plate 10), enlarge, and grow in an irregular pattern along the iris surface. Overlying these fragile new vessels is a transparent fibrovascular membrane. The new vessels grow toward the anterior chamber angle, transverse the

TABLE 17-6. Conditions Associated with Neovascularization of the Iris and Neovascular Glaucoma

Ocular vascular disease

Central or branch retinal vein occlusion

Central or branch retinal artery occlusion

Diabetic retinopathy

Extraocular disease

Carotid artery disease/ligation

Assorted ocular diseases

Retinal detachment

Sickle cell retinopathy

Ocular neoplasms

Malignant melanoma

Retinoblastoma

Ocular inflammatory disease

Chronic uveitis

Endophthalmitis

Sympathetic ophthalmia

Ocular surgery

Cataract extraction (especially in diabetic patients)

Vitrectomy (especially in diabetic patients)

Retinal detachment surgery

Source: Modified from B Fisch. Gonioscopy and the Glaucomas. Boston: Butterworth–Heinemann, 1993;99.

scleral spur, and arborize into the trabecular meshwork (see Color Plate 11). The fibrovascular membrane also covers the trabecular meshwork, causing a reduction of aqueous humor outflow.[21] If the membrane contracts, it acts like a zipper, which pulls the peripheral iris into the trabecular meshwork, leading to the formation of PAS (Figure 17-7). The pigmented layer of the iris becomes pulled tangentially, which causes the pupillary border to bow forward (ectropion uvea). This gives the stroma of the iris a uniform, compact appearance. This is evident in the late stage of neovascular glaucoma, once the angle is permanently occluded.[20]

Careful high-magnification biomicroscopic examination with bright illumination of the iris, especially at the pupil margin, is important in patients at risk for rubeosis irides. Gonioscopy should be done at every follow-up visit in patients who have experienced central vein occlusion or in patients with severe nonproliferative or proliferative diabetic retinopathy. Fluorescein angiography of the iris may detect iris neovascularization before it can be visualized with the biomicroscope. This may be useful in the differentiation of iris tufts from early neovascularization.[22]

A patient with neovascular glaucoma typically presents with acute onset of pain, redness, and decreased vision, although this is not a clear-cut rule. Patients may present with neovascular glaucoma with good vision and a fairly benign-appearing eye. Biomicroscopic examination may reveal conjunctival hyperemia, corneal haze, a deep anterior chamber with flare, and possible hyphema. New vessels can be observed on the iris and in the angle. Bullous keratopathy is often present and makes iris and angle examination difficult. Topical glycerol in a 50–100% solution may be used to acutely reduce the edema and allow examination of the cornea, angle, and other ocular structures.[21] However, iris neovascularization and ectropion uvea can usually be visualized despite corneal edema. Clinical examination of the iris should make the diagnosis of neovascular glaucoma straightforward.

The management of neovascular glaucoma is extremely difficult once closure of the angle occurs. It is far more effective if angle neovascularization and PAS can be prevented. Panretinal photocoagulation (PRP) is efficacious at halting the growth of the new vessels and leads to regression in most instances. PRP should be performed at the first sign of iris or angle neovascularization to prevent PAS formation. After PRP, the vessels can begin to regress within days to weeks. Additional fill-in PRP sessions may be required. Continued medical therapy may be needed, despite an open angle, to treat residual trabecular meshwork damage. Success of PRP is related to the amount of PAS present. For example, if PAS are present in more than 270 degrees of the angle, adjunctive medical or surgical therapy for glaucoma is usually required to control IOP.[23] Panretinal cryotherapy to the peripheral ischemic retina is used when PRP fails or the retina cannot be visualized (e.g., an opaque media), although it carries the risk of additional potential complications (e.g., increased inflammation, vitreous hemorrhage, or retinal detachment). Goniophotocoagulation, the application of laser burns directly onto the new vessels, is a controversial treatment for angle neovascularization that may salvage the remaining open angle and halt the progression of the angle vessels, thus providing temporary treatment before PRP or filtering surgery.[22]

Medical management (Table 17-7) of neovascular glaucoma includes aqueous suppressants (topical nonselective beta blocker, α_2 agonists, oral or topical carbonic anhydrase inhibitors), cycloplegics, anti-inflammatory agents, and, if needed, an oral hyperosmotic agent. Miotics and epinephrine drugs should be avoided because they increase the permeability of the blood-aqueous barrier, cause conjunctival congestion, and exacerbate pain.[22] Topical prostaglandins are generally not used in the treatment of neovascular glaucoma because they can exacerbate the inflammatory component of the condition.

Full-thickness filtering surgery with the use of antimetabolites (e.g., mitomycin C or 5-fluorouracil used during surgery, or 5-fluorouracil injected subconjunctivally after surgery) or seton devices (e.g., Molteno implant) may be required if the IOP is uncontrolled on

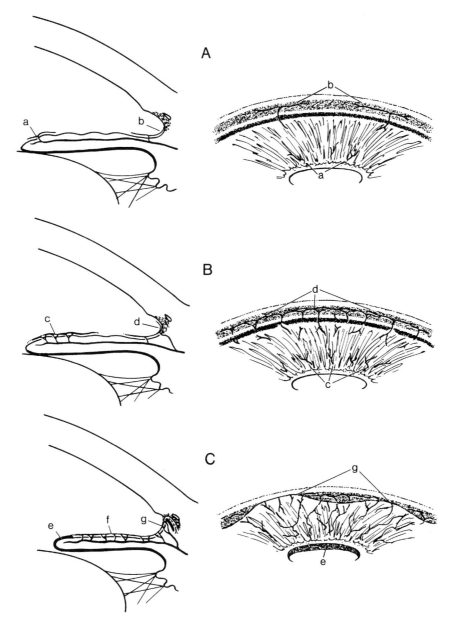

FIGURE 17-7. The stages of neovascular glaucoma. (**A**) Preglaucoma rubeosis iridis. New vessels on the surface of the iris (a) and anterior chamber angle (b). (**B**) Open-angle glaucoma stage. Neovascularization increases and a fibrovascular membrane forms on the iris (c) and anterior chamber angle (d). (**C**) Angle-closure glaucoma stage. Contraction of the fibrovascular membrane results in corectopia, ectropion uvea (e), flattening of the iris (f), and peripheral anterior synechiae (g). (Reprinted with permission from MB Shields. A Study Guide for Glaucoma [3rd ed]. Baltimore: Williams & Wilkins 1982;264.)

medical therapy and useful vision remains.[22,23] If the glaucoma is refractory to medical and surgical treatment and useful vision is lost, the main management goal is to keep the eye free of pain. This is achieved with topical cycloplegics (homatropine 5% or atropine 1% b.i.d.), which help to decrease ocular congestion and increase uveoscleral outflow, along with topical steroids (prednisolone acetate 1% topically q.i.d.) to help reduce inflammation. If total synechial angle closure has occurred, cataract and bullous keratopathy are usually

inevitable consequences. A bandage contact lens may be used to control pain secondary to bullous keratopathy. If this is ineffective, retrobulbar injection of alcohol or enucleation may be necessary to reduce the pain associated with endstage neovascular glaucoma.[20,23]

Iridocorneal Endothelial Syndrome

Iridocorneal endothelial (ICE) syndrome includes several previously named corneal disorders, which probably rep-

TABLE 17-7. Management of Secondary Angle-Closure from Neovascular Glaucoma

1. Panretinal photocoagulation (if media clear)*

    Panretinal cryotherapy (if media opaque)*

2. Aqueous suppressants:

    • Acetazolamide 250 mg q.i.d. orally or topical carbonic anhydrase inhibitor, 1 gtt b.i.d.–t.i.d.

    • Nonselective beta blocker, 1 gtt b.i.d. topically

    • α_2 Agonist, 1 gtt b.i.d.–t.i.d. topically

    Cycloplegic agent:

    • Homatropine 5% or atropine 1% b.i.d.–t.i.d. topically

    Anti-inflammatory agents:

    • Prednisolone acetate 1%, 1 gtt q.i.d. topically

    Hyperosmotic agents (e.g., p.o. 50% glycerin solution, 2–3 ml/kg or 45% isosorbide solution, 1.5 ml/lb of body weight)

3. If intraocular pressure/inflammation remains elevated/ severe and useable vision remains:

    • Filtration surgery with antimetabolite (e.g., mitomycin C or 5-fluorouracil)

or

    • Filtration surgery with drainage implant (e.g., Molteno) and antimetabolite

    • Cycloablative procedures to the ciliary body (if IOP remains increased) or

    • Endolaser photocoagulation of the ciliary body (if the patient is aphakic)

4. To treat a blind, painful eye:

    • Cycloplegic/mydriatic agents: atropine 1%, 1 gtt qd–t.i.d. topically

    • Anti-inflammatory: prednisolone acetate 1%, 1 gtt q.i.d. topically

    • Bandage contact lens (for bullous keratopathy)

    • Retrobulbar injection of alcohol

    • Enucleation

*If retinal ischemia is the underlying cause.

TABLE 17-8. Iridocorneal Endothelial Syndrome

Progressive (essential) iris atrophy

Marked iris atrophy*

Holes in the iris (stretch and melting holes)*

Variable degrees of corectopia and ectropion uvea

Peripheral anterior synechiae (membrane covering angle)

Abnormal corneal endothelium

Chandler syndrome

Abnormal corneal endothelium

Corneal edema and haze*

Corectopia

Mild iris atrophy

Peripheral anterior synechiae (secondary to corneal membrane)

Cogan-Reese syndrome (iris-nevus syndrome)

Pigmented pedunculated iris nodules*

Abnormal corneal endothelium

Corneal edema

Iris atrophy

Peripheral anterior synechiae

*Prominent clinical feature.

resent a broad clinical spectrum of a single disorder (Table 17-8). The ICE disorders are usually unilateral, nonhereditary, and more common in women than men, and in white individuals than non-white.[24] The ICE syndromes include progressive iris atrophy, Chandler syndrome, and Cogan-Reese (iris nevus) syndrome. Each of the ICE syndromes has prominent features. The main clinical characteristics of progressive iris atrophy are iris holes and PAS. Chandler syndrome is the most common of the ICE syndromes. Corneal anomalies are the primary abnormalities, but iris malformations may also be noted. It is characterized by a fine beaten-silver appear-

ance to the corneal endothelium, and corneal edema is an early and prominent sign.[25] Cogan-Reese (iris nevus) syndrome has the prominent feature of iris-pigmented nodules. In this disorder, glaucoma occurs early, whereas corneal decompensation occurs late in the disease.[25]

Common to all of the ICE syndromes is an underlying disorder of the corneal endothelium. The corneal endothelium of patients with an ICE disorder has a fine, beaten-silver appearance to some degree.[23,24] The effects of this endothelial defect can range from an asymptomatic clinical finding to corneal edema with a subsequent decrease in visual acuity. PAS, extending to or beyond Schwalbe's line, and a glassy cellular membrane may cover parts of the angle structures in all the ICE syndromes (see Color Plate 9).[26] Contraction of the membrane may be associated with progressive synechial angle closure, corectopia, ectropion uvea, iris atrophy, and iris hole formation (Figure 17-8). The cellular membrane may also lead to a decrease in outflow facility by blocking the trabecular meshwork.[26]

The differential diagnosis of secondary angle-closure glaucoma associated with an ICE syndrome includes other endothelial dystrophies. Posterior polymorphous dystrophy usually is bilateral and does not involve the iris, and only 20% of patients develop glaucoma. Fuchs' endothelial dystrophy is usually bilateral, presents in the fifth or sixth decade (women more than men), and is not associated with glaucoma. It also does not have iris involvement, and central guttatta are

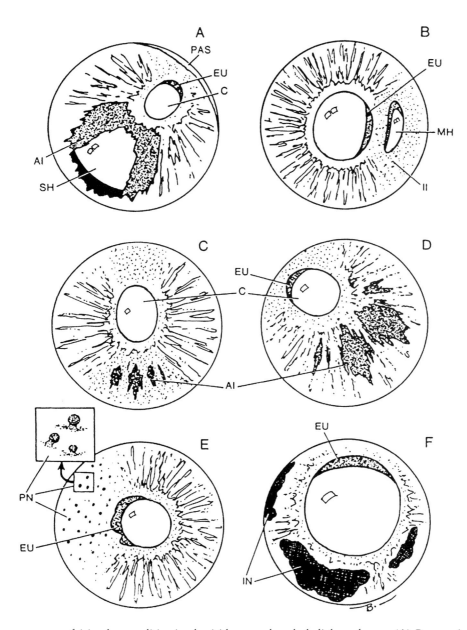

FIGURE 17-8. The spectrum of iris abnormalities in the iridocorneal endothelial syndrome. (**A**) Progressive iris atrophy with peripheral anterior synechiae (PAS) visible on the peripheral cornea, marked corectopia (C), ectropion uvea (EU), and a stretch hole (SH) surrounded by atrophic iris (AI). (**B**) Progressive iris atrophy with a melting hole (MH) surrounded by ischemic iris (II). (**C**) Chandler syndrome with mild corectopia and atrophy of the iris. (**D**) Intermediate variation with more advanced corectopia and atrophy of the iris than in the typical Chandler syndrome, but no hole in the iris. (**E**) and (**F**) Cogan-Reese (iris nevus) syndrome with pigmented, pedunculated nodules (PN) or diffuse iris nevi (IN). (Reprinted with permission from MB Shields. A Study Guide for Glaucoma [3rd ed]. Baltimore: Williams & Wilkins 1982;282.)

noted on the endothelium. Rieger syndrome, aniridia with glaucoma, and malignant melanomas of the iris are also included in the differential diagnosis, but these other conditions usually do not cause secondary angle closure.[24,26]

Patients with angle closure glaucoma secondary to ICE syndrome may present with pain, decreased vision, and iris abnormalities. The pain and decreased acuity may be a result of corneal edema or elevated IOP.

In the majority of cases, the severity of the secondary glaucoma with an ICE syndrome is proportional to the extent of the PAS. Management of these patients is therefore case specific. The main treatment goals are to reduce the IOP and corneal edema. Because of the wide spectrum of clinical manifestations, successful management (Table 17-9) may require topical aqueous suppressants, oral aqueous inhibitors, and filtering surgery.[26] Epinephrine and miotics are ineffective. Argon laser tra-

TABLE 17-9. Management of Iridocorneal Endothelial Syndrome and Secondary Angle-Closure Glaucoma

1. Medical management—secondary glaucoma:

   Aqueous suppressants:

   - Nonselective beta blocker, 1 gtt b.i.d.

   - α_2 Agonist ophthalmic solution, 1 gtt b.i.d.–t.i.d.

   - Carbonic anhydrase inhibitors (e.g., acetazolamide, 250 mg p.o. q.i.d., or topical carbonic anhydrase inhibitor, 1 gtt b.i.d.–t.i.d.)

   Medical management—corneal edema:

   - Topical hypertonic solutions (e.g., sodium chloride 5% ophthalmic solution)

2. Surgical management—angle-closure glaucoma

   - Filtering surgery with antimetabolite

   - Repeat filtering surgery with antimetabolite or with seton

   Surgical management—irretractable corneal edema

   - Penetrating keratoplasty

TABLE 17-10. Management of Secondary Angle-Closure Glaucoma Caused by Uveitis/Chronic Inflammation

1. Angle closure secondary to peripheral anterior synechiae (PAS)

   Primary goals: reduce the inflammation, prevent optic nerve damage from elevated intraocular pressure, prevent further PAS

   Uveitis treatment:

   - Anti-inflammatory agent: e.g., prednisolone acetate 1% ophthalmic solution, 1 gtt q1h, then tapered

   - Mydriatic-cycloplegic agent: e.g., homatropine 5% ophthalmic solution, 1 gtt t.i.d.

2. Glaucoma treatment:

   - Aqueous suppressant: nonselective beta blocker, 1 gtt b.i.d.; acetazolamide, 250 mg p.o. q.i.d. or topical carbonic anhydrase inhibitor, 1 gtt b.i.d.–t.i.d.; α_2 agonist ophthalmic solution, 1 gtt b.i.d.–t.i.d.

   Surgical management:

   - Filter with antimetabolite, with or without seton

beculoplasty is not considered a treatment option in these cases.[25,27] If corneal edema is not managed by decreasing the IOP, topical hypertonic agents may be added.

Filtration surgery is indicated when the IOP cannot be controlled medically. Filtering surgery is often successful, but over time, the fibrous membrane may grow over the sclerostomy and necessitate further surgery. Full-thickness procedures, along with the use of cytotoxic agents (e.g., mitomycin C or 5-fluorouracil used during surgery, or 5-fluorouracil injected subconjunctivally after surgery) increases the success rate.[25,27] Corneal edema may also remain, despite controlled IOP, because of endothelial dysfunction. Penetrating keratoplasty may be indicated in such cases.[24]

Angle-Closure Glaucoma Secondary to Uveitis and Inflammatory Conditions

Surgery, trauma, and idiopathic or specific inflammatory conditions (e.g., sarcoidosis, ankylosing spondylitis) can lead to secondary angle-closure glaucoma through the deposition of inflammatory cells and debris in the angle and PAS formation.[28]

In a patient with angle closure secondary to inflammatory conditions, evidence of chronic inflammation can be seen on examination. This may include keratic precipitates, corneal opacification, cells and flare in the anterior chamber, and lenticular opacification (see Color Plate 7). The vitreous may have cells, haze, or other evidence of posterior inflammation. In addition, the retina, choroid, and optic disc may exhibit evidence of inflammation in cases of posterior uveitis.[4] Primary angle-closure glaucoma may also present with cells and flare in the anterior

chamber, but no evidence of more extensive inflammation will be present (e.g., keratic precipitates), and a narrow angle is seen in the fellow eye.[4] A complete laboratory evaluation is indicated in chronic, recurrent, or recalcitrant uveitis to determine the presence of an underlying systemic disorder (see Table 15-3).

Management of secondary angle closure from uveitis or chronic inflammation is usually through medical therapy (Table 17-10). Aqueous suppressants (e.g., topical nonselective beta blocker, topical α_2 agonist, oral or topical carbonic anhydrase inhibitor) are used to reduce the IOP. Miotics are contraindicated because they further induce ciliary spasm, increase inflammation, and enhance the formation of posterior synechiae. Topical prostaglandins should be avoided because they can exacerbate the inflammatory component. Oral hyperosmotic agents may be used with acute elevations in IOP, but they may not be as effective if the blood-aqueous barrier is broken, and they fail to produce an osmotic gradient. Topical corticosteroids (e.g., prednisolone acetate) are used to decrease the amount of inflammation and improve outflow facility. However, the patient must be monitored carefully because steroid use may cause a further increase in IOP in steroid responders.[28] Rimexolone (Vexol) may be useful in such cases because it has a potency similar to that of prednisolone acetate but there is a delay in the development of raised IOP.

If the glaucoma cannot be managed through medical therapy, then filtering surgery should be considered. The success rate of conventional filtration surgery in uveitic glaucoma is poor because of the increased tendency for postoperative inflammation and scarring of the filtering bleb.[18,29] Trabeculectomy with the use of antimetabolite agents in conjunction with releasable

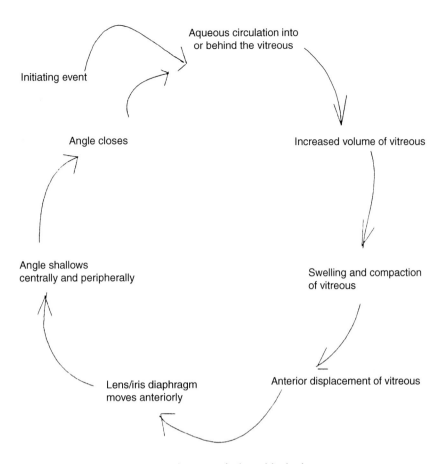

FIGURE 17-9. Mechanism of ciliary block glaucoma.

scleral flap sutures increases the success rate. Seton devices (e.g., Molteno implant) are considered when filtration surgery with antimetabolites has failed.[18]

SECONDARY ANGLE-CLOSURE GLAUCOMA WITHOUT PUPIL BLOCK CAUSED BY A FORWARD DISPLACEMENT OF THE CILIARY BODY

Ciliary Block Glaucoma

Ciliary block glaucoma, also known as *malignant glaucoma*, is a rare type of secondary angle-closure glaucoma that most often results as a complication from intraocular surgery for angle-closure glaucoma, especially when part of the angle remains closed at the time of surgery. The name *malignant glaucoma* has been used because of the poor prognosis and response to medical treatment in patients with this disease.[30] It has also been reported to occur after Nd:YAG capsulotomy, laser iridotomy, and cataract or filtering surgery, and it has occurred spontaneously and after trauma, inflammation, the use of miotics, and exfoliation syndrome.[30]

Ciliary block glaucoma is the result of a cascade of events (Figure 17-9). It usually begins in an anatomically

predisposed eye that has a decreased space between the ciliary body and adjacent lens. This may exist in several situations, including an eye with a smaller globe and normal-sized lens (nanophthalmos), increased lens size caused by an aging or cataract formation, a decrease in the anterior-posterior lens position as the result of weakened or slackened zonules (e.g., secondary to pseudoexfoliation of the lens capsule or trauma), or after contraction or swelling of the ciliary body (e.g., caused by inflammation or vascular engorgement). Any of these factors helps lead to a seal between the anterior hyaloid and ciliary body. As a result of this bond, aqueous humor flow is diverted posteriorly, which leads to entrapment of aqueous humor within the vitreous or posterior vitreous space. The anterior hyaloid becomes inflamed and less permeable as it becomes compacted. Eventually, the posterior lens surface attaches to the vitreous face (Figure 17-10). This causes further diversion of aqueous humor posteriorly into the vitreous, contributing to increased pressure and forward displacement of the lens and iris, which accelerates the cycle of events.[30,31]

Factors that may be present and also contribute to ciliary block include a thicker, less permeable vitreous face and swollen tips of ciliary processes caused by inflammation. Ciliary body spasm or prolonged angle closure cause the zonules to slacken, thus allowing the

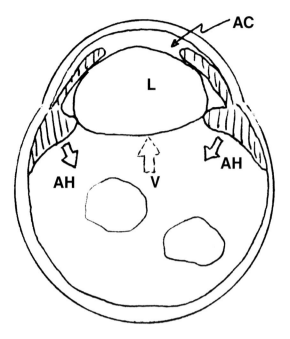

FIGURE 17-10. In ciliary block glaucoma, aqueous humor (AH) accumulates within the vitreous cavity (*black arrow*). This results in forward displacement of the anterior hyaloid and capsule (*open arrow*). (AC = anterior chamber; L = lens; V = vitreous.)

lens to be further pushed forward. Pockets of aqueous humor are formed throughout the vitreous and posterior to the vitreous where it has detached from the retina. These pockets cause increased posterior segment pressure, further condensing the vitreous, and additionally increase the posterior segment pressure.[30]

The classic type of ciliary block glaucoma occurs immediately to months after ocular surgery (e.g., cataract extraction or filtering surgery). Predisposing factors include pupillary block glaucoma or pre-existing ciliary block glaucoma.[30] A milder type of ciliary block glaucoma may occur spontaneously or after inflammation or the use of miotics. Examination reveals central and peripheral shallowing of the anterior chamber along with a mild to moderately elevated IOP. If an iridectomy is present, it will be patent.

Pupillary block glaucoma and wound leak must first be ruled out when diagnosing ciliary block glaucoma. In ciliary block glaucoma, the pressure in the vitreous cavity is greater than in the posterior and anterior chambers, which causes the lens-iris diaphragm to be pushed forward. The entire anterior chamber is shallow, and cornea-lenticular touch may be present. In pupil block glaucoma, the defect exists between the anterior and posterior chambers. Therefore, the anterior chamber is shallow peripherally but relatively deep centrally (Figure 17-11). To distinguish

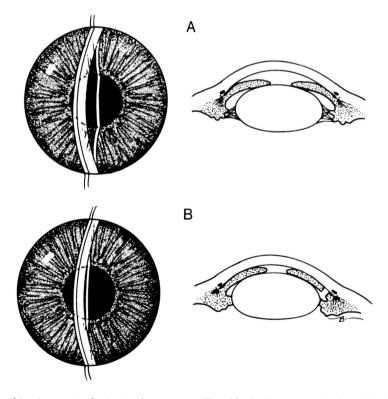

FIGURE 17-11. The slit-lamp biomicroscopic distinction between pupillary block glaucoma and ciliary block glaucoma. (A) In pupillary block glaucoma, the central anterior chamber shows moderate depth with a bowing of the peripheral iris. (B) In ciliary block glaucoma, the entire lens-iris diaphragm is shifted forward with marked shallowing or loss of the central anterior chamber, despite a patent iridectomy. (Reprinted with permission from MB Shields. A Study Guide for Glaucoma [3rd ed]. Baltimore: Williams & Wilkins 1982;338.)

TABLE 17-11. Management of Ciliary Block Glaucoma

Phakic eye

Medical therapy

- Atropine 1%, 1 gtt t.i.d.
- Phenylephrine 2.5%, 1 gtt q.i.d.
- Topical nonselective beta blocker, 1 gtt b.i.d.
- Topical α_2 agonist, 1 gtt b.i.d.–t.i.d.
- Carbonic anhydrase inhibitor, acetazolamide 250 mg q.i.d. or topical carbonic anhydrase inhibitor b.i.d.–t.i.d.
- Oral hyperosmotic agent (e.g., 50% glycerin solution, 2–3 ml/kg, or 45% isosorbide solution, 1.5 ml/lb of body weight)

Failure to halt attack:

- Argon laser to ciliary processes or neodymium:yttrium-aluminum-garnet (Nd:YAG) laser to anterior hyaloid

Attack still not reversed, or in lieu of laser:

- Suprachoroidal tap and anterior chamber deepening, vitreal disruption, cataract removal with hyaloidectomy and capsulotomy

Post–cataract removal (pseudophakic) eye: no remaining posterior capsule

Medical therapy as above

Laser management:

- Multiple laser iridotomies; argon laser to ciliary processes; Nd:YAG hyaloidotomy

If laser fails to reverse attack:

- Surgical treatment as above

Post–cataract removal eye: with capsule intact

Medical therapy as above

Laser management

- Multiple laser iridotomies; argon laser to ciliary processes, YAG capsulotomy; Nd:YAG hyaloidotomy

If laser fails to reverse attack:

- Surgical treatment as above

between ciliary block and pupillary block glaucoma, a PI is created. Patients with ciliary block glaucoma are not cured with a PI. Patients with pupillary block glaucoma have a shallow or flat peripheral anterior chamber that deepens after the PI is performed.[31]

Other elements of the differential diagnosis include choroidal detachment and suprachoroidal hemorrhage. Choroidal detachment is common after filtration surgery in a hypotonus eye. A suprachoroidal hemorrhage is characterized by a flat or shallow anterior chamber in the presence of normal or elevated IOP. Single or multiple dark reddish-brown elevations of the choroid can be visualized in the peripheral retina when

indirect ophthalmoscopy is performed. Ultrasonography can also assist in the diagnosis.

Initially, ciliary block glaucoma is treated medically (Table 17-11). Mydriatic-cycloplegic agents are used to relax the ciliary body, contract the zonules, and pull the lens posteriorly. Oral or intravenous hyperosmotic agents are given to shrink the vitreous and reduce pressure from the posterior pole. Medications that reduce the amount of aqueous humor secreted (nonselective beta blockers, α_2 agonists, and carbonic anhydrase inhibitors) may be used. Anti-inflammatory agents can be used even if inflammation is not contributing to the process because the high IOP and contact of intraocular structures trigger an inflammatory response. Early diagnosis and intervention with proper medications play important roles in the success of treatment of ciliary block glaucoma. Miotics are contraindicated because they cause the ciliary muscle to contract, which allows the lens to move forward, further narrowing the angle.

The purpose of surgical intervention in ciliary block glaucoma is to open the barrier created by the anterior hyaloid and allow aqueous humor to be redirected back to the anterior chamber. Argon laser photocoagulation can be used to shrink the ciliary processes if they are visible through an iridectomy.[32] This, along with aggressive medical treatment as outlined in Table 17-11, can restore the normal flow pattern of aqueous humor. Nd:YAG laser may be used in phakic and aphakic eyes with ciliary block glaucoma. The laser is aimed at the anterior hyaloid face, usually through an iridectomy. This creates an opening for the flow of aqueous humor forward to the anterior chamber.[30] If laser surgery fails, surgical aspiration of vitreous or anterior vitrectomy may be performed to release the ciliary block. The fellow eye is also at high risk of developing ciliary block glaucoma, and therefore prophylactic laser iridotomy and avoidance of miotics is indicated.[30,33] If intraocular surgery is required in the fellow eye, care must be taken to assure that the IOP remains low and the angle is open before surgery.

Iris Cysts and Ciliary Body Cysts

Iris or ciliary body cysts may infrequently cause a forward displacement of the peripheral iris and secondary angle-closure glaucoma. Multiple cysts precipitate angle closure more often than those existing in isolation. Cysts of the iris and ciliary body are fluid-filled nodules, arising primarily from epithelial tissue.

Iris cysts are usually dark brown in color and produce smooth elevations of the iris, giving it an undulating appearance. These cysts, which develop from the posterior epithelial layer of the iris, may be classified as either *primary* or *secondary*. Primary cysts are congenital and develop without an associated condition.[34] Shields[34] divided these cysts into four types: (1) those that appear at the pupil margin and are multiple and bilateral; (2) those that are located in the mid-zonal portion of the iris, have a smooth appearance, and block the transmission of light; (3) those that are located in the peripheral iris at the base of the ciliary body; and lastly, (4) those lesions that have dislodged into the anterior or vitreous chamber.

Secondary cysts result from surgical or nonsurgical trauma, the use of miotics, inflammation, or parasite infection.[35] Secondary cysts are more likely to cause secondary angle closure, but this can occur with both types.[23] A hereditary component may be present in patients with multiple, bilateral iris, or ciliary body cysts.[36]

Ciliary body cysts may or may not be pigmented and are usually more difficult to detect. Peripheral cysts may be visualized on biomicroscopic examination as a subtle anterior displacement of the iris stroma. A vertical slit beam is most useful to highlight the elevated areas. In cysts that are very difficult to detect, it may be helpful to rotate the slit lamp to the side opposite the elevation, use a horizontal beam, and have the patient look in an extreme field of gaze, toward the side of the elevation. The clinician looks obliquely into the suspicious area, with the pupil widely dilated. Three-mirror gonioscopy, with and without tilting of the lens, can be used to further visualize lesions of the peripheral posterior chamber.[23,35] They are observed more readily with gonioscopy when they are posterior to the iris, through a dilated pupil.[36] Iris and ciliary body cysts must be differentiated from malignant melanoma or other tumors of the iris or ciliary body. Documented growth, prominent vascularity, and alteration of adjacent structures (e.g., acquired heterochromia) are some characteristics that should make these lesions suspicious.[23]

Because most iris and ciliary body cysts remain stationary and produce no symptoms, they are treated only when necessary. Secondary angle-closure glaucoma may rarely occur because of a forward displacement of the peripheral iris. If the cysts are visible, argon laser therapy is used to collapse them.[36] When they are not visible, it may be necessary to first create a laser iridotomy to allow visualization of the cysts; then, argon laser is directed through the iridotomy to puncture them. Argon laser photocoagulation ruptures pigmented cysts easily and therefore is used to treat iris cysts and pigmented ciliary body cysts.[23,36] Multiple, clear ciliary body cysts carry a poorer prognosis. Nd:YAG laser appears to be promising in puncturing nonpigmented ciliary body cysts.[36]

Angle-Closure Glaucoma Secondary to Intraocular Tumor

Intraocular tumors can lead to secondary glaucoma through various mechanisms, and secondary open-angle glaucoma is more commonly encountered than angle-closure glaucoma. Angle closure can occur via a posterior mechanism, if the tumor, subsequent retinal or choroidal detachment, or suprachoroidal hemorrhage pushes the lens-iris diaphragm forward (see the section Angle-Closure Glaucoma Secondary to Ciliochoroidal Effusion).[37] Also, direct invasion of the angle structures, the formation of PAS or posterior synechiae, and neovascularization of the angle can lead to angle closure.[23] Tumors may be primary in origin or present via metastasis. Secondary open- and closed-angle glaucoma may also coexist.[38]

Secondary angle-closure glaucoma is more common in posterior uveal melanoma than in angle tumors. Anterior melanomas more often cause secondary open-angle glaucoma if the trabecular meshwork is invaded by the tumor or other types of cells (e.g., macrophages, red blood cells) and blocks aqueous outflow.[38] However, ciliary body melanomas have been reported to cause angle closure.[23] With posterior lesions, tumor size and the presence of retinal detachment are more significant factors relating to angle closure than tumor location or the presence of scleral invasion.[37,38] In these cases, the large mass effect of the tumor causes a total retinal detachment and a forward displacement of the lens, which results in pupillary block.

As is true with all types of secondary angle closure, the clinician should be suspicious when angle-closure glaucoma is found and the angle of the opposite eye does not appear to be closeable on gonioscopy. The patient's medical history must include any previous diagnosis of cancer. Ciliary body melanomas may cause refractive changes, cataracts, ocular inflammation (e.g., episcleritis, uveitis, endophthalmitis), and vitreous or anterior chamber hemorrhage.[23] When performing biomicroscopy, the clinician should also look for iris and ciliary body lesions. Local iris heterochromia or dialysis of the iris root may be visible on biomicroscopy.[23] Once the pupil is dilated, careful fundus and three-mirror gonioscopic examination is necessary to look for lesions of the ciliary body, choroid, or retina. If other mechanisms for secondary angle closure are not found or in the presence of an opaque media, transillumination, in addition to ultrasonography, should be performed to help identify the presence of a choroidal or ciliary body mass that cannot be directly visualized.[39] A melanoma shows low internal reflectivity on A-scan ultrasonography, and metastasis has medium to high internal reflectivity.[40] Fluorescein angiography of the iris or retina may be useful in some cases. Fine-needle aspiration biopsy of the anterior chamber with cytologic examination may also be helpful to distinguish a melanoma from a benign lesion.[39] Radioactive phosphorus (^{32}P), although used less frequently today, may also be useful in the diagnosis of uveal melanoma.[41]

Management of a patient with intraocular tumor (Table 17-12) varies with the tumor type, location in the eye, level of IOP elevation, patient's age, and medical

TABLE 17-12. Management of Angle Closure Secondary to Intraocular Tumor

1. Medical therapy:

    Aqueous suppressants:

    • Nonselective beta blocker, 1 gtt b.i.d.

    • α₂ Agonist ophthalmic solution, 1 gtt b.i.d.–t.i.d.

    • Carbonic anhydrase inhibitor (e.g., acetazolamide, 250 mg p.o. q.i.d. or topical carbonic anhydrase inhibitor, 1 gtt b.i.d.–t.i.d.)

2. Small, anterior lesion without neovascularization:

    • Laser iridotomy

    • If intraocular pressure remains uncontrolled, cyclocryotherapy to ciliary body

    • Sector iridectomy to remove lesion

    • Iridocyclectomy if the lesion involves the adjacent ciliary body

3. Small, anterior lesion with neovascularization:

    • Laser goniophotocoagulation

    • Panretinal photocoagulation

4. Large posterior lesion: enucleation

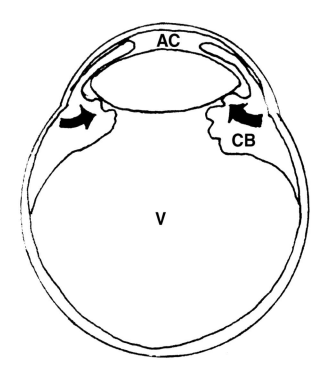

FIGURE 17-12. Ciliochoroidal effusion is characterized by a shallowing of the peripheral and central anterior chamber (AC) because of the swelling or detachment of the choroid and ciliary body (CB), which, in turn, causes the lens-iris diaphragm to be rotated forward. (V = vitreous.)

status.[41] The patient is initially managed medically through the use of aqueous suppressants (topical nonselective beta blocker, α₂ agonist, and carbonic anhydrase inhibitor) in an attempt to acutely reduce the IOP and halt the angle closure attack. Oral hyperosmotics may be added if the IOP remains acutely elevated.

Because most posterior lesions that cause secondary angle closure are large at the time of diagnosis, enucleation is the usual mode of treatment.[39,41] The Collaborative Ocular Melanoma Study (COMS) found neither benefit nor harm from radiation treatment before eye removal in patients with large melanomas.[42]

Smaller anterior lesions (e.g., ciliary body, iris melanoma) without neovascularization usually carry a more favorable vision prognosis. In these cases, a laser iridotomy should be considered. If this is unsuccessful and the IOP remains uncontrolled, a cyclodestructive procedure (e.g., cyclocryotherapy) may be attempted. If neovascularization is present, laser goniophotocoagulation and PRP may be necessary. Surgical iridectomy is avoided because of the risk of tumor dissemination. In some cases, a sector iridectomy is performed to remove small iris melanomas (less than 3 clock hours in size). If an iris melanoma involves the adjacent ciliary body, iridocyclectomy may be necessary.[41]

Angle-Closure Glaucoma Secondary to Ciliochoroidal Effusion

Ciliochoroidal effusion is a condition associated with an accumulation of fluid from the choriocapillaris in the

suprachoroidal space (the potential space between the sclera and choroid/ciliary body). It may lead to angle closure through choroidal detachment, swelling of the ciliary body, and forward rotation of the lens-iris diaphragm (Figure 17-12). Ciliochoroidal effusion may be idiopathic or the result of a number of conditions, both ocular and systemic. The largest categories of associated conditions include inflammatory, vascular, postoperative, and neoplastic mechanisms.[43,44]

Various types of inflammation may lead to secondary angle-closure glaucoma from ciliochoroidal effusion. For example, posterior scleritis, a granulomatous inflammation of the sclera, can result in a swollen ciliary body and choroidal detachment, which leads to a forward displacement of the lens-iris diaphragm and subsequent angle closure.[40]

Nanophthalmos may be associated with uveal effusion, nonrhegmatogenous retinal detachment, and secondary angle-closure glaucoma. Angle closure is the result of choroidal congestion from increasing resistance to vortex venous outflow secondary to the decreasing elasticity of the extremely thick sclera found in this condition. Nanophthalmos with ciliochoroidal effusion and secondary angle-closure glaucoma also has some common clinical features: a familial predisposition, small equatorial diameter of the globe and horizontal corneal diameter, high hyperopia, and normal lens size are usually seen.[42]

TABLE 17-13. Management of Ciliochoroidal Effusion

Primary goal: Reduce the swelling of the ciliary body to allow it to rotate posteriorly and relieve pupillary block

Medical management:

- Mydriatic-cycloplegic agent: e.g., homatropine 5% ophthalmic solution, 1 gtt t.i.d.

- Anti-inflammatory agent: e.g., prednisolone acetate 1% ophthalmic solution, 1 gtt q1hr, then tapered

- Oral corticosteroids or nonsteroidal anti-inflammatory agents, to control posterior inflammation

- Aqueous suppressants (beta blockers, α agonists, carbonic anhydrase inhibitors)

Surgical management:

- Goniosynechialysis when many peripheral anterior synechiae are present

- Posterior sclerectomy with drainage of suprachoroidal fluid

Intraocular surgery has also been known to precipitate ciliochoroidal effusion and secondary angle-closure glaucoma. PRP may initiate a large inflammatory response and a breakdown of the blood-retina barrier. Angle closure may occur during or after treatment and usually resolves spontaneously over the next few days. Scleral buckling procedure for retinal detachment may also rarely cause ciliochoroidal effusion with secondary angle closure. In these cases, the vortex veins may be blocked if the buckle compresses them. Blockage of these drainage channels leads to increased transmural pressure in the ciliary process capillaries, ciliary body swelling, and forward rotation.[45,46]

Idiopathic ciliochoroidal effusion is a condition marked by swelling and anterolateral rotation of the ciliary body, with no obvious underlying etiology. The shift of the ciliary body causes relaxation of the zonules, a thickening of the lens, and myopic shift. The swollen ciliary body may be visualized on gonioscopy, or the typical quadrilobed annular choroidal detachment may be seen with indirect ophthalmoscopy.[47]

The biomicroscopic appearance of angle-closure glaucoma secondary to ciliochoroidal effusion includes an extremely shallow central anterior chamber with a flat peripheral chamber. The iris surface is very convex and the lens-iris diaphragm is anteriorly displaced. No angle structures are seen on gonioscopy. IOP is moderately to severely elevated. Blurred vision caused by an acute myopic shift may be observed. The induced myopia occurs from the relaxation of the zonules and forward movement of the ciliary body, causing the lens to become thicker and rounder. B-scan ultrasonography may show a choroidal or ciliary body detachment. Indirect ophthalmoscopy usually confirms the presence of the ciliochoroidal detachment. Scleral depression may or

may not be necessary to visualize the detachment; in fact, the ora serrata is much more evident than usual, without indentation.

Angle closure from ciliochoroidal effusion must be differentiated from primary angle-closure and ciliary block glaucoma. Primary angle-closure glaucoma is a bilateral condition, and the central anterior chamber depth is only slightly shallow. Ciliary block glaucoma has a similar presentation to ciliochoroidal effusion, but ultrasound and indirect ophthalmoscopy fail to show choroidal thickening or detachment.[44]

The management of secondary angle-closure glaucoma from ciliochoroidal effusion is primarily through medical therapy. It is basically the same for all causes of ciliochoroidal effusion (Table 17-13), but it becomes case specific if an underlying systemic condition needs to be treated. In all cases, cycloplegics are necessary to relax the ciliary muscle, break any pupillary block, deepen the anterior chamber, and open the angle. Pilocarpine therapy is contraindicated. Aqueous suppressants (e.g., nonselective beta blockers, α_2 agonists, carbonic anhydrase inhibitors, hyperosmotics) are used to lower the IOP. Steroids (topical, oral, or both) or nonsteroidal anti-inflammatory agents are used to decrease inflammation.[44] The resolution of angle closure may take from 48 hours to 2 weeks. It is important to realize this so that the appropriate treatment is not abandoned too early.[40,44,46] Refractory cases may require surgical drainage of the suprachoroidal space.[44]

SUMMARY

The causes and mechanisms of secondary angle-closure glaucoma are many and diverse. A patient presenting with angle-closure glaucoma must be evaluated very carefully to differentiate secondary from primary angle-closure glaucoma. The importance of evaluating the anterior chamber of the fellow eye to distinguish between these two conditions cannot be overemphasized. If fellow eye is phakic and the angle appears open, then the diagnosis of primary angle-closure glaucoma is highly unlikely. In general, the depth and appearance of the fellow eye along with accompanying features of the involved eye help to establish the diagnosis. It is also imperative to accurately diagnose the type of secondary angle-closure glaucoma because management differs according to the underlying condition.

REFERENCES

1. Ritch R, Shields MB. Classification and Mechanisms. In R Ritch, MB Shields (eds). The Secondary Glaucomas. St. Louis: Mosby, 1982;3–7.

2. Tomey Karim F, Al-Rajhi AA. Neodymium:YAG laser iridotomy in the initial management of phacomorphic glaucoma. Ophthalmology 1992;99:660–665.

3. Ritch R. Glaucoma Secondary to Lens Intumescence and Dislocation. In R Ritch, MB Shields (eds). The Secondary Glaucomas. St. Louis: Mosby, 1982;131–149.

4. Fourman S. Diagnosing acute angle-closure glaucoma: a flowchart. Surv Ophthalmol 1983;33:6:491–494.

5. Chandler PA. Choice of treatment in dislocation of the lens. Arch Ophthalmol 1964;71:765–786.

6. Murrill CA, Stanfield DL. Primary Care of the Cataract Patient. Norwalk, Conn.: Appleton & Lange, 1994;94–104.

7. Tomey KF, Traverso CE. Neodymium-YAG laser posterior capsulotomy for the treatment of aphakic and pseudophakic pupillary block. Am J Ophthalmol 1987;104:502–507.

8. Cohen JS, Osher RH, Weber P, Faulkner JD. Complications of extracapsular cataract surgery. The indication and risks of peripheral iridectomy. Ophthalmology 1984;91:826–830.

9. Aphakic and Pseudophakic Pupillary Block. In NS Jaffe, MS Jaffe, GF Jaffe (eds). Cataract Surgery and Its Complications (5th ed). St. Louis: Mosby, 1990;385–399.

10. Samples JR, Bellows AR, Rosenquist RC, et al. Pupillary block with posterior chamber intra ocular lenses. Arch Ophthalmol 1987;105:335–337.

11. Van Buskirk EM. Pupillary block after intra ocular lens implantation. Am J Ophthalmol 1983;95:55–59.

12. Willis DA, Steward RH, Kimbrough RL. Pupillary block associated with posterior chamber lenses. Ophthalmic Surg 1985;16(2):108–109.

13. Schadler PW, Eitzen EM, Truxal AR. Acute pseudophakic pupillary block glaucoma. Ann Emerg Med 1990;19:330–332.

14. Shrader CE, Belcher CD, Thomas JV, et al. Pupillary and iridovitreal block in pseudophakic eyes. Ophthalmology 1984;91:831–837.

15. Hardten DR, Lindstrom RL. Complications of cataract surgery. Int Ophthalmol Clin 1992;32(4):131–155.

16. Ritch R. Pathophysiology of glaucoma in uveitis. Trans Ophthalmol Soc U K 1981;101:321–324.

17. Krupin T, Dorfman NJ, Spector SM, Wax MB. Secondary glaucoma associated with uveitic glaucoma 1988;10:85–90.

18. Kotas-Neumann R, Lee DA. Glaucoma and Uveitis. In EJ Higginbotham, DA Lee (eds). Management of Difficult Glaucoma. Cambridge: Blackwell Scientific Publications, 1994;125–143.

19. Weinreb RN. Management of uveitis and glaucoma. J Glaucoma 1994;3:174–175.

20. Wand M. Neovascular Glaucoma. In R Ritch, MB Shields (eds). The Secondary Glaucomas. St. Louis: Mosby, 1982;162–193.

21. Cavallerano AA, Alexander LJ. The Secondary Glaucomas. In JG Classe (ed). The Secondary Glaucomas in Optometry Clinics—Glaucoma. Norwalk, Conn.: Appleton & Lange, 1991;127–164.

22. Higginbotham EJ, Yang CB. An approach to the management of neovascular glaucoma. In EJ Higginbotham, DA Lee. Management of Difficult Glaucoma. Cambridge: Blackwell Scientific Publications, 1994;113–124.

23. Fisch B. Gonioscopy and the Glaucomas. Boston: Butterworth–Heinemann, 1993;77–92.

24. Arffa RC. Grayson's Diseases of the Cornea (3rd ed). St. Louis: Mosby, 1991;417–438.

25. Ritch R. Cases in controversy: management of ICCE. J Glaucoma 1994;3:154–159.

26. Shields MB. Glaucoma associated with primary disorders of the corneal endothelium. In R Ritch, MB Shields (eds). The Secondary Glaucomas. St. Louis: Mosby, 1982;69–83.

27. Wilson MR. Cases in controversy: management of iridocorneal endothelial syndrome. J Glaucoma 1994;3:154–159.

28. Hoskins HD, Kass M. Becker and Schaeffer's Diagnosis and Therapy of the Glaucomas (6th ed). St. Louis: Mosby, 1989;208–237.

29. Patitsas CJ, Rockwood EJ, Meisler DM, Lowder CY. Glaucoma filtering surgery with postoperative 5-flurouracil in patients with intraocular inflammatory disease. Ophthalmology 1992;99:594–599.

30. Lieberman MF. Diagnosis and Management of Malignant Glaucoma. In EJ Higginbotham, DA Lee (eds). Management of Difficult Glaucoma. Cambridge: Blackwell Scientific Publications, 1994;183–194.

31. Dueker D. Ciliary-block glaucoma—differential diagnosis and management. J Glaucoma 1994;3:2:167–170.

32. Simmons RJ, Maestre FA. Malignant Glaucoma. In R Ritch, MB Shields (eds). The Glaucomas (2nd ed). St. Louis: Mosby, 1996;841–853.

33. Simmons RJ, Thomas JV. Malignant Glaucoma. In R Ritch, MB Shields (eds). The Secondary Glaucomas. St. Louis: Mosby, 1982;331–344.

34. Shields JA. Primary cysts of the iris. Trans Am Ophthalmol Soc 1981;79:771–809.

35. Shields JA, Kline MA, Augsburger JJ. Primary iris cysts: a review of the literature and report of 62 cases. Br J Ophthalmol 1984;68:152–166.

36. Vela A, Rieser JC, Campbell DG. The heredity and treatment of angle-closure glaucoma secondary to iris and ciliary body cysts. Ophthalmology 1983;91:332–337.

37. Yanoff M. Glaucoma mechanisms in ocular malignant melanomas. Am J Optom 1970;70(6):898–904.

38. Shields CL, Shields J, Shields MB, Augsburger JJ. Prevalence and mechanisms of secondary

intraocular pressure elevation in eyes with intraocular tumors. Ophthalmology 1987;94:839–846.

39. Shields MB. Glaucoma Associated with Intraocular Tumors. In R Ritch, MB Shields (eds). The Secondary Glaucomas. St. Louis: Mosby, 1982;194–206.

40. Litwak AB. Posterior scleritis with secondary ciliochoroidal effusion. J Am Optom Assoc 1989; 60(4): 300–306.

41. Goldstick BJ, Weinrab RN. Glaucoma Associated with Intraocular Tumors. In EJ Higginbotham, DA Lee (eds). Management of Difficult Glaucoma. Cambridge: Blackwell Scientific Publications, 1994; 274–281.

42. Collaborative Ocular Melanoma Study Group. The Collaborative Ocular Melanoma Study (COMS) randomized trial of pre-enucleation radiation of large choroidal melanoma. II: Initial mortality findings COMS report No. 10. Am J Ophthalmol 1998; 125:779–796.

43. Brockhurst RJ. Vortex vein decompression from nanophthalmic uveal effusion. Arch Ophthalmol 1980;98: 1987–1990.

44. Fourman S. Angle-closure glaucoma complicating ciliochoroidal detachment. Ophthalmology 1989;96: 646–653.

45. Michaels RG, Wilkerson CP, Rice TA. Retinal Detachment. St. Louis: Mosby, 1990;1008–1012.

46. Schepens CL. Retinal Detachment and Allied Diseases. Philadelphia: Saunders, 1983;988–1023.

47. Phelps CD. Angle-closure glaucoma secondary to ciliary body swelling. Arch Ophthalmol 1974; 92:287–290.

Glaucoma Case Study Analysis

Glaucoma Case Study Analysis

Anthony B. Litwak and Paul C. Ajamian

CASE 1

A 38-year-old African-American man comes into the clinic with acute bilateral red eyes and is diagnosed with epidemic keratoconjunctivitis (EKC). After his EKC resolves, he is evaluated for a complete eye examination. He has no past medical or ocular history, and there is no family history of glaucoma. His best-corrected acuity is 20/20 in each eye. Pupils are equal and round, and respond to light without an afferent pupillary defect. Extraocular movements (EOM) are full, and confrontation fields are full to finger counting. Slit-lamp evaluation is unremarkable. Tensions as measured by Goldmann applanation are 23 mm Hg in both eyes at 2 PM. Gonioscopy shows grade 4+ open angles without evidence of angle recession or peripheral anterior synechiae. There is 1+ pigment in the trabecular meshwork. Dilated fundus examination shows relatively large optic nerves and a cup-to-disc ratio of 0.9 in the right eye (Figure 18-1A) and 0.9 in the left eye (Figure 18-1B). The rim tissue appears equal between the superior and inferior poles compared with the temporal pole in the right eye. An inferior notch is seen in the neuroretinal rim tissue of the left eye. Nerve fiber layer (NFL) evaluation shows multiple slit defects in the superior arcades and a single slit defect in the inferior arcade of the right eye (see Figure 18-1A). An inferior wedge defect is present in the left eye (Figure 18-1B). The macula, vessels, and peripheral examination are unremarkable. Stereoscopic disc photographs are taken.

Diagnosis

At this point, the patient is diagnosed with glaucoma based on the optic nerve and NFL appearance. No evidence is found of a secondary component, so the diagnosis is primary open-angle glaucoma in both eyes. A large cup might be expected because of the large optic nerve, but the rim tissue should be greater in the superior and inferior rim than the temporal rim tissue. This is not the case in the right eye. In the left eye, a notch is present in the inferior rim tissue that is pathognomonic for glaucoma damage.

Management

The patient is scheduled for a 30-2 Full Threshold (Swedish Interactive Thresholding Algorithm [SITA] was not available) visual field test and another intraocular pressure (IOP) check (morning) to establish the baseline pressures when the patient is not on medicines. One week later, the patient has the visual field, and the IOP is 25 mm Hg OU at 10 AM. The visual field test shows a nasal cluster in the inferior field on the pattern deviation plots in the right eye (Figure 18-1C). The glaucoma hemifield test (GHT) in the right eye is outside normal limits, and the corrected pattern standard deviation (CPSD) has a P value of <2%. The left eye shows a superior nasal step and a superior paracentral scotoma in the graytones (Figure 18-1D). Fewer than ten points are flagged on the pattern deviation plots, but several of the points have P values <.5% and are close to fixation. The GHT is outside normal limits and the CPSD is <.5%. Although the number of flagged points on the pattern deviation plots is minimal, this is clearly an abnormal visual field. The field loss correlates with the optic nerve and NFL appearance in both eyes.

The next step is to quantify the amount of glaucoma damage based on the optic nerve and visual field

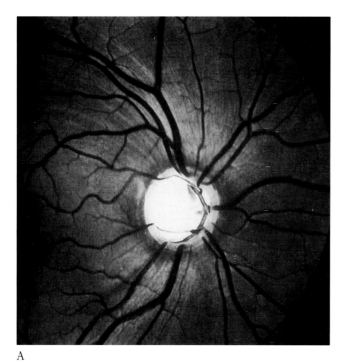
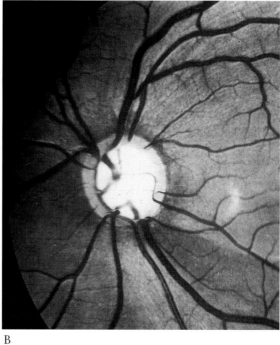

A

B

FIGURE 18-1. Right optic nerve (**A**) shows a vertical C/D ratio of .9 with thinning of the neuroretinal rim tissue in the superior and inferior poles. Nerve fiber layer (NFL) shows multiple slit defects in the superior arcades and a single slit defect in the inferior arcades. Left optic nerve (**B**) shows a vertical C/D ratio of .9 with an inferior notch in the neuroretinal rim tissue. NFL shows an inferior wedge defect.

(see Table 11-1). The classification of the visual field loss in the right eye is mild based on the mean deviation value of –1.82; the number of flagged points on the pattern deviation plot is 12; and the four points off of fixation have values of 31, 32, 34, and 31 dB. The optic nerve shows thinning of both the inferior and superior neuroretinal rims, making the classification one of moderate damage. The NFL loss is mild based on slit defects in both hemifields. The final classification is based on the most advanced of the three, which would be moderate, based on the optic nerve appearance (Table 18-1).

In the left eye, the classification of damage would be severe (Table 18-2). This is based on the inferior complete notch of the optic nerve, the inferior complete wedge defect, and one of the four points off of fixation on the visual field, which has a dB value of 3. This patient should also be followed with a 10-2 visual field in the left eye to monitor for fixation loss.

Based on these findings, the patient is diagnosed with moderate damage in the right eye and severe damage in the left eye; the target pressure is set at a decrease of 30–40% in the right eye and 40–50% in the left eye (see Table 11-3). Another significant factor in setting the target pressure for this patient is his age. This patient is only 38 years old and has more than 40 years to become visually impaired from his disease, if he lives a normal life span. The target pressure is set for 40% reduction in the right

eye and 50% reduction in the left eye. The patient is asked to come back in a few days for a third IOP reading while he is off medications to complete the baseline IOP. On the third reading in the early morning, the IOP is 27 mm Hg in the right eye and 28 mm Hg in the left eye.

The target pressure is set from the highest of the three IOP readings, in this case 27 mm Hg right eye (OD) and 28 mm Hg left eye (OS). The target pressure is 16 mm Hg in the right eye and 14 mm Hg in the left eye. The patient denies any breathing problems and is not taking any breathing medicines. The pulse is 72 beats per minute and the blood pressure is 130/80. The patient is started on timolol 0.5% b.i.d. OU with punctal occlusion and asked to return for two IOP readings in the next month. The patient is instructed to take his medication first thing in the morning and then 12 hours later. On follow-up morning visits (these are chosen because the patient exhibited higher morning pressure readings), the IOP is 17 mm Hg and 18 mm Hg on one day, and 19 OU on another. Little change in pulse rate or blood pressure is seen, and the patient reports no complaints with the eye drops. Compared with the baseline readings of 23–28 mm Hg, the timolol is effective, but the target pressures are still not met. Latanoprost (Xalatan) is added at bedtime to the left eye only as a monocular trial, and the patient is asked to return in 1 month. The morning IOP is 17 mm Hg OD and 14 mm Hg OS. The pressure is significantly lower in

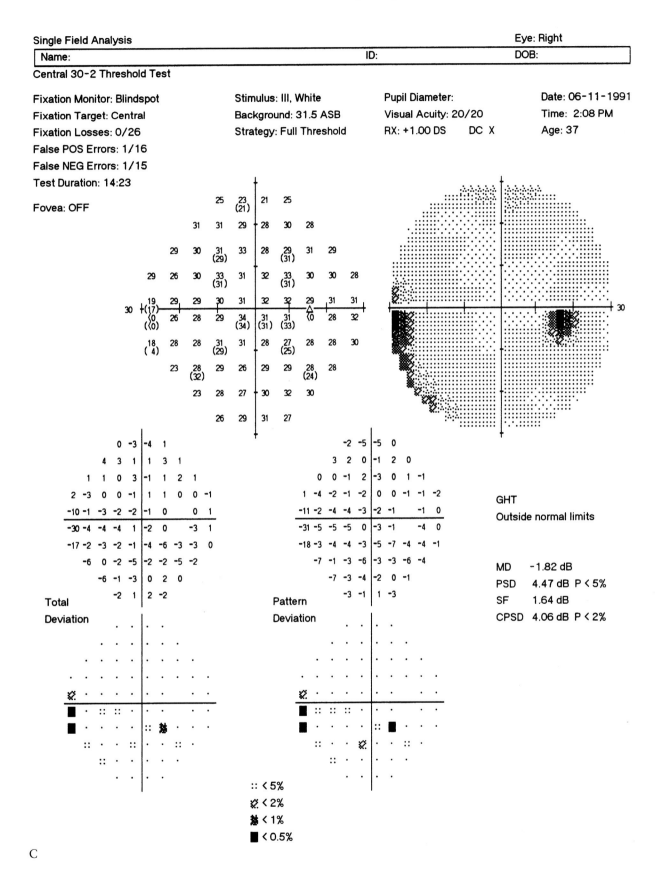

Single Field Analysis
Eye: Right

Name: | ID: | DOB:

Central 30-2 Threshold Test

Fixation Monitor: Blindspot
Fixation Target: Central
Fixation Losses: 0/26
False POS Errors: 1/16
False NEG Errors: 1/15
Test Duration: 14:23

Fovea: OFF

Stimulus: III, White
Background: 31.5 ASB
Strategy: Full Threshold

Pupil Diameter:
Visual Acuity: 20/20
RX: +1.00 DS   DC X

Date: 06-11-1991
Time: 2:08 PM
Age: 37

GHT
Outside normal limits

MD   -1.82 dB
PSD   4.47 dB P < 5%
SF   1.64 dB
CPSD 4.06 dB P < 2%

Total Deviation

Pattern Deviation

:: < 5%
⌖ < 2%
▨ < 1%
■ < 0.5%

C

FIGURE 18-1. (*continued*) Right visual field (C) shows an inferior nasal defect in the graytones and pattern deviation plots. The glaucoma hemifield test (GHT) is outside normal limits and the corrected pattern standard deviation (CSPD) shows a probability value of <2% (*see next page*).

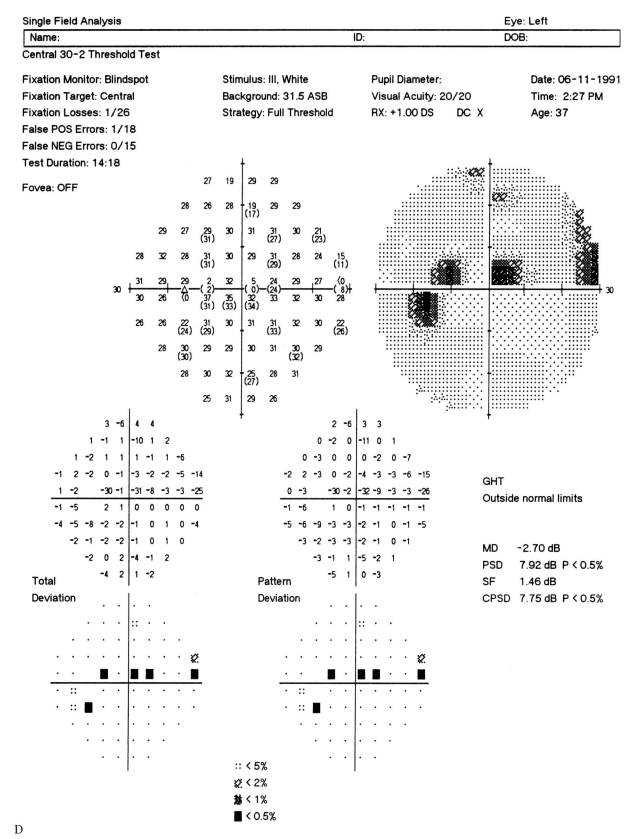

FIGURE 18-1. (*continued*) Left visual field (**D**) shows a superonasal step and a superior paracentral scotoma in the gray-tones. There are less than 10 points being flagged on the pattern deviation plots; however, several of points have P values <.5% and are close to fixation. The GHT is outside normal limits and the CPSD is <.5%.

TABLE 18-1 Classification of Glaucoma Damage for Right Eye

Right eye damage*	Optic nerve	Nerve fiber layer	Visual field mean defect	Visual field pattern deviation	Four central visual field points off fixation
Mild		X	X	X	X
Moderate	X				
Severe					

*See Table 11-1 for explanation of classifying the degree of glaucoma damage.

TABLE 18-2 Classification of Glaucoma Damage for Left Eye

Left eye damage	Optic nerve	Nerve fiber layer	Visual field mean defect	Visual field pattern deviation	Four central visual field points off fixation
Mild			X	X	
Moderate					
Severe	X	X			X

the left eye compared with the right eye, so the latanoprost is probably effective and the patient is instructed to use latanoprost in both eyes. One month later, the IOP is 14 mm Hg OU. The patient is at target on this particular day; however, he showed a 5-mm diurnal range while off of medicines, and it is not known whether the IOP is being measured at a peak or trough.

The patient comes back in another month, and the IOP is 14 mm Hg OD and 16 mm Hg OS. The patient is slightly above target in the left eye. He is given the option of a third medication for the left eye or argon laser trabeculoplasty (ALT). The patient elects for ALT. ALT is performed 180 degrees in the left eye after instilling one drop of apraclonidine (Iopidine 0.5%). One hour postoperatively, his pressures are 14 mm Hg OD and 15 mm Hg OS. A mild anterior chamber reaction is present in the left eye. The patient is instructed to continue his current glaucoma drops with the addition of prednisolone acetate (Pred Forte) to use q.i.d. for 4 days and then taper by one drop per day. One week later the iritis has resolved and the IOP is 14 mm Hg OD and 12 mm Hg OS. The prednisolone acetate is discontinued, and the patient is asked to return in 5 weeks so the effect of the ALT can be judged. At this time, his pressures are 15 mm Hg OD and 12 mm Hg OS. The ALT appears to be effective, and the patient is at target pressure in both eyes. A 3-month follow-up appointment is scheduled with repeat visual field testing.

Six months after the initial diagnosis, repeat 30-2 Full Threshold visual field testing is performed, and the patient is dilated so that the optic nerves can be re-evaluated. The visual fields and optic nerves are unchanged, and the patient is tolerating the medications well and is at his target pressure. At this point, the medications are continued and the patient is scheduled for 3-month IOP checks and 6-month repeat visual field.

Clinical Pearls

This case shows that the only reason the patient was diagnosed with glaucoma was because he sought care for an acute viral conjunctivitis. Glaucoma is an asymptomatic disease, and even patients with advanced damage rarely exhibit symptoms.

This is an African-American patient who has a field defect that is close to fixation in the left eye and is only 38 years old. This patient is probably at high risk for progression and becoming visually impaired during his lifetime from glaucoma. This is the type of patient for whom I would consider filtering surgery early in the course of treatment if the target pressure is not met or the visual field loss shows progression. This patient needs to be followed closely with repeat visual fields every 6 months, with 10-2 field tests also performed in the left eye to monitor fixation.

CASE 2

A 50-year-old white man reports to the clinic with a complaint of reduced reading vision. He has a medical history of hypertension and is taking verapamil. His ocular history is unremarkable. He states he has a brother with glaucoma who is taking eye drops, but he does not know the severity of the glaucoma.

Best-corrected visual acuity is 20/20 in each eye with a slightly hyperopic correction. With a +1.50 reading add he reads .37M print. EOM are full. Confrontation fields are full to finger counting. Pupils are equal, round, and reactive to light without an afferent pupillary defect. Slit-lamp biomicroscopy is unremarkable. Tensions by Goldmann applanation are 18 mm Hg OU at 10 AM. Gonioscopy reveals grade 3+ open angles with 1+ pigment in the trabecular meshwork. No evidence of angle recess or peripheral anterior synechiae is present.

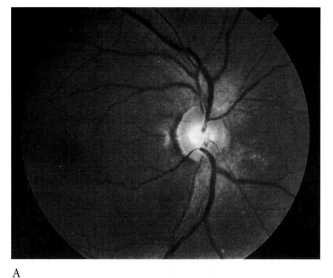

A

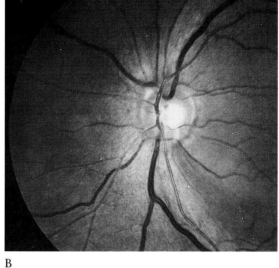

B

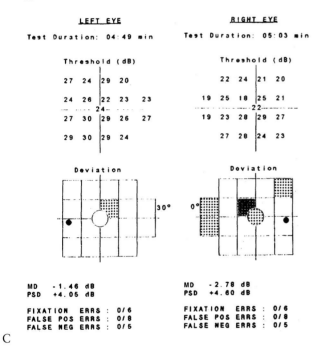

C

FIGURE 18-2. Right optic nerve (**A**) shows a vertical cup-to-disc ratio of .55 with slight thinning of the inferior rim tissue compared to superior. Nerve fiber layer (NFL) examination uncovers an inferior wedge defect. Left optic nerve (**B**) shows a vertical cup-to-disc ratio of .5 with slight thinning of the inferior rim tissue compared to superior. NFL examination reveals a smaller inferior wedge defect compared to the right eye. (**C**) Frequency doubling perimetry using the Full Threshold N-30 program shows bilateral superior defects greater in the right eye than the left eye (*see next page*).

Dilated slit-lamp evaluation of lens reveals clear lenses without sign of cataract. Dilated fundus evaluation shows a cup-to-disc ratio of 0.55 vertically in the right eye and 0.50 vertically in the left eye. The rim tissue is noted to be slightly thinner inferiorly compared to superiorly. NFL examination uncovers inferior wedge defects that are greater in the right eye than in the left (Figures 18-2A and B). The macula, vessels, and periphery are normal.

Visual field testing using frequency-doubling technology using the N-30 threshold program reveals a superior defect in the right eye and one P value <5% superiorly in the left eye (Figure 18-2C). Visual field defects are confirmed with Humphrey 30-2 Full Threshold perimetry (Figures 18-2D and E). Note that just a few points are flagged on the pattern deviation plots, but both fields show abnormal GHT.

Diagnosis

At this point, sufficient evidence is present based on the NFL abnormality and corresponding visual field defect to diagnose glaucoma. As with any newly diagnosed glaucoma patient, we should obtain three baseline IOP readings. Subsequent IOPs are 16 mm Hg OU and 19 mm Hg OU.

The diagnosis is normal-tension glaucoma (NTG), although an IOP spike can never be ruled out. I typically perform a diurnal curve before starting treatment for this type of patient. In this case, the diurnal curve was relatively flat in an IOP range of 17–20 mm Hg. It is also

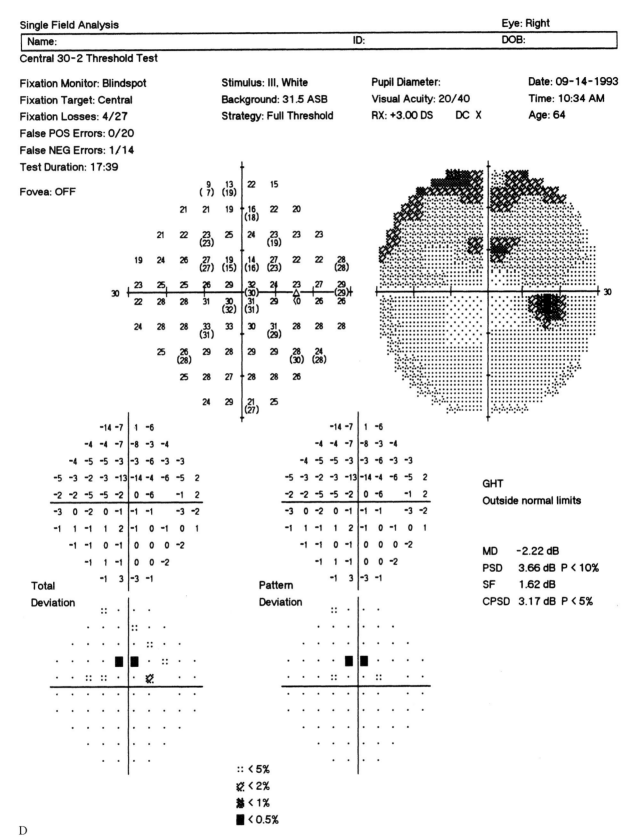

Single Field Analysis   Eye: Right

Name: ID: DOB:

Central 30-2 Threshold Test

Fixation Monitor: Blindspot   Stimulus: III, White   Pupil Diameter: Date: 09-14-1993
Fixation Target: Central   Background: 31.5 ASB   Visual Acuity: 20/40   Time: 10:34 AM
Fixation Losses: 4/27   Strategy: Full Threshold RX: +3.00 DS   DC X   Age: 64
False POS Errors: 0/20
False NEG Errors: 1/14
Test Duration: 17:39

Fovea: OFF

GHT
Outside normal limits

MD   -2.22 dB
PSD   3.66 dB P < 10%
SF   1.62 dB
CPSD 3.17 dB P < 5%

Total Deviation

Pattern Deviation

:: < 5%
▨ < 2%
▩ < 1%
■ < 0.5%

D

FIGURE 18-2. (*continued*) (**D**) Humphrey Full Threshold 30-2 visual field testing confirms a small superior paracentral scotoma in the right eye. Note outside normal limits glaucoma hemifield test (GHT) (*see next page*).

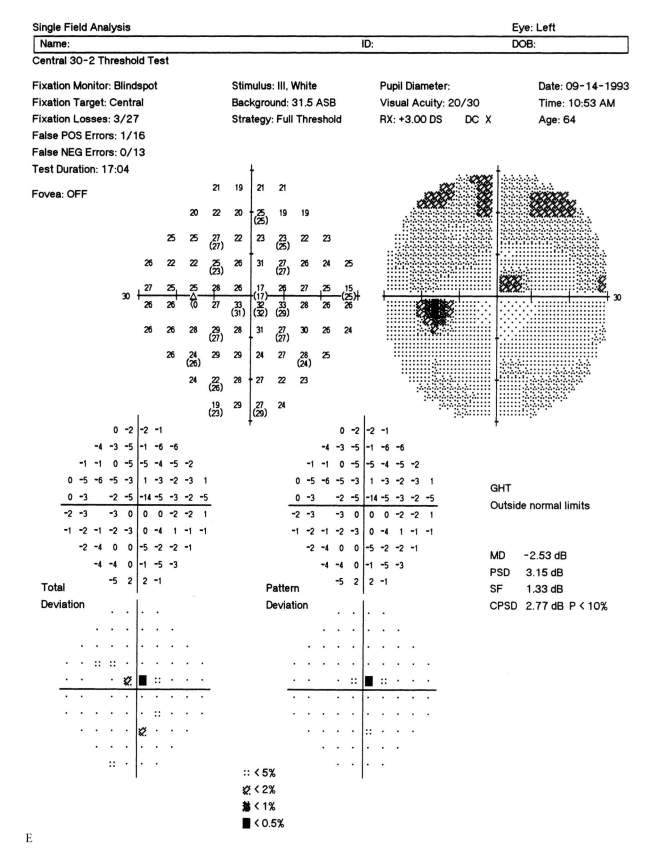

Single Field Analysis   Eye: Left

Name: ID: DOB:

Central 30-2 Threshold Test

Fixation Monitor: Blindspot   Stimulus: III, White   Pupil Diameter: Date: 09-14-1993
Fixation Target: Central   Background: 31.5 ASB   Visual Acuity: 20/30   Time: 10:53 AM
Fixation Losses: 3/27   Strategy: Full Threshold   RX: +3.00 DS   DC X   Age: 64
False POS Errors: 1/16
False NEG Errors: 0/13
Test Duration: 17:04

Fovea: OFF

GHT
Outside normal limits

MD   -2.53 dB
PSD   3.15 dB
SF   1.33 dB
CPSD 2.77 dB P < 10%

Total Deviation

Pattern Deviation

:: < 5%
⬚ < 2%
⬚ < 1%
■ < 0.5%

E

FIGURE 18-2. (continued) In the left eye (E), the graytones look relatively good; however, the pattern deviation plot shows a superior cluster with one of the four central points having a value of 17 dB. The GHT is outside normal limits.

possible that the patient's oral calcium channel blocker may be lowering his IOP. Systemic beta blockers and clonidine drugs can also lower IOP and mask true primary open-angle glaucoma.

Management

Should this patient be treated? Data from the Collaborative Normal Tension Glaucoma Study found that lowering IOP by 30% reduced the risk of glaucoma progression from 35% to 12%.[1] However, 65% of the patients diagnosed with NTG did not progress in 5 years without treatment. In this case, the degree of visual field loss appears mild, but the location causes concern. Both the frequency-doubling technology (FDT) and standard perimetry show that points right off fixation are being affected. In the left eye, one of the central four points has a dB level of 17. This finding and the results of the Normal Tension Glaucoma Study would convince me to begin treatment in this patient.

The first therapeutic agent to use in NTG is controversial. In the Normal Tension Glaucoma Study, no adrenergic agents, such as beta blockers, were used because of their potential affect on blood supply to the optic nerve. The agents used in this study were pilocarpine, ALT, and filtering surgery. Topical carbonic anhydrase inhibitors, α_2 agonists, or prostaglandins were not available at the time of the study.

I would start this patient with a monocular trial of latanoprost q.h.s. Latanoprost is a drug that can be evaluated with monocular trials because it does not have a contralateral effect (unlike beta blockers and α agonists). Latanoprost has been shown to lower IOP in NTG and can also lower IOP below the patient's episcleral venous pressure. I would set a target pressure of 30% below the highest baseline IOP, or $20 - (0.3 \times 20) = 14$ mm Hg.

Four weeks later, the IOP in the eye being treated with latanoprost was 11 mm Hg, and IOP in the fellow eye was 16 mm Hg. The patient was instructed to take the drop in both eyes at bedtime. One month later, the IOP was 12 mm Hg OD and 13 mm Hg OS. Because the patient is at target pressure, the follow-up is 3 months for an IOP check and 6 months for repeat visual fields and dilated fundus examination.

Second-line treatment options would include brimonidine, topical carbonic anhydrase inhibitors, or ALT if the patient's IOP rises above the target levels. Filtering surgery should be contemplated only if glaucoma progression is confirmed by optic nerve (by disc photos) or visual field loss progression occurs despite medical and laser therapy.

Clinical Pearls

NTG should not be considered to be a rare entity. It probably accounts for 20% of open-angle glaucoma, and as many as 50% of open-angle glaucoma patients exhibit an IOP in the statistically normal range at some time (below 22 mm Hg).

This case shows the importance of careful optic nerve and NFL evaluation for every patient because a significant number of glaucoma patients have statistically normal IOP. It also highlights the potential use of frequency-doubling technology as a screening device for glaucoma detection.

NTG patients do not require a neurologic workup when the clinical findings match glaucoma except for the lack of elevated IOP. Evidence of optic disc pallor or swelling, visual field loss that respects the vertical meridian, or visual acuity or visual field out of proportion to the optic nerve appearance are reasons to consider additional neurologic testing.

CASE 3

A 49-year-old white man reports for a second opinion for glaucoma. He has a medical history of asthma and uses an oral inhaler. His ocular history is unremarkable, and no family members have glaucoma. Review of his prior ocular examinations reveals 20/20 visual acuity, IOP pressures of 15–20 mm Hg (symmetric between the two eyes) based on several readings, and cup-to-disc ratios of 0.6 in both eyes with normal white-on-white visual field test results.

Visual acuity is measured at 20/20 in each eye. EOM, pupils, and confrontation fields are normal. Slit-lamp biomicroscopy is unremarkable. Tensions by applanation are 17 mm Hg OD and 18 mm Hg OS at 10 AM. Gonioscopy reveals grade 3 open angles with trace pigment in the trabecular meshwork. There is no evidence of angle recession or peripheral anterior synechiae. The lenses are clear.

Stereoscopic dilated fundus examination reveals a vertical cup-to-disc ratio of 0.8 OD and 0.85 OS (Figures 18-3A and B). The neural-retinal rim tissue is symmetric between the superior and inferior rim and between the two eyes. The retinal NFL is intact (Figures 18-3C and D). The macula, vessels, and peripheral fundus examination are within normal limits. Full Threshold visual field tests using the 30-2 pattern are normal (Figures 18-3E and F).

Diagnosis

The one suspicious finding in this patient suggestive of glaucoma is a large cup-to-disc ratio. Furthermore, the previous eye notes from 2 years prior recorded a smaller cup-to-disc ratio. Does this patient have glaucoma? If so, is the glaucoma progressing?

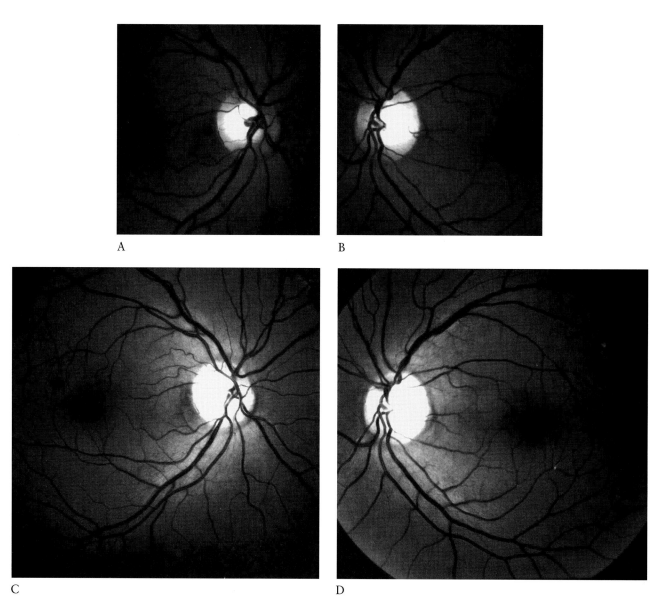

A   B

C   D

FIGURE 18-3. Right eye (**A**) and left eye (**B**). Optic nerve reveals a vertical cup-to-disc (C/D) ratio of 0.8 OD and 0.85 OS; however, the patient also has a very large optic disc. The vertical disc diameter measures 2.5 mm OD and 2.6 mm OS with a Volk 60 D lens (Volk Optical, Mentor, OH). The neuroretinal rim tissue is symmetric between the superior and inferior rim and between the two eyes. In this case, the large cup is physiologic. Right eye (**C**) and left eye (**D**). The nerve fiber layer is intact in both eyes, indicating that the large cupping is probably secondary to the large physiologic disc size. Right eye (**E**) and left eye (**F**) show a normal visual field result, suggesting that the large C/D ratio is physiologic.

Clinical Pearls

The interobserver agreement of cup-to-disc ratio grading has been proven in clinical studies to be poor. This discrepancy results from different levels of clinical training, observation skills, and type of instrumentation used to examine the optic nerve (stereo versus monocular technique). Because of these factors, the cup-to-disc ratio should not be assumed to have changed when different observers are grading the cup-to-disc ratio. This emphasizes the value of taking ste-

reoscopic optic disc photographs to use for future comparisons.

Another important clinical pearl is to differentiate patients who have large physiologic cupping from glaucoma. Large physiologic cups occur in patients with large physiologic discs. One way to determine the size of the disc is to measure the vertical disc diameter with a 60-diopter Volk lens (Volk Optical, Mentor, OH) (see Chapter 5). This patient had a measured vertical height of 2.5 mm OD and 2.6 mm OS, which is more than 2 SD

Single Field Analysis   Eye: Right

Name:	ID:	DOB:

Central 30-2 Threshold Test

Fixation Monitor: Blindspot   Stimulus: III, White   Pupil Diameter: Date: 05-02-1995
Fixation Target: Central   Background: 31.5 ASB   Visual Acuity: 20/20   Time: 11:54 AM
Fixation Losses: 1/24   Strategy: Full Threshold   RX: +2.50 DS   DC X   Age: 48
False POS Errors: 0/12
False NEG Errors: 0/12
Test Duration: 14:42

Fovea: OFF

```
                    23   25   23   27
                        (21)
                 23   25   21   26   26   28
            27   24   27   27   24   31   25   29
                     (29)          (31)
         25   26   28   27   33   30   27   28   28   28
                     (29)          (25)
      27   29   31   30   33   32   32    4   33   33
 30 ─────────────────────────────── (32) ─△─────────── 30
      26   28   30   33   34   31   29    0   22   28
                     (34) (31)          (32)
         26   28   28   31   31   30   29   28   28   26
                     (31)               (29)
            25   28   31   30   27   27   28   28
               (28)                   (32)
                 25   28   25   28   30   28
                    26   23   27   27
```

```
        -1  -1   0   4                     -2  -2  -1   3
      -3  -2  -6   0   0   2             -4  -3  -7  -1  -1   1
    0  -4  -1  -2  -5   3  -3   2       0  -5  -2  -3  -5   2  -4   1
 -1  -2  -2  -3   2   0  -4  -1   0   0   -2  -3  -3  -4   1  -1  -5  -2  -1  -1
  0   0   0  -2   1   0   1       3   4   -1  -1  -1  -3   0  -1   0       2   3
 -1  -1  -1   1   2  -1  -2      -3  -1   -2  -2  -2   0   1  -2  -3      -4  -2
 -1  -1  -2  -1  -1  -1  -2  -2  -2  -3   -1  -2  -3  -2  -2  -2  -3  -3  -3  -4
    -3  -1   1   0  -3  -4   0  -1        -4  -2   0  -1  -4  -4  -1  -2
      -3   0  -4  -2   0  -1             -4  -1  -5  -2   0  -2
        -1  -4  -1  -1                     -1  -5  -2  -2

Total                               Pattern
Deviation                           Deviation
```

GHT
Within normal limits

MD   -0.92 dB
PSD   2.03 dB
SF   1.18 dB
CPSD   1.53 dB

```
::  < 5%
▩  < 2%
▨  < 1%
■  < 0.5%
```

E

FIGURE 18-3. *(continued)*

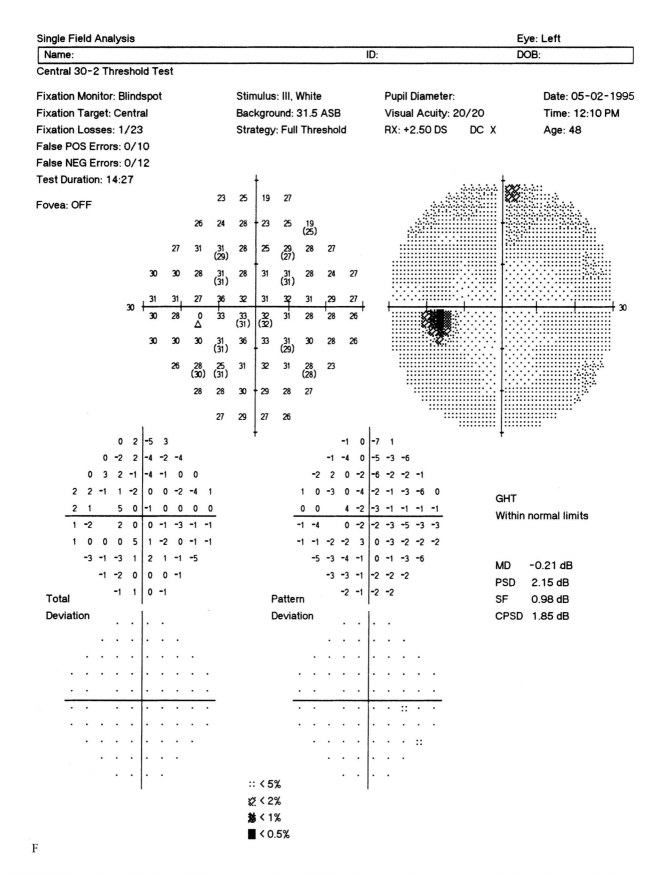

FIGURE 18-3. (*continued*) Left eye (**F**) shows a normal visual field result, suggesting that the large C/D ratio is physiologic.

larger than the average-sized optic nerve (see Figure 5-10). Based on the disc size, this patient would be expected to have a large physiologic cup. Given the large disc size and the normal IOP, NFL, and visual field tests, this patient is diagnosed with a large physiologic cup with a low suspicion of glaucoma. The management would be to photograph the optic nerve and NFL and repeat the visual field examination every 1–2 years. IOP checks should be scheduled at 6- to 12-month intervals.

If this patient develops signs of glaucoma damage, beta blockers should be avoided because of the history of breathing problems. Also, carbonic anhydrase inhibitors should not be used with a history of sulfa allergy. Latanoprost or brimonidine (Alphagan) would be good choices for initial therapy.

CASE 4

A 74-year-old white man comes in complaining of blurred vision. His medical history is significant for hypertension for 5 years, which is well controlled. His ocular and family history is unremarkable. Visual acuity is 20/40 in both eyes, which improves to 20/25 with refraction. EOM, pupils, and confrontation fields are normal. Slit-lamp examination shows a normal anterior chamber with 2+ nuclear sclerosis of the lens. The media equals the vision. Tensions by applanation are 22 mm Hg OU at 9 AM. Gonioscopy shows grade 2 open angles without pigment or peripheral anterior synechiae. The iris contour is slightly convex.

Dilated fundus examination shows a cup-to-disc ratio of 0.5 OU (Figures 18-4A and B). The NFL is intact OU. The macula, vessels, and peripheral examination are unremarkable. Postdilation IOP is 24 mm Hg OU, and gonioscopy shows grade 3+ open angles. Visual field testing is shown in Figures 18-4C and D. How should this patient be managed? Does he have glaucoma?

Diagnosis and Management

This patient has mildly elevated IOP and an abnormal visual field. He also has moderate cataracts, which can cause an overall depression of the visual field, but this can be accounted for by evaluating the pattern deviation plots, which are abnormal. However, the optic nerve and NFL still do not match the severity of visual field loss. Furthermore, the visual field is plagued with fatigue artifacts. There is a generalized reduced sensitivity in the peripheral points which are tested towards the end of visual field examination. The left visual field shows an increase in false-negatives and a cloverleaf pattern indicative of a lack of response after the first few minutes of the test. This patient should have the visual field test repeated with a shorter testing strategy (SITA Fast or frequency-doubling technology) and given more breaks during the examination. If the visual field test still suggests poor correspondence with the optic nerve and NFL, then the patient should be followed with serial optic nerve and NFL photographs. I would not recommend treatment in this patient, given the healthy appear-

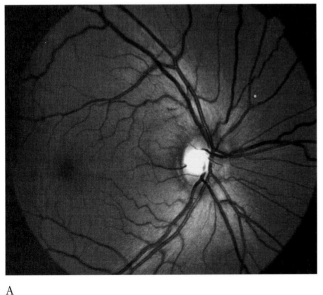

A

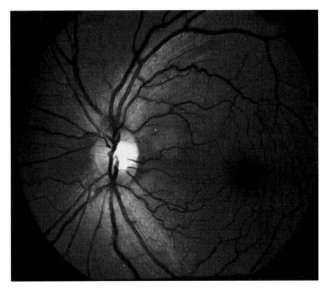

B

FIGURE 18-4. Right (**A**) and left (**B**) optic nerves show a vertical cup-to-disc ratio of .5 with symmetric neuroretinal rim tissue between the superior and inferior poles and between the two eyes. The nerve fiber layer is intact in both eyes (*see next page*).

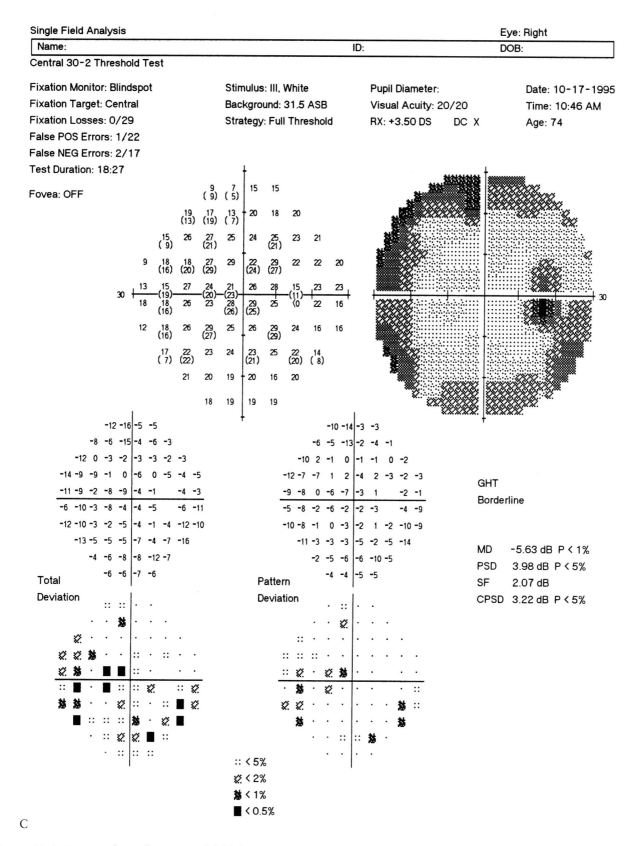

Single Field Analysis　　　　Eye: Right

Name:	ID:	DOB:

Central 30-2 Threshold Test

Fixation Monitor: Blindspot　　　Stimulus: III, White　　　　Pupil Diameter:　　　　Date: 10-17-1995

Fixation Target: Central　　　　Background: 31.5 ASB　　　Visual Acuity: 20/20　　Time: 10:46 AM

Fixation Losses: 0/29　　　　　Strategy: Full Threshold　　RX: +3.50 DS　　DC X　　Age: 74

False POS Errors: 1/22

False NEG Errors: 2/17

Test Duration: 18:27

Fovea: OFF

GHT
Borderline

MD　　-5.63 dB　P < 1%

PSD　　3.98 dB　P < 5%

SF　　　2.07 dB

CPSD　3.22 dB　P < 5%

Total Deviation

Pattern Deviation

:: < 5%

▨ < 2%

▩ < 1%

■ < 0.5%

C

FIGURE 18-4. (*continued*)　Right (C) visual field shows generalized constriction on the graytones, several clusters of P values <5% on the pattern deviation plots, and a borderline glaucoma hemifield test (GHT). None of the reliability indexes is flagged.

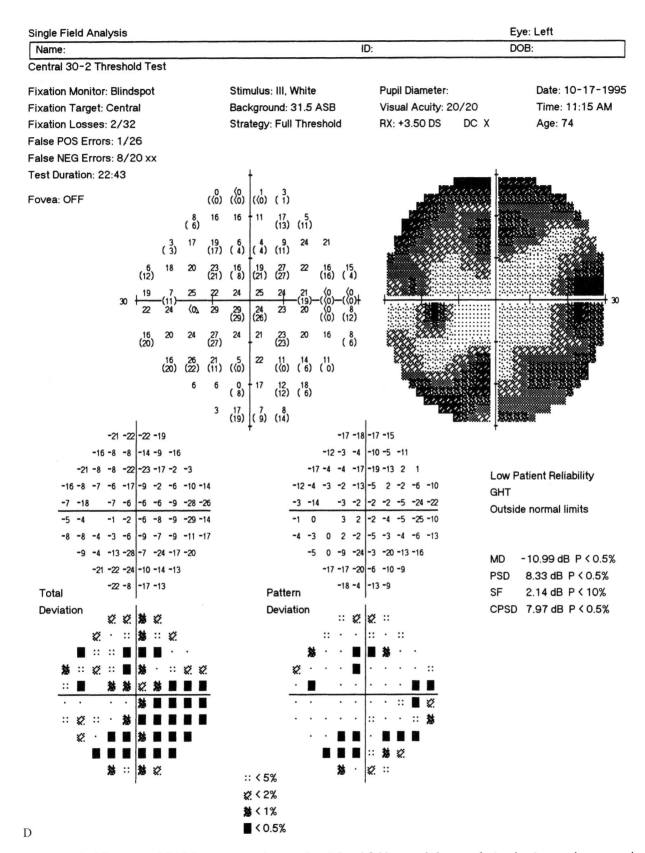

Single Field Analysis   Eye: Left

Name: ID: DOB:

Central 30-2 Threshold Test

Fixation Monitor: Blindspot   Stimulus: III, White   Pupil Diameter: Date: 10-17-1995
Fixation Target: Central   Background: 31.5 ASB   Visual Acuity: 20/20   Time: 11:15 AM
Fixation Losses: 2/32   Strategy: Full Threshold   RX: +3.50 DS   DC X   Age: 74
False POS Errors: 1/26
False NEG Errors: 8/20 xx
Test Duration: 22:43

Fovea: OFF

Low Patient Reliability
GHT
Outside normal limits

MD   -10.99 dB P < 0.5%
PSD   8.33 dB P < 0.5%
SF   2.14 dB P < 10%
CPSD   7.97 dB P < 0.5%

Total Deviation

Pattern Deviation

:: < 5%
▨ < 2%
▩ < 1%
■ < 0.5%

D

FIGURE 18-4. The left (D) visual field shows a more depressed peripheral field, several clusters of missed points on the pattern deviation plots, and an outside normal limits GHT. However, the left eye also has flagged false negative errors, indicating patient fatigue. In this case, both visual fields do not match the optic nerve; therefore, the visual fields are not accurate. The patient is more alert toward the beginning of the test, when the central points are being tested, and then fatigues toward the end of the test, when the more peripheral points are tested. The fields should be repeated with a faster testing strategy and the patient given more breaks during the test.

ance to the optic nerve and relatively low risk for developing glaucoma.

This patient also shows slightly narrow anterior chamber angles. However, they are probably not a significant factor in this patient because they are open to trabecular meshwork, no signs of intermittent closure are present, and the angles do not narrow further (but actually increased in depth) on dilation. This patient should be monitored with gonioscopy every 6 months and educated on the symptoms of angle closure.

Clinical Pearls

Many first-time field testers exhibit an abnormal visual field that improves with subsequent testing; this is referred to as a *learning curve*. A significant number of patients also are poor visual field testers no matter how many tests are performed. This is why it is extremely important to always correlate the visual field test results to the optic nerve examination.

CASE 5

A 66-year-old African-American man comes in who was diagnosed with glaucoma in 1998 and was transferring his care from a private physician to the VA because he could not afford to pay for his medications. He is currently taking timolol, brimonidine, and latanoprost. His IOP has been poorly controlled, his C/D ratio is .9 OU, and his visual fields have gotten progressively worse over the last year.

Clinical examination reveals visual acuity of 20/20 in each eye. His refractive error is +4.50 – 1.00 × 90 in the right eye and +3.50 sphere in the left eye. EOM are full, confrontation fields are full, and pupils are normal. Slit-lamp examination reveals a clear cornea, shallow

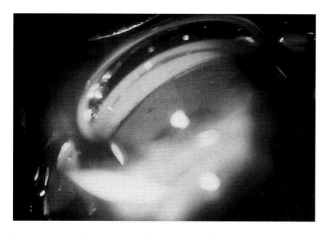

FIGURE 18-5. Gonioscopy photograph of patient with chronic narrow-angle glaucoma with the development of peripheral anterior synechiae in the angle. After a peripheral iridotomy was performed, part of the angle (right) opens to ciliary body.

anterior chamber by Von Herick, and a convex iris contour. Tension by applanation is 28 mm Hg OD and 22 mm Hg OS. Gonioscopy shows grade 1 angles inferiorly and nasally and closed angles superiorly with peripheral anterior synechiae on pressure gonioscopy. The lens shows 2+ nuclear sclerosis.

Diagnosis and Management

At this point, the diagnosis is chronic angle-closure glaucoma. This type of glaucoma can mimic primary open-angle glaucoma, but over time the IOP becomes more difficult to control as the angle slowly starts to close up. The superior angle is typically the first affected because it is anatomically the shallowest. The patient is treated with neodymium:yttrium-aluminum-garnet (Nd:YAG) laser peripheral iridotomies OU. After the procedure, marked deepening of the anterior chamber is seen, but peripheral anterior synechiae remain in the superior angle (Figure 18-5). IOP improves to 15 mm Hg OD and 12 mm Hg OS when the patient is on timolol 0.5% b.i.d. OU alone. The patient should be followed with serial IOP checks and gonioscopy every 3 months. Dilated optic nerve examination of the optic nerve and visual field tests should be performed at 6- to 12-month intervals. His target pressure is set ≤ 15 mm Hg due to his severe glaucoma damage.

Clinical Pearls

This case exemplifies the need for gonioscopy for all glaucoma and glaucoma suspect patients. Acute angle-closure glaucoma is rare in African-American patients, but chronic angle-closure glaucoma occurs with equal frequency between whites and African Americans.

Once a peripheral iridotomy is performed and the angle opens, it is important to follow the patient closely for a concurrent open-angle glaucoma (mixed-mechanism glaucoma). This patient had one-fourth of the angle occluded from peripheral anterior synechiae. Appositional closure can also damage the trabecular meshwork despite opening of the angle. Patients with acute or chronic angle closure require constant monitoring and may require antiglaucoma medication to control the IOP because of visible or subclinical damage to the trabecular meshwork.

CASE 6

A 66-year-old white man with no medical history reports for a routine eye examination. The patient reports a brother with glaucoma who is taking eye drops.

Best-corrected visual acuity is 20/20 in each eye with a slightly myopic correction. EOM are full. Confrontation fields are full to finger counting. Pupils are

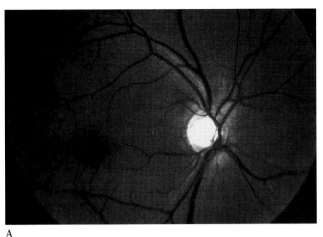
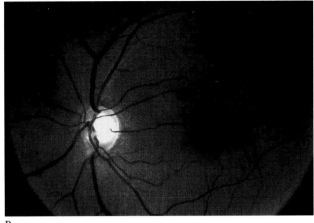

A   B

FIGURE 18-6. Dilated stereoscopic fundus evaluation of the optic nerves shows a vertical cup-to-disc ratio of .7 in the right eye (**A**) and .8 in the left eye (**B**). The rim tissue is slightly thinner superiorly in the left compared to the inferior and the superior rim tissue in the right eye. An acquired pit of the optic nerve is also noted in the superior portion of the optic cup in the left eye. Nerve fiber layer (NFL) evaluation shows some mild relative thinning in the 7–9 o'clock position in the right eye (**A**) and from the 1–2 o'clock position in the left eye (**B**). (*continued*)

equal, round, and reactive to light without an afferent pupillary defect. Slit-lamp biomicroscopy is unremarkable. Tensions by Goldmann applanation are 23 mm Hg OU at 9 AM. Gonioscopy reveals grade 3+ open angles with 1+ pigment in the trabecular meshwork. No evidence is seen of angle recess or peripheral anterior synechiae. Lenses show trace nuclear sclerosis OU.

Dilated stereoscopic fundus evaluation of the optic nerves shows a vertical cup-to-disc ratio of 0.7 in the right eye and 0.8 in the left eye. The rim tissue is slightly thinner superiorly in the left eye compared with inferior and compared with the superior rim tissue in the right eye. An acquired pit of the optic nerve is also noted in the superior portion of the optic cup in the left eye. NFL evaluation shows some mild relative thinning in the 7 o'clock to 9 o'clock position in the right eye (Figure 18-6A) and from 1 o'clock to 2 o'clock in the left eye (Figure 18-6B). Full Threshold 30-2 visual field tests are normal in both eyes (Figures 18-6C and D). A cluster of points is seen in the inferior nasal quadrant of the left eye, but none of the points in the cluster has a P value <1% (see Figure 18-6D). The GHT and CSPD are normal. Does this patient have glaucoma?

Diagnosis

There is objective evidence based on the optic nerve and NFL examination that this patient does have glaucoma in his left eye. The right eye is also suspicious because primary open-angle glaucoma is a bilateral dis-

ease and mild NFL loss to the inferior arcade has occurred.

This type of patient is a good candidate for short wavelength automated perimetry (SWAP), because a strong suspicion for glaucoma damage exists even though the white-on-white perimetry is normal. This patient also does not have significant cataracts, which can taint the result of SWAP perimetry. SWAP testing shows nasal defects by graytone analysis (Figures 18-6E and F). However, because of the wide variability in SWAP testing, it is recommended that clinicians use the SWAPPAC analysis of the pattern deviation plots to look for abnormalities. Here, an inferior nasal cluster in the left eye correlates with the superior rim tissue and nerve fiber thinning, and also the location of the acquired pit of the optic nerve. The right SWAP pattern deviation plot is normal. This patient has increased fixation losses; however, the technician recorded good fixation.

Management

Based on the clinical findings just described, I would diagnose primary open-angle glaucoma in the left eye and probable primary open-angle glaucoma in the right eye. I would classify the amount of damage as mild and set a target pressure of 20% reduction in the right eye and 30% in the left eye. I would obtain three baseline IOP readings and start treatment in both eyes. I would follow the patient with serial white-on-white visual field testing because of the higher variability of blue-yellow perimetry.

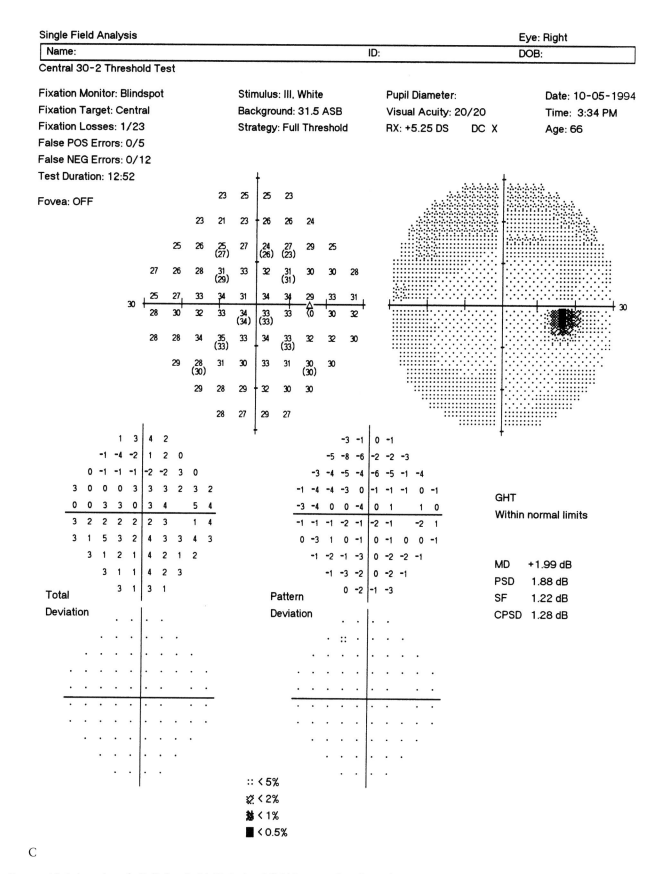

FIGURE 18-6. (*continued*) Full threshold 30-2 visual field is normal in the right eye (**C**).

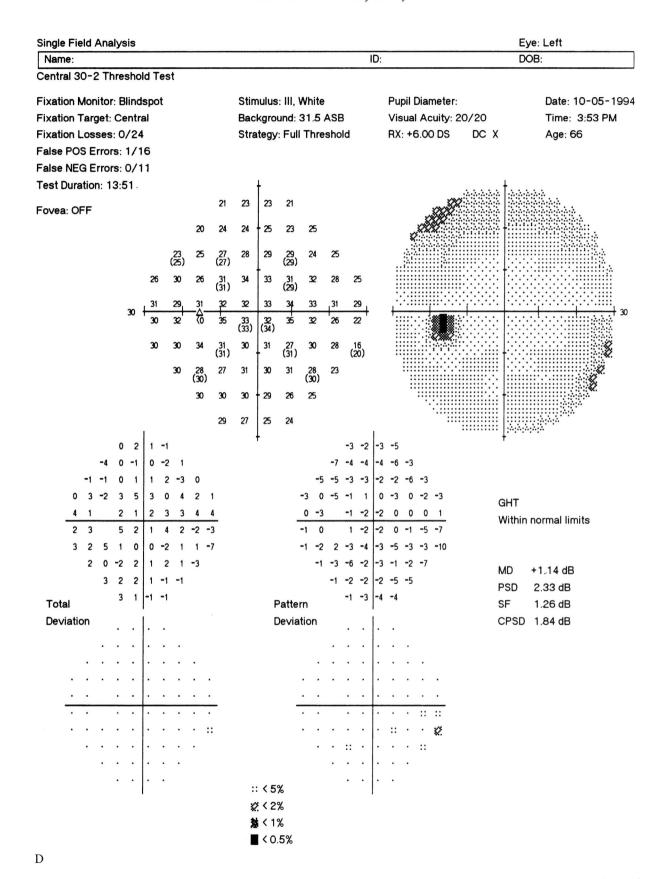

D

FIGURE 18-6. (*continued*) There is a cluster of points on the pattern deviation plots in the inferior nasal quadrant of the left eye (**D**); however, none of the points in the cluster has a P value <1%. The glaucoma hemifield test (GHT) and corrected pattern standard deviation (CSPD) are normal. (*continued*)

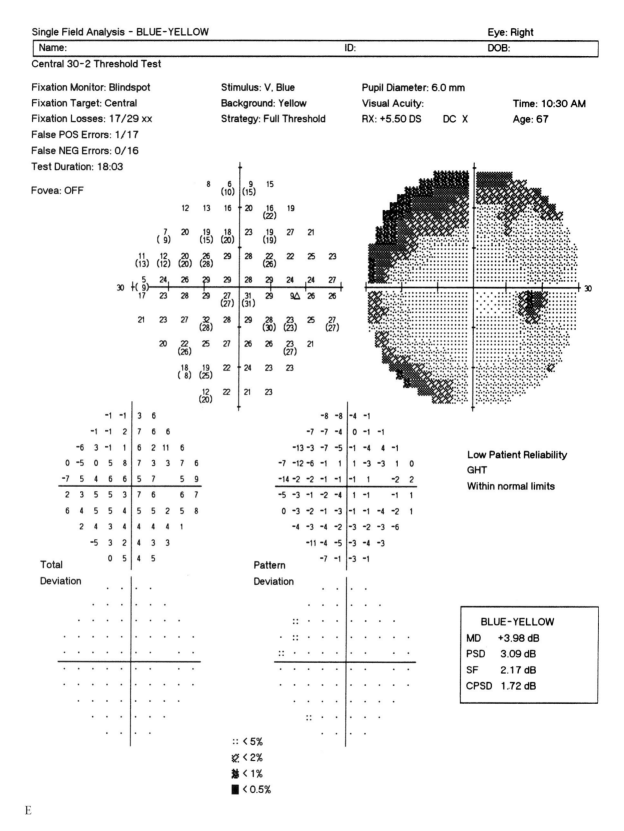

Single Field Analysis - BLUE-YELLOW   Eye: Right

Name:	ID:	DOB:

Central 30-2 Threshold Test

Fixation Monitor: Blindspot   Stimulus: V, Blue   Pupil Diameter: 6.0 mm

Fixation Target: Central   Background: Yellow   Visual Acuity: Time: 10:30 AM

Fixation Losses: 17/29 xx   Strategy: Full Threshold   RX: +5.50 DS   DC X   Age: 67

False POS Errors: 1/17

False NEG Errors: 0/16

Test Duration: 18:03

Fovea: OFF

Low Patient Reliability

GHT

Within normal limits

Total Deviation

Pattern Deviation

BLUE-YELLOW

MD   +3.98 dB

PSD   3.09 dB

SF   2.17 dB

CPSD   1.72 dB

:: < 5%

< 2%

< 1%

■ < 0.5%

E

FIGURE 18-6. (*continued*) (**E** and **F**) Short wavelength automated perimetry (SWAP) shows nasal defects by graytone analysis in both eyes. However, because of the wide variability in SWAP testing, it is recommended to use the SWAPPAC analysis of the pattern deviation plots to look for abnormalities. The right SWAP pattern deviation plot is normal. (**E**) There in an inferior nasal cluster in the left eye (**F**), which correlates with the superior rim tissue and NFL thinning and also the location of the APON. The visual field technician reported good patient fixation despite increased fixation losses in both eyes.

Single Field Analysis - BLUE-YELLOW   Eye: Left

Name:		ID:		DOB:

Central 30-2 Threshold Test

Fixation Monitor: Blindspot   Stimulus: V, Blue   Pupil Diameter: 6.0 mm

Fixation Target: Central   Background: Yellow   Visual Acuity: Time: 10:53 AM

Fixation Losses: 7/29 xx   Strategy: Full Threshold   RX: +6.00 DS   DC X   Age: 67

False POS Errors: 0/20

False NEG Errors: 1/15

Test Duration: 17:53

Fovea: OFF

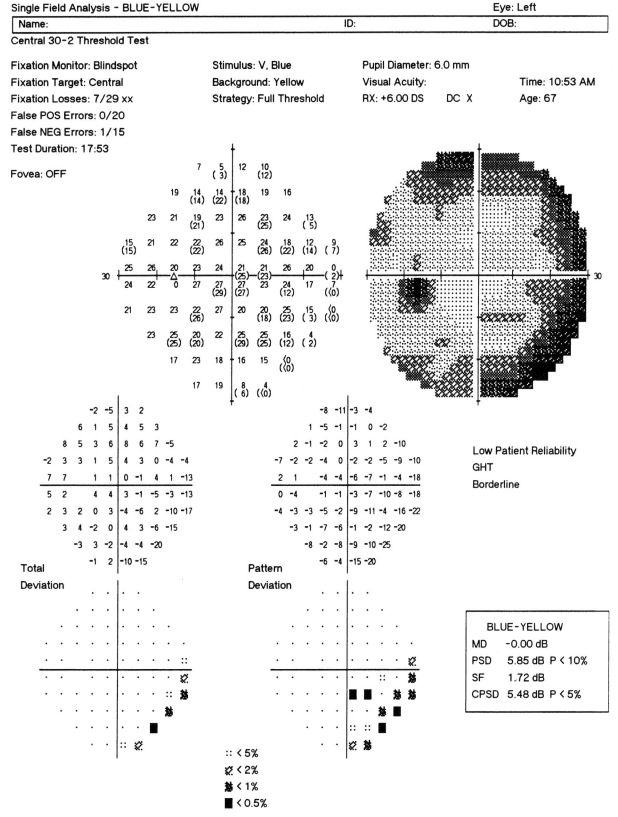

Low Patient Reliability

GHT

Borderline

Total Deviation

Pattern Deviation

:: < 5%

⊘ < 2%

▓ < 1%

■ < 0.5%

BLUE-YELLOW	
MD	-0.00 dB
PSD	5.85 dB P < 10%
SF	1.72 dB
CPSD	5.48 dB P < 5%

F

Clinical Pearls

SWAP has a relatively limited use in the diagnosis and management of glaucoma. I use SWAP for high-risk glaucoma suspects (based on risk factors or suspicious optic nerves or NFL) who test normal on white-on-white perimetry. I do not use SWAP in patients who already show white-on-white defects, in patients with cataracts, or in patients who are poor or fatiguing visual field testers. SWAP is used to diagnose early glaucoma and can be used to follow for early glaucoma progression.

CASE 7

A 38-year-old African-American man reports to the clinic for a routine eye examination. He has no significant medical history. There is no family history of glaucoma. His best-corrected acuity is 20/20 in each eye. Pupils are equal and round, and respond to light without an afferent pupillary defect. EOM are full and confrontation fields are full to finger counting. Slit-lamp evaluation is unremarkable. Tensions as measured by Goldmann applanation range between 20 mm Hg and 25 mm Hg on three separate readings. Gonioscopy shows grade 4 angles without evidence of angle recession or peripheral anterior synechiae. The lenses are clear without cataracts. Optic nerves show large discs with vertical cup-to-disc ratios of 0.80 in the right eye and 0.85 in the left eye. NFL exhibits mild thinning inferiorly greater than superiorly in both eyes (Figures 18-7A; only right eye is shown). Visual field testing shows a repeatable superior defect in both eyes.

Diagnosis

The patient is diagnosed with primary open-angle glaucoma with mild to moderate damage. His target pressures are set 30% below baseline or 17 mm Hg. During 3 years of follow-up, the patient is presently on three glaucoma eyedrops (timolol, latanoprost, and dorzolamide). He has developed allergy to brimonidine. He has had 360 degrees of ALT in both eyes. His IOP readings during follow-up range between 11 mm Hg and 21 mm Hg, with an average of 17 mm Hg. His serial visual fields for the right eye are shown in an overview and glaucoma change probability printout (Figures 18-7C and D; only the right eye is shown). The question is whether the visual fields appear stable or are showing enough progression to warrant filtering surgery.

Visual Field Interpretation

There is a marked learning curve from the first to second field (see Figure 18-7C). After the second field, a new defect in the inferior field appears to be present. However, all subsequent fields show marked long-term fluctuation with some points getting worse and some getting better. In the glaucoma change probability plot (see Figure 18-7D), the program automatically discards the first visual field because it recognizes the learning curve. The next two visual fields are averaged to form the baseline, and then each subsequent field is compared with the baseline. Scattered points on the change probability plot show declines with P values <5% (*dark triangles*), but only two or three points were flagged on all three tests. Has this patient's glaucoma gotten worse?

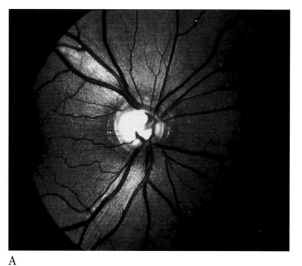
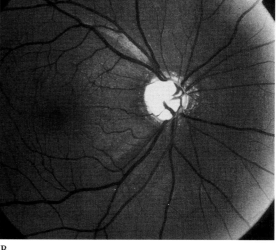

A   B

FIGURE 18-7. Initial photograph of the optic nerve and nerve fiber layer (NFL) (**A**) shows a cup-to-disc ratio of .8 in the right eye with mild NFL thinning inferior. Photograph taken 3 years later (**B**) shows marked loss of neuroretinal rim tissue in the superior and inferior poles and severe NFL loss inferior and moderate NFL loss superior. Comparing photographs confirms glaucoma progression.

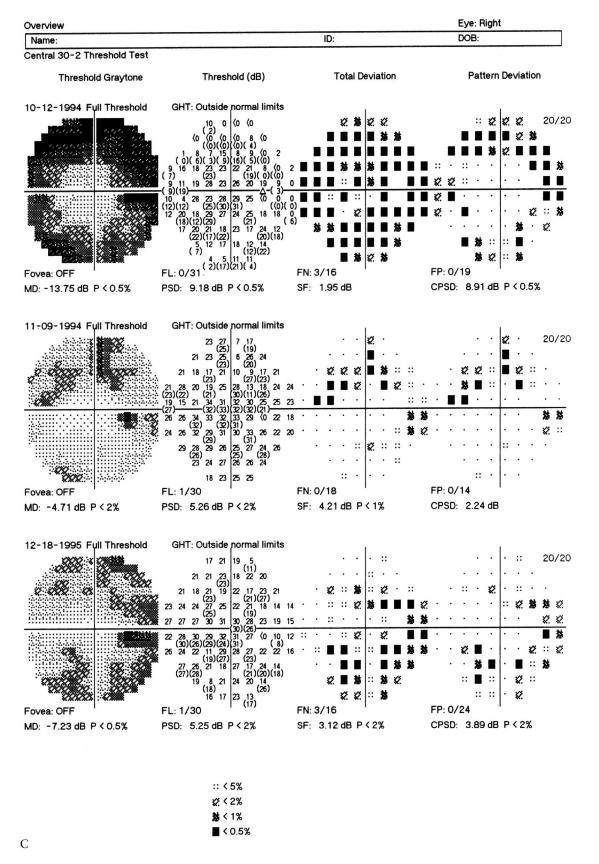

FIGURE 18-7. (**C**) Overview printout of the right visual field. There is a marked learning curve from the first to second field. After the second field, there appears to be a new defect in the inferior field. However, all subsequent fields show marked long-term fluctuation with some points getting worse and some getting better (*see next page*).

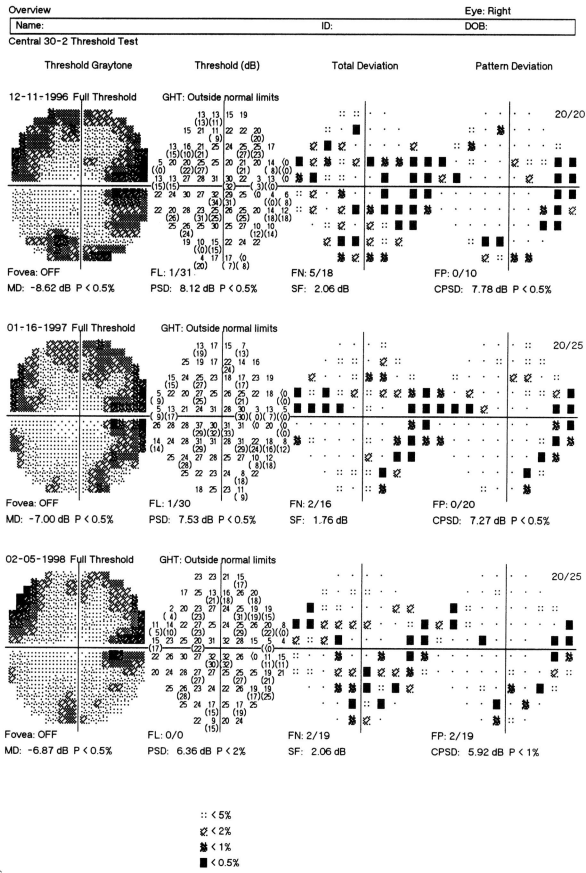

C

FIGURE 18-7. (*continued*)

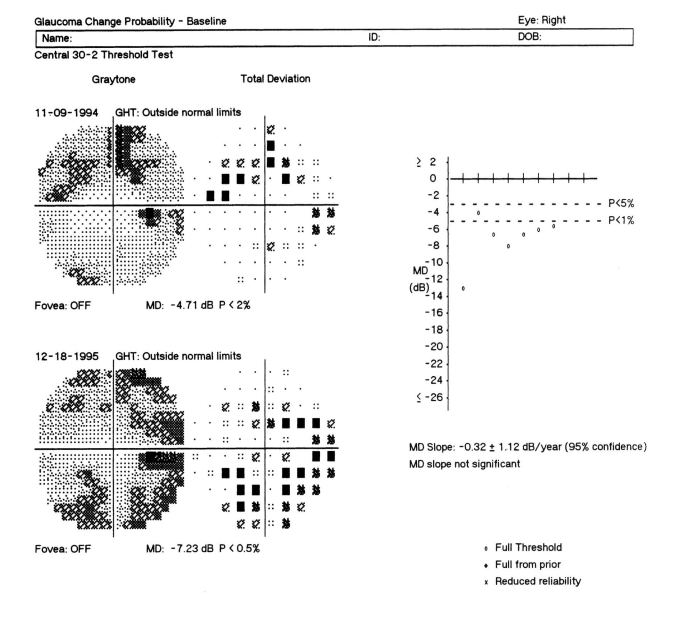

D

FIGURE 18-7. (*continued*) (**D**) Glaucoma change probability (GCP) printout of the right eye. In the GCP, the program automatically discards the first visual field because it recognizes the learning curve. The next two visual fields are averaged to form the baseline and then each subsequent field is compared to the baseline (*see next page*). There are several superior nasal points in the "deviation from baseline" that have declined by 10 dB. There are scattered points on the change probability plot that show declines with P values <5% (*dark triangles*); however, there are only two or three points that flagged on all three tests. In this case, the glaucoma progression is much more obvious by comparing the optic nerve/NFL photographs (**A** and **B**) than by the visual fields. (*continued*)

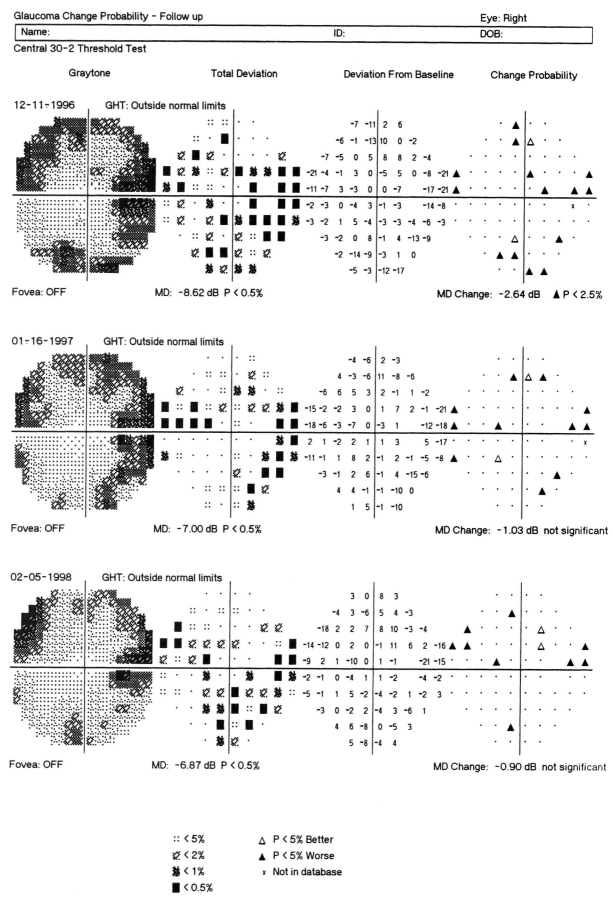

FIGURE 18-7. (continued)

D

A large degree of long-term fluctuation can occur in individual visual field points that are damaged by glaucoma. It is over this long-term fluctuation that the clinician must decide whether the visual field is stable or progressing (see Chapter 7). This patient also had serial optic nerve and NFL photography. When the most recent NFL photograph (see Figure 18-7B; only the right eye is shown) is compared with the initial NFL photograph (see Figure 18-7A), marked loss of the NFL is seen in both the superior and inferior arcades. The left eye showed a similar appearance. This is objective evidence that the patient's glaucoma has progressed. The patient had mitomycin C filtering surgery in both eyes. Mitomycin C was used as an adjunct because the patient was young and African American (two risk factors for filter scarring and failure). Post-filter IOPs have remained consistently in the low teens without medications.

Clinical Pearls

This is a young patient with a clear media. In this case, it is important to evaluate the total deviation plots rather than the pattern deviation plots on the visual field.

This patient's rapid glaucoma progression was not readily apparent on the visual field tests. Long-term fluctuation can be difficult to differentiate from glaucoma progression. Optic nerve and NFL serial photography can also be helpful in determining progression. However, it is important to note in the Normal Tension Glaucoma Study that 89% of the patient's glaucoma progression was identified by visual field testing and only 11% by serial photography.[1] Even so, with the difficulty of interpreting progression with visual fields, serial photography is recommended for all glaucoma patients and glaucoma-suspect patients.

Only a minority of patients (approximately 10%) with glaucoma go blind from the disease. It is important to identify which glaucoma patients are progressing (and likely to become impaired from the disease) and to institute aggressive therapy (e.g., filtering surgery) for these patients. Clearly, looking at the serial change in the photographs over 3 years, this patient was rapidly progressing. Also, this patient is young and needs to preserve vision for many years. It is best not to wait until the patient has tunnel visual fields to recommend filtering surgery.

CASE 8

A 72-year-old woman was seen in the Omni Eye Service for the first time in February, requesting a second opinion on the status of her glaucoma. On questioning, she had an 8-year history of glaucoma and had been put on two medications by the first doctor, and then a third medication 1 year ago by a different practitioner. She was not sure whether she had ever had a visual field test, and she was vague when we asked about the frequency of follow-up visits. However, she seemed confident when we asked about her medications and even produced the bottles of three different glaucoma drops, including dorzolamide (Trusopt), pilocarpine 2%, and a beta blocker. All bottles were at least one-half full. When asked whether she was using her medications, she said, emphatically, "yes." We reviewed exactly how she used each drop. I asked when she last used her drops, and she replied "this morning at 8 AM." Her visual acuity was 20/30 OD and 20/40 OS from brunescent nuclear sclerotic cataracts. Pupils revealed moderate reaction to direct light OU and a trace afferent defect OS. A slow response on confrontation fields in the superior nasal quadrant OS was noted. IOP by Goldmann applanation was 24 mm Hg OD and 32 mm Hg OS. Gonioscopy revealed grade 4 open angles OU. Optic nerve evaluation revealed significant cupping (.9+) in both eyes, with significant notching of the inferior temporal rim greater OS than OD. Automated threshold fields showed advanced glaucomatous loss, OS greater than OD.

On completing the examination, I asked her to once again review her medication regimen with me. I reviewed each bottle again, holding one up at a time and asking how often she used it. The discussion then took an interesting turn. When we got to the pilocarpine and the dorzolamide, she admitted to not having used those particular drops since last September and December, respectively. I asked why, especially since there were plenty of drops left in the bottle. It was then and only then that she told me she was simply following instructions. The expiration dates on the bottles were September and December of that previous year, respectively, and she interpreted that to mean that the drops should not be used beyond that time! Obviously she had used the drops very sparingly up until then, allowing the medication to expire before it ran out.

I gently brought up the issue of cost, saying, "if the medications were less expensive, would you have an easier time refilling them?" She responded affirmatively, and we discussed alternatives (ALT) and patient assistance programs. I procured some samples for her, and gave her a glaucoma medication dosing schedule (see Figure 11-2). On multiple follow-up visits, her IOP pressure has been in the mid teens.

The lesson here is that persistence pays, and compliance can sometimes only be assessed by asking the same questions in different ways. Just because a patient tells you something once does not always mean it is so. Care must be taken not to scold or appear annoyed, and you will gain the patient's trust for many years to come.

REFERENCE

1. The Collaborative Normal Tension Glaucoma Study Group. Comparison of glaucomatous progression between untreated patients with normal-tension glaucoma and patients with therapeutically reduced intraocular pressure. Am J Ophthalmol 1998;126:487–497.

Index

Note: Page numbers followed by *f* indicate figures; numbers followed by *t* indicate tables.